W9-CAV-678

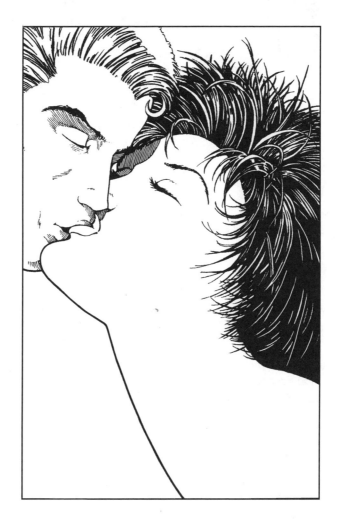

Welcome!

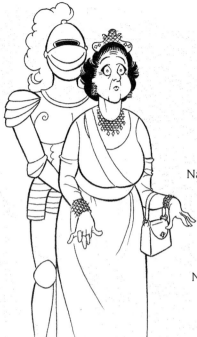

North American Distribution

National Book Network
Lanham, Maryland
(800) 462-6420

Canada

National Book Network
Toronto, Ontario
(877) NBN-BOOK

United Kingdom

NBN International
Plymouth, UK
44 (0) 1752 202301

New Zealand

Addenda
Newmarket, Auckland
64-9-529-9571

Australia

Tower Books
Frenchs Forest NSW
02 9975 5566

Elsewhere In the Federation

Brazilian Edition by
Editora Landscape
Sao Paulo, Brazil

Croatian Edition by
Mozaik Knjiga
Zagreb, Croatia

Czech Edition by
Alpress
Prague, Czech Republic

German Edition by
Goldmann (Bertelsmann)
Munich, Germany

Hebrew Edition by
Babel Publishing House
Tel Aviv, Israel

Hungarian Edition by
Athenaeum 2000
Budapest, Hungary

Italian Edition by
Nuova Pratiche Editrice
Milan, Italy

Korean Edition by
Darimedia Publishing House
Seoul, South Korea

Norwegian Edition by
Pax Forlag
Oslo, Norway

Polish Edition by
Swiat Ksiazki
Warszawa, Poland

Russian Edition by
Eksmo
Moscow, Russia

Serbian Edition by
Alfa-Narodna Knjiga
Belgrade, Serbia

Slovenian Edition by
Presernova Druzba
Ljubljana, Slovenia

Guide To Getting It On

for adults of all ages

author & publisher
Paul Joannides, Psy.D.

illustrator
Dærick Gröss Sr.

editor
Toni Johnson

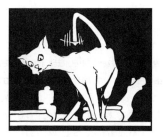

Goofy Foot Press
Oregon, U.S.A.

Guide To Getting It On!
Sixth Edition

V. 6.0   2009

Copyright © 2009 by Goofy Foot Press
All rights reserved. More or less.

Publisher's Cataloging-In-Publication
Joannides, Paul N.
Guide to getting it on! / Paul Joannides, author;
Daerick Gross, illustrator.-- 6th ed.
p. cm.
Includes bibliographical references and index.
ISBN: 1-885535-33-3
ISBN-13: 978-1885535337
1. Sex instruction. 2. Sex. 3. Man-woman
relationships. 1. Gross,Daerick. 11. Title.

HQ31.J63 2009   613.9'6

Goofy Foot Press
Oregon, U.S.A.
www.goofyfootpress.com

printed in
Saline, Michigan
McNaughton & Gunn
Made in the U.S.A.

Fair Use

Feel free to copy up to 250 words of this book, except for quotations and song lyrics, as long as the title, author and publisher are cited. That's called fair use. Reproducing more than 250 words by any means (electronic, Internet, mechanical, photocopying, recording or otherwise) without written permission from the publisher is theft. It is illegal. The only exception is if you are writing a legitimate book review. Copy the illustrations from this book without written permission, and we will send Guido to break your kneecaps.

Bed of
CONTENTS

How to & Then Some

Your First Time

Technology & Culture

Orientation & Gender

Sex & the Human Condition

Beyond Vanilla

Below the Belt

Pregnancy (or Not) & Parenting

Sex in History & Popular Culture

(continued...)

Technology

Page Layout Software : Adobe InDesign CS3
Operating System : Mac OSX on a really old Sawtooth Mac
Website & Podcast Engineer : Braxton Sherouse • Tech Consultant : Cyrus Farivar
Book Interior Consultant : Dmitri Siegel • Copy Editing : Jennifer Ashley
Cover Graphic Consultant : Rose Reed/Newport Lazerquick
Prepress/Press : McNaughton & Gunn

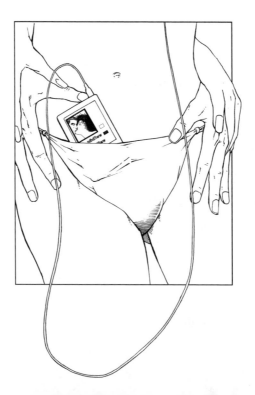

Warning & Disclaimer

Hard as we tried, this Guide isn't perfect, nor was it intended as a final authority on sex. There will be times when it is better to consult your beautician, bartender, or best friend. You might also speak to a physician or licensed sex therapist. Ultimately, it is your body and your sexuality—venture beyond the bounds of common sense at your own peril.

This book talks about sex acts which are illegal in some parts of the planet. Know your state or nation's laws about sex and break them at your own risk; prison sentences, public stonings or beheadings could result.

No one involved with the writing or publishing of this book is a physician or licensed sex therapist, although members of these professions have been consulted on thorny issues. The people who have contributed ideas to this book are mostly psychologists, psychoanalysts, social workers, lawyers, teachers, writers, a couple of surfers, and even a prostitute and a priest. The actual writing was done by a mental-health professional. Just because some of these people have college degrees doesn't mean they know any more about sex or sexual relationships than you do. They all struggle at times. Still, their perspective might be helpful and even refreshing.

While the techniques mentioned in this book work well for some people, they might not be good for you. Check with a physician or licensed sex therapist before attempting any sexual act that you are unfamiliar with, or do so at your own risk and with the understanding that bad things might happen. Consult with a physician if you have any condition which precludes strenuous exercise or erotic activity.

All readers, except those who are trying to get pregnant, are encouraged to use birth control and to adopt a medically-sound strategy for avoiding sexually transmitted infections. However, no form of birth control is foolproof, and diseases have been known to outsmart even the finest of barriers. These are normal consequences of having sex and are not the fault of this book.

This book was written to help expand the consciousness of its readers. Neither Goofy Foot Press nor any of its minions shall be liable or responsible to any person or entity for any loss, damage, injury or ailment caused, or alleged to be caused, directly or indirectly, by the information or lack of information contained in this book.

This book contains anatomical illustrations which are at best simple approximations. If your anatomy differs from what is shown, take heart. Hopefully there is at least some similarity with what's beneath your clothes and what's between these covers.

If you do not wish to be bound by this disclaimer, please return this book with a photocopy of the sales receipt to the publisher for a full refund.

for Toni Johnson

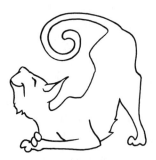

1
In The Beginning

There are a number of excellent books on sex that are much thinner than this one. They don't release expanded and updated editions every two years, but they can clearly help you to be better in bed.

So why *The Guide*?

For starters, each of the lovers you have in life will want something different from you. Some will want you to touch them between their legs, others will want you to touch their soul. This book tries to help you with both.

The Guide encourages you to explore dimensions of sexuality that people usually aren't told about—from the emotional part of getting naked together to why a guy who takes his penis too seriously might have trouble pleasing his sweetheart. It covers subjects like hand jobs and heart throbs, kisses above and below the waist, friendship, and sex in Cyberspace.

But most important of all is the *Goofy Foot Philosophy* which says that it doesn't matter what you've got in your pants if there is nothing in your brain to connect it to.

Do With It What You Want

Since this is a book about sex, it might be a good idea to include a definition of what sex is. But trying to define sex is a lot like trying to insert a diaphragm: just when you think you've got it in, the thing turns ninja on you. Here are a few of the issues that need to be addressed if you are trying to define "sex:"

💡People think of intercourse as the ultimate sex act, the real thing–*ipsum fuctum*. But if intercourse is the ultimate act, then how come making out or holding hands is sometimes sweeter and more meaningful?

🔆Almost all sex acts can be painful, obnoxious, or boring unless you do them with someone who turns you on. Does this mean that the mental part of sex is more important than the physical part?

🔆Why does one couple find a particular sex act to be highly erotic while another couple finds the same act to be disgusting?

🔆A person has sex and an orgasm, but doesn't feel sexually excited. The next afternoon he or she catches the brief but intense gaze of a sexy stranger and nearly bursts with feeling. How can a brief glance take your breath away more than sex with a long-term lover?

🔆You are getting a physical exam. You are naked, and your genitals are being touched. Neither you nor the examiner is aware of any sexual excitement. However, if you were naked and being touched in this way after a romantic date, it might be incredibly sexual. How much do we rely on the context or situation to tell us what's sexual and what isn't?

🔆How can a song, car, or piece of clothing be sexy?

Needless to say, we have given up on trying to pin a tail of definition on the big donkey of sex. It seems that any definition of sex needs to fit who you are as an individual as well as your particular situation. Instead of pretending to know what that might be, consider this:

> Learning about sex and intimacy is a lifelong task. Even with years of experience, we still blow it on occasion. The best we can do in the pages that follow is to tell you what we wish we had known about sex many years ago. Do with it what you want.

Morality & What's in Your Pants

In much of America we still try to equate morality with whether you keep your pants on. We also associate morality with religion. But the truth is, there are Christians, atheists and Jews who are moral people, and Christians, atheists and Jews who are immoral people. The same is true for people who are sexually active and for those who aren't. Morality, from this Guide's perspective, is respecting and caring for your fellow human beings. It has little to do with the way you enjoy your sexuality, unless what you do breaks a special trust or violates the rights of others.

Hmmm. A Book on Sex

Consider the books on sex that were written between 1830 and today. Some of these books gave a girl a psychiatric diagnosis if she masturbated or wanted to be on top, and the theories about boys could be contradictory and bizarre. Some of today's sex books make strange claims as well. Yet the writers of these books consider themselves to be paragons of reason and truth. So please be aware that books on sex don't often pass the test of time and this is a book on sex.

While there are plenty of sexual traditions, there are no *Ten Commandments of Sex*. Sex books are merely a reflection of the time and culture that spawn them. Sexual fashion will change many times between now and when you are a resident of the old folks' home.

Birth Control & Gnarly Sex Germs

The chapters on birth control and sex germs talk about everything from scruffy sex rodents to things you can do to make a rubber feel right. Hopefully, their perspective on sex will help you avoid things like unwanted pregnancies and an early funeral. In the meantime, it might be helpful to remember that just about anything in this world that's worth doing will kill you if you're stupid about it. Having sex can be far less risky than driving on the freeway or even driving across town. It just depends on how smart you are about sex and how badly you drive.

How It Fits In

Back when your mother was in school, she couldn't sneak a cell-phone between her legs during a lecture, snap a picture of her pre-mom crotch, and send it to one of your potential fathers with CU2NITE, Wet4U or IWSN ("I want sex now!").

Although today's technology might be more interesting than before the reasons why people have sex are pretty much the same. Love and infatuation still top the list, but satisfying animalistic passions and having fun are frequent motivators. People also have sex to make babies, to make money, or to help them feel more desirable and less lonely.

Sex with the same person can mean different things at different times. Early in a relationship, it might excite you and rev you up; later it might be a source of comfort and calm. In most relationships, there will be times when the sex is boring or when it makes you feel more distant than close.

For those of you who are younger: people sometimes refer to matters of the younger heart as puppy love and treat it with disrespect. That's silly. The most powerful feelings in life are often puppy love. Cherish them. As for having sex with your puppy love, far be it from this Guide to say yes or no. It might be wonderful, but then again, maybe not. Just be aware that there's usually more to a good carnal experience than the hydraulics of sticking hard into wet. For some people, what separates good sex from bad are intangibles like fun, friendship, love and caring.

As you get older, your expectations about sex may change. For instance, if you just turned 17, getting laid in and of itself can be a huge thing. But by the time you turn 34, you'll have more experience under your belt. By then you might want your sex life to take you some place different than when you were younger. Perhaps you will be searching for different qualities in a partner as well. Hopefully, you will want sex to be special no matter what your age.

A Red Flag—Matters of the Heart

Sex can be as emotionally powerful as you want to make it. But good luck if you are trying to have sex without it becoming emotional.

The emotions that accompany sexual relationships can be magical, enchanting and wonderful. Then again they can be really awful. A cherished relationship can fizzle and go flat, leaving you empty and hollow. Or it can cause you so much heartache that you might wish you were dead. The tears can pour from a place so deep that you'll wonder if they will ever stop.

Fortunately, lovemaking can be a way of working through fears and crises, as well as a place for growth, forgiveness, fun and friendship. If you make it a priority and keep working at it, sex can help you be fully present, honest, and emotionally naked and alive with yourself and your partner.

No Assumptions Here

Most of us make assumptions about the sex lives of other people. For example, consider Tim, a quiet, college-aged computer geek, and Jake, a well-liked 27-year-old shortstop on his company's baseball team. Tim is bicep-challenged while Jake looks like he just leapt from the pages of *Men's Health*. Yet Tim the geek has a creative and fulfilling sex life with his girlfriend, while Jake the god is a virgin. Jake lives in fear that someone will discover that his sex life consists of one-handed surfing in cyberspace.

This book is just as much for Tim and his girlfriend as it is for Jake and Rosie. It makes no assumptions except that you are curious about sex and might want to enjoy it even more.

Charts, Graphs & Sex Surveys

This book has no charts or graphs. If you are the type who's bamboozled by such things, consider the following: how do you graph the value of a loving glance or heartfelt hug? Yet try to enjoy sex in a relationship without them. Rather than assuming which graph is best for you, this Guide tries to accommodate a full range of sexual tastes and beliefs, be they conservative, eclectic, or kinky. Are any of us just one or the other?

This book also avoids the latest in popular surveys, such as one recently done by the BBC. This study found that the top seven traits women find most important in a male partner are humor, intelligence, honesty, kindness, values, communication skills and dependability. That sounds well and fine, until you realize that things like "loves me," "shares my interests," "exciting sex partner," and "acceptable to parents and friends" were not on the list of desirable characteristics that women could check. And while the attractiveness of a partner's teeth came in 16th out of 23 on the BBC study, do you honestly believe that teeth would have been ranked that low if the study had been funded by a huge company that makes dental products?

Final Alpha Note

Most people would probably agree that sex is best when it's honest, caring and fun. The same should be true for books on sex. Hopefully, you will find *The Guide's* attempt at explaining love and sex to be honest and true, and with a colossal amount of respect for anyone who reads it.

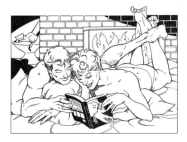

Dear Paul,

In my intro psych class, they wanted us to take a detailed survey about sex. My boyfriend and I really like sex, but I didn't feel comfortable doing the survey and left most of it blank. Does this mean I'm weird?

Athena from Mt. Holyoke

Dear Athena,

My own suspicion about sex surveys was born two days before I took my first intro-to-anything class in college. Perhaps some background will help.

I had spent my first 18 years in a small town that didn't have a lot of stop lights or two-story buildings. It did, however, have a large number of bars and churches, and girls who if they didn't get knocked-up by the end of high school feared a life of loneliness and isolation.

So I had spent the totality of my life in the nape of America's red neck, and suddenly found myself as a freshman at UC Berkeley, where there were Krishnas instead of cows, and "weed" was no longer the hallmark of poor pasture management.

Back then, I had no idea that the nice, neanderthal-looking guy who lived upstairs in my dorm would become a founder of Apple computer, or that I would someday write a book on sex that people like yourself would have on their shelves.

What I did know is that I had to show up at the student health center to take a physical exam. That's when I became one of hundreds of guys in their boxers or briefs, waiting in a mile-long line to pee on command. But first, we got to stand in front of a row of doctors who pulled our briefs down and reported what they saw to the young nursing students who were sitting next to them with charts in hand. Not being ones to take it on faith, the young nursing students looked up and checked as well.

When I got back to the dorm there was a thick survey sitting on my desk. It wanted to know about my personal sexual habits. Being barely a man and just two days in the big city, I wasn't ready to confess "how many times I masturbated during the past week." What I did know is that no matter how far from home you are and no matter how fast of a lane you have fallen into, what's personal is personal, and nobody has a right to take that from you.

So, like you, I left the survey blank.

As I think back over the sex survey from my first few days in college, I am reminded of how complex and personal sex is for some of us, as it seems to be for you. At the same time, I appreciate that your best friend might be posting clips of herself having sex on the Internet. And what about all of the people who post the most intimate details of their private lives on their blogs?

Are you "weird?" Perhaps. But I'm not so sure how many of us aren't.

CHAPTER
2
Romance

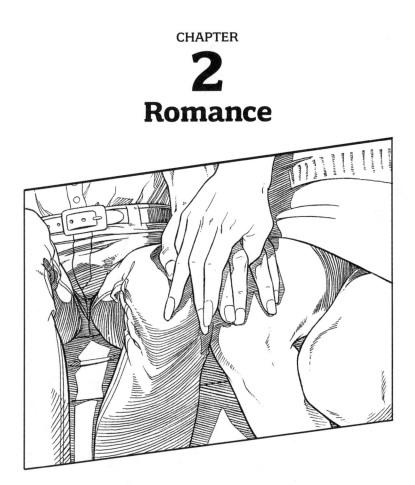

Romance is something thoughtful that you do for someone you love. It's the Gorilla Glue that holds a relationship together. It's lube for above the belt instead of below.

Romance can be as simple as leaving a note on the refrigerator that says "I love you" or giving an unexpected hug. It can also include heroic gestures, like helping your partner do his taxes, or scouring the tile in her skanky-looking shower, or taking a whole day to organize your lover's Nightmare-on-Elm-Street closet.

Contrary to what the ads in newspapers and television tell you, romance does not need to cost a thing. There's not a single thing about being romantic that should require the folks at MasterCard to increase your credit limit.

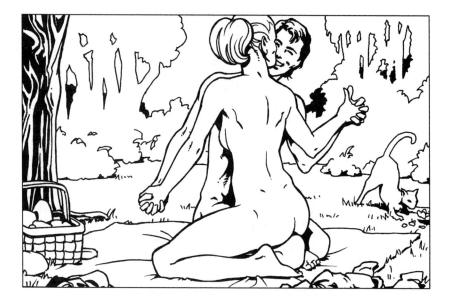

You are deluding yourself if you think that the only way you can be wildly romantic is by increasing the national debt.

Romance vs. Sex

Try not to assume that romance will result in sex. Romance resides in a special universe somewhere between Platonic love and carnal lust. Romance can evolve into sex, and the sex can be wonderfully romantic, but it's just as possible to have a perfectly romantic evening and end up in bed alone. When that happens, you do what the rest of us have done since the beginning of time: you lather up Little Willy with his favorite brand of lotion and romance him yourself, or you pull out your trusty vibrator and caress the front of your thong with it.

Romance When You Are Dating as Opposed to When You Are Married

Getting the oil on your partner's car changed and having it washed can be a romantic thing if you are just dating. However, if you are married, she might smile and say, "Looks nice," but it's one of those things that's migrated from the romance column to being one of your jobs.

On the other hand, when you were just dating, going to a movie might not have been all that romantic, given how you would do it at the drop of a hat a couple of times a week. But once you have kids, going to a movie involves hiring a baby sitter and picking her up, getting dinner made for the

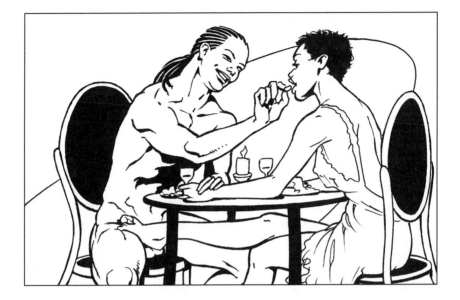

little ones, and finding some way to defy the laws of parenting and get to the theater on time. By virtue of the wedding ring and your most excellent breeding skills, going out to see a movie has gone from routine to romantic.

Likewise, your partner may have loved receiving stuffed animals before marriage, but after having children, the population of stuffed animals in your household has reached critical mass. She's thinking, "How do I sneak this bag of stuffed animals to Goodwill without little Ally having a meltdown?"

Married or not, getting a lover her favorite chocolate is almost always romantic regardless of the number of notches on the side of her uterus. Chocolate works on the same part of the brain as cocaine and heroin.

Getting Your Romance Meters in Sync

When it comes to being romantic, people can have very different styles. If the person feels like a keeper, try to figure out what is romantic to him or her. This might be different from what's romantic to you.

Things that make a big splash might be what catches your romantic eye, while your partner prefers the understated. Just because his or her romantic style is different from yours doesn't mean you can't be wonderfully romantic in each other's eyes. It might help to make an ongoing mental list of romantic things that your partner goes "Wow!" over. That way you won't be caught scratching your head when the need for romance arises.

It can be harder to connect with a partner romantically when one or both of you feels overwhelmed. Romance during stressful times can require shifting gears. It might include anything from digging in and just being there, to quietly taking up the slack when your partner isn't able to do what he or she usually does. If your partner has a huge project coming up, or is dealing with a gnarly life stressor, plan ahead for things you can do to help make it better.

Romance in Long-Term Relationships

In long-term relationships, all the romantic gestures in the world are meaningless if you aren't trustworthy or don't do your share of the housework. Cooking a special dinner or sending an unexpected card won't get you far if you didn't do the chores that your partner was counting on you to do.

For romance to work in a long-term relationship, it helps if both of you are reliable and do as you say. Then, the kind and thoughtful gestures have a footing on which to stand. On the other hand, when you hear people who have been together for a long time say that the sparkle is gone in their relationship, they have sometimes worked so hard on being reliable that they have forgotten about the little gestures that help make a relationship hot.

There's a balancing act in any long-term relationship, given how "reliability" means going to work and keeping your commitments, while "erotic" is more about dropping everything and having sex in the moment.

The Thrill Is Gone

Neurobiologists are finding that we use at least two different brain responses to process how we feel about our lovers. When a relationship is new, during the first six months to a year, we process our lovers in the wild'n'crazy part of the brain. Our good judgment is mostly shot to hell, and even a lover's most annoying habits seem endearing. We pine over them, obsess about them, and want to have lots and lots of sex with them.

Then, after nine months to a year, many of us start to process our long-term partners with the "long-term relationship" parts of the brain. To protect your sex life from being lost in the kids-and-a-mortgage part of your brain, it helps to add novelty. Novelty is a way of lobbing your relationship back into the sexually-exciting part of the brain.

So if you find yourself thinking more about getting new matching recliners for in front of the TV instead of interesting places and positions for having sex—it is important for the two of you to do fun and interesting things together, or to visit new and different places. Without tempering the familiar with the new, your relationship might be doomed to reside in the grandma/grandpa part of your cranium.

So, let's say your husband of fifteen years is the most trustworthy and hard-working man on the face of the earth. He's a great father to your kids, and you love him dearly, but the romance in your relationship is kaput. And let's say you have been noticing the pool man a lot more than you did before. By the time he leaves each week, you are wetter than the pool deck. How do you get that kind of passion back with your husband?

It's quite possible that in your husband's mind, his way of being romantic is by working his tail off for you and the kids. Worse things have happened. Be sure that at least a couple of times a week you tell him how much you appreciate how hard he works. Do this from now until the end of time. Then, think back over the past fifteen years and come up with things the two of you have enjoyed doing together—without the kids. Maybe it's river rafting, maybe it's shopping for antiques or going to a carnival. Maybe it's working in the garden together. If it's possible, find ways for the two of you to start doing some of these things together again. (Of course, if you and he are locked into some kind of unconscious struggle where you are acting out stuff from your respective pasts, it is best to get marital or individual counseling.)

Keep in mind that this kind of approach is a traditional one that doesn't reach too far into the world of sexual novelty. Someone less traditional might recommend that you broach the subject of trying a threesome with your husband and the pool boy. But swinging is more apt to work if the primary couple has a solid and satisfying sexual relationship to begin with. Unless your husband is secretly lusting after the pool boy as well.

What Readers Have to Say about Romance

"Romance is being kind, gentle, and thoughtful. Sometimes intense as when making love, sometimes only on pilot light, but never off."
male age 70

"Romance is being naked in the sun." *male age 42*

"Romance is when she and I can absolutely forget that the rest of the world exists. Just today we both had a million things to do to prepare for the coming workweek, but I turned on the CD player and played a great Spanish song about a bull that falls in love with the moon. Soon we had dropped our work and were spinning each other around the living room like two people who had no idea how to dance flamenco." *male age 25*

"What is romance? Stroking my hair, holding my hand, helping me with the housework, cooking, talking, sharing the day with me."
female age 43

"Romance is waking up in my partner's arms and being told that he loves me." *female age 27*

"Romance is when we go Rollerblading at the beach." *male age 32*

"Romance is sitting on a hammock together reading our books."
female age 26

"It's bringing home a single rose or a little something to say I was thinking of you today." *female age 34*

"Doing things that show he values me as a life partner and not just a bed partner." *female age 45*

"For romance, I enjoy a great bubble bath together with candles and wine, lots of great smelling scents whether it's perfume, incense, or just the smell of my man." *female age 36*

"If he brings you flowers or jewelry and he's not there in any other way, it's not romance." *female age 45*

RESOURCES for when romance is gone in an otherwise loving relationship: Sure, there are couples who manage to buy houses together, raise a family and negotiate the nastiness of everyday life and still have hot and sizzling sex. There must be some in your own city or state. But the ability to trust that a partner will pick up the kids on time, or won't spend the day gaming when you don't have enough money to pay the rent—that kind of stability and trust becomes way more important than sex. On the other hand, predictability and steadfastness aren't always the hallmark of hot times in bed. In her well-written book *Mating in Captivity: Reconciling the Erotic and the Domestic* (Harper Paperbacks, 2007), therapist and author Ester Perel looks at whether it is possible to keep sex alive in a long-term relationship. She does so in a way that is thoughtful, intelligent and helpful.

A Highly Evolved Thanks to Anthropologist Helen Fisher from Rutgers.

3
Kiss Me!
Lip-Smacking Good

This chapter is about kissing on the upper body as opposed to kissing on the genitals, although one often leads to the other. A lot of couples mix the two together—a little peck, a little suck, a little peck, a little suck. Sometimes kissing is used as a starter, to help stir up your body fluids for what's to follow. Other times, kissing is all there is.

Kissing can be awkward at times, especially at the start. But even if your lips are so experienced they could dock space shuttles for NASA, you might find some helpful reminders in the pages that follow.

The Power of Talking in Tongues

It's funny how kissing a partner on the lips usually makes more of an emotional statement than kissing him or her on the genitals, even if the latter sometimes feels better. For instance, one of the Goofy-Foot advisors, who makes her living by having sex with different men, reports that she won't let anyone other than her husband kiss her on the lips.

It's also interesting how when a relationship starts to go sour, couples usually stop kissing on the lips long before they stop having intercourse.

There are reasons why lip-locking is sometimes more intimate than getting into a partner's pants. Much as we might hate it, from the moment we are born, most of us are kissed constantly by moms, dads, aunts, uncles, grandparents, and anyone else whose approaching lips we can't successfully dodge. Being kissed on the lips, cheeks and top of the head symbolizes a profound love that we hopefully come into the world experiencing.

Another reason for the added power of kissing is so many of the major senses have their outlets on the human face. There is vision, smell, hearing, and taste. And the lips and skin are exquisitely sensitive to touch. There are, in fact, so many sensory centers located on or near the human face that we have terms such as "You're in my face" or "Get out of my face" to express annoyance or social discomfort. (Interestingly, the ability to have an orgasm is not considered one of the basic senses, although it overwhelms the other senses when it happens.)

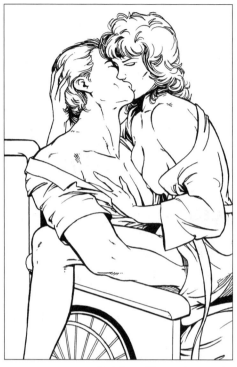

When Kissing Is the Main Course

Kissing is often a prelude to other things, but there are plenty of times when kissing is all you get. Like when you are sixteen and necking all night long. Or when you are older but want to feel like you are sixteen. Don't for a moment think that monster make-out sessions are kids' stuff. Some people experience these as hotter than much of the intercourse they've had.

If all you plan on doing is making out, be sure to put your gum in a safe place where you can find it afterward. It will help take the edge off until you can go home and masturbate.

Readers' Smooch Advice: The Basics

"Please don't eat my mouth. A good kiss can make me wet with desire, with only the softest touch." *female age 23*

"Kissing is not just a preliminary to fucking. Gently explore with your tongue, lightly suck on her lips and tongue. If she is into it as much as you, kiss with good suction, not lazily." *female age 45*

"When you're kissing, be gentle; don't swallow a woman's entire face into your mouth or dig your teeth into her cheeks." *female age 36*

"Start really light. Barely brush your lips against hers. Be very aware of her response. Increase the pressure ever so slightly when she begins to meet your lips. Eventually, touch the tip of your tongue to her lips. If she opens her mouth, you can let your tongue enter just the smallest bit, but try not to force her mouth open." *male age 25*

Be Sure to Ask

Kissing is such a powerful thing, yet we seldom take the time to ask a partner how he or she likes to be kissed. Maybe he or she is turned on more by delicate little butterfly kisses than by some overly dramatic lip-lock that you saw at the movies. You'll never really know unless you ask, and it's a shame not to ask.

Breathe or Die, and Don't Forget to Swallow

When you are new to kissing, you might find yourself holding your breath. Sometimes there are good reasons for this, but usually it's a bad idea. When you are kissing, your mouth is often busy, while your nose is mostly in the way. Breathing through your nose gives it a purpose and keeps your partner from feeling like you are attempting mouth-to-mouth resuscitation.

People who are new at kissing sometimes ask what to do with their noses when they smooch. They also ask if they should kiss with their eyes open or closed. We don't know. As for the issue of serious salivary action, take these comments to heart:

"Turn off the water works! There is nothing worse than a big slobbery wet kiss." *female age 27*

"Try not to slobber!" *female age 25*

"An overly wet mouth is a turn-off." *female age 32*

"Girls love slobber. At least that's what they tell me. Maybe that's 'cause I slobber, though. Hey, wait a second!" *male age 22*

Flossing, Brushing & Garlic

It is raunchy to kiss with pieces of food stuck in your teeth. Flossing and brushing can make you far more attractive than wearing cologne or sucking on breath mints. If you are concerned about bad breath, check with your dentist. Dentists know all about bad breath, as many of them seem to have it. Ask if you should scrape the surface of your tongue with the edge of a spoon. The white gooey stuff that the spoon picks up is said by some to cause certain kinds of bad breath.

If you are eating food with garlic or onions, make sure the person you plan to smooch shares some big bites. Flossing and brushing won't put a dent in breath that is laced with garlic. Your only defense is to share the offense.

If You Are Wearing Braces

For people who have braces with rubber bands, consider taking the rubber bands out ahead of time. One reader barely escaped mid-smooch tragedy when a rubber band on his sweetheart's braces came unhooked and nearly shot him in the uvula. A direct hit would have triggered the same reflex that causes projectile vomiting.

Also, be aware that an incoming tongue might get scratched or caught on metal edges that don't pose a problem for you. You might tell a new partner that you are concerned about this and would feel better if he or she slowly and thoroughly explored the inside of your mouth with his or her tongue.

Great Kissing Advice

"The best thing you can do during a good kissing session is to ask your partner to kiss you the way he or she likes to be kissed. It really works. Just sit back and let him or her take over; you'll learn all kinds of things." *male age 26*

French Kissing

French kissing is the oral version of spelunking. The reason it is called "French kissing" is because French women found it to be an effective way to make French men stop talking.

French kissing is not a tongue-to-tonsils regatta. Try swallowing first, and don't go shoving your tongue down your partner's throat. Pretend your tongue is Baryshnikov instead of Vin Diesel, and you will do just fine. There is always time for tonsil-sucking later.

When you are French kissing, keep in mind that mouths enjoy variety. Don't cling to your partner's mouth like it's a New York City parking space. Bring your tongue out for air, and change the pace with a little lip-neck action before re-probing the deep.

"Take it slow and easy, but not too easy." *female age 26*

"Don't jam your tongue down someone's throat until she invites you in." *female age 38*

"Getting deep throated for fifteen minutes at a whack is no fun." *fem, 48*

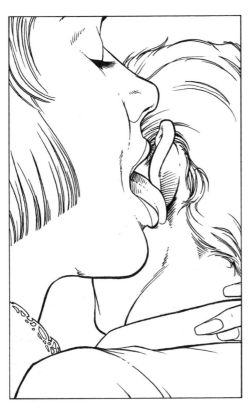

Putting the "Neck" in Necking

In hundreds of sex surveys, both male and female readers of *The Guide* have said that they wished their partner spent more time kissing them on the neck. Lots more time.

So while lips, eyelids, ears, noses, cheeks and foreheads are excellent areas to kiss, don't forget the neck. We're not talking vampire action, but something this side of raising a hickey might help create a welcome reception in parts of the body that are further south.

What about Hickeys?

Hickeys are what happen when a lover sucks on your neck or other body parts with enough force to cause internal bleeding. The hickey is the resulting bruise. Some people are proud of their hickeys and display them the way bikers do tattoos. Other people feel mortified when they discover a brownish or bluish blotch that wasn't there the day before. They even wear turtlenecks in the middle of summer to cover the things up.

Keep in mind that people with certain skin types hickey-up worse than others. As for hickeys between the legs, who much cares unless you are going to the beach or having an extramarital affair?

One woman who called a radio talk show said that her boyfriend had given her a hickey in the middle of her forehead. How do you explain that one, unless you lucked out and got it the night before Ash Wednesday?

How to Hide a Hickey

Concealing a hickey with make-up is by no means a straight-forward procedure. The first thing to understand is that you need green to neutralize red. So if the hickey is reddish in color, dab a green concealer directly over it

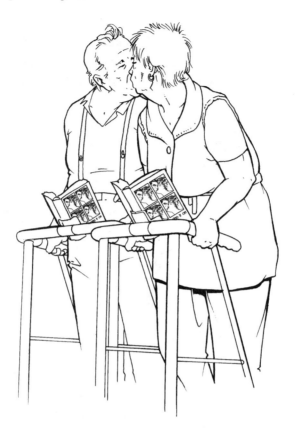

first. Then use your regular skin-color foundation or concealer and powder on top. If you don't neutralize the reddish blotch with green, the hickey will usually triumph.

Be sure to dab the concealer on rather than rubbing it in. If you don't have green, use an oil-based concealer that is lighter than your natural skin color, as the hickey color will cause it to look darker. But focus the lighter concealer only on the hickey area. Otherwise, the area around the hickey will look like a big smudge, and everyone will know. Scarves and high-necked collars can help.

The Real Estate between Your Ears & Knees

This guide places way too much emphasis on the standard blue chip kissing zones—lips, nipples and genitals. Lovers who enjoy each other will often go from head to toe, discovering and rediscovering where a partner loves to be kissed. Here are a few areas to consider:

Skin Folds The places on the body where the skin folds or creases tend to be very sensitive and love to be kissed. These include the backs of knees, the fronts of elbows, the nape of the neck, under breasts, on eyelids, armpits, crotches, between fingers and toes, and behind ears.

Lower Back & Buns The lower back and rear end can be exquisite places to kiss and kiss again.

Bellies & Navels Think of the navel as a little vulva rather than a collecting point for lint. Some people love to have their navels licked and caressed. Others become seriously annoyed.

Long Licks Don't hesitate to get your tongue really wet and take a long lick up your partner's body, from hip to armpit or tailbone to neck (known as "Australian" in some circles.)

Human Serving Tray Fruits, dessert foods, and certain liquors can be served on various parts of the body with pleasing results.

Love Bites Teeth on skin can feel really nice or really ugly. If this is what you would like to try, lube your lover's skin with oil or saliva so your teeth glide along the surface. Then raise your lips up and gently run your teeth back and forth. You might try a little biting action on large muscle groups such as the shoulders or buns. Be sure to get lots of feedback from the bitee, and for heaven's sake, stop short of violating cannibalism statutes.

Eskimo Pies & Eskimo Kisses: Kissing in Other Cultures

You may have heard that Eskimos don't kiss like we do. Instead of kissing on the lips they allegedly rub noses. What's closer to the truth is that Eskimos put their noses in close proximity to inhale the breath of a loved one. Perhaps they do this to keep their lips from freezing together. They may avoid oral-genital contact for the same reason.

Eskimos find that inhaling the breath of a lover is erotic; those of us from more temperate climates prefer exchanging wads of saliva. People raised in different cultures don't always agree on what's sexy.

Kissing on the Edge of Town

In nearly every community where people have lips, there tend to be special places where the locals go to make out.

In the town where your author grew up there were two favorite places where people went to kiss and grope—well, three if you counted the local drive-in, but that was more like an extra bedroom. One of those places was at the river, which was in the mountains that were east of town. Another was in the orange groves.

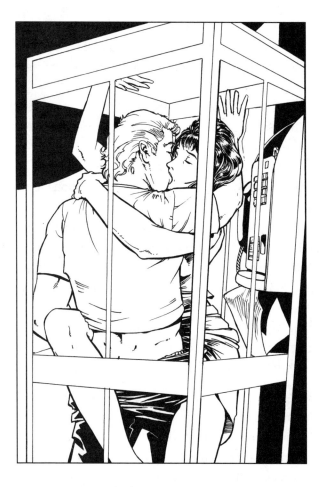

Perhaps there were places where you grew up that lovers went to for making out. Maybe there still is one where you and your sweetheart go.

Passion Pits & the Phone Booth—Symbols of the Past

Not long ago, there were more than 4,000 drive-in theaters or *passion pits* in America where younger couples kissed, groped and petted themselves into a Friday-night frenzy. While the population is nearly double today what it was then, there are now fewer than 500 drive-in theaters in America.

If the loss of the drive-in has led to less making out, it wouldn't hurt to occasionally have a "Drive-In Night," where all you do is grope and make out in front of a big-screen TV. You might visit the iTunes Music Store to download a copy of The Tubes' song *Don't Touch Me There* (3:30 version). Crank it up whenever fingers start creeping below a girl's beltline. And don't forget the popcorn.

4
The Importance of Getting Naked

In human relationships, there are different kinds of nakedness. Sometimes, we just get physically naked. Other times, we get emotionally naked as well. Whatever your situation or inclination, this chapter talks about taking your clothes off, and suggests a kind of nakedness that has emotional as well as physical grit. It also talks about different ways of getting naked, and the things we cover ourselves with that entice but keep us just this side of wearing nothing.

Getting Naked—An Overview

For some people, getting naked in front of a lover is as easy and natural as drinking a glass of water. Some even send naked pictures of themselves over their cellphones. For others, getting naked can cause distress or embarrassment. Some people even engineer situations where they can get it on without taking their clothes off in front of a partner. Perhaps this gives you an idea of how powerful getting naked can be, and how vulnerable we can feel about our bodies.

As a culture, we are so uptight about nakedness that we don't have street-corner fountains with fat marble cherubs peeing into large pools of water or public paintings of naked Botticelli babes. A bare crotch on network television is about as common as a snowstorm in Siam, and even the suggestion of body parts beneath a person's blue jeans on the public airwaves can result in a massive fine from the FCC. No wonder why a free-for-all of nakedness has evolved over the Internet!

No matter what our culture's public stance, we are clearly interested in nakedness, given how so many ads and images in our society drip with prurient fury. Perhaps we have learned to cope with all of the mixed messages by becoming more aroused by near-naked images than by actual nakedness. Or near-nakedness might simply allow more space for our fantasies to imagine what's under the skimpy wrappers. Whatever the case, with their suggestion of impending nakedness, the pictures in this chapter may have more intrigue than if the couples in them were buck naked.

The Naked-Nipple Rule

In North America, we believe that a woman isn't really naked unless her nipples are showing. This was particularly obvious after the famous Superbowl half-time show. Even though the woman's crotch was well covered, the fact that her nipple saw the light of day caused a major furor. In Europe, they still don't understand what the big fuss was all about.

Hopefully you will feel free to do your own half-time show at home, violating the naked-nipple rule as often as you please.

Getting Naked — Hidden Possibilities

If you and your sweetheart are in the process of becoming more physical, you might consider some of the hidden possibilities that getting naked has to offer. A lot of honesty and trust can be generated when you are naked together, something that rarely develops if the sole purpose of taking your clothes off is to have intercourse. It's how you can learn to relate physically with more than just your crotches. It's how a guy can learn to have his penis resting on a woman's soft, warm skin without feeling like he has to perform with it, and how her vulva and breasts can be pushing against him while she dozes off.

Naked Logistics

If it feels like your relationship is ready, you might consider planning a time and place where the two of you can work on getting naked. Some couples enjoy undressing each other, while others make a game out of taking their clothes off, from playing strip poker to lighthearted wrestling. There are occasions where one partner blindfolds the other before undressing him or her.

Sometimes getting naked happens naturally if you go skinny-dipping or hot-tubbing, and some couples enjoy undressing each other while dancing. If you try this, be sure to have birth control handy in case you suddenly find yourselves doing the polka.

Occasionally, people find it helpful to tell each other some of the things that they do and don't like about their bodies. Some women worry their butts are too big or their breasts are too small. Some guys worry they aren't hung well enough, or they might be hung too well, or that their penis might bend the wrong way when it gets hard. Just getting your fears out in the open will usually help you feel more comfortable.

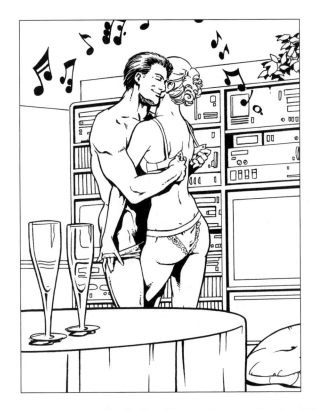

For couples who are particularly self-conscious, writer Jay Wiseman suggests getting naked in total darkness. Each partner then takes turns examining the body of the other with a small flashlight—one of those little penlight things that excites just enough photons to light up an area the size of your thumbnail. This can be a fun game that taps into all sorts of fantasies as well as helps decrease the anxiety of being seen naked all at once. Another way for the shy to share their nakedness is by getting a fun top or T-shirt to wear with nothing on underneath. Or maybe you'd like to try a pair of silk boxers.

Guys Worry: Wood Good, Wood Bad?

When it comes to getting naked, men sometimes worry whether they should or shouldn't have a hard-on. It doesn't matter. It's fine if you have one, it's fine if you don't. The point is learning to associate nakedness with something other than just sex or taking a shower.

Some people don't have the slightest hesitation to get naked for sex, but if it's getting naked just to talk or hold each other, good luck. They sometimes become fidgety and fire off a rapidly dismissive, "Sure, we'll have to try that sometime...." Perhaps that kind of nakedness feels too intimate.

Naked & Getting Off

While getting naked together doesn't need to include orgasms, some couples find it uplifting to have one or two somewhere along the way. So plan your naked time to include lots of holding and touching, try an orgasm or two, and then even more holding and touching afterward. (One reader comments, "Good luck on this one. I've spent a lot of lonely time while my partner sleeps immediately after orgasm.")

Coming is usually the last thing that couples do when they are having sex. Yet it might be nice to spend extra time holding and touching each other after you have orgasms, rather than simply rolling over and falling asleep or running off to work. Coming clears the senses in a way that allows many of us to share a special kind of warmth and tenderness.

Sex Tips with a Cranky Marxist Edge

Sometimes a half-peeled banana is more exciting than one with no peel at all, or so we've been led to believe. This type of philosophy has helped fuel the multimillion-dollar lingerie business, which for years has made a handsome profit selling flimsy wisps of underwear to women under the name of lingerie. Now manufacturers are gouging men with similar intent. They embroider the name of some fancy clothes designer or tennis-shoe manufacturer into the elastic waistband of men's briefs and suddenly charge $10 to $20 for a pair that you could otherwise buy at Sears for $2.50. **Counterpoint:** "I have read portions of *The Guide* out loud to my girlfriend, and we are enjoying it very much. I have but one complaint: stop the lingerie bashing. It is perhaps the only good thing about American consumerism."

If you find underwear to be erotic, here are a couple of possibilities:

 Women who wear nylons and garters might consider putting their panties on over the garter belt instead of under, so their panties can come off while leaving the stockings and garters intact. Fine tips such as these can be found in Cynthia Heimel's classic *Sex Tips for Girls*. Her lingerie chapter offers insight about women's underwear that no male writer short of a transvestite would ever get right.

 A common garter *faux pas,* according to Los Angeles' Trashy Lingerie, is wearing the rear garter all the way back instead of to the side. On the right leg, the front garter should be worn at dead center (12:00), and the

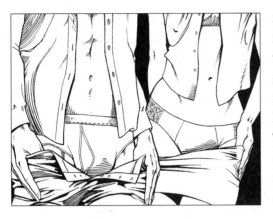

rear garter should attach to the nylon at 3:30 to 4:00 as opposed to 6:00. On the left leg the front garter attaches at 12:00 and the rear garter at 7:30 or 8:00. This helps keep the seams straight. The "western woman" pictured on page 811 almost has it right, although her rear garter is closer to 5:00 than 3:30-4:00.

Another Trashy Lingerie tip: if you wear a push-up bra, put it on, and then reach across your chest with your right hand. Grab your left breast from under your armpit, lifting it up and dropping it into the bra cup. Do the same thing with your left hand and right breast. Another bra misdemeanor: incorrectly adjusting the straps so the bra rides up too high or droops down too low. See pages 803-804 for info on how to make sure your bra fits right.

Here's a piece of shagadelic seduction advice from the 1960s: When going out, a woman might let a man know that she is not wearing any underwear, or reach into her purse and pull out a pair of panties while saying, "Oops, guess I forgot to put these on!"

When sitting down to lunch or even for a long plane flight, some women briefly hike up their dress and intentionally adjust a garter in view of a man whose salivary glands they hope to make flow. The art of doing this is in the ability to disguise the purposefulness of the act. Reaching for something in the overhead compartment can achieve similar results if you are wearing a dress or skirt that's short enough.

Here's a way to add a bit of variety and challenge when doing oral sex: Go down on your partner while she or he is still wearing underwear. You can reach under the material with your tongue, push it to one side for proper access, or pull it off with your teeth. You'll probably need a fingertip assist, but the gesture is what counts!

If you are having a quickie, you might keep your underwear on and try working your way around it. Also, some couples enjoy having oral sex and intercourse while one or both partners is wearing crotchless underwear.

Dry humping with only your underwear on can be fun. So can taking a shower or bath while still wearing your underwear. Plenty of dry humping gets done at the beach when it's not very crowded and people are wearing swimsuits.

Women shouldn't hesitate to take their lovers with them when shopping for lingerie. Shopping for a new bra or skivvies might seem mundane to a woman, but it could be a fun treat for a man. It will also help give him ideas for when he wants to get you a special gift. If it's possible, ask him to accompany you into the dressing room. A drawback, unfortunately, is that a man's presence might cause other women who are shopping for bras and panties to feel self-conscious.

For guys, the next time you are in a big department store with your sweetheart, nudge her into the men's underwear department and ask her what style and colors she thinks might look best on you. This can make for added pleasure the next time she pops the buttons on your blue jeans.

Men's Underwear

Men have a choice of wearing briefs, boxers, boxer-briefs, men's G-Strings thongs, nothing, or even women's underwear if they're of that ilk. Most of us end up wearing whatever our mothers bought for us as kids, usually briefs or boxers. Each provides a different kind of feeling that a man gets used to, thus casting him for life as either a briefs guy or a boxer guy, although there are probably some men who are switch-hitters. More and more men find that boxer-briefs offer the best of both worlds.

While a briefs guy might experiment with boxers for a couple of months or even years, there is a tendency to go back to what he started with. Same with a boxer guy. A woman shouldn't push the issue one way or the other, unless the man doesn't care or is the type who tells her when to wear a bra.

Cramped Penis Alert

A guy's penis usually hangs downward when it's soft, but as it stiffens it needs extra head room to accommodate the expansion. If a man is wearing jeans, the expanding penis often gets trapped in a downward position (ouch!) or gets stuck in a horizontal pickle. So if you are fooling around with your clothes on, the penis will usually need a quick assist to rise above it all. While it might be a bit presumptuous for a woman to lend a helping hand if you are making out on a first date, this can be a really nice gesture once you are on groping terms. When the bulge starts to grow, just reach inside his pants and pull the penis up so its head is pointing toward the man's chest, unless it naturally bends down.

Jocks

Some men like to wear athletic supporters for erotic purposes. Perhaps one reason for this is the athletic supporter emphasizes a man's rear end by keeping it naked while highlighting his genitals by keeping them covered. Some women get turned on by seeing a lover in an athletic supporter, as long as it isn't wringing wet from playing four hours of rugby. It never hurts for lovers to ask each other about these things.

Learning from Lady Lawyers

During the 1970s and 1980s, lady lawyers suddenly began to penetrate the traditional male lair. Being confused about how to be taken seriously, most of these women started wearing boring wool suits with blouses that had floppy bows (the "lady lawyer" uniform). The intent was to look as non-sexual and unalluring as humanly possible, as femininity was considered to be a liability when arguing matters of law. Short of wearing a body bag to court, most of the women succeeded handily. Some of these lady lawyers made it a point to wear steamy lingerie under their boring suits. It was a way of saying to themselves, "At least some part of me is still feminine."

In our society, wearing lingerie has been an important way for women to feel feminine. In fact, some women feel sexier wearing lingerie than they do being naked. Some women feel better masturbating while wearing lingerie or underpants.

As for guys feeling more masculine while wearing boxers, briefs, or jockstraps, some do and some don't. What feels best of all is when a lover pulls off whatever it is you are wearing.

Girls UnderGear

In case you had trouble getting the Stargate open and have been on another planet for the past couple of years, here's a brief list of what today's earth girls are covering their celestial crotches with:

Thong—A narrow piece of material that passes between the legs and up through the butt where it attaches to a waistband. Thongs have traditionally been the underwear of strippers. Then, women in Brazil started wearing them, and it was only a matter of time before they worked their way under North American dresses and jeans. There are different types of thongs, including G-strings or T-backs, which are the underwear equivalent of dental floss; the Tanga, which has more material in the seat; and the Rio, which has straps on the sides. [Sorry, but our gyno-experts say thongs cause your puss to chafe. Also, the butt-floss part of the thong provides a super-highway for butt bacteria to get into your vagina and cause an infection.]

Hipsters or *Boy Shorts*—The comfort favorite of many girls, hipsters and boy shorts are like low-rise briefs that offer full coverage without looking like granny panties. Materials can range from cotton to lace. *Hipsters* stop higher on the thigh while *boy shorts* have the start of leg.

Bikini—The modern bikini was born in 1946. It was named after the island Bikini Atoll, which is part of the Marshall Islands in the Pacific Ocean where nuclear weapons were tested. It was so daring that the only model who would originally wear it was a nude dancer. It did not become popular in the US until Brian Hyland's song *Itsy Bitsy Teenie Weenie Yellow Polka Dot Bikini* hit the charts, and American women suddenly started gearing up—or down. Who knew that bikini panties would become commonplace and seem conservative when compared to today's popular G-strings? *String bikinis* have a strings on the sides that connect the front and back panels.

Granny Panties—These occupy the women's underwear niche that's between the bikini and Depends.

Visible Panty Line—No matter what a girl wears underneath, *VPL* or *Visible Panty Line* is one of the more serious of the female fashion felonies. The biggest cause is panties that are too tight. Some thongs and boy-shorts can help, but not if what you are wearing is extremely tight or transparent.)

Bras—Bra styles run from shock-absorbing sports bras to the massive range at Victoria's Secrets. Given the cultural significance of the breast and what holds it up, see Chapter 70, "The Historical Breast and Bra" in the "History and Popular Culture" part of this book.

Stripping

Until the advent of Chippendales, stripping was something that only girls did, and it usually fell into one of two categories. The first was the playful, private stripping that a woman does for her significant other. Even evangelical marriage manuals nod and wink when a good Christian wife puts on a show to get her man's baby-making gears going. The other kind of stripping is for pay in front of strangers. Society frowns on women who do this. If you doubt that, try telling your mom you are dating someone who strips at the Kitty-Kat Lounge.

Contrary to what you might think, it's the girls in the audience at the male strip shows who go wild and get aggressive, while men at girlie strip shows are expected to be more subdued, even when they pay for lap dances. And hard as this is to believe, the *US News and World Report* says that Americans spend more at strip clubs than at the opera, ballet, Broadway and Off-Broadway theater, and classical-music performances combined. So if you are into it, why not try it at home? For guidance, consider *The Stripper's Guide to Looking Great Naked* by Jennifer Axen and Leigh Phillips, Chronicle Books.

The authors interviewed strippers from all over the country for suggestions that could be helpful to girls who want to make an impression in front of their partners.

An important cornerstone of a stripper's appeal is how each one needs to adopt her own unique look. It does you no good to try looking like someone else. It's all about attitude and having your own style rather than sporting the perfect bod. Forget buying expensive products, going on strange diets and spending hours at the gym.

The Stripper's Guide offers a number of tips based on general body types a woman might have. For instance, when it comes to trimming your pubic hair, women with a voluptuous or well-endowed body might try a landing strip. The vertical line balances the curves and draws the eyes downward. A woman with an I-shaped body might go for a more natural-looking pubic bush, one that makes a wide oval that tapers at the bottom but doesn't stray below the bikini line. This helps make her hips look more round and curvy.

And what if you find yourself in a game of strip poker but haven't trimmed your pubes in a month and are wearing a granny bra? According to *The Stripper's Guide,* head for the bathroom for your three minutes of ABT "allowable bathroom time." Stuff the granny bra in your purse or into a drawer (better to be totally topless than shirtless with an ugly bra). Then run your fingers under cold water, and tweak your nipples with them. If the cards aren't running your way, and you lose your pants, make a show of taking them off, but sit with your legs crossed.

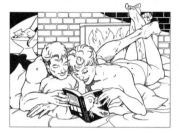

Dear Paul,

I get seriously turned on when my girlfriend is wearing pantyhose. There's something about the feel of them on her legs that makes Mr. Winky pop straight in the air. Any advice about this?

Seamless in Seattle

Dear Seamless,

Given how most of our mothers wore nylons or pantyhose, and considering how often our toddler selves stood next to them with arms wrapped around their legs, it's a wonder more guys aren't stirred into action by the feel of a woman in pantyhose.

Assuming your girlfriend is understanding and willing, ask her to cut out the cotton crotch on a pair of pantyhose. Thanks to the new ventilation system, you'll be able to go down on her as well as have intercourse while she is wearing her customized pantyhose. Make sure she cuts out the crotch on the inside of the seam so they don't unravel. Also, consider helping her to arrive orally before slipping your penis in, because it isn't likely that you will be lasting for long if nylons are your thing. If she isn't handy with scissors, she can purchase crotchless pantyhose in some stores, but probably not at places like Wal-Mart.

For those of you who are wondering about the difference between a guy with a healthy appreciation of girls in pantyhose versus one with a serious fetish, see the chapter on kink.

Thanks to the writings of Barbara Keesling, Linda Levine, Lonnie Barbach, Cynthia Heimel, and Jay Wiseman for naked inspiration. Ditto to the folks at Los Angeles' Trashy Lingerie, and to Katherine Liepe-Levinson, author of *Strip Show*. Thanks also to Leslie Davisson who was involved in the original launch of *The Guide*.

5
On the Penis

This chapter was written for women readers, although the men who have seen it claim to be amused. The topic is boys and their toys. Hopefully the following pages provide some insight into the love, and sometimes hate, relationship between a man and his weenie.

Toys, Pain & Pleasure

As a woman, the first thing you will find out about penises and testicles is that most guys take them way too seriously. There are reasons for this:

The penis is the only childhood toy that a guy gets to keep and play with throughout his entire life. It is the only toy he will ever own that feels good when he tugs on it, that constantly changes size and shape, and is activated by the realm of the senses. Try to find that at Toys'R'Us.

One of the first things a man does when he wakes up in the morning and the last thing he does at night is to touch his penis and testicles. It's a male ritual of self-affirmation that has little to do with sexual stimulation. A daytime extension of this is known as pocket pool.

The average male pees between five and seven times a day. Each time he pees he has a specific ritual, from the way he pulls his penis out to how he wags it when he's done. When he is peeing alone a guy will often invent imaginary targets in the toilet to gun for. An especially fine time is had when a cigarette butt has been left behind. Floating cigarette butts are the male urinary equivalent of the clay pigeon. While this may be a difficult concept for a woman to fully grasp, it does make for a certain amount of familiarity, friendship, and even self-bonding between a man and his penis.

🔆Another bathroom-related matter has to do with visual reinforcement. How many women look down when they are peeing to see what's coming out of their bodies? Guys look down often. As a result, we males get visual reinforcement for the feelings we have in our genitals when we pee. While women experience a hand-eye-genital experience when they use tampons, it's usually not all that visual, and it doesn't start until after puberty. Between erections, corrections, pocket pool and peeing, guys have far more sensory experience with the penis than most women have with their vaginas. This must be why women sometimes call us "Dicks!"

🔆You wouldn't believe how often the human male experiences a jolt of pain in his testicles. It is a discomfort that gives a guy the kind of extra-personal relationship with his reproductive equipment that menstruating women have with theirs. The source of agony can be anything from an elbow during a game of basketball to simply bending over and having your pants crimp the very life force out of you. One of the great culprits in male testicular angst is the horizontal bar on the bicycle frame. Why is it that girls' bicycle frames are V-shaped when it is guys who need the V? Not only did this confusion among bicycle makers result in our younger selves not getting to look up girls' dresses when they were mounting their bikes, but many of us still have the word Schwinn engraved on the underside of our testicles from each time a foot slipped off the pedal.

🔆This may be difficult to fully appreciate, but there is the matter of the unwanted hard-on. The unwanted hard-on usually strikes with predictable ferociousness first thing in the morning. Not only does it interfere with the ability to relieve a full bladder, but it provides logistical problems for a guy who has to traverse shared hallways to get to the bathroom. The unwanted hard-on can be excruciating and even painful for its most frequent victim, the adolescent male. The unwanted hard-on is much less of a problem after a man turns thirty, and by the time he's forty it is an event accompanied by a sigh of relief and a moment of thanks.

🔆Our society teaches us that sexual pleasure between a man and a woman depends on the man's ability to get hard and stay hard. What a demented view of sex. This puts a lot of pressure on guys to be consummate cocksmen. It makes us more dick-centered than necessary, at the expense of everyone.

When life is full of despair, the one thing that a guy can usually count on for a good feeling is his penis, unless matters are totally out of hand, in which case he needs to consider something stronger like tequila or prayer.

These items aside, the most important thing for a woman to know about a penis is how it figures into a man's concept of his own manliness. Ridiculous, but important.

Weirdness in the Locker Room

You might think that a man's primary concern about penis size has to do with what a sexual partner likes. But how he stacks up among his buds is just as important, if not more. When we asked men if they feel comfortable about being naked in the locker room, the majority answered the question as if we'd asked about penis size, even if the words "penis" and "size" were never part of the question. These are the exact answers men gave when asked:

"How do you feel about being naked in the locker room?"

"I used to feel uncomfortable back in my freshman year of high school. Then I realized that I was really a little bigger than average."

male age 21

"I used to think that my penis was really small, and so I was shy about it. As it turns out, I'm on the high end of average when erect: I'm just not a hanger." *male age 32*

"I have an inferiority complex about the size of my penis. I don't care how many studies tell me that I am right in the middle of the curve, I will always feel small." *male age 25*

"I was raised in a fairly strict and religious environment, so nudity of any kind was a no-no. My equipment is pretty small, and I was a late bloomer. All this adds up to being very shy about my own appearance. In junior high and high school, when 'naked locker time' was mandatory, I would arrive as early as possible and change quickly so that others wouldn't see me. If others were around me without clothes on, I gave myself tunnel vision or imaginary blinders so I wouldn't see other guys' equipment. I didn't want to be perceived as gay, and glancing around was a good way to get yourself taunted at least, beat up at worst." *male age 41 (And this guy was straight!)*

The men who said they were comfortable in the locker room often made reference to their penis size as well, indicating they were well hung. You can almost predict how a man feels about being naked in the locker room by asking how he feels about the size of his penis. Hopefully, the following from a Marine who has been in combat helps provide perspective:

'The tradition of group showers is still strong in the Marine Corps. It makes us more comfortable with each other, and if you are trusting a guy to save your life, do you really think penis size is that big a deal? Before the military though, I worried I didn't 'measure up.'" *male 27*

As for guys checking out other guys, you would think this curiosity would decrease as they get to be adults. Not so, according to a study by a group of Ph.D. students. These students hung out in rest rooms at a San Diego Padres game and secretly studied a hundred different men who were peeing. They claim that many of the men made an attempt to check out the equipment of whomever was peeing next to them. Furthermore, men who were well-endowed went out of their way to show their bigger units to the other men who were peeing. Of course these tendencies might be more true of Padres fans than, say, Kansas City Royals fans, who are usually too busy weeping in the men's room to check out the size of the other boys' bats. So if you are a man who has ever glanced down at another man's penis when you are peeing, take comfort in knowing that you are probably normal.

Size, Shape, Plumbing & The Goofy Dick Game

Ads like those below have flooded the backs of newspapers and magazines since the 1800s (see page 870). We now have TV infomercials and e-mails promoting products for "natural male enhancement." The products don't work—they never have—but the scams still do.

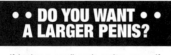

• • DO YOU WANT • •
A LARGER PENIS?

If having a small penis makes you self-conscious, you can now add up to 3" in just minutes. No matter what size you are, you can add inches & make it thicker & firmer. An amazing new product! Not a pill or drug: not weights or a pump but a natural way to prosthetically increase your penis to its maximum potential. Increases your power & makes you the stud you always

SMALL PENIS?
ERECTION PROBLEMS?

LINGA-100 is the pure, natural laboratory blend designed to actually enlarge the penis and induce & maintain multiple, long term erections. LINGA-100 allows a more intense, deeply satisfying male climax while developing sexual power, physical strength and mental awareness. LINGA-100 was developed by top Swiss scientista involved in natual sex hormone research. Thousands of

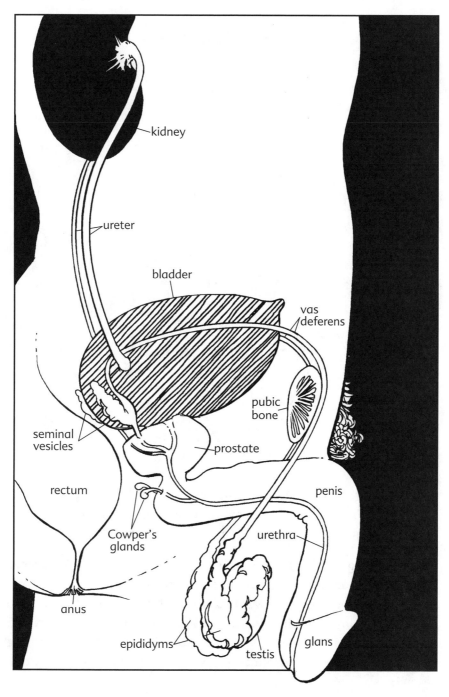

What's Inside a Guy

The Bone Yard

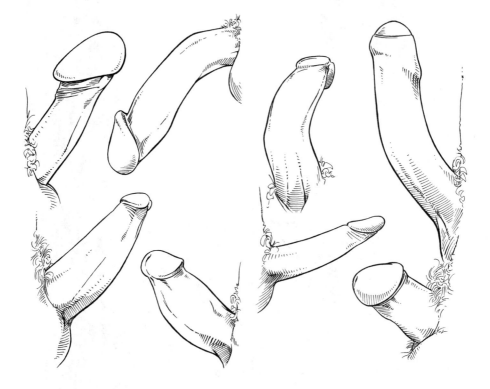

Shape From these drawings of real-life erections, you can see that terms like "6 inches" or "normal" are somewhat meaningless. All of these erect penises are normal, yet very different from each other. One even points down.

Size According to a study at the University of California at San Francisco, the average length of a flaccid penis is 3.4 inches, while the average length of an erect penis is around 5 inches. Most guys are within 2 inches of these figures. However, the way researchers in San Francisco measure a penis might be different from the way researchers in Rome do it. The exact same penis might be 6" in the City By the Bay, but only 5.75" when measured in the City of the Seven Hills.

Plumbing See the illustration on page 63 for all the gory details.

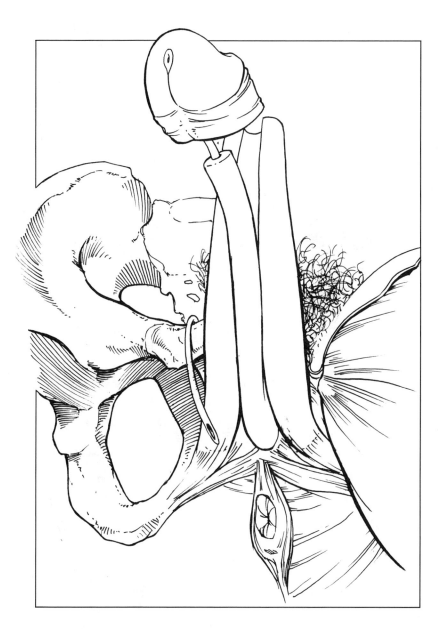

The Wrecking Yard

THE GOOFY DICK GAME
Real Penises of Real Guys

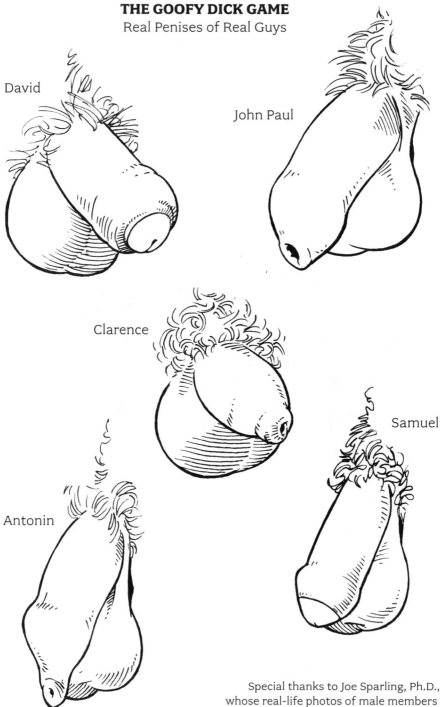

David

John Paul

Clarence

Samuel

Antonin

Special thanks to Joe Sparling, Ph.D., whose real-life photos of male members were used to make these illustrations.

You Be the Judge!
Match Each Soft Penis On
The Other Page With Its Erection
On This Page

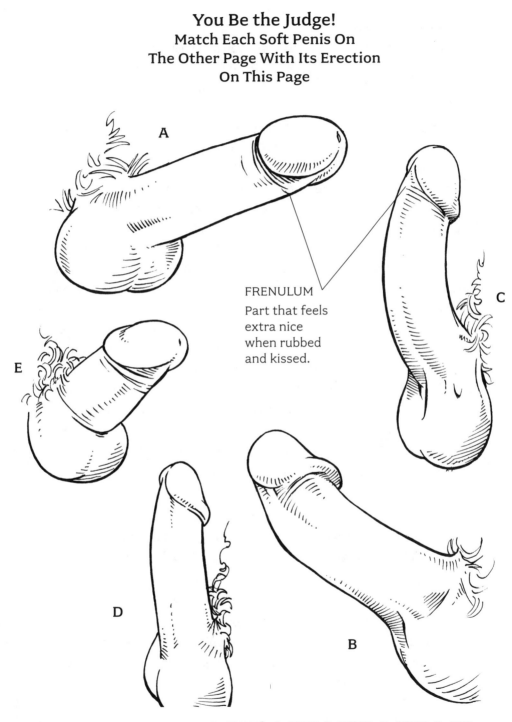

FRENULUM
Part that feels
extra nice
when rubbed
and kissed.

David—A   Antonin—C   Clarence—E   Samuel—D   John Paul—B

Manliness—What Is It?

In our culture, being manly means you don't act gay. It also means if you have girly parts to your character, you keep them well hidden. So when we are trying to define what's manly or masculine, what better place to start than with a quote from a man who is smart, good-looking, brawny, (6'2" and 195 lbs.), buff, and successful. He's no wimp with a hammer and table saw, and he has an 8" penis that most guys would be happy to own. If you found yourself out-numbered in a bar-room brawl, you could do worse than to have this man by your side. Here's what he recently said about being manly:

"The first time I heard my voice on a tape recorder when I was a kid I was mortified—I sounded so, well, gay. I wondered how my family had been able to live with the shame of having such a publicly identifiable invert in their own home. But then I started listening to other men; men who I knew were straight, and it turns out there are a lot of nellie-sounding breeders in the world (Orrin Hatch, anyone?)."

OK, the name of the straight-looking, manly guy who made this obser-vation is Gus Mattox. He was recently named the Gay Male Porn Star of the Year. He embodies the perfect combination of sensitivity and rough-guy manliness that most straight women would be thrilled to sleep with.

So what is being masculine, anyway? Is it a physical way of being? Is it a state of mind? Is it having the right politics? Is it what your dick gets hard over? Can you still be manly if you sound like a prissy snap-queen?

This Guide's definition of masculinity keeps evolving. Here it is in its current state:

Masculinity is mostly an invention of modern culture. It doesn't have a huge foundation in science or nature, yet it remains a pow-erful force in the way we view ourselves and each other.

To be manly or masculine in American culture, a guy should be a fairly responsible person who can be independent when the occa-sion demands. As often as not, he should be caring, comforting, and kind. He should be able to give and receive physical and emotional tenderness without being too controlling. He should have values and work ethics, and he shouldn't need to prove his masculinity by trying to scare or intimidate others.

He doesn't need to have a pussy-seeking sensor at the end of his penis, and his physical appearance can range from Bill Gates geek to porn-star perfect. Showering should be a priority.

There are plenty of males who have none of these qualities, but appear to be total studs nonetheless. These are guys who usually take their penises way too seriously. That is because the only way they can convince themselves that they are real men is by performing manly activities or drinking lots of beer or doing drugs, and then having a vagina or hole nearby that they can stick themselves into. They tend to be more show than substance.

Penis As Camouflage: Why It's Difficult to Be Satisfied By a Guy Who Takes His Penis Too Seriously

A hard penis is sometimes used to camouflage what's missing inside a man, as well as what's missing in a relationship between a man and a woman. If a guy is all hung up about his penis being a symbol of his manliness or demands that it have a disproportionate amount of attention, then it gets in the way of his being at one with a lover. The same is true for a guy who needs to always play a manly role. He sometimes feels more warmth for his car or computer than for his partner.

Unfortunately, a lot of women grew up thinking that a distant, self-involved, dick-centered type of guy is what manhood is all about. As a result, they end up being attracted to males whom they can never really get close to, and spend the rest of their lives bellyaching about what duds men are.

Narcisso 'Gasms

Biologically, most women can have a couple of orgasms to the average man's one. This is fine with most men, since most of us would like to see our partners have as much pleasure as their hearts and loins desire. But for a man who takes his penis too seriously, orgasm giving can becomes too important. A partner's orgasms become reassurance that he is a total guy. We all do this to some extent, but for some it's a matter of narcissistic life and death.

If your man is like this, you may discover that your main function in life is to look good and have lots of loud orgasms. Or maybe it's just to look good. Consider yourself an offering to the great Dick God.

The Penile-Pumping Regatta

Some men lose emotional connection once intercourse begins. The woman starts to feel like she's become a masturbation machine. Sex becomes a pumping regatta in order to prove dick-worthiness. This can be really boring for both partners.

To give you an idea of how much insecurity is involved in all this, consider the words of a 29-year-old man who is starting to question why he takes his penis so seriously:

> "It's like, I attack sex. I'm afraid of slowing it down. If I'm gonna be fucking, I'll fuck like crazy, gotta have a huge dick and fuck like crazy to avoid dealing with whatever's making me anxious. Women have always said to me, 'God, you can't get enough.' But I think the reason I can't get enough is that if I slow down, the fears start to crowd in on me. Does this woman really want to be with me? Is she going to leave? Is my cock good enough? It's hard for me not to use sex as a seal of approval."
>
> —From Harry Maurer's *Sex: An Oral History,* Viking Press.

Of course, there are plenty of women who have their own insecurities. Is getting breast implants or wearing a padded bra all that different from this guy's need to have a big penis?

The Diagnosis & Cure

How do you distinguish a man who takes his penis too seriously from one who doesn't?

The man who doesn't take his penis too seriously doesn't beg out when it comes to doing the dishes. He may have various passions in life, often sports, music, business, or trying to fix things (sometimes successfully), but these usually help to center rather than isolate him. Sex with him is a natural extension of your friendship that makes all the sense in the world.

As for "curing" the kind of man who takes his penis too seriously, you can't. Hard as you might try, no human being has ever changed just because someone else wanted him or her to. It's something that has to come from within. Friends and lovers can sometimes help if they are willing to call the guy on his nonsense, but they can't make the changes for him.

Sexual Awareness: Hood Ornaments vs. Wet Triangles

When it comes to sexual awareness, the penis is positioned like the hood ornament on a car. It's difficult to ignore what your hood ornament is telling you when it's making a tent in the front of your pants. Sometimes we guys aren't even aware that we are sexually aroused until we feel ourselves start-ing to get hard.

Women are not conditioned from early childhood to associate sexual arousal with specific body cues in the way that men are. While their genitals often swell and lubricate, no flags get waved. Most of the changes happen on the inside and can be chalked-up to a nice tingly sensation between their legs. Besides, "good" girls are often taught to ignore their body's sexual cues.

While the penis can be a reliable indicator of sexual excitement, it does have its share of false positives, and occasional negatives.

Unwanted Wood

"For some reason, out of nowhere, your penis starts to get hard, and it is extremely difficult to stop." *male age 25*

"It's totally embarrassing. You just want to get up and go, but you can't. So you start pulling on your shirt or sweater to try to cover up the bulge. You become very self-conscious; you think everyone is looking at your crotch." *male age 43*

"It's like being in an elevator with an umbrella that will not go down." *male age 42*

"It can physically hurt when your penis is trapped in your jeans pointing downward and it suddenly gets hard for no reason what-soever." *male age 26*

"Most of my memories of unwanted erections were at school, gener-ally during class, and I was terrified that someone would notice." *male age 24*

"I travel a lot for business and sometimes wake up erect after a flight. It's terribly embarrassing. If I can't think the damn thing down, then I have to go through the tricky maneuver of flipping it up, trapping it under my waistband without being noticed, and then keeping my briefcase in front of me when I stand." *male 25*

Women usually assume that the presence of a hard-on means that a man is sexually aroused, and that no rise in his pants means he isn't. If only it were that simple. Consider the occurrence of the unwanted hard-on. The average teenage male is capable of getting a totally unwanted hard-on in the middle of an algebra test for absolutely no reason, unless he is a member of that rare breed who finds polynomial equations sexually arousing. When you are a young man, hard-ons just happen; nobody is more befuddled than the possessor of the penis. To say that all hard-ons are a sign of sexual arousal badly overstates the case. One reader took a bad grade in an early-morning high-school class because he couldn't go to the chalkboard due to his unwanted erections. His only thoughts were of frustration, not sex.

In addition to getting unwanted hard-ons, there are times when a man can feel highly aroused, yet either fail to get hard or have it go limp when he needs it the most (floppus erectus).

False Negatives: When Gravity Dings the Dong

Confucius says
*If limp dick is worst thing that happens to your relationship,
you live charmed life.*

Hopefully your lovemaking isn't solely dependent on the man's ability to get hard. If it is, your sexual relationship might be somewhat limited. It's also disconcerting to think that your entire sex life might be centered on the whims of the average penis, hard or soft.

Regarding the biology of erections, it is perfectly normal for a hard penis to partly deflate every fifteen minutes or so. Regarding the psychology of erections, be aware that hard-ons have been known to fly south for varying periods of time, from a single day to who knows how long.

The most unhelpful thing a woman can do when a guy can't get it up is to become defensive. Women often assume that erection failures mean the man doesn't find them attractive or that he might be gay. These are possibilities. But there are a billion other reasons for not being able to get an erection, from fearing that you won't be good in bed to what just happened on Wall Street. Physical problems like diabetes can also be a factor.

Given the stress of living in the modern world, it's a wonder we men are able to get it up as often as we do. And given the lack of tenderness or excitement in some relationships, an unerect penis might be a signal that the man and woman need to get closer emotionally.

While most of us have been raised to think of a limp penis as a sign of failure, perhaps it might be more productive to view it as an opportunity to bring a man and woman together. (For a more complete discussion of male hydraulic failure, see Chapter 58: "When Your System Crashes.")

Betty on Dick

The following passage is from Betty Dodson's classic *Sex for One* from Harmony Books. In addressing the issue of misbehaving penises, Ms. Dodson speaks with welcome concern:

"Although I ran only a dozen men's groups, the experience helped me to let go of my old conviction that men got a better deal when it came to sex.... I thought they could always have easy orgasms even with casual sex, and I envied their never having to worry about the biological realities of periods or pregnancies. But the truth is that not all men are able to be assertive studs who make out all the time.... The most consistent sex problem for many men in the workshops was owning a penis that seemed to have a will of its own. An unpredictable sex organ that got hard when no one was around and then refused to become erect when a man was holding the woman of his dreams in his arms...."

If this situation sounds familiar, tell your man that there probably isn't a woman alive who wouldn't be happy to receive a long, lingering back rub and oral sex in the place of intercourse. Or what about a go at an extended orgasm from the "Zen of Finger Fucking" chapter? In other words, if his woody won't work, let him know in no uncertain terms that there are plenty of other ways to please you sexually.

This Guide's philosophy:

Never, ever let a recalcitrant penis ruin your time or his!

Dick at Dawn

Guys often wake in the morning with erections, which are usually left over from dream sleep. Contrary to what you might think, a man's first feelings upon waking with an erection aren't necessarily sexual. They are more along the lines of "I wish this stupid hard-on would go down so I can pee," or "Damn, I hate having to wake up this early."

While some men enjoy having sex first thing in the morning, not all men associate early-morning erections with horniness. In fact, a man who wakes up in a grumpy mood might feel seriously annoyed if a woman assumes that his early-morning wood is for sitting on. She may need to coax him into having sex, although his penis is rock hard.

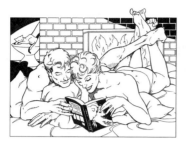

Dear Paul,

My boyfriend always wakes up in the morning with an erection. But when we start having intercourse, it goes down. He doesn't have this problem any other time. What's up?

Gretta in Marietta

Dear Gretta,

Sometimes a dog barks when he's happy; sometimes he barks when he's upset. It is a wise owner who knows the difference. Contrary to how it seems, the kind of erection your boyfriend has when he first wakes up is little more than a limp penis trapped inside of a raging hard-on. It happens because he wakes up while in the middle of a dream.

Dream-sleep erections occur no matter what a man is dreaming about. He could be dreaming that he's being chased by a pack of hungry wolves, and his dick would be hard as a rock. Although his penis looks hard and feels hard, it's not the kind of erection that the boy gets when he's been thinking about you all day. In fact, I recently read some research suggesting that sleep erections don't involve the same neurology as erotic erections. So even if it seems like your man is ready for action, treat his penis like it's a floppy one that needs to be aroused. Try kissing or playing with it before jumping your boyfriend's bone(s). This will help turn it into a waking-state erection and might help prevent it from going down.

Since his erection was not born from sexual desire, don't assume that your boyfriend feels like having sex. He might feel better if he could pee and brush his teeth. On the other hand, he may be just fine boning the babe of his dreams with a full bladder and dragon breath.

A Wet Warning—Ain't Love Grand!

Every once in a while a girlfriend will ask a guy if she can stand behind him and hold his penis while he pees. This is a completely normal request born of completely normal curiosity. But be forewarned that you are sometimes giggling so hard that the entire bathroom becomes a target. On the other hand, women sometimes do a better job of aiming the thing than we men. As for penile calligraphy skills, one female friend of this Guide loves grabbing her husband's penis and writing their names in the snow with its amber stream.

First Ejaculation

Before starting puberty, a guy can stroke his little pecker until it falls off, and his orgasms will mostly be dry except for maybe a few drops of clear, slick, slightly viscous fluid. During puberty, this changes until he produces an adult-sized wad when he has an orgasm. Instead of being clear and thin, it's white and thick. Instead of being a drop or two, it's a teaspoonful or two that oozes all over the place.

The process of going from a few drops to a full wad can be quite wonderful if you know what to expect and know it's normal. It can be disturbing if a guy doesn't have a clue, especially if he hasn't been told about ejaculation and masturbates for the first time after entering puberty. By then he's fully loaded and ready to shoot. Perhaps porn on the Internet is so prevalent these days that some young guys might be better prepared for their first wad than some of these readers were:

> "I didn't really know what I was doing. I was about eleven and discovered this new feeling when I rubbed this silky part of my blanket over my penis, so I kept doing it. Eventually, I got this intense feeling in my groin and then there was this goop everywhere. I was completely freaked and grossed out. I thought that I broke myself, but was too afraid to tell my parents." *male age 24*

> "I had heard about masturbation while sitting in the back of the school bus. When I tried it just the way the kids told me, it was almost like pain. For weeks I would stop short of actual orgasm for fear that I would do some sort of internal damage to myself. Finally, one day I kept rubbing through my fear and found that I enjoyed the hurting tremendously." *male age 25*

The Couch-Potato Penis

As things get older, they start to petrify or harden. This is true for logs, fossils and the human brain. Unfortunately, it is not true for the human penis. As a penis approaches its fifth decade, it tends to petrify less fully than it did earlier in life. It also squirts less fluid during ejaculation. Some women will cling to this information like a ray of hope, while others will be disappointed. Whatever your situation, it shouldn't make much difference. As the bearer of the penis gets older, he becomes wiser in the ways of love. By then, he can compensate with wit and wisdom for what he loses in hardness and volume.

Also, older men seldom make an effort to stay in good shape. It's being out of shape, rather than increasing age, that often causes the couch-potato penis and decline in libido. However, age alone is responsible for changes in ejaculation, with the middle-aged man sometimes feeling nostalgic for his teenage genitals, which, in some guys could propel ejaculate three feet.

Bebop & Squirt — Men & Multiples

Most males experience orgasm as an overlapping two-part process—sensation and ejaculation. Some guys have learned to separate the two events, experiencing a series of orgasmic sensations before they finally ejaculate. According to Dr. Marian Dunn, who interviewed a number of men with this ability, the one common thread was that their partner remained in a state of high sexual excitement after the man's first feeling of orgasm. This seemed to provide an essential path of feedback that the man could feel in his penis as it remained inside her vagina.

Some of the men had small ejaculations with each orgasm, while others didn't ejaculate until the end. Some of these men had been able to do this all of their lives; others had learned it recently. The men who had always been able to do it assumed that all men could and were surprised when a sexual partner pointed out the difference.

This should not be confused with delayed ejaculation, a situation where the man wants to have an orgasm but is unable to.

Hormone Advisory

Plenty of people feel that testosterone influences sexual behavior as well as aggressive behavior. Since males have higher levels of testosterone than females, and since males commit the lion's share of aggressive criminal acts, this connection might make sense. However, researchers have found that low levels of testosterone are associated with higher levels of aggression in men, and higher levels of testosterone have been associated with calmness, happiness and friendliness.

In both men and women, at least some testosterone is thought to be necessary to have a sex drive. Since men have as much as five times more testosterone than women, people who don't know much about physiology assume this means that men have a higher sex drive than women. Wrong!

While women may have less testosterone, their testosterone receptors are more sensitive than men's. So the same amount goes further in women than in men. As for the notion that women have a lower sex drive than men, good luck proving that generalization on women in this day and age.

In working with mice in the lab, researchers are starting to explore the possibility that it's the male mouse's ability to respond to estrogen that causes his natural aggressiveness. This has interesting implications with humans. While both men and women have estrogen, it's possible that men's estrogen receptors are more sensitive than women's. It could be that Mighty Mouse gets his "might" from the hormone that we associate with Minnie Mouse's female features. Plus, it seems that estrogen might be necessary for a man to ejaculate.

While this doesn't solve anything, hopefully it helps you to appreciate the complexity involved in hormones and sexual behavior. Just because this hormone or that is circulating in the body doesn't mean a whole lot. There's the matter of hormone receptors, and of how the person has been socialized to behave when he or she gets a rush of this or that. It is also possible that hormone levels rise or fall in response to a social situation. So with sexual behavior, it might be our hormones that respond to the sexual feelings we are having, rather than hormones causing the feelings.

On Men's Hormones

Research indicates that men have mood shifts every bit as strong as women's. This makes nonsense of the myth that men are more emotionally stable than women. Researchers are also finding that sex hormones affect the moods of different men in different ways. Some men become irritable or depressed when their testosterone level is elevated. Others appear to become calmer. How men respond to changing hormone levels is an individual matter which may have more to do with social conditioning than with biology.

As for hormones and sexual desire, a certain level of male hormone is necessary for sexual arousal, but it isn't very high. Increasing the amount of male hormone above this level doesn't make men any hornier. The only time added hormone increases a man's horniness is when his testosterone level is below the minimum to begin with. Hopefully this is a message for you to not take things like testosterone and DHEA without first having your blood levels tested, and only then under the direction of a skilled physician if lab results show a deficiency.

Guys & Horniness

It is sometimes assumed that the average male wants to have sex each and every hour of the day as long as the opportunity presents itself. There are some guys for whom this axiom simply doesn't apply, at least around here, anyway. Maybe it's a problem with our masculinity, maybe we are latent homosexuals, or maybe we have nervous systems that are sensitive enough to be impacted by some of the really disturbing things that happen in the world. Or maybe we are really tired and need a good night's sleep. Whatever the case, it is sometimes difficult to drop everything and have sex. There are plenty of times when it's just as nice to cuddle up close to a sweetheart and enjoy falling asleep in each other's arms.

The Vicissitudes of Mercy Sex — Making a Man Come Sooner

Let's say you are getting your man off as an act of kindness and aren't particularly into it, or you really need a good night's sleep but won't be able to get one until your guy's glands have sneezed. Here are a few suggestions that might be helpful in making a man come sooner. The latter suggestions, which deal with increasing his level of mental excitement, will likely be more effective, but they might be more taxing on you if you are not particularly into it.

Tighten the Foreskin Pulling the foreskin taut around the base of the penis can cause a man to feel more sensation when his penis is stimulated.

Focus on the Frenulum The frenulum is the most sensitive part of the penis. It's just below the head of the penis, on the side where the seam runs up the shaft. During oral sex, you might focus on this area. If doing him by hand, make sure that your fingers run over this part of the penis with a fair amount of pressure during each stroke. Pumping too quickly may numb out the penis and be counterproductive. Also, using a well-lubricated hand rather than masturbating him dry might help to speed up his ejaculation.

Visuals If the man is turned on by your naked body, for heaven's sake, crank up the lights and park the parts he enjoys most in full view. If there's a particular bra that gets him going, wear it during the sex.

Adding a Squeeze or Twist Try giving a well-lubricated hand job where your entire hand wraps around the penis and twists up and down it as though it were following the red stripe on a barber's pole. Try a similar twisting motion with your head during oral sex. Just a slight turn of the neck is all that's needed, nothing to give you whiplash. At the same time, work the area between his testicles with one of your hands.

Play with Yourself Never hesitate to play with your nipples or vulva. Some men will be so turned on by watching you play with yourself that they will begin to masturbate and finish themselves off with their own hand.

Pleasure Toggles Some men have a spot along the part of the penis that is buried beneath their testicles or all the way back to the rim of their anus which deepens the degree of sensation when pressed upon. Knowing your man's sexual anatomy and keeping a finger on this spot may help move up launch time. Women who give superb blow jobs often work these areas with one hand while tending to the end of the penis with their tongue and lips.

Nipples Some guys' nipples are quite sensitive; others aren't. If your man's are, tweaking them with your fingertips or caressing them with your lips and tongue can speed up arrival time.

On or Up His Rear It doesn't matter if it's your bum or his, the human anus is probably the second-most sensitive part of the body. A wet finger on it, swirling around it, or pushed into it can speed some men up considerably.

Extras If he gets turned on by you talking dirty to him, do it if you are in the mood. If he likes X-rated movies, load his favorite one in the DVD player. If you are having intercourse, try slowing down the thrusting rather than speeding up, or change his pace. If he is thrusting shallow, have him thrust deep. If you usually do it in the bedroom but are able to switch to the kitchen or living room, a change in routine can help increase the level of excitement and speed of launch time.

If His Weenie Goes Pop

So let's say you are riding your cowboy in a sexual way, and you suddenly fall off, or you rise up a little too high and slam his penis on the way down or you are trying one of those ridiculous intercourse positions that some artist put on some Pharaoh's tomb. Or perhaps you've had a wicked week at work, and the kids have the flu, and the last thing in the world you want sticking inside of you is your partner's penis, but he has the nerve to insist nonetheless. Whatever the cause of the calamity, should your man's erection suddenly bend in a direction that nature didn't intend and makes a cracking sound or goes "POP," get it to a hospital right away. Although rare, the pop might be from the snapping of a ligament in the penis that acts like the suspension cables on the Golden Gate Bridge. If it breaks, internal bleeding that might permanently damage the penis can result. Urologists can usually save the wounded soldier within the first few hours post-pop, but wait more than a day, and your guy could end up going to the grave with a penis that's shaped like a deflated circus balloon, or worse yet, an Allen wrench.

An erect penis can also be damaged if it is repeatedly bent mid-shaft. This sometimes happens during sloppy intercourse and might eventually lead to Peyronie's disease. Peyronie's disease can cause painful and/or bent erections. Some physicians believe that Peyronie's disease results from patches of calcium that collect on the penis at points where it has been tweaked. Peyronie's disease can be very disfiguring and very difficult to treat.

Warning The intercourse position that can cause the most potential damage to the penis is when the woman is on top (e.g. page 117). Be sure her vagina is plenty wet and understand that bad things can happen if the penis pulls out too far and then gets sat on it when the head is not inside the vaginal opening (or anus, if that's your sport). Any kind of genital pain that lasts more than ten minutes needs to be tended to by a physician. Serious long-term damage can often be averted if you get medical help right away.

Dear Paul,

Why are guys always touching and grabbing at their genitals?"

Eva from Evanston

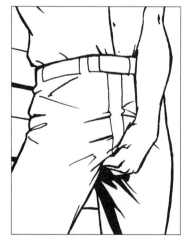

Dear Eva,

When the skin on the balls sticks to the thighs, and the skin on the penis sticks to the skin on the balls, you get a claustrophobic feeling. It's like if you had to keep your arms pressed against your sides all the time. Try it for just five minutes without lifting them. When this happens with a guy's penis and scrotum, he's gotta dig to lift and separate or it starts to feel like he's going to go nuts. Body powder can sometimes help. Underwear that doesn't fit right can make matters worse.

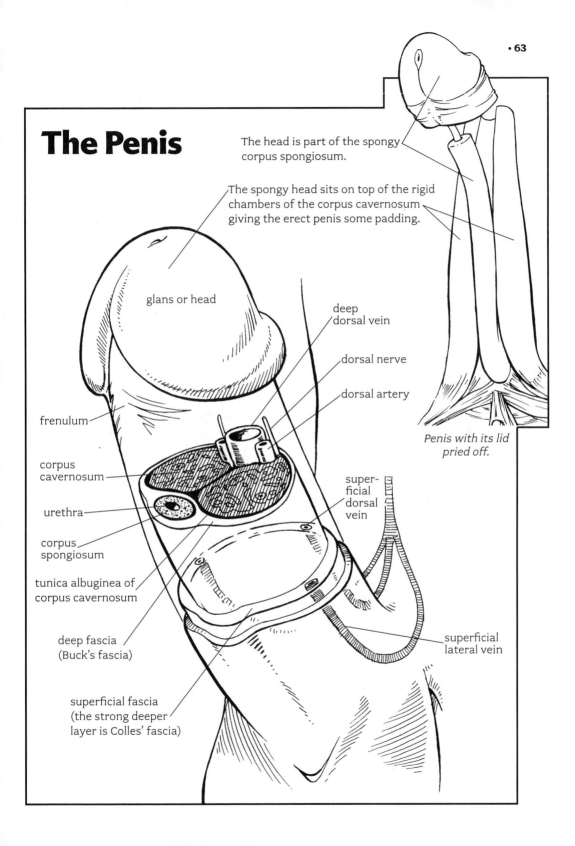

The Penis

The head is part of the spongy corpus spongiosum.

The spongy head sits on top of the rigid chambers of the corpus cavernosum giving the erect penis some padding.

glans or head

deep dorsal vein

dorsal nerve

dorsal artery

frenulum

corpus cavernosum

urethra

corpus spongiosum

tunica albuginea of corpus cavernosum

deep fascia (Buck's fascia)

superficial fascia (the strong deeper layer is Colles' fascia)

superficial dorsal vein

superficial lateral vein

Penis with its lid pried off.

Dear Paul,

When guys are peeing, why can't they aim it right? Would it kill them to get all of it in the bowl?   *Nancy in Niagara Falls*

Dear Nancy,

The problem is not with the aim, but with the unpredictable nature of the stream. It breaks up about as often as the signal on a cell phone. Sometimes a rebel tributary appears and shoots off to the side, sometimes a healthy stream will suddenly turn into a spray, and sometimes it goes exactly where you aim it, but the toilet water splashes up and makes a mess on the rim.

This is no reason why a guy shouldn't grab a wad of toilet paper and clean up after himself (bowl, floor, walls, shoes, ceiling). This is something that parents should teach their sons. Also, I don't know if you are aware of the first law of fluid dynamics, but a man never pees on his pants leg unless it is one minute before an important meeting, first date, or job interview.

Dear Paul,

The skin on the shaft of my husband's penis is a lot darker than the skin on the rest of his body. Is this normal?   *Amber from Brownsville*

Dear Amber,

It's perfectly normal. Penises vary as much in skin tone as they do in size and shape. One man's penis might be darker than his normal skin color, another's might be lighter, and a third might even have freckles or blotches. You can't predict the tone of the bone until the pants are down.

Dear Paul,

When my husband's penis is erect, it almost points down instead of up. Is this normal?   *Diane in Bend*

Dear Diane,

Penises often point up, at approximately a 30-degree angle from the stomach, assuming the guy doesn't have a big beer belly. But plenty of erect penises stick straight out, and others point down. You might try an intercourse position where you are on top but facing his feet. From this position, his funky rooster may be able to tickle parts of you that a man with an "uppie" would miss. Most important is that you and he experiment with positions that feel good for both of you.

Dear Paul,

When it comes to pleasing guys, why are they so focused on their penises? There's so much of the body that feels good when it's kissed and touched, yet they seem to want everything to focus on the penis.

Flabbergasted in Frankfurt

Dear Flabby,

Let me start by asking you a few questions. Let's say you've just cooked your lover a romantic, candlelit dinner. You've gone to the gym, feel really good about your body, and you are wearing a killer dress with your sexiest lingerie underneath. You want him to want you more than he wants his car, a new computer or Monday-Night football.

But when the lights finally go down, much to your surprise, his willy is nilly. No matter what you try, he's not able to have an erection. So tell me, what's going through your mind? Are you thinking that he's not interested? Are you worried that he doesn't find you attractive? Let's say you call it a wash and go for it another time. If he still has no erection, are you thinking maybe he's a wimp? Gay? If you are married, do you start to wonder if he's having an affair?

The sad truth is, you are just as focused on his penis as he is—as the ultimate indicator that you are attractive and that he is excited about you. So once a penis gets hard, a guy figures he'd better start doing something with it ASAP. If the thing suddenly goes down, especially if it deflates while your legs are wrapped tight around his waist and you've just cried out, "Fuck me harder," heaven help the poor boy. He'll be a big disappointment to you and an even bigger disappointment to himself. All of your hard work—the day, the beautiful dinner, the romantic evening—will be ruined because of the focus that you, he, and the rest of us place on his penis. So while you make a point that I clearly laud, there's more to it than meets the eye.

I'm still simplifying this way too much. There are plenty of other issues involved, like the way many of us have learned to focus on our penises since it wouldn't be manly to do otherwise. Honestly, if you heard about a woman taking a leisurely bath and playing with her nipples for half an hour, you'd probably say, "cool." So would most men. But what if you heard about a guy taking a leisurely bath and playing with his nipples for half an hour? I know what you'd be thinking. While male nipples might be wired the same as yours with the same potential for sensation, we certainly don't think of them in the same way. Besides, unless it's a hottub, men are supposed to take showers.

And finally, whether it's due to our biology or simply the things we teach ourselves about sex, a man sometimes feels a strong need to ejaculate once he becomes aroused. This need is much more pronounced in the teens or twenties than later in life. It makes us focus on having to do something with that darned penis rather than being able to enjoy what's going on around us.

In Praise of Geeks!

What better way to end this chapter than with the following sentiment that a female reader e-mailed to us:

> "I don't know about other women, but I have discovered that the *geek* crowd which doesn't often get laid in high school has a great deal of time to contemplate what they'd do if they ever got their hands on a woman. They are far better lovers because they've taken the time to contemplate something other than *scoring*. As a friend of mine used to say, 'Nine-tenths of sex happens in your mind; the rest is all in your head.' Geeks think, while jocks avoid it at all costs because in high school, thinking is not cool. Besides, geeks know how to be passionate rather than just *stoked*. Give me a geek any time."

CHAPTER

6

Semen Confidential

Ayoung woman in Utah asked, "Why does male ejaculate smell vaguely of cleaning products?" It's funny how one question can lead to an entire chapter—about semen, not cleaning products. Analyzing the Clorox smell led to more questions about semen stains, semen allergies, upset stomachs after swallowing, and finally finding the answer to a question a reader submitted several years ago: "Why does my boyfriend's jizz burn when it gets in my eye?"

You'll find answers to these questions in the pages that follow.

Lock and Load

Semen doesn't come out the end of a penis fully homogenized like milk from a carton, even if the guy has been bouncing on a trampoline for an hour. The first squirt has secretions from the Cowper (bulbourethral) and Littre glands. The prostate gland manufactures the next wave of man chowder, which is 15% to 30% of the total volume. This is followed by the relatively small but potent contribution of sperm from the balls below. And the seminal vesicles hold up the rear of each ejaculation, producing 65% and 80% of every man's wad. Total volume: about a teaspoon or less (see also Chapter 16 on the prostate, pages 204-206).

Why Semen Smells Like Clorox

When Ms. Utah asked why male ejaculate smells vaguely "of cleaning products," we assume she is referring to the Clorox smell, unless semen in Utah smells like Windex, 409 or Janitor in a Drum.

After performing countless biopsies of testicles, urologists discovered that testicular fluid and sperm are odorless. It's the part of the semen that comes from the seminal vesicles and the prostate that add the odor. The characteristic cleaning-product smell of male ejaculate is the fault of spermine, which is made by the prostate. Spermine is a member of a chemical family known as polyamines.

Changes in the pH of semen and the variations in a chemical balancing act known as buffering explain why some boy's batter smells more like cleaning products than others, or why one guy might smell more like Clorox one day and Janitor in a Drum the next.

For science and history buffs, spermine phosphate crystals were first found in sperm by Leeuwenhoek in 1678, which is where the name "spermine" came from, although women since the time of Aristotle have known about the cleaning-product smell. After a guy ejaculates, the phosphate is pried off the molecule and the free base of spermine is released which gives off the chlorine-bleach smell. Semen stops smelling after it's been out for a while due to the free bases linking to form something else.

When A Penis Spits in Your Eye

As for the reader's question about why her boyfriend's ejaculate burns so much when it gets in her eye, we'd given up on it after receiving a particularly curt and nasty response from an optometry professor at a leading university. Fortunately, it's true what they say: Persistence is the twin sister of excellence, and persist we did.

While the concentration of spermine in semen isn't nearly as high as when you order it from a chemical supply house, pure spermine carries some seriously harsh warnings. The material safety data sheet for it says:

> **Danger!** Corrosive. Causes eye and skin burns. May cause severe respiratory-tract irritation with possible burns. May cause severe digestive-tract irritation with possible burns. May cause central-nervous-system effects. May cause cardiac disturbances. **Causes eye burns.** May cause chemical conjunctivitis and corneal damage. Causes skin burns.

While there might be other chemicals in semen that cause your eyes to burn, the number one culprit on anyone's list should be spermine.

Why the Upset Stomach?

Some women report getting a tummy ache after swallowing their lover's splooge. This is usually blamed on the prostaglandins that are in semen, which might make it similar to the kind of stomach upset that some people get after taking aspirin. However, after reading spermine's material safety data sheet, you can't help but wonder if spermine is involved as well.

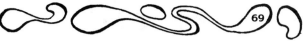
What Makes Boy Batter Taste Like It Does

A thorough explanation of why male ejaculate tastes the way it does is beyond the scope of this book, and probably beyond that of any other. However, in looking at the chemicals in semen, the amount of citrate ions stick out a bit. These ions help semen to be a strong buffering agent; they also make for a lot of calcium citrate, which tastes both salty and sour.

Semen also has a number of other ions, namely magnesium, potassium, sodium, and zinc. As for how zinc tastes, there's a fairly well-known taste test that's used to determine if people have low levels of zinc. You are given a solution of zinc to drink, and if you can't taste anything, it's because your body has a zinc deficiency. However, if you've got an acceptable level of zinc, the zinc solution tastes "strong and unpleasant." This might indicate that semen would taste better to people who have a zinc deficiency, although it's probably not wise to phone your healthcare provider and say, "My boyfriend's cum tastes really yummy to me. Does this means I'm zinc-deficient?" Let's just say there's a fair amount of zinc in spunk, and zinc doesn't taste very good unless you have a zinc deficiency, or maybe his semen is low in zinc. Ditto for magnesium, and we all know what sodium tastes like.

On the good side, semen does contain fructose and glucose. However, in their "Review of the Physical and Chemical Properties of Human Semen," Owen and Katz discovered that the amount of fructose and glucose can vary as much as four-fold from man to man.

Semen is also home to low concentrations of other polyamines by the names of putrescine and cadaverine. These compounds are essential for cells to live. They also like to announce themselves when cells die. Both putrescine and cadaverine are well-named and are responsible for the rotting flesh smell that the formerly-living start to have soon after they die. They are used by the food industry as important indicators of spoilage in food.

Most cheeses that are really smelly and sharp-tasting are high in putrescine, but so is fermented soy sauce, shrimp, and certain citrus fruits. Putrescine and cadaverine are what bring us the fishy smell when women have bacterial infections in their vaginas. One reason why semen doesn't ordinarily smell fishy is because it has a very low concentration of cellular matter in it.

When Semen Smells Bad Rather than Just Bleachy

After being with a couple of men, most women have a baseline sense of what semen normally smells like. However, semen occasionally has an extra pungent edge to it that our andrology-urology consultant says can be the result of a hidden prostate infection—he's talking a combined strong-bleach smell and fishy odor. The fishy part comes from the polyamines that are released from the decaying white blood cells.

Semen normally has some white blood cells in it, but at a very low level. When a man has a prostate infection, the white blood cell count in his semen increases, which results in more polyamines like putriscene being liberated:

> "Since I do a lot of semen analysis in my office, I can tell the semen that has lots of white blood cells when we open the container. It has a really strong, bad odor—to the point that my research assistant is able to suspect that men have infection just from the odor of semen when we are preparing slides to be examined."

Men who have prostatitis might notice yellowish, jellylike globs in their semen. Suspicions also rise when semen has a honey-like sweet smell. This can be the result of a staph infection. Whatever the case, healthy happy man-jam tends to be mostly white and has the smell of clean, fresh bleach.

Out, Damn Spot

Ever notice that some boys' semen stains worse than others? Semen contains a lot of protein, much of which is albumin. This is the same kind of protein that is in egg whites, although we don't recommend baking with it.

As protein dries it changes optical qualities and color. Men who have a lower volume of ejaculate with white blood cells in it may have more of a tendency to leave yellowish semen stains in their underwear and on sheets.

How Thick is Splooge?

Viscosity is a measure of how fast or slow a given liquid flows from a container. According to one study, the viscosity of male ejaculate fresh from the penis can vary from 1.3 cP to 23.3 cP at room temperature. For reference, the viscosity of water at room temperature is around 1.0 cP. Such a wide range means some guys shoot a wad that is almost as thin as water while others need a grease gun to get it out. Young men who ejaculate frequently tend to have semen that is a bit watery.

Also, the viscosity of semen starts to change as soon as it is ejaculated. That's because during ejaculation, PSA from the prostate joins the part of the semen that's made by the seminal vesicles and starts a reaction that makes it become watery. If a man ejaculates in a clear glass, within 5 to 30 minutes his semen will become almost like water. This tends to happen much faster when semen is in the vagina than when it is out in the open, and it's why liquid drips out of a woman's vagina when she stands up after intercourse.

Volume and Why You'll Probably Never Shoot Like a Porn Star

When sperm researchers are between grants and have way too much time on their hands, they appear to do a lot of jerking off. You would come to this conclusion as well if you could see how many studies have been done on the volume of human ejaculation.

These studies found that the average volume of each wad is between 2.3 ml and 4.99 ml. For reference, a teaspoon is a pubic hair shy of 5.0 ml. So it's safe to say that the average guy shoots between half a teaspoon and a full teaspoon each time he ejaculates. (The average bull weighs between 1,000 and 2,000 lbs, and ejaculates between 4 ml and 8 ml.)

Also, given that these studies were averages of groups of men, the range of 2.3 ml and 4.99 ml seems awfully wide. So there were clearly differences in protocols or the way the ejaculations were collected.

Is Male Ejaculate an AntiDepressant?

Researchers have come up with fascinating observations about semen absorption and mood in women. They found that women whose partners did not use condoms scored lower on tests for depression than women whose partners did use condoms. This has led them to believe that hormones in semen are absorbed into the women's bodies through the vagina, and that those hormones have an anti-depressive or a possible mood-elevating effect.

We know that hormones are absorbed through the walls of the vagina. This is what makes the birth-control method NuvaRing work. We also know that components in semen can be found in a women's bloodstream hours after intercourse. But we didn't know that the hormones in semen might act as antidepressants. Semen contains estrogen, testosterone, follicular-stimulating hormone, luteinizing hormone, prolactin and prostaglandins.

The authors of this study wisely looked for other factors that could explain the differences in depression, such as the length of the relationships, birth-control pill use, not being in a relationship vs. being in a relationship, and high-risk behavior vs. low-risk behavior. None of these could explain the differences in the women's depression. All roads led to semen in the vagina.

Could this be an unconscious factor in why so many women don't insist that their partners use condoms, when it would otherwise make sense?

In this study, women whose partners were using condoms showed similar amounts of depression as women who weren't having intercourse at all. And women who were having intercourse without condoms had sex more often than their safe-sex sisters. There were also differences in scores of depression among the women in the condomless couples. Women who had most recently received a semen deposit had the lowest levels of depression among all subjects who were studied.

The authors of this study were the first to caution that their findings were only preliminary and suggestive. However, if semen does have the ability to help a woman keep depression at bay, it could help offset the decline in raw sexual excitement that often happens as a relationship matures. Instead of being the exciting lover that he may have been in year one, by year ten, a husband and his penis might be his wife's mood-elevating drug.

Other researchers who are studying how the brain processes sexual attraction have cautioned about the possible "dangers" of casual sex: that it might cause people who are hooking up for convenient sex to have unintended romantic feelings for each other. Perhaps the absorption of the man's sperm adds to the unexpected romantic feelings. All the more reason to use a condom if you are having sex with someone who is more physically attractive to you than emotionally attractive.

Semen Allergies

A semen allergy is caused by an allergic reaction to a particular protein in semen. The onset can vary. A woman could have been just fine with a partner's semen for a couple of years, and then suddenly start having an allergic reaction to it for no good reason. On the other hand, a semen allergy can be there from the start. Symptoms include burning and itching.

While a semen allergy isn't totally rare, it's not particularly common. One way to decide if the reaction you are having is to semen or chronic vaginitis is to use a condom during intercourse. (It's best to use a polyurethane condom or perhaps one of the new Lifestyles Skyn condoms, given how your

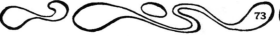

symptoms might also be from a latex allergy.) If the symptoms appear only after intercourse without a condom, it's time to consider a semen allergy.

Aside from a complete gynecologic exam, you will need to get intradermal testing to see if you have an allergy to semen. This is where a small amount of semen is injected under the skin.

Fortunately, there is a desensitization treatment for semen allergy that is safe and effective. You need to do it under the supervision of an allergist or immunologist. It is called a "graded challenge" where diluted solutions of semen are placed in your vagina every twenty minutes until you are able to tolerate undiluted semen. The downside is that the couple has to have intercourse at least once every 48 hours to maintain the desensitization!

Another fascinating thing about semen allergy is you don't get a bad reaction to the semen of just one guy. If you did, switching partners would be a treatment option, although not always a desired or practical one. If you get a semen allergy, it's to a protein in semen that all guys have. Also, once you develop a semen allergy, it's not just in your vagina. The burning and itching can occur any place where semen touches your skin, including in your mouth or up your bum. As is the case with food allergies, a semen allergy might go as fast as it came.

Spying on Sperm

We strongly encourage you to look at your own or your partner's semen under a microscope. You won't believe how cool millions of sperm can look. Here's how you do it:

Materials: You'll need access to a microscope that has 100x and 400x magnifications, a microscope slide and coverslips, and a human male with a hard-on. Make sure the microscope has a good light and that you can focus on the edge of a coverslip that's on a glass slide.

Producing the sample: This is the funnest part! If you don't know how to produce semen in the bottom of a glass, there are plenty of chapters in this book that can help. If you need lube, only use saliva. Most commercial lubricants do evil things to sperm.

Timing: You'll want to have the guy's semen under the microscope within 60 to 90 minutes after it is produced.

The Container: As you might recall from the start of this chapter, semen doesn't squirt out pre-mixed. So you'll need to collect the entire ejaculation in the same container, because if you don't, you might not be collecting the squirts that have sperm. Be sure to use a container large enough to fit the head of your penis into while you splooge. (Do not collect your specimen in a condom. The materials in most condoms are not sperm friendly.)

The Semen: While it tends to come out thick, your semen will liquify within 15 to 20 minutes—so much that it will become almost as thin as water. After it has liquified, give it a close look with your naked eyes. According to our sperm consultant:

"If it is clear (transparent), the sperm count is probably low. If it is cloudy but you can see through it (translucent), it is a medium sperm count. If it is creamy white or yellowish and you can not see through

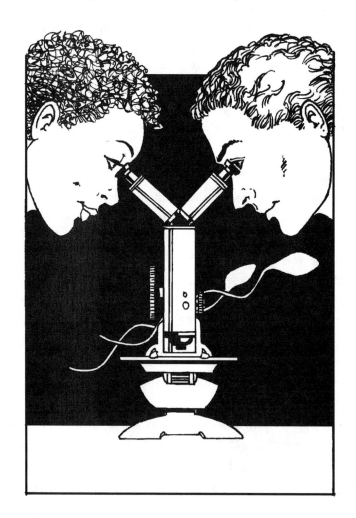

it, it is probably a fairly high sperm count. This is not a measure of fertility, just something interesting. Besides, it only takes one sperm for paternity, and the number of sperm depends on many things, including how often you ejaculate, if you've been in hot tubs or hot baths, what medications you are taking, etc."

The temperature: Keep your specimen between body temperature and room temperature. Any colder or hotter, and sperm start dropping like flies. If you're taking it from your dorm to the biology lab, keep it warm and safe.

Slide Prep: Lightly swirl the semen in the container to mix it. Put a drop or two on the slide, and then place a cover slip over it.

Look-See: Put the slide on the microscope's platform and look at it with the 10x objective (at hopefully a 100x magnification). The sperm are going to be very small and difficult to see. Once you spy sperm, change to the 40x objective, but don't make any significant changes in focus or you risk breaking the slide with the lens. If you need to make changes in the focus, go back to the 10x objective and do it that way.

Other Gunk in Your Junk: Semen has more than 300 constituents, including proteins, fats, immature sperm cells, old dead parts of sperm, and occasionally blood cells. Given the less-than optimal conditions you are probably working under, it wouldn't be surprising if 50% or more of your sperm were dead as little doornails before you look through the microscope. Also, only about 15% of sperm are the beautiful type with flowing tails, the rest are not like you see in the textbooks.

Dear Paul,

When I have an erection, it starts dripping like I've come before I actually come. Is something wrong with my penis?
Marty from Manitoba

Dear Marty,

It sounds like precum, which is one of nature's finer sex lubes. Unlike your regular ejaculate, precum is clear and oozes out gradually instead of shooting across your chest. It makes the head of your penis slippery and more disposed to slide kindly into the vagina of the love of your life. It may also help make the urethra less acidic so your ejaculate is more likely to get a girl pregnant. You can tell precum from urine by touching it with your fingertip and then pulling your finger away. Precum will stay connected to your finger, making a clear, cool-looking spindle, like bubble gum when you pull part of it out of your mouth. Precum can also drip out with a morning erection or when you've got unwanted wood in the middle of a class or at work. Any other fluids of an unknown origin that drip out of your penis, especially if they are a bit green or pus-like, should be checked out by your healthcare provider.

Readers' Comments

*What did you think
the first time you saw a guy ejaculate?*

"I was a little shocked. I was young, 15, and I don't think I understood exactly what was going on. It's also when I realized that tissues weren't just for noses anymore." *female age 27*

"I did it right! Good job! I was proud of me. Then I thought, 'Geez, I hope my mom doesn't come home early.'" *female age 22*

"I remember being disgusted and oddly fascinated at the same time, and I couldn't believe how far that stuff could shoot out!" *female 32*

"It just kind of oozed out. For some reason I thought there was supposed to be more of a stream." *female age 37*

"I was jealous he could actually project it from his body and I couldn't." *female age 23*

"I was kinda grossed out by the whole thing." *female age 45*

"I was proud that I made him ejaculate, but I couldn't believe that people actually would let that go in their mouths. I was a senior in high school." *female age 25*

"I wondered what it felt like. I wondered what it tasted like. Also, I wondered what it would feel like to have that happen inside of me." *female age 25*

"I vaguely remember thinking, it's amazing how their bodily process is. Also, there is what is needed to help form a human being." *female age 36*

A Very Special Thanks: to Darius A. Paduch, MD., PhD, Urology & Reproductive Medicine, Weill Cornell Medical College, Steven "Dr. Sperm" Schrader, Ph.D., NIOSH, and Jennifer Collins, MD, Albert Einstein School of Medcine.

7
What's Inside a Girl?

Most books on sex present female genitals as though they were a static entity that is easy to comprehend. They give you a few carefully illustrated diagrams and proceed to speak of women's genitals as one would a carburetor. This is a big mistake.

Since you can't hardly see them, women's genitals are more of a mystery than men's. And although men's and women's genitals are made from many of the same cells, if a man approaches a woman's genitals in the same way he does his own, he and his partner might be missing out on a lot of fun.

This chapter approaches women's genitals differently than most books on sex. It begins with a boy's quest to discover what's between a woman's legs.

Instant Pussy

What follows is an experience that the author of this book had with women's genitals when he was 11-years-old and very, very curious.

He had been in the city visiting relatives and it was time to return home. He was at the bus depot early. The northbound bus didn't leave until noon, so he had time to kill. He also needed to use the rest room.

The men's bathroom in the Greyhound depot was a far cry from the one-seater he had grown up with. It was massive, not too nice on the nose, and it had three vending machines that called to him like giant aluminum Sirens.

One of the machines had men's colognes in it; you could spritz yourself with Old Spice or Brut for a dime. Next to that was a machine with a product that was totally baffling. And next to the mystery machine was one that said *Instant Pussy—2 Quarters*.

To put this into proper perspective, back then candy bars weren't much more than a nickel, and two quarters amounted to a near fortune. But then again, the front of the machine promised a facsimile so exact that you couldn't tell the instant pussy from the real thing.

For the next hour, the young boy pondered the ultimate existential question: ten candy bars or instant pussy, ten candy bars or instant pussy, ten candy bars or instant pussy. A rush of guy hormones apparently kicked in, and he returned to the smelly porcelain palace with two shiny quarters.

The rest of the day was spent in quiet anticipation, with thoughts of instant pussy overwhelming whatever interesting sights and sounds the big city had to offer. Finally, after he had arrived home and done his chores, he anxiously opened the small box and read the instructions. "Place capsule in a large glass of warm water." He spent the next half hour trying to decide just how warm the water should be. He even took out the thermometer and tried to make it a perfect body-heated 98.6. Then came the big moment. He crossed himself and revved up his courage. With an Enola Gay-like swoop, his trembling fingers dropped the capsule into the glass. Then he waited for the hidden mystery to unfold. And he waited. And he waited.

Forty minutes went by before the gelatin capsule finally melted and revealed a thin piece of sponge in the shape of a cat.

A grown man would have known to go for the candy bars. But the young boy was still clinging to the hope that there were answers to questions that felt so much bigger than him.

What's Inside a Woman?

A fine way to learn about what's inside a woman is to hold her. For hours. Your skin against hers, the weight of her body and emotions pressing against yours. And if you really want to learn about a woman, consider having babies and raising them together. Hopefully you will like what you discover, although there are no guarantees for either of you. As for understanding a woman's sexuality, some women will let you deep inside of them; others will only have sex with you. It's no different than with men.

The Myth That Men Are Hornier than Women & Men Peak Sexually In Their Late Teens While Women Peak in Their Late Thirties

There is a silly notion in our society that young men are hornier than young women and that the cause is biological (hormones, chromosomes, or the will of God). It is also said that women don't reach their sexual peak until they are in their late 30s.

It is interesting that these myths don't exist in cultures that are more accepting of women's sexuality than our own. Perhaps it's not until women in North America get into their thirties that they start to realize what a crock they have been swallowing all their lives about themselves and their sexuality. But by that time, many of their male contemporaries have gotten fat or are out of shape, which makes them less receptive to anything that requires physical effort and stamina.

Wrestling with the Concept of "Womanhood"

People make all kinds of assumptions about womanhood, yet not many of these assumptions hold up to scrutiny. Consider some of the contradictions we have about womanhood:

💡 Intuition is said to be a defining element of womanhood. Yet there is not a single respectable study on intuition that has ever shown women, as a group, to be any more or less intuitive than men. Besides, you don't have to know too many women who date and marry total jerks to have serious doubts about the assumption that women are the more intuitive gender.

💡 In the past, motherhood was thought to be an essential element of womanhood. Yet we all know plenty of women without children who are far from deficient in the area of womanhood, whatever womanhood might be.

💡 It is often assumed that women are the less aggressive gender and that men's aggression makes them more bullying or controlling than women. While women don't always do it with bullets and knives, there is no shortage of aggressive, controlling, and unpleasant females. When you adjust for the number of miles driven by each sex, there are just as many aggressive female drivers as male drivers, and researchers have found that when women don't think anyone is watching, they can be even more aggressive than males. Aggression, or the lack of it, is not a defining element of womanhood.

💡 One female professor-type penned a bestseller that claims there are big differences in the ways men and women express themselves. Perhaps this is a defining element of womanhood. Yet when an interviewer noted that this woman's own style was more like the men she describes in her book, she fully agreed and added that her husband's style is more like a woman's. It's a good thing she didn't include herself and her husband in her studies.

💡 There are women who equate womanhood with their ability to create desire in a man's eyes or a bulge in a boy's boxers. Others don't view womanhood as having anything to do with being attractive to men.

Some of today's women feel challenged in trying to define womanhood. Hopefully you and your sexual partners will feel safe enough to be whatever you need to be, whether it is society's stereotypes of manly, womanly, boy-like, girl-like, passive, active, or bits and pieces of each.

Women's Sexual Anatomy — The Nerve of It All

In the late 1950s, a scientist named Kermit Krantz dissected the genital regions of eight dead women. He explored how women's genitals are wired. It is difficult to find a single research report on the topic of women's sexuality that is of more value than the one produced by Kermit Krantz.

He found a great deal of variation in the way the nerve endings are distributed throughout the different women's genitals. While there tended to be a higher concentration of nerve endings in the clitoris, the amount varied significantly among the different women; that is, some had more nerve endings in the labia minora (inner lips) than in the clitoris, and some women's nerve endings were highly concentrated in one area while other women had nerve endings that were spread out over a larger area. To quote Dr. Krantz:

"The extent of innervation in different females varies greatly."

What this suggests is that no two women get off sexually in the exact same way. Each woman needs to explore her own unique sexual universe, from where to touch to the kinds of fantasies that get her off. One woman might love oral sex and be so-so about intercourse, while the next craves a penis between her legs.

A man won't know exactly what a woman likes in bed until she tells him. It's not the sort of awareness he is going to assimilate during a one-night stand. The most important thing that experience can do is to help him feel comfortable asking for and taking direction.

Show & Tell

"While women speak to each other in graphic terms about things like menstruation, blow jobs, and the ratio of penis size to male ego, we usually don't talk to each other about what our crotches look like; not that we'd necessarily want to." *female age 34*

Most guys know what other guys' penises look like. That's because male genitals stick out. You can't help but notice when you shower or pee together. But women have no subtle way of looking at each other's genitals. Perhaps

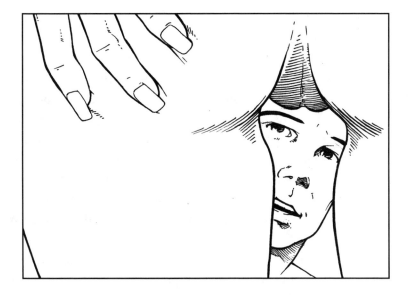

that's why some women find it reassuring to see pictures of other women's vulvas. They are often surprised to find that there is so much variation.

There are even photo books on vulvas which have been published by feminists. But the muff shots in the politically-correct beaver books have a sterile edge that's not particularly arousing. Perhaps it's because there are no visual cues that the women are having fun. The new-age beaver books are missing an attitude that says, "What we have between our legs is a good thing. It's cool, it's nice, we like it." Perhaps there is something reassuring about a woman who finds her genitals to be sexy. Perhaps it's why some men nearly ejaculate on the spot if a partner enjoys masturbating and lets him hold her or watch while she's doing it. Maybe it explains some of the allure of lingerie. It's in knowing that a woman finds her genitals sexy enough to cover them in a sensual or erotic way.

Dear Paul,

My girlfriend thinks her genitals are ugly. Is there anything I can do to help her change her mind?

Bobby in Beaver Falls

Dear Bobby,

It's the strangest thing how women can harbor negative feelings about the way their crotches look. A lot of girls don't even look at their own genitals until they are older, and even then, they refer to them as "down there."

Men end up knowing more about women's genitals and how they look than a number of women do.

Then again, our society has never wanted girls to be curious about their genitals. While it is natural for a child to fall asleep with a hand between her legs, parents often assume that this kind of self-comforting will turn an innocent girl into a slut-in-the-making. Heaven help a young girl who is caught bringing her fingers to her mouth or nose after touching herself "down there."

As I mention in Chapter 51: Keeping Your Kitty Happy, a number of young women won't use OB tampons or the NuvaRing because they find it disgusting to put their fingers inside their own vagina. What are we doing when we raise intelligent young women to think it's "icky" to stick their fingers inside their vaginas?

I recently received a video showing one of Betty Dodson's workshops where women check out each other's equipment. One of the women here at the Goofy Foot Press, who prides herself on her independence and liberation, felt uncomfortable when she first saw the tape. Then she remembered that she is just fine with porn tapes where men's penises are wagging all over the place, so she made a serious effort to relax and watch the tape. She had never realized her own discomfort with women's genitals.

How can you help your girlfriend be more positive about her genitals? First, begin by realizing this is part of a cultural disease. Then, perhaps with patient and creative encouragement on your part, maybe her own eyes will start to reflect the delight that's in yours when you look between her legs.

Busy Little Beavers

People refer to everything between a woman's legs as her vagina. Yet this is far from true. What sits between a naked woman's legs is her vulva.

You might ask, "What difference does it make if you call it a vulva or vagina?" One female educator answered this question by asking: "What if parents taught their children that they had no eyes, ears, nose or mouth, but instead gave them one word for their entire face and called it 'tongue'?" This would be confusing. It might suggest that parents are afraid of faces and all the wonderful things they can do.

Some men see no need to learn about the different structures that are between a woman's legs. They figure, "My penis goes in there just fine. She likes it, I like it, what's more to learn?" And some women are more concerned

The Vulva

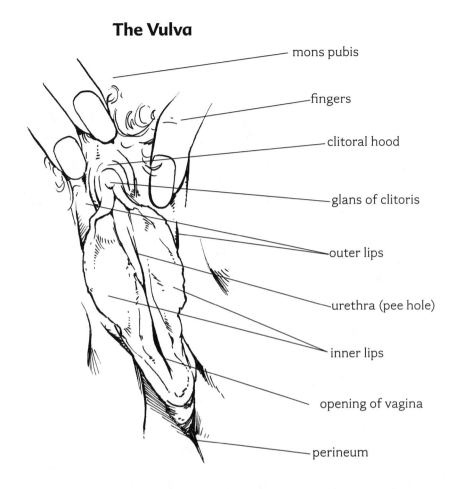

mons pubis

fingers

clitoral hood

glans of clitoris

outer lips

urethra (pee hole)

inner lips

opening of vagina

perineum

with how to wax the outside of their genitals than in knowing what's inside of them. Hopefully you'll want to know what's inside a girl's genitals. It really can made a difference in the pleasure you are able to give and receive.

The Mons: Love-Making Ally Due To The Ligaments Within

The mons pubis is a fleshy mound that sits on top of the pubic bone. It is usually covered by pubic hair, unless the woman has been trying to wear a thong with grace or likes the look and feel of being bare.

The suspensory ligament of the clitoris has its base in the mons pubis.

Some women enjoy it if a partner pushes his fingers against the mons and rubs the fleshy mound in a circle, or if he pulls it upward. This kind of movement might apply pressure to the deeper parts of the clitoris. Other women enjoy having the pubic hair tugged that grows from their mons.

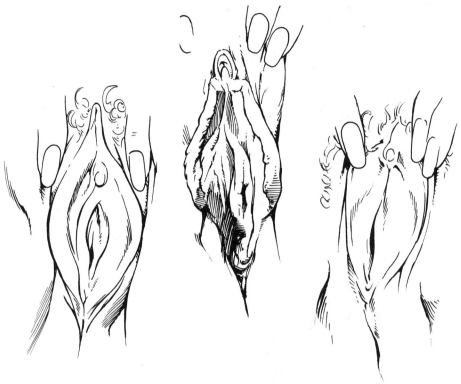

Lips, Lips, Lips

Even the ancient Romans got it wrong. They named the outer lips "labia majora" (big lips) and the inner lips "labia minora" (small lips). They should have called them "inner" and "outer," given how the inner lips are often more major than the outer lips. The inner lips usually give vulvas their unique personalities. They fan out in different ways and shapes, and when a woman is aroused, they perk up and deepen in color.

The outer lips often have hair on them and are mostly made up of fatty tissue. Their skin is similar to that of the male scrotum.

The inner lips are bald. Their tissue has a rich supply of blood vessels and nerves. It is sexually reactive, and expands when a woman is sexually aroused. Their skin is more like the skin on the penis.

The inner lips attach to the glans of the clitoris. Some women play with them or stroke them when they are masturbating. Caressing the inner lips or gently tugging on them can provide a neat way of stimulating the clitoris.

During intercourse, the inner lips are pushed and pulled with each stroke of the penis, which can tug and stimulate the glans of the clitoris.

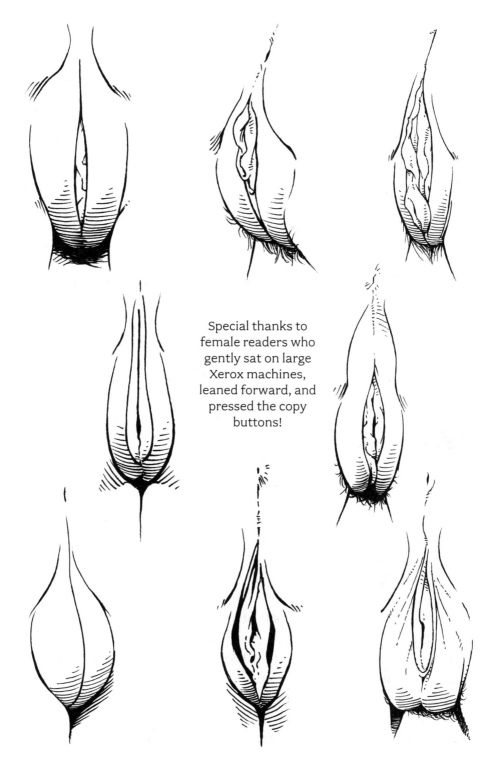

Special thanks to female readers who gently sat on large Xerox machines, leaned forward, and pressed the copy buttons!

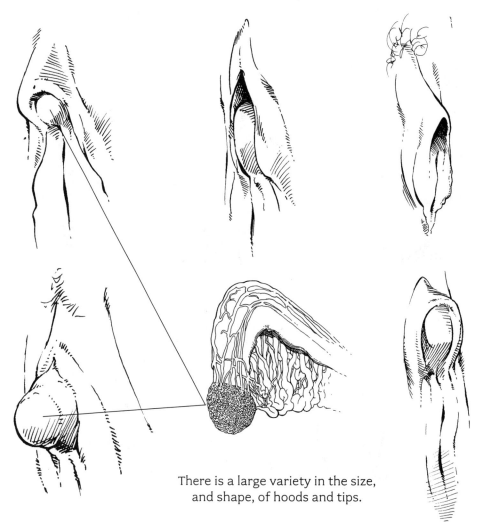

There is a large variety in the size,
and shape, of hoods and tips.

Clitoris: Point Guard for Women's Genitals

Most people think a clitoris is the little knob you see when a woman spreads her legs. But as you can see in the illustration to your right, it is much bigger and more involved than that.

The glans or tip is a small but potent part of the entire clitoris. The hood-like structure that drapes over it is just that—the hood. It's like the foreskin on a penis. When women masturbate, they often press a fingertip against the hood and rub it in a small circle or back and forth. The glans and shaft beneath the hood seldom complain.

The size of the tip or glans of the clitoris can range greatly. In some women, it nearly pops out to shake your hand; in others it can hardly be seen.

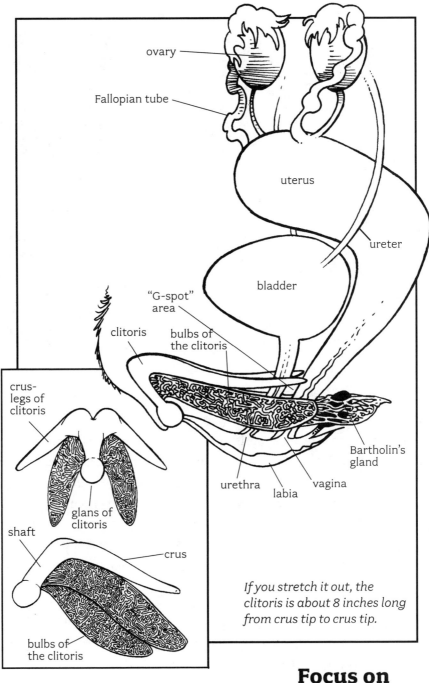

ovary

Fallopian tube

uterus

ureter

bladder

"G-spot" area

clitoris

bulbs of the clitoris

Bartholin's gland

crus-legs of clitoris

glans of clitoris

shaft

crus

bulbs of the clitoris

urethra

labia

vagina

If you stretch it out, the clitoris is about 8 inches long from crus tip to crus tip.

A "crus" is an individual leg of the clitoris. "Crura" refers to both of them.

Focus on the Clitoris

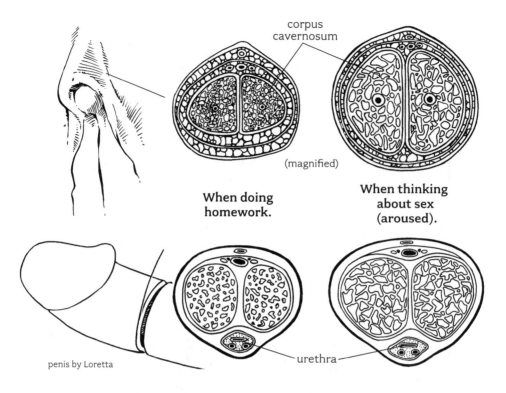

corpus
cavernosum

(magnified)

**When doing
homework.**

**When thinking
about sex
(aroused).**

penis by Loretta

urethra

X-Section of a Clitoris Glans and a Penis

When the glans is really large, it can look like a mini penis, complete with a head and shaft. No matter what its size is, it can often be quite sensitive.

The hood of the clitoris can usually glide back and forth over the glans without it feeling abrasive. However, some hoods are permanently attached or bonded to the clitoris. This is perfectly OK and sexual sensation feels fine. Surgery to separate the hood from the glans is seldom necessary or wise.

Some women find their clitoris changes sensitivity with the time of the month, in others it keeps an even keel.

As a woman approaches orgasm, it can seem like the tip of her clitoris disappears or retracts. This can be confusing for the man who is trying to stimulate the clitoris by hand or mouth. Should he play Hercule Poirot and give chase, or wait until the clitoris returns?

The mystery could be due to pelvic muscle contractions that cause the shaft and glans to straighten out. If you are stimulating the clitoris with your finger or tongue, it might feel like it suddenly starts to hide or retract. If whatever you were doing managed to get it to throb or spasm, don't change now unless the lady requests. Let it play its game of cat and mouse.

The Crura of the Clitoris

The clitoris proper has three different parts: the glans or tip, the shaft, and the crura or legs. The crura look like the legs of a wishbone. They run beneath the labia. The shaft and crura contain bodies of erectile tissue that are called the corpus cavernosum, just like the cylinders that are in the penis.

The Bulbs of the Clitoris aka "Vestibular Bulbs"—Clitoris Adjacent

Mother Nature planted a pair of bulbs inside her favorite garden. They are called the bulbs of the clitoris, and they swell and blossom each time a woman is sexually aroused. They are close to the clitoris and communicate with it through blood vessels, but they are made of slightly different tissue. (See the bulbs on pages 87 and 188.)

The bulbs of the clitoris are more elastic than the clitoris glans or tip. Since they don't have a tough skin encasing them like the chambers of the penis do, the bulbs can expand proportionally more than the clitoris or penis when a woman is sexually aroused. (It's the chambers pushing against the tough outer casing that helps the penis get hard as opposed to just bigger.) The bulbs of clitoris also have larger spaces that blood can rush into

The Axis of Arousal—Clitoris, Clitoral Bulbs & Labia Minora

When a woman becomes sexually aroused, her clitoris, clitoral bulbs and inner lips become engorged with blood. This is similar to what happens to a penis when a man becomes aroused.

These structures communicate with each other when a woman is becoming sexually excited. It's not like they text-message each other, but all three are highly involved when sexual excitement is in the air. (Researcher Helen O'Connell might suggest that we include the urethra, making the axis of arousal a quartet of pleasure.)

Suggestion: take a moment and look at the diagrams of the clitoris in this chapter. See the placement of the crura and the bulbs? Some women enjoy it when a partner does a deep fingertip massage of the tissue that's beneath their labia. It may seem like it would be painful since you are reaching almost to the pelvic bone, but what you are really doing is stimulating the rich vascular beds in the hidden parts of the clitoris (see page 188). With plenty of feedback, you'll learn what feels good and what doesn't.

The Clitoris during Intercourse

"I rub the heck out of my clitoris during intercourse. I do it to reach an orgasm when my partner is almost there." *female age 25*

"I almost always rub on my clit during intercourse. I usually make small circular motions, which is not how I move my finger when I masturbate. I love when he does it too, although sometimes I have to move his hand into the correct spot." *female age 24*

"I have tried rubbing my clit once or twice, but prefer to focus my attention on his dick inside of me." *female age 20*

The glans of the clitoris is seldom positioned to rub noses with an incoming penis. Some women enjoy the added stimulation of a finger or vibrator during intercourse, or they sometimes push the clitoris against the shaft of a sweetheart's thrusting penis or grind it against his pubic bone. Other women do just fine with thrusting alone.

A Final Note on the Clitoris — How Do You Pronounce It?

One day, the author of this book had to address a classroom of students and he needed to say "clitoris." There he was, with almost thirteen years of college under his belt, not knowing how to pronounce the word "clitoris." To prepare, he wrote "clitoris" on one card and "penis" on another. He then asked friends of both sexes to say the two words out loud.

No one had any hesitation in pronouncing penis, but almost everyone approached clitoris with a perplexed look and said, "Well, here's how I have always pronounced it." Some said cli-TOR-is, others said CLIT-or-is. As he was exploring his own usage of the word, he realized that the only time he had referred to it was in bed with a woman, and then he called it "it." Either pronunciation is correct.

Urinary Meatus, More Fun Than It Sounds

There is a small circle of firm tissue around the end of the urethra. It is between the inner lips (east and west) and the tip of the clitoris and the mouth of the vagina (north and south). It is sensitive enough that some women rub it when they are masturbating. It is called the "urethral meatus," which is Greek for "pee and play."

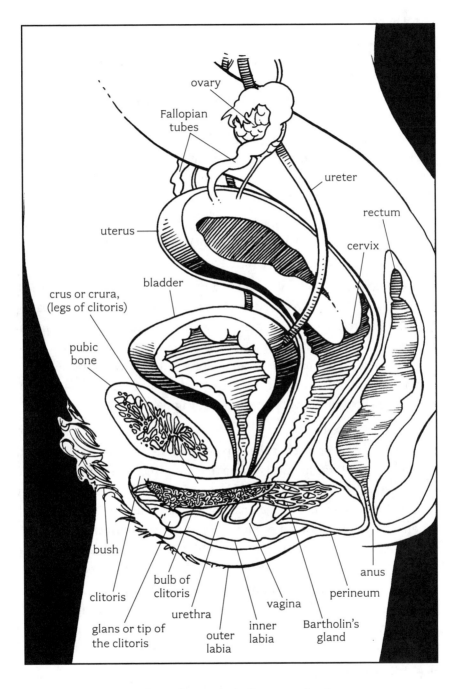

ovary

Fallopian
tubes

ureter

rectum

uterus

cervix

crus or crura,
(legs of clitoris)

bladder

pubic
bone

bush

anus

clitoris

bulb of
clitoris

perineum

glans or tip of
the clitoris

urethra

vagina

outer
labia

inner
labia

Bartholin's
gland

What's Inside a Girl

The Vagina

The human body is made up of many different tubes. The favorite tube of many straight males and lesbians is the vagina, a hollow canal with walls that contain four layers of tissue, nerves and blood vessels. When not aroused, the walls of the vagina lie flat against each other like a firehose without water. When aroused, a vagina straightens out and puffs up a bit.

When sexually aroused, the first third of the vagina becomes narrower while the back part expands and sometimes balloons open, a little like the bottom half of an hour glass. Some women particularly enjoy stimulation at the opening of their vagina:

> "The main request I ask of my partner is to tease me with his cock. That's because most of the sensitivity in my vagina is at the opening."
>
> *female age 25*

The first third of the vagina is often sensitive to touch, while the back two-thirds are more sensitive to pressure. For some women, the back part expands before orgasm and then contracts. This might cause a longing to have something inside the vagina which the rear walls can grasp.

We could try to map out a vagina for you, but why not make your own vaginal love maps? What nicer way to spend an afternoon than exploring the tender shoals of a lover's warm, moist vagina.

Sponges in the Vagina?

There is a spongy area above the walls of the vagina called the urethral sponge. The urethral sponge is tissue that surrounds the entire length of the urethra, which is the tube that takes urine from the bladder to the blowhole. It runs along the roof of the vagina. The sponge is a little like the foam insulation that protects hot-water pipes. If you put your finger in a vagina and make a "come here" motion, you are pushing into the urethral sponge. Some women find that this feels very, very good. Others find it to be annoying.

The tissue of the urethral sponge contains tiny periurethral glands that have an embryological and histological similarity to the prostate. But it should not be called a "female prostate," as this would be confusing and incorrect. There is no prostate gland in the female pelvis.

Papa Freud & The Viennese Vagina

Not too long ago, Freudian psychiatrists proclaimed that women had defective egos if their orgasms didn't originate from deep inside the vagina.

Sex researchers in the 1960s did society a huge service in showing that the majority of women's orgasms involve the clitoris rather than the vagina. But this wasn't meant to discount the vagina as a source of pleasure.

Some women find that having something in the vagina when they come helps their orgasm feel more like "full-body." For other women, orgasms from clitoral stimulation alone light up their bodies from head to toe.

Sex has its variations and its possibilities. One woman might prefer oral sex to intercourse, another might enjoy masturbating while her partner holds her or masturbates with her. A third woman might not feel satisfied unless her lover's penis is deep inside her vagina. A fourth woman might prefer oral sex with John, but intercourse with Bill.

Four Scores & Seven Vaginas Ago

If you have had the good fortune to experience sex with a number of women and were of a clear mind when doing so, you may have noticed that not all vaginas are created equal. Not all penises are created equal, either.

For instance, you might get weak in the knees at the sight of a certain woman, but after having intercourse with her your penis complains that jerking off in the shower feels better. At the same time, a woman who seems quite plain on the surface may be the one whose vagina you remember most throughout life.

Vaginal Farts

> "My boyfriend was performing oral sex on me and fingering my vagina. When I sat up, all of the air in my vagina came rushing out and made a huge fartlike noise. I was totally embarrassed; it was completely unexpected. I looked at my boyfriend with shock on my face, and then we both started laughing." *female age 25*

Occasionally, air gets trapped inside a vagina and makes a fartlike noise when it comes out. This happens all the time. Both of you created the situation and hopefully you had a fine time doing so. It's just normal room air that is seeping out, nothing that's going to corrode the finish on the door hinges.

Vaginal farts are more likely to happen after you have had an orgasm and the rear part of your vagina ballooned open. The noise can happen when it is returning to its normal resting state. The Irish utilized this principle to create the foghorn.

A Tipped Uterus

Women with a tipped uterus sometimes feel uncomfortable discussing the ins and outs of intercourse with their gynecologist. So if you have a tipped uterus, this section was written for you.

The uterus is an upside-down pear-shaped organ that is located between a woman's bladder and her rectum. It is where human infants spend their first 40 weeks. Many people consider it to be the strongest muscle in the body.

Up to 30% of women have a uterus that is tipped, retroverted or tilted. These terms more or less mean the same thing—that the uterus points backwards and sits on the assward side of your vagina instead of on the belly-button side.

Think of the standard, factory-equipped female pelvis as having a vagina and uterus that more or less make a "p." The vagina is the straight part of the P, and the uterus sits above it like the round part of the P, pointing toward the woman's belly button. If the uterus is tipped, the arrangement becomes more like a "q", where the uterus points the opposite way.

This might be why some women with a tipped uterus experience period pain more as a back ache than a pain in their abdomen, and why they tend to have more back pain and diarrhea when they are menstruating. In fact, some women with a tipped uterus know when their period is coming because they start having loose stools that might be caused by a release of prostaglandins.

Given how the penis slides up the straight part of your "p" or "q", intercourse positions that work well for a woman with a "p" alignment might not work as well for a woman with a "q" alignment. What you are trying to maximize is a smooth sliding path where the penis can make it all the way in without banging into your cervix, uterus or ovary. Significant factors will include the size of your boy's piston, the way it points when erect, and the position you are in. Another factor will be if your uterus shifts when you are sexually aroused.

If you have a tipped uterus and experience pain during rear entry intercourse, it might be due to the penis banging into your uterus or your ovaries. The pain might also come from extra air that can accumulate during intercourse in the vagina of a woman with a tipped uterus. So your lover needs to realize that while his former partner might have been the Reverse Cowgirl Queen, this position might cause you a lot of pain.

Here's what three women who took our sex survey say, but what works for you may be very different than this.

> "My uterus is tilted. It makes doggy-style intercourse painful. I prefer to be on top of my boyfriend."

> "I have a very tipped uterus. Unless I'm pregnant they can't pick it up on a regular ultrasound because it leans so far backwards. Intercourse feels best with me on top or missionary. I've found that doggie style isn't very comfortable for me, nor is me being on top while facing his feet. As long as we are close to each other, belly touching belly, deep thrusting is fine. If we are separate, like if I'm laying down and he is in an upright position, deep thrusting can be uncomfortable. Where I'm at in my cycle also plays a role in how comfortable or uncomfortable things are."

> "I have a tipped uterus, and this may be why it hurts when my partner thrusts too deep. It may also be why I don't like to be penetrated from the rear. Being on top is the most comfortable position for me and the one that provides the highest likelihood of orgasm."

As for birth control and conception, there is a popular myth that women with tipped uteruses can't conceive as easily as other women. Don't believe it. Also, some women with a tipped or tilted uterus refer to it as an "inverted uterus." However, an inverted uterus is a rare event that happens when your uterus turns inside out right after you've given birth. Also, the uterus can sometimes become tipped due to a problem such as endometriosis, so if you start having discomfort with intercourse, be sure to tell your doctor. As with all questions regarding matters of health, the information in a book can never take the place of an exam from a gynecologist.

The Cervix

The cervix is a small, fleshy dome in the rear of the vagina near the top. Nature put it there as a valve or gatekeeper that joins the uterus and the vagina. The cervix can be as small as a cherry in a woman who has not delivered a baby through her vagina, or it can be much bigger. It has a dimple in the center that menstrual fluids flow down and male ejaculate flows up.

The cervix sometimes feels softer during ovulation, when mucus passes through it and bathes the vagina. This keeps it clean and more acidic, conditions which encourage conception. At the point when conception is most likely to occur, the mucus becomes clear and slippery, like raw egg-whites.

The cervix has a space around it that is called the fornix. This is a delightful area to explore with a finger. It is also a good space to know about when the woman's vagina isn't particularly deep or her lover has a long penis. Couples in this situation might want to find intercourse positions that encourage the penis to slither under the cervix and into the rear fornix. This will add an extra inch or two of runway space. Some women find stimulation of the space around the fornix to be quite pleasing; others will surely hate it.

From a sex therapist: Women often report feeling pain during sex that is deep in their vagina. In many cases it is because they are not aroused so their vagina is not fully tilted. What they feel is the pain of their partner's penis hitting the cervix. They should slow down and get aroused or change position, then continue with intercourse. You have no idea how many women are surprised about this and don't realize that what they feel is their cervix!

There are at least two ways to see a cervix. The first is by using a speculum. This is a metal or plastic device that physicians insert into a woman's vagina to help push the walls apart. It allows the physician to see parts of a woman that most boyfriends and husbands never do. If you have a healthy

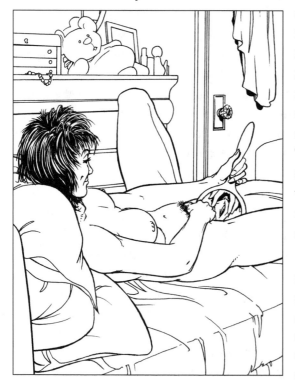

curiosity, get a speculum from your physician or medical-supply store. Lube it with KY jelly, gently insert it into the vagina and add the krypton beam of your favorite flashlight. This will give your partner a bird's eye view of the cervix. You'll need to incorporate a hand-held mirror to see it yourself.

When people see how small the slit in the cervix is, they sometimes exclaim, "A baby is supposed to fit through that?" It clearly expands and stretches.

Another way of seeing inside a vagina is to get an acrylic dildo with a view port that is optically designed to give you 5X magnification. These aren't cheap. Once you insert it, the cervix should be in there somewhere.

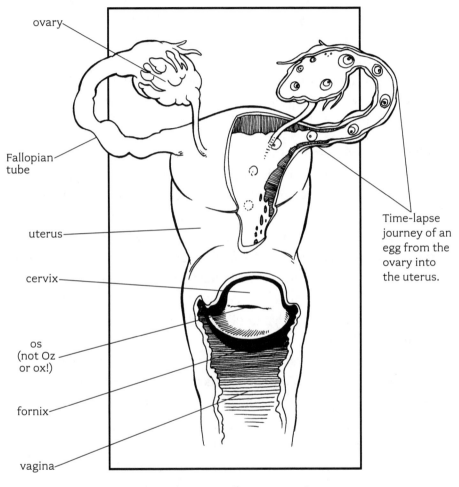

ovary

Fallopian tube

uterus

cervix

os
(not Oz
or ox!)

fornix

vagina

Time-lapse journey of an egg from the ovary into the uterus.

Focus on the Cervix

Science doesn't yet understand the role of the cervix in sexual response. While it seems that the cervix should be a player, there are women who have had their cervixes surgically removed who have a robust sexual experience.

Ovaries

A man's testicles announce themselves wherever he goes. Not so with a woman's ovaries. It's possible to have a long-term relationship with a woman and not even know her ovaries are there, except indirectly through events like pregnancy or menstruation.

Assuming you want to, the best time to feel a woman's ovaries is when she is lying on her back and is in an "It's OK if you feel my ovaries" mood. Otherwise, don't even try. Rest one hand on her lower abdomen below her belly button. Place a lubricated finger or two from your other hand deep into her vagina. When you encounter the rear wall of her vagina, veer to the left or right and push up gently while pushing down with the hand that's on her abdomen. You will need to rely on her instructions. If a woman doesn't know where her ovaries are, she might ask her gynecologist to show her.

G-Spot vs. G-Spot Area

Over the past ten years, the G-spot has become a major industry, complete with G-spot books, G-spot vibrators, G-spot toys, and G-spot videos.

While researchers don't question the fine orgasms that some women have with G-spot stimulation, there isn't any special wiring or trigger-tissue in the G-spot area that would make its stimulation universally wonderful for all women. So what is it about stimulating that area that give some women some of their finest orgasms?

One of the problems is that until recently, we've mainly been limited to doing research on cadavers. And while some of these dead women might be orgasming through the cosmos or having some righteously good sex in the afterlife, you can't see how different parts of a person sexual anatomy interact when they're dead. We're talking permanent stop-action.

However, with some of the newer technologies, researchers can see inside the sexually active pelvis of a live human. And to that end, researchers in France have suggested that the internal structure of the clitoris gets displaced during intercourse, and it might actually be the internal structure of the clitoris that's helping create the extra-intense orgasmic experience. While the work that these researchers are doing is in its infancy and may prove to be fruitless, it is still quite fascinating. Whatever the case, these researchers refer to it as the G-spot area rather than the G-spot, which is how *The Guide* has been referring to it for years. That's because the wiring just doesn't seem to be there for a specific "spot" or trigger point.

Another idea has been proposed by one of our gynecology consultants. She says, "I always felt that the G-spot was actually a stimulation of the area that corresponded to the trigone of the bladder and that was why many women felt even greater sensations when their bladders were slightly full during sex. I have some patients who intentionally drink fluids to fill their bladder prior to sexual play because it 'feels better'. When they do this, I think the trigone presses down more on the anterior vaginal wall and is more easily stimulated." This corresponds with the experience of many women who find that G-spot area stimulation causes a feeling of bladder fullness.

> "When my partner is going down on me and inserts his finger, placing pressure upwards on the top wall of my vaginal canal, it feels really really good if I ignore that it also feels like I need to pee."
>
> *female age 24*

G-spot aficionados recommend the woman relaxes and stops worrying about peeing all over the place. Hopefully you'll try it for yourself to see if it's a good or bad thing for you. One way to find the G-spot area is to put a finger part way into the vagina and make a "come here" motion with it.

The G-Spot Bottom Line

With all of the media hype and sex-store attention about G-spot stimulation, some readers will be thinking, "Why waste so much time with her clit when I could be stimulating her G-spot?" The answer should depend totally on what it is your partner wants rather than what someone else tells you. Mercifully, one of the world's top researchers in women's sexual anatomy has provided readers of *The Guide* with an answer to these burning questions. The following is from Claire Yang, M.D., a neurophysiologist and researcher in the Department of Urology at the University of Washington:

> "I think that because the sexual response is so closely linked to emotions, the experience of pleasure, and in particular sexual pleasure, it is not going to be tied directly to anatomical structure, even during sexual arousal. For instance, why do women not feel sexual stimulation when those same areas that you describe are being examined during a gyn exam? The bottom line is: the entire genital area has nerves (as does the entire body), and in the context of sexual arousal, the processing of the messages is what makes the

experience, not just the manual stimulation. I think the cortical processing of sexual stimulation by the female brain is extremely variable, and to pin down a particular area (or situation) that is universally arousing is not possible at this time. That is why the concept of the G-spot has not gained universal acceptance. That is why the pursuit of a female sexual-arousal drug has been elusive. That is why the female sexual response will remain a mystery for a little while longer."

As for any consensus from Goofy Foot Press, the writers at the major women's magazines routinely call the author of *The Guide* to ask about this spot or that spot—the G-spot, the C-spot or the X-Y-Z-spot. It's never enough for them if he says, "That might feel good for some women, but not so good for others." These writers are hellbent to write a story that will sell magazines. It's a rare day when one of them values the idea of a woman exploring for herself and finding what does and doesn't work for her.

Variations in Wetness

When sexually aroused, some vaginas get so wet that the woman needs to wring out her underwear. Other women can be every bit as aroused, but their vaginas remain dry. And some women can be very wet, but not be sexually turned-on. Wetness also varies during certain phases of your cycle. (Our gyno consultant says that too many women think there's something wrong with their pusses just because they are normally moist during the day.)

Men shouldn't be so silly as to gauge a woman's level of sexual arousal on vaginal wetness alone. And a woman shouldn't feel there's anything wrong with her if she puddles her pants during the day from thinking about sex, or needs to add lube before intercourse. There are great lubes including saliva and a number of vegetable oils for when a vagina is too dry, and towels for when it's a fountain.

As for extra wetness during or just before orgasms, some women have a little, others have a lot. Collectively, his and her sex fluids have been known as the wet spot on the mattress. Its diameter can vary from couple to couple.

The biggest problem with expelling extra fluid at orgasm is that women who do it sometimes feel embarrassed and try to prevent it. As a result, they keep themselves from fully relaxing, and this can inhibit orgasms. Most guys are happy to have a partner who drenches them or the mattress, especially when they realize it means she may have had a really nice orgasm.

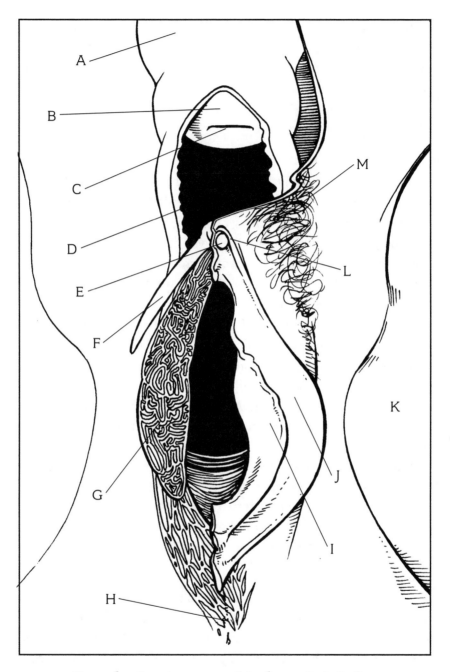

Female-Anatomy-as-Modern-Art Quiz

A—uterus; B—cervix; C—os; D—vagina; E—glans or tip of clitoris;
F. crus or leg of clitoris; G—bulb of clitoris; H—perineum;
I—inner lip or labia minora; J—outer lip or labia majora;
K—inner thigh; L—hood of clitoris ; M—pubic hair

If you happen to be a gusher or a bed-drencher, please don't think that any man in his right mind is going to have a problem with it. Why not have fun shopping together for sets of towels that are just for sex? And if you are worried about the mattress, take solace in knowing that they now make waterproof mattress-pad covers that feel and sound like normal mattress-pad covers. They are wonderful!

Is PseudoScience All Wet?

It's unfortunate how little real science there is on sexual pleasure. But this does not justify attempts to invent science in the name of sexuality.

Science knows next to nothing about the male prostate gland, yet it is large, and you can actually feel it. We haven't found anything in the female body other than the bladder that would produce several ounces of female ejaculate, yet some writers are claiming that women have a prostate gland, and that it can do this and more.

Since the male prostate gland produces less than a teaspoon of fluid for each male ejaculation—this female prostate must be a whopper!

If women readers do have a prostate gland, take some sound advice and keep quiet about it. Otherwise, surgeons will start cutting yours out as fast as they are trying to cut ours out. And if you don't have a prostate gland, be glad. You won't believe the problems a prostate gland can cause as you get older.

Women were having some pretty outrageous sex for centuries before Grafenberg discovered his spot. And female sex fluids have been around since the Tigris and Euphrates started flowing through the Fertile Crescent. Whatever you want to call it, and however you want to describe it, enjoy exploring your body's sensations, and cherish them.

Menopause

Menopause is what naturally happens to a woman's body when she is over 40 and stops having her monthly periods and no longer has to worry about getting pregnant. People have always believed that a woman's sex drive goes down as she enters menopause. Yet researchers have discovered that when a menopausal woman gets into a new relationship, she can be as horny as her 20-something self. Seems that it's the excitement in her relationship, rather than her gonads, that often determines how much she wants sex.

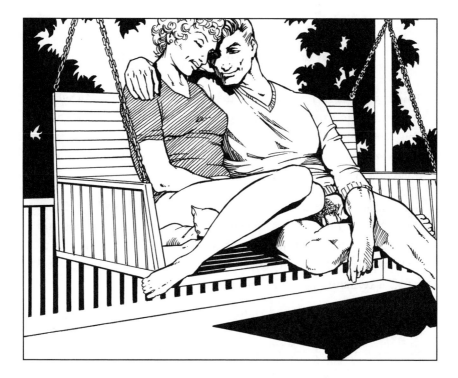

As for vaginal lubrication, some menopausal women find that they get less wet when sexually aroused. In some women, the skin in their vagina starts to feel less elastic or more sensitive during menopause. While there are certainly hormonal creams that can help, the women from Touch of a Woman strongly recommend that you or your partner massage your vulva and opening of your vagina every day with a moisturizer to help keep it more elastic. If you are approaching menopause, please give their totally free, drug free program a look. And keep in mind that the woman who has written this protocol is an MD and a very fine one. The title is "Still Juicy: Maintaining Sexual Health through and beyond Menopause." As of presstime, the link was hideously long:

www.a-womans-touch.com/article/37/63/Still_Juicy_Maintaining_
Sexual_Health_through_and_beyond_Menopause.html

As for other concerns, stress can impact a menopausal woman more than before she was menopausal. This can be extra difficult if her own mom and dad are in declining health and she has to deal with their situation. On the plus side, her children might be starting to live on their own, so she and her partner can have more time to do as they please.

Reader Comments

What does it feel like in your genitals when you are sexually aroused?

"Tingling starts in my clitoris and spreads to my labia. My whole vulva starts to throb, literally. The throbbing is extremely pleasurable. Then my vulva gets swollen and almost hot. Once it is swollen, every slight touch sends lightning bolts of pleasure all around my whole body." *female age 23*

"Sometimes it's an ache not unlike having a full bladder. Other times, a sensation of heat and congestion in my labia, clitoris and vagina. If I'm highly aroused, or if my clothing is tight, I'll be able to feel my pulse between my legs. Sometimes I'll feel my tendons and muscles twitching as well." *female age 36*

"My labia feel swollen and tight; my clitoris becomes hard. Sometimes my clitoris feels like it's huge, and it sort of throbs. If I am extremely aroused, my whole vulva feels as though it's pounding, with my clitoris as the center." *female age 26*

"You know the feeling you get right before your leg or arm falls asleep? I mean, before it's annoying or hurts. It's a really intense tingling feeling. It makes my whole body feel warm and excited. There are moments, however, right before my partner enters me, when my vagina actually aches." *female age 27*

When did you first make the connection between being sexually aroused and being wet?

"When I was around 10 or 11, while watching a sex scene in a film. My panties got wet, and I realized that was why. If I'm really turned on, I'll drip down to my ankles." *female age 25*

"I first connected being wet with sexual arousal when I was 13. I was watching a silent, vintage erotic film with a friend. When I went to the bathroom, I was soaked!" *female age 26*

"The first time I connected wetness with sex was when I was 9 or so and got all wet and throbby when I was watching a couple kissing at the beach. But I don't always get wet when I feel aroused; it isn't an indicator for me." *female age 38*

"When I first masturbated, I only touched myself on my clitoris, so I was very surprised when I eventually felt my vagina and it was dripping fluid." *female age 23*

About being wet…

"Being wet is hard to explain. I don't know if I can offer insight because it just happens. The most annoying thing is that if you don't wear panties and get wet, it tends to be very messy, but arousing!" *female age 36*

"For me, the degree of my wetness varies greatly from time to time and seems to be largely affected by how mentally 'into' having sex I am at that given time." *female age 34*

"If my boyfriend just starts kissing me and wants to have sex, I am not automatically wet. I need to be turned on. This could be my way of slowing down and paying attention to my body, or it could be by talking sexy, reading, looking at, or listening to erotica." *female age 26*

"It does not work when my partner concentrates solely on doing mechanical things to get me wet. Yet a simple, very tender kiss can do it." *female age 48*

"I enjoy sex a great deal, but seldom get wet." *female age 32*

A Very Special Thanks to the following for their generous help and advice:

• Claire Yang, MD, Department of Urology, University of Washington

• Alessandra Rellini, Ph.D., University of Vermont

• Marca Sipski, MD, Director of Neuroscience Rehabilitation Research, University of Alabama at Birmingham

• William W. Young, MD, Department of Obstetrics and Gynecology, Dartmouth Medical School

• Maureen Whelihan, MD, Gynecology

• Carol Tavris, Ph.D. and Leonore Tiefer, Ph.D.

Some of the illustrations in this chapter were strongly influenced by:

Atlas of Human Sex Anatomy, Second Edition, Robert Latou Dickinson, The Williams & Wilkins Company, Baltimore, Maryland, 1949

A New View of a Woman's Body by the Federation of Feminist Women's Health Centers, Illustrations by Suzann Gage, West Hollywood, California. If you found the drawings in this chapter helpful, you are encouraged to purchase the classic *New View* directly from the authors at:

www.progressivehealth.org

8

The Hymen

The hymen is a collar of tissue around the opening of the vagina. It is the source of myth and legend, and it remains a mystery to much of modern medicine. Not that many primary care physicians can even accurately locate the hymen. When we recently polled a group of gynecologists and women's sexual health experts, few could say what happens to the hymen of a sexually-active woman over time.

Some of the better studies on the hymen have only been done in the last couple of years, and some of these contradict each other. The research that's been done on hymens is mostly related to investigating sexual abuse, so it's not particularly helpful if you are trying to understand the hymen in a context of healthy sexual activity.

In this chapter we will present much of what is known about the sexually-happy hymen. If there are holes in our knowledge, it pretty much goes with the territory.

How Your Hymen Came to Be

There are a few very helpful things to know about hymens—and just knowing these two things will help you to understand more about this little collar or ring of tissue than—oh—99% of the population knows.

But first, we need to get our anatomy right.

The hymen is located just inside the opening of the vagina. Unfortunately we often refer to everything that's between a woman's legs as her vagina, which is like saying "New York" without specifying whether you mean New York City or upper state. So to see the hymen, you need to pull apart the labia or lips and look inside the opening of the vagina.

In understanding how the hymen came to be and why it is where it is, you need to know the difference between the vulva and vagina, because each had a hand in the development of the hymen while the woman was still in her mother's womb.

VULVA: This is the part of a woman's genitals that are on the outside—the part that you actually see and that's been the focus of many a magazine centerfold. It includes the mound that's covered with pubic hair, the tip of the clitoris, and the lips or labia. Some people think the vulva is what they named the car known as the Volvo after.

VAGINA: This is the part of women's sexual plumbing that's on the inside. The vagina itself is a tube-like structure that's located inside a woman's body. It's where a tampon and penis slide into, although hopefully not at the same time. The vagina starts just inside the vulva, where the hymen is, and runs all the way back behind the cervix.

The Hymen—Where East Meets West

The vulva and vagina did not come from the same kind of embryonic tissue. So what you have are two different kinds of tissue, with the hymen being the border or checkpoint between the two.

While this analogy might be stretching it a bit, think of when two different land masses collide and a mountain range is created at that spot. The Himalayas are a case in point—a fine example when you consider that both *hymen* and *Himalayas* both start with an "H."

What's particularly interesting about this embryonic junction is that the tissue on the inner side of the hymen comes from the vagina which is estrogen-sensitive. So when the girl begins to go through puberty and her estrogen levels rise, the hymen changes considerably.

How the Hymen Changes—It's Puberty and Not the Penis That Does It

As the body changes, so does the hymen. Before puberty, a girl's hymen is often crescent-shaped, although there are certainly variations. The hymen is stretched across the opening of the vagina and it is almost translucent. You can actually see some of the capillaries in it and it covers much of the opening of the vagina.

By the end of puberty, the hymen no longer drapes across the opening of the vagina, but becomes more like an O-ring or collar, allowing a penis (or tampon) to have full entry. This is from the impact of estrogen on the hymen tissue, which has estrogen receptors in it just like the walls of the vagina.

Adult Woman
Stretching her lips apart to show
the opening of her vagina and her hymen.

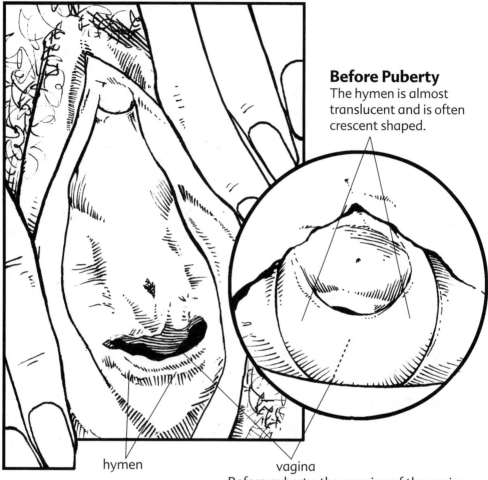

Before Puberty
The hymen is almost
translucent and is often
crescent shaped.

hymen   vagina

Before puberty, the opening of the vagina
is often hidden behind the hymen.

Estrogen Effects from Puberty
Due to the effects of estrogen, the walls of the hymen
become thicker, shorter and more elastic. Far from making
hymens that pop, nature seems to have made them ready
for intercourse by changing them during puberty.

The changing HYMEN

Since the estrogen makes the hymen more elastic, our modern notion that the hymen "pops" like a cherry during the first intercourse is silly.

The estrogen that comes with the start of puberty causes the hymen to become shorter and thicker, more like a hedge or collar than the former drape or a wall that it was during childhood. With this thickening comes elasticity.

So it is puberty that changes the hymen, not the first intercourse. In fact, it's as if nature is changing the girl's hymen to make it ready for intercourse.

From Saran Wrap into Spandex

Researchers often have trouble distinguishing between the hymens of teenage girls who are sexually active and hymens of teenage girls who are still virgins. That wouldn't be the cause if hymens were like the tops of pop bottles or "Cherries that pop."

Still, it's hard to dispel the myth that the hymen is a disposable seal of virginity, like the sheet of plastic that's fused onto the top of a frozen dinner or a cup of yogurt that is torn to shreds after the first intercourse. Think of football players running onto the field and bursting through a wall of painted butcher paper that cheerleaders are forever holding the sides of— that's how we think of the first intercourse.

In actuality, the hymen of a woman who is past puberty looks a lot more like the stargate in Stargate Atlantis, minus the cool-looking chevrons that are embedded within it.[1]

Your First Intercourse

We also assume that there will be blood after the first intercourse. Yet way more than half of the women who take our sex survey say there wasn't any blood.

As an indicator that the cherry-popping myth has simply morphed rather than gone away, a number of the women who answered our survey felt that the reason they didn't bleed during their first intercourse was because they had already torn their hymen while riding a horse or doing the splits, or while their boyfriend was feeling them up.

---

[1] If you are a diehard sci-fi fan, you might be better off whispering into your lover's ear that you're hot to jump through her Stargate than referring to her vagina as the wormhole. While you would be technically correct in Stargate terms, calling a puss a wormhole is asking for a world of hurt.

Researchers who were investigating athletic injuries in girls' crotches, including splits- and inline-skating related truma, found that it wasn't the hymen that was bleeding. In cases where the hymen most certainly should have torn if it were going to tear, it was the vagina itself that split and bled rather than the hymen. And why horseback riding would wear away a hymen is anyone's guess, unless there's a question of who was riding whom.

While a hymen will most likely be stretched during a first intercourse, it shouldn't ordinarily tear. If it does, or if there is pain, there are at least two possible causes:

Not Fully Estrogenized: In some women, the hymen doesn't become fully estrogenized or elasticized during puberty. One healthcare provider who does premarital exams told us that she sometimes prescribes a bit of estrogen cream for her abstinent patients who are getting married whose hymens haven't become very elasticized yet. So if you haven't had intercourse and are concerned, this would be a good question to ask a gynecologist—Does your hymen appear to have been adequately estrogenized for intercourse? (As for the effect of hormonal birth control on the hymen, we don't know. No research has been done.)

Clumsy or Not Aroused Enough: Another reason for why a first intercourse can be painful is when the male partner is inexperienced, rough, has poor aim, is really big, or there's not enough lubrication. As a result, the hymen might tear or bruise, in the same way your gum might when you chomp on it mercilessly. There is an entire chapter on your first intercourse later in the book. Hopefully it can help prevent a painful first time.

Another thing researchers have discovered is just how quickly the hymen heals itself. Medical examiners have been surprised at how normal the hymen can appear to be in girls who they know have been sexually molested. The latest research has found that tears in a hymen usually heal quickly, often within 24 to 48 hours.

So if your hymen does split or tear during intercourse, the bleeding gum example is a pretty accurate comparison. Your hymen should heal as fast.

Tag

A hymen can start bleeding for the first time years after a woman has been having intercourse. This might be due to a tear in a "hymenal tag," which is a remnant of the hymen. These tags are like any of the other folds of skin inside the vagina, except they might look like pointy bits where there would otherwise be smoothness. Hymen tags are fairly common, but most women never detect them because they don't feel any different from other parts of the vagina.

What Happens to the Hymen Over Time

One of our gynecology consultants said that the hymen wears away with intercourse. The larger the penis, the more it wears. She believes she can accurately guess the size of a woman's boyfriend or husband's penis based on how worn the hymen appears to be. Another gynecologist disagreed, saying that you can't predict anything about the number of sexual partners or their girth by the appearance of the hymen.

Needless to say, a bit of research might be nice, but one would need to examine the hymens of young women before they had ever had intercourse, and then a few years later. You would also need to know the dimensions of their partners' penises, approximately how many thrusts they would receive per average intercourse, and how often they had intercourse. (We're right on it—have the grant applications ready to file as soon as this edition of *The Guide* goes to press.)

All of the groin experts who we consulted with did agree that it's not unusual to see fronds of the hymen protruding from the vagina. These might have been tags from the hymen that became stretched. They also agreed that childbirth would be a hymen's worst nightmare, causing a fair amount of stress on the hymen as an infant passes by.

Warranty Repair: Revirginization

"Revirginization surgery," is when a surgeon takes the tattered edges of a hymen and purse-strings them together. None of our consultants were too excited about it. In fact, the explicatives that some of them used in describing the wisdom of "revirginization surgery" are not appropriate for a family book like this. However, if the alternative is being stoned in the village square...

Hymen Issues

If you have trouble removing tampons and intercourse is uncomfortable and your gynecologist says you have a septate hymen, a bit of local anesthetic and a small snip can often do wonders. A septate hymen is one that hangs vertically through the center of the vagina and looks a bit like the uvula at the back of your throat except it usually attached at both the top and the bottom. The ridge around the head of the penis can catch on this kind of hymen on the out stroke.

An "imperforate hymen" is more rare than a septate hymen. It is where the hymen completely covers the opening of the vagina. If you really do have an imperforate hymen, having it taken care of surgically is essential.

However, if you are having discomfort during sexplay, don't automatically assume the problem is your hymen. One thing to discuss with your gynecologist is whether the pain is at the opening or the back of your vagina. Before assuming your hymen is to blame, you might want to rule out things like vaginismus, vulvar vestibulitis syndrome, chronic constipation, certain infections, adhesions under the clitoral hood, or when the woman is not adequately aroused or there's not enough lubrication.

Vaginsimus is when the ring of muscles around the opening of the vagina automatically clamps shut. Vulvar vestibulitis is where the vestibule and the hymen are very tender when touched lightly with even a cotton swab, not to mention a big old incoming penis or somebody's fingers.

NOTE: No matter what your symptoms are, if a hymenectomy is suggested, getting a second opinion is not only wise but important.

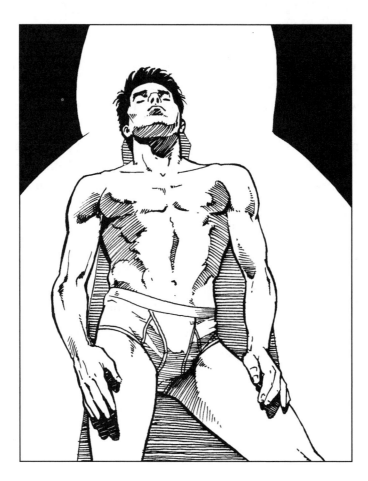

He's waiting for you at
www.GuideToGettingItOn.com

9

Orgasms

" Define orgasm? It's somewhere between a hand grenade and a sunset."

—Mr. Billy Rumpanos, lifetime surfer and
early friend of Goofy Foot Press

One of the many nice things about sharing sex is having orgasms, also known as coming. But orgasms are not without their mystery. Perhaps it might be helpful to consider a few comments about orgasm from Dr. Frieda Tingle, the world's leading expert on sex:

Q. Dr. Tingle, what do you think of sex in America?
A. I think it would be a good idea.

Q. Do you think Americans are too concerned about orgasms?
A. Whose? Their own or their neighbor's?

Q. In general.
A. Orgasm is very important for many Americans because it tells them when the sexual encounter is over. Most of these people enjoy competitive sports, where some official is forever blowing a whistle or waving a little flag to let them know the event has ended. Without orgasm, they would be fumbling around, never knowing when it was time to suggest a game of Scrabble or a corned-beef sandwich.

Q. What kind of things affect a person's ability to have an orgasm?
A. One important factor is diet. Many times I have been told that it is impossible to have an orgasm after eating an entire pizza. I assume this has something to do with the Italian religious taboo against sexual abandon. Another factor is the weather. Many patients have told me that if the window is open and they are being rained on, it is particularly difficult to have the orgasmic experience....

(Dr. Frieda Tingle is the alter ego of Carol Tavris and Leonore Tiefer.)

Orgasm Defined

The best way to define orgasm is to put your hand in your pants and give yourself one. But this assumes that you are able to give yourself orgasms and that you don't have six different kinds when you do. Perhaps you will find the following definition to be helpful:

💡 Orgasms are extra-special sensations that people sometimes experience while being sexual, either alone or with a partner. They occur after a certain threshold of excitement has been crossed and can last from seconds to minutes or longer. A sense of well-being or relief often follows. This might be due to a release of pain inhibitors following orgasm. For instance, studies have shown that people with arthritis sometimes get pain relief for three to four hours after having an orgasm.

💡 Orgasms often feel as if they are being broadcast from the genitals or pelvic floor, although there is no reason why they can't come from other parts of the body.

💡 Some people experience orgasm as a single, tidal-wavelike surge of sensation with a couple of brief aftershocks; others experience it as a series of waves, genital sneezes, or bursts of light, color, warmth, and energy. Some describe orgasm as creeping up on them and slowly flooding their senses. Some of us experience it as an explosion while others call it a whisper.

💡 Some orgasms make you feel great; others can be wimpy and disappointing. Some orgasms are strictly physical; others are physical and emotional. Some reach into the body; others reach into the soul. Some are intense and obvious; others are diffuse and subtle.

💡 The way an orgasm feels can vary with different types of sexual activity; for instance, oral sex orgasms might feel different from intercourse orgasms. Masturbation orgasms are often the most intense, but not necessarily the most satisfying.

💡 Orgasms with the same partner are likely to run the gamut from totally spectacular to downright disappointing. It depends on the particular day, and whether your worlds are colliding or are in sync.

💡 Some people have orgasms when a lover kisses them on the back of the neck; others need a stick or two of dynamite between the legs. The amount of stimulation needed to generate an orgasm has nothing to do with how much you enjoy sex.

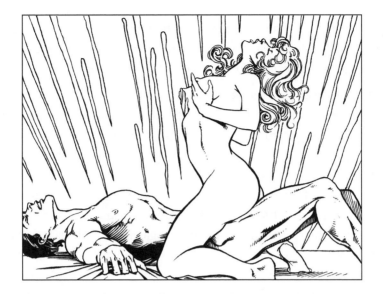

💡 When shared with someone you love, the feelings that follow orgasm can make it possible to experience a special kind of intimacy.

💡 Some people feel pleasantly amped or energized following orgasm, while others feel mellow and might want to sleep. For some people, one orgasm begs for another. For others, it calls for hugging and tenderness.

💡 Genitals can become extremely sensitive after having an orgasm. Stimulation that may have felt wonderful moments before orgasm often feels painful or abrasive immediately after. It never hurts to ask your partner about this, since it's true for some but not all.

💡 Some people are easily derailed on the road to orgasm. For others, the phone can ring, the earth can shake, and a dam can break—they come no matter what.

💡 A philosopher named Sartre noticed that as he was having an orgasm he entered his own private orbit which caused him to lose awareness of his partner. Some philosophers make up for this temporary separation by feeling extra-close right after orgasm.

💡 It is not necessary or even desirable for partners to come at the same time. For instance, it can be wonderful to feel or watch your partner have an orgasm, which is difficult to do if you are coming simultaneously. On the other hand, it might be nice to occasionally blast off together. Just be aware that not many couples are able to pull this off.

💡 Some people have orgasms with their legs squeezed together, while others come with their legs wide apart (innies vs. outies). People who prefer coming one way sometimes find it difficult to come the other way.

Does Orgasm Alter Your Consciousness?

When people are coming, they often experience a change in consciousness. Some of the latest brain research suggests why.

Doing high-tech scans on orgasming brains is very new and fraught with technical difficulties. They are highly suspect for technical reasons that are not the fault of the researchers. That said, PET scans of the brains of orgasming people show that several parts of the conscious brain are shut down or turned off when a person is having an orgasm. From the scans, it appears that people enter into a deep, emotionless state while coming—with women going into an even deeper state than men.

Past editions of this book described some women's orgasms as transporting them into another dimension that incorporates aspects of Disneyland and perhaps an orbit or two around the moons of Jupiter. The new brain-scan data suggest that this might result from a combination of what's being shut down in the orgasming person's mind, in addition to what's being lit up.

Your Partner's Orgasms

We often assume that a partner who has an orgasm is fully satisfied, while one who doesn't is somehow disappointed. This assumes that you want nothing more from sex than orgasms. For instance, most of us can give ourselves really intense orgasms when we masturbate, but not many of us can get feelings of closeness, friendship, and love when we do ourselves solo. For some people, these latter feelings are the most important part of lovemaking. So try to be sensitive, but not too paranoid, about your partner's orgasms.

Women, Orgasms and Intercourse

If wanting orgasms were the sole reason for doing a particular sex act, not that many women would bother with intercourse. Only about 30% of women have orgasms from intercourse alone. Plenty of women who have orgasms during intercourse need extra clitoral stimulation in addition to thrusting, or they need the guy to ride high so his pubic bone rubs against them in the right places. Lots of women prefer having an orgasm before intercourse. They say that the intercourse feels better after they've come.

Things that increase the chance of orgasm: being seriously into your partner, exercise and a healthy diet, reading romance novels and seeing erotic images, and anything else that turns you on or increases your level of excitement. (Going to college increases the chance of a woman orgasming from masturbation; guys have never needed a degree to figure that one out.)

Things that decrease the chance of orgasm: being annoyed or angry with your partner, smoking (chemicals in tobacco constrict blood flow to the genitals and may lower the level of testosterone in both men and women), stress (notice how you tend to have more sex while on vacation), not sleeping enough and taking certain drugs. Antihistamines will dry up more than just your nose, and there's a huge list of drugs that will dent your libido or seriously delay your orgasm, especially SSRI anti-depressants such as Prozac, Zoloft and Paxil. Hormonal methods of birth control can have sexual side effects in some women, as is reported in the chapter on birth control.

Being Catholic also makes it less likely that women will have orgasm during intercourse. Almost twice as many Protestant women as Catholic women report they orgasm during sex. Perhaps one problem for Catholic women is the Catholic church's strident prohibition against touching yourself, which is how a lot of women learn to have orgasms. Information on how Catholic males learn to have orgasms is still under litigation in many dioceses throughout the land.

Expressions, Decibels & The Way People Come in the Movies

Some people worry about how they behave when they are having orgasms. Some are self-conscious because they lose control, others because they don't. The answers? There are none. There is no correct way to come. Sexuality is an altered state of mind; what you do with it is strictly a matter of personal choice.

Some people fear that they will look weird if they allow themselves to be overwhelmed by an orgasm. They fear that their partner will laugh or find them ugly. Quite to the contrary. It is far more likely that a partner will think something like the following:

> "WOW! Her face got all twisted and contorted when she came. She looked like she was on an extreme acid trip. She must have had a major orgasm. Maybe I'm not so bad in bed after all...."

Of course, there are plenty of people who have sensational orgasms but hardly show it at all. Their orgasms are an internal phenomenon that remains hidden from the outside world. Unfortunately, many of us assume that women are supposed to make noise when they are coming, even though there is no correlation between decibels and delight. Some women sound like freight trains when they orgasm; others become completely quiet except for an occasional twitch and sigh. The same is true for men. If your partner comes in a quiet way and you would like to know more about it, why not ask?

Keep in mind that many of us learned to come quietly at a very young age. That's because there might not have been much privacy where we masturbated; letting out a large bellow would have informed the entire household. This was particularly true if you shared a room with siblings, and even worse if you had the top mattress in a bunk bed. The same difficulties are faced by people living in dorms, sororities, fraternities, and military barracks, where roommates often sleep only a few feet away. In these situations, we pretend to be asleep when masturbating—a funny notion when you consider that our roommates are probably pretending that they are sleeping as well.

The great sex-noise dilemma is also faced by parents while making love (or trying to) when there's a household full of kids. Depending on the ages of the children, their response to hearing mom and dad can range from "Mommy sounds upset" to "That's SO gross, turn up the stereo!"

Is It Possible to Have Too Many Orgasms?

Some of the Tantric types nearly hemorrhage at the notion of a man ejaculating more than twice every ten years. They think that the male body is depleted when it ejaculates. As a result, they hoard the white sticky stuff like generals do weapons-grade plutonium. Some even teach themselves to have dry orgasms.

Is there much reality to this seed-spilling fear? It has been written that the Nazis pondered this same question. To test it out they forced a prisoner of war to masturbate every three hours, day and night, for the duration of World War II. Thanks to the Allied invasion, the prisoner finally got to stop jerking off. He apparently went on to father several children and lived to a ripe old age, certainly as old as most seed-retaining monks if they didn't fib about being 128 when they are really only 55. As for other living examples, one friend of Goofy Foot Press is now in his early 70s, but his mind is incredibly sharp, and he doesn't look a day over 50. He currently has at least five ejaculations per week, down from the ten or so he had been having since he was a teenager. According to semen-retention theories, he should either be dead or a zombie. On the other hand, Doug Abrams, one of the healthier-looking guys on the planet, has co-authored a book on the Tantric position of coming without squirting. Doug practices what he preaches, and it is our hope that his prostate doesn't suddenly explode one day.

Regarding women and orgasm: nobody in his or her right mind has ever worried about a woman having too many orgasms, except for the people who live next door or in the apartment below.

Where Does Coming Come From?

The following quote is from a woman who had a spontaneous orgasm while riding public transit — a rather scary thought if you have ever taken the bus in places like Los Angeles or Detroit:

> "I've perfected this wonderful ability to orgasm without touching myself. It started one day on the commuter train when I was ovulating, and I felt myself throbbing. I started running a fantasy in my mind and discovered I could bring myself to orgasm. The only trouble with a public place is you have to control your breathing...." [A former high-school homecoming queen from the Midwest, as found in Julia Hutton's *Good Sex,* Cleis Press.]

Sex therapist Herbert Otto writes about the time in college when he and his friends were talking about different ways of masturbating. One fellow said that he could ejaculate without touching his penis. Naturally, bets were made. The room became quiet, and Mr. Spontaneous Combustion whipped his penis out of his pants. After his eyes were closed for a while, his penis became erect. Eventually, he began breathing faster, and suddenly he had an ejaculation.

Not only is it possible for some people to have an orgasm without genital stimulation, but it can even happen without sexual thoughts. For instance, some women have spontaneous orgasms during highly charged debates or intellectual discussions that have nothing to do with sex. One female reader had her first orgasm as a teenager while her hair was being brushed, and as a 40-year-old she still has orgasms when her hair is brushed.

While not many of us are able to have orgasms without genital stimulation, the existence of hands-free orgasms does suggest that there is more to orgasm than genital contact. For instance, there are plenty of people who have suffered nerve injuries and can no longer feel sensation in their genitals, yet they learn to have orgasm feelings in other parts of their bodies, such as their faces, arms, necks, lips, chests, and backs. This indicates that the power to experience an orgasm resides somewhere in the senses and not simply in the groin. (One woman whose clitoris and vagina were removed due to cancer was able to experience the same kind of intense multiple orgasms after the surgery as before.)

People who have lost one of their senses do not suddenly grow new ones to compensate. Rather, they are forced to better use the senses that remain. This suggests that many of us could achieve greater sexual pleasure from other parts of our bodies if we learned to allow it. One way of doing this is mentioned later in this Guide, where the woman stimulates her partner's penis with one hand while using her other hand or lips to caress another part of his body not normally associated with sexual feelings.

Orgasm-Chapter Letdown

One of the failings of this book is that it doesn't define "orgasm" more broadly. For instance, in talking about male orgasm, it is assumed that this happens when a penis is squeezed, stroked, fucked or sucked. But what if a man has an intense full-body orgasm when his partner kisses his neck for hours? In assuming that an orgasm needs to squirt out of our genitals, we keep ourselves from exploring other possibilities. But to include the full range of possibilities would add another hundred pages to this book, and if that doesn't make you cry out in horror, nothing will.

Pain Next to Pleasure

Receptors for pain and pleasure are located next to each other throughout our bodies. These receptors often fire at the same time. It is our brain's job to decide whether the overall experience feels good or bad. To make such a decision, our brain will sort through its data base of everything from whether we are ticklish to how we feel about people with brown hair and green eyes who are trying to get us off. As a result, our brains each make their own decisions about what is pleasurable and what is painful.

For instance, while one person might enjoy masturbating to the fantasy of seeing Johnny or Amber naked, the mere hint of Johnny or Amber's presence might make another person feel sick to his or her stomach. Or one person might find spanking to be painful and a turn-off, while another might find spanking to be painful and erotic. The stimulus is the same, but how we feel about it depends on how our brain interprets it.

The way we interpret pain is also impacted by our level of sexual arousal. For instance, people who enjoy an occasional slap on the rear during sex usually don't like the pain unless it's done when they are sexually aroused. Being aroused can cause the brain to throw routine caution to the wind, converting feelings that are otherwise painful into feelings of pleasure.

Possible Assist for Women's & Men's Orgasms

When women are about to come they often pull in or tighten their pelvic muscles. Yet doing just the opposite, pushing out, might make their orgasms more intense. Some women will hesitate to do this from fear that it might cause them to pass gas, but what the heck, you'll both live if she does. And if you consider the gas-passing habits of most couples, chances are she owes him a few.

Whether you are male or female, you might occasionally experiment with relaxing the muscle tone in your pelvis when you come. For instance, some men find that they can prolong the feelings of orgasm if they relax their crotch and anus as orgasm is about to come.

What Was It Like?

Lovers sometimes ask each other if they came, but not what coming feels like. Granted, sexual experiences are hard to put into words, since they often exist on the cusp between physical and emotional sensation. But asking a partner to describe what an orgasm feels like might lead to some interesting insights and discussions.

Guys Faking Orgasm?

Back when the first edition of the Guide was published, the section on faking orgasms assumed that it was women who did the faking. Not anymore. It seems that up to 30% of young adult males have faked orgasms at one time or another. These are men in the middle of their so-called sexual prime.

Researcher Karen Yescavage found that guys fake orgasm for reasons like: "I was tired," "I faked it so she wouldn't see me go limp," "So she would think she was doing a good job," or "I wanted to get it over with." The reasons women gave for faking tended to fall into the—"I-was-tired-bored-or-it-was-hurting"—category.

The good news is that even the people who admitted to faking orgasms didn't fake them very often. Also, a number of people who faked felt it helped increase the intimacy in sex. For them, the intimacy was more important than whether they really came or not. Other people feel that deceiving a partner is wrong no matter what the justification. They can't see how you can lie and feel more intimate at the same time.

Interestingly, lesbians faked orgasms as often as straight white women, while straight white women faked orgasms twice as often as Hispanic women. One possible conclusion is that lesbians and white males may expect their partners to have more orgasms than Hispanic males do, and so the white females and lesbians felt more compelled to fake orgasms.

If Your Partner Fakes Orgasms

One of the worst things you can do when a partner fakes an orgasm is to go on a mission to help him or her have real orgasms. This usually makes matters worse.

When it comes to orgasms, there is sometimes a fine line between helpful concern and obnoxious fretting, especially if the reason you need your partner to have an orgasm is for your own reassurance that you are a good lover.

Rather than trying to help your partner have an orgasm, why not try to discover the things that give him or her pleasure and comfort? Contrary to what you think, this might simply be holding each other for an extended time or not grabbing for your lover's crotch the minute you feel horny. If your partner has suggestions about technique, all the better, but this might not be where the issue lies.

Far more relationships crumble from a lack of emotional pleasure than from a lack of orgasms. As long as you are able to give each other emotional pleasure, there are plenty of ways to achieve orgasm. This book lists several hundred of them.

Orgasm Dementia

Sometimes it's fun to count orgasms and go for it like pigs to mud. But for some people, orgasm production and/or procurement has a suspicious edge. Here are a few reasons why:

Some people get a sense of smug superiority by claiming how many orgasms they either had or "gave" a partner. They confuse sex with pinball.

Some people use pleasure-giving as a way of controlling a partner. They might hardly come at all while making sure that a partner comes several times. While this might not sound like such a bad problem, keep in mind that partners who won't surrender the reins sexually are sometimes very controlling in other aspects of life as well.

There are people who expect their partners to supply them with constant orgasms. This can breed resentment over time, as the other partner starts to feel used.

Some people need to have sex or masturbate several times a day to help numb a chronic sense of anxiety or ease feelings of deadness. Having a constant stream of orgasms can be their way of keeping an emotional funk at arm's length. Do not confuse this with sexual pleasure, even if they do.

How Do I Give a Girl an Orgasm?"

One of the worst things that ever happened to sex was the idea that we needed to give a partner an orgasm. It would have been much better if we had simply set our sights on trying to please each other. Lord knows, that would have been challenging enough.

Wanting to give a partner an orgasm seems harmless enough on the surface. It's only when she doesn't cooperate that we start to get frustrated and our good intentions turn into something like "You'd better have this orgasm or it's going to make me feel like I didn't please you." Likewise, guys who boast, "I never come before my partner does!" don't realize the subtle pressure they are putting on their partner to hurry up and come!

Another problem with the concept of giving a girl an orgasm has to do with ownership. If you are the one who is giving the orgasm, then it's not really her orgasm until after you have given it to her. So whose orgasm is it anyway? Hers or yours?

And finally, what if you feel the need to give her an orgasm, but she would rather you stroked her hair or gave her a long, loving foot rub? What if she would rather that the two of you took a long shower together, and lathered each other up and hugged and kissed while your bodies are soapy and slick? But you can't do that. You've got to give her an orgasm!

Reinventing the Sexual Wheel — Marketing & Orgasm

In order to sell books and tapes on sex, publishers want us to feel sexually inept if we don't buy whatever sexual experience they are hawking. For instance, during the last couple of years we were supposed to buy books and DVDs on G-spot orgasms, female ejaculation, extended orgasms, one-hour orgasms, Tantric-sex orgasms, extraordinary orgasms for boring people, and now, orgasms through herbal enhancement. It's only a matter of time before publishers start to sell *Better Orgasms for Your Dog and Cat,* and try to make you feel like a pet sadist if you don't plunk down $29.95 for the DVD.

Many of us would enjoy having bigger and better orgasms if we could. But sometimes the consumer simply has to say, "Enough is enough."

Readers' Comments

For men: What does an orgasm feel like?

"My knees get weak and I tingle everywhere. It feels like I am numb all over." *male age 21*

"Like an energy emanating in the soles of my feet, up the back of my legs, in and through my rear end, to my belly button, and out through my balls and penis. Awesome, warm, exhausting." *male age 26*

"When I'm getting close, it feels like every ounce of fluid in my body has been forced into my penis. My whole body is in anticipation of the moment when my penis can no longer take the incredible pressure and bursts. Flames envelope the entire thing and the shock reverberates throughout my entire body." *male age 25*

"Orgasm makes me feel very connected to my lover, like I'm becoming a part of her." *male age 39*

"It feels like all your vital matter collects in your penis and then shoots out of you!" *male age 22*

For women: What does an orgasm feel like?

"Every orgasm I have is different! Sometimes I feel like I'm just melting, floating away. Sometimes I feel like I'm running or pushing into the orgasm. Sometimes an orgasm will sneak up on me; other times I will be able to control its arrival and duration." *female age 45*

"All my orgasms seem to be the same beast, but with varying levels of intensity from 'Gosh, was that it?' to an ache so sharp it's almost hard to bear. My most intense orgasms tend to come from using a vibrator but, oddly enough, they're not always the most satisfying."

female age 36

"Orgasms range for me from a simple response in my genitals, without much sensation and even some numbness, to a mind-blowing, explosive force of nature that permeates my whole body, mind, and emotions, encircles my partner and fills the room around us. Sometimes it's the physical sensations that are the most intense part of orgasm; other times it's the emotional quality and being with my partner that take top billing. Even when the physical sensation isn't very intense, I generally feel much more whole and integrated after an orgasm."

female age 47

Your first orgasm?

"With a vibrator at age 38. Finally!!!" *female age 49*

"It didn't happen until seven months after my first sexual experience. I had no idea what was happening. We were through having sex. When I began to put my clothes back on, I started to tingle and fluids started flowing out. It felt great, but I was actually kind of scared and embarrassed." *female age 21*

"I had an electric shaver that had an attachment which was a massager. After about an hour of moving it around on my clit (and praying that the pillow between my legs was muffling the sounds so my parents didn't hear) I had an orgasm. I'd already had sex many times with my boyfriend, but I felt like I was really sinning now!" *female age 25*

"I didn't really know what I was doing. I was about 10 or 11 and discovered this new feeling when I rubbed this silky part of my blanket over my penis, so I kept doing it. Eventually I got this intense feeling in my groin and then there was this goop everywhere. I was completely freaked and grossed out. I thought that I broke myself, but was too afraid to tell my parents." *male age 24*

"My first orgasm took place at age 18, when my fiancé introduced me, despite my initial revulsion and disbelief, to the delights of cunnilingus. I thought he was depraved. I was sure I was going straight to hell. I couldn't wait for it to happen again!" *female age 55*

"I had my first orgasm during one of my first menstrual periods. The feeling of a clean pad against my genitals made me feel a warmth I had never experienced before. I rubbed against it to see if I could prolong the sensation, although I had no idea what the sensation was. I just knew it felt good!" *female age 45*

"I didn't know what was going on. My body felt like it was convulsing. I tried not to let the guy know this was happening. I didn't know at the time I was supposed to let myself go and enjoy it." *female age 26*

"The first one I had was clitoral—it tickled (I was probably 10). The second type of orgasm I had was when I was 20. I felt it more in my vagina. It was overwhelmingly emotional and I came in a flood, and I do mean flood. I thought I had peed all over my partner. Now I have both kinds of orgasms. I get to pick, let's see, lobster or steak?"

female age 26

"My first orgasm was when I was making out in the back seat of a car. I was on top of my boyfriend and there was a lot of bumping and grinding going on, and I just climaxed, with my clothes on." *female age 49*

"I was surprised by how sensitive my clit was, but I wasn't sure the actual orgasm was an orgasm because it didn't seem nearly as explosive as what happened in the bodice-rippers I'd been reading. I couldn't believe I'd gone through all this work for that. Happily, many years of practice improved the results!" *female age 36*

"Age 20. One morning before arising I was idly rubbing my clit and fantasizing, and from out of nowhere excitement began building more intensely than it ever had before. I rubbed myself quite vigorously and for a very long time, until suddenly there was a mind-blowing explosion. I was certain that everyone in the house figured out what I was doing. I was very embarrassed. However, I repeated the experience every night—it took over an hour of heavy-duty stimulation at first."

female age 51

"My first orgasm was by a male friend (not a lover). I told him that sex was not that great. He used his fingers to teach me what it could feel like. I remember thinking 'Oh God, this is an orgasm!'" *female age 48*

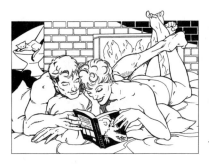

Dear Paul,

My girlfriend doesn't like me to play with her breasts, and the only way she can have an orgasm is when I give her oral sex. My former girlfriend didn't like me to give her oral sex, but sometimes had an orgasm from breast stimulation alone. Both women enjoy sex, but seem so different. How come?

Confused in Kalamazoo

Dear Confused,

For some people, you play with their breasts, and BOOM! their genitals are on fire. For others, you are better off reading them their constitutional rights than tweaking their titties.

As for why the different responses, I'd like to share with you an idea that is being proposed by Herbert Otto, author of *Liberated Orgasm.* He feels that the kind of orgasms we experience are in part determined by what our culture teaches us to expect.

For instance, in the 1950s, a lot of teenagers enjoyed extended kissing and petting sessions, but intercourse before marriage was seriously frowned upon. So a woman who was a teenager in the 1950s might have learned to have orgasms from necking and nipple-play sessions in the front seat of a car—without a single touch or lick below the belt. This same woman's unmarried granddaughter pays no social price for messing around with her pants off. She has read *Cosmo* since she was 12 and feels that nothing short of a partner's mouth welded to her clitoris is going to give her an orgasm. And so her body responds differently than her grandmother's. Of course, this doesn't explain why your former girlfriend doesn't like oral sex, unless she's your current girlfriend's grandmother.

There are dozens of other reasons why one partner might prefer attention above the waist while another prefers it below. In responding to your question, I've focused on some of the less-obvious factors that sometimes play a role.

Now, did you ever wonder if your girlfriend has written in asking why YOU like something one way while her former lover liked it another way?

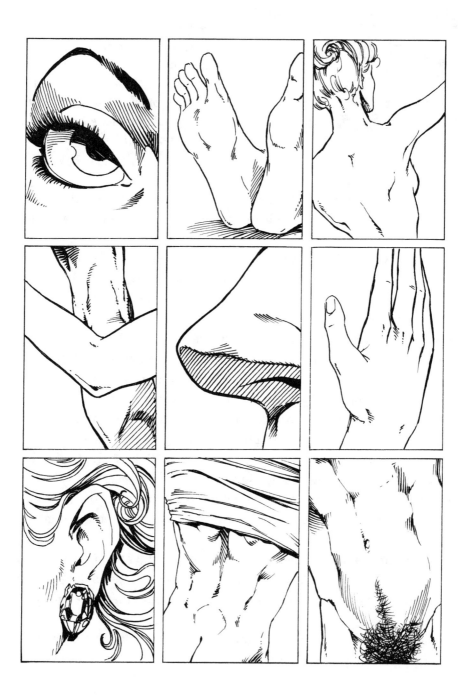

10

Talking to Your Partner about Sex

There's one way that dogs do it, and one way that sheep do it. This is also true for elephants, lemurs and wildebeests. Unicorns need to be extra-careful when it comes to oral sex, and the female praying mantis eats her male sex partners—to death.

The animal with the greatest potential for a varied sex life is the human. Human brains are beefier, which means that our minds have extra room for thoughts about sex. But when it comes to putting those thoughts and feelings into words, all bets are off.

This wouldn't be so bad if we weren't the only animals who do our sex indoors and in private. We could watch our neighbors do it, and have plenty of clues about what to do ourselves. Instead, getting it on can be a mystery.

The upcoming chapters attempt to shed light on the how-to part of that mystery. They describe tips and techniques for giving your partner monster amounts of pleasure. Hopefully you will find these techniques useful. But first, it might be a good idea to mention a few things about what makes sex good, and how to talk to your partner about those things.

Give and Take

Author Julia Hutton interviewed eighty people to find out how each person defined "good sex." Needless to say, she got eighty different answers. According to Ms. Hutton, "The interviews suggest that sexual savvy depends less upon how-tos than on self-knowledge, which evolves slowly, awkwardly and through many different routes."

People usually assume that if both partners are sexually amped, then all they need to do is get naked and good sex will follow. If only it were that easy. Consider the following quote from a 29-year-old kindergarten teacher (Chris is her husband):

"With Chris, I like having him in me, that warm good feeling. I've discovered I can ask for what I like, that there's nothing wrong with wanting your nipples pulled taut. I've learned that keeping a vibrator by the bed is not a crime. I've learned that Chris can come, and then I can come, and we can both enjoy watching each other come— as opposed to having this simultaneous orgasm that's supposed to move the world. If we have intercourse that's fine, if we don't that's fine. Sometimes we come home weary from work and it's: what do you want? Do you want to masturbate? Do you think you can focus enough for intercourse? It's negotiation, which I never thought it would be. I always thought it would be this mystic experience, but it's become a verbal experience." From Julia Hutton's *Good Sex,* Cleis Press

While some couples have good sex from the start, other couples take months and sometimes years to find a satisfying groove. Most couples report that their sexual desire for each other waxes and wanes, although sometimes it just wanes.

Shame between the Sheets

Because Ford never learned to say his original name, his father eventually died of shame, which is still a terminal disease in some parts of the Galaxy.
From Douglas Adams's *A Hitchhiker's Guide to the Galaxy*

Guilt and shame are fascinating emotions. We become sloppy and unmotivated without them, yet with too much guilt and shame we are at war with ourselves.

Plenty of us might do better in bed if we felt less guilt and shame about what turns us on sexually, assuming it does no harm to others. This is especially true for people who are too bashful to tell a partner what does and doesn't feel good. Hopefully, this book can help with that score.

Naked & Tongue-Tied

Consider the following conversation between two people who are about to have intercourse together for the first time:

"Uh, should I...?"

"I guess."

"OK."

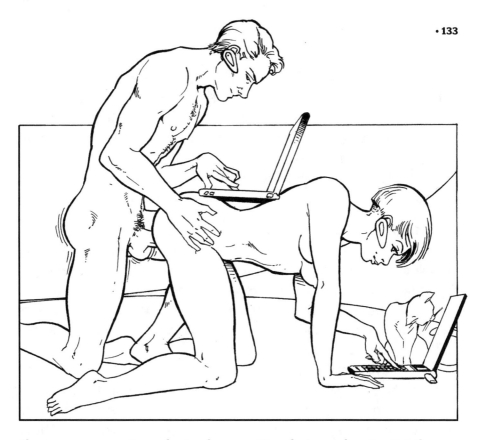

The way we connect our devices keeps getting faster and easier. But the way we connect emotionally is still smoke signals and knuckles dragging on the ground. Matters of the heart often require us to power down before we pucker up—to unplug before we unzip.

That's it. The intercourse begins. Fewer than ten words, most of them single syllables. Grunting cavemen were probably more expressive. And then there's the prolific verbal exchange at the end of the event:

"That was really good."

"Me too."

While most of us aren't too ashamed to have sex, plenty of us approach critical mass when it comes to talking about it. One problem has to do with the lack of a comfortable, shared vocabulary about sex. Many of us feel stuck between the rock of stiff Latin terminology and the hard place of sexual slang, e.g., "When I was giving you cunnilingus..." or "When I was eating out your pussy..." Neither feels particularly special or comfortable.

When talking to your partner about sex, it may help if you have a comfortable name or term for your genitals. For instance, a husband and wife who had a seriously contentious relationship were in sex therapy, and the wife was asked to give her vagina a special name. She called it "jewel box." How sweet. Considering how vicious they were with each other, she should have named it "Jaws." Whatever you want to name your special spots is fine. Hopefully you will both be comfortable calling them that.

After Marriage — Grow, or It May Die

Plenty of couples talk even less about sex after they've been married for a couple of years. Things like the interest rate on your credit cards or replacing the kitchen cabinets garner more excitement than finding new things that turn each of you on. Sexual desires start becoming hidden, and we sometimes feel embarrassed or shy about mentioning things that we would have stayed up all night trying a few years earlier.

After a while, sex has no room to grow. "I don't want him to know THAT about me" becomes more powerful than "It might be exciting if he knew that about me!" Perhaps we have too much to lose if a partner disapproves, or maybe we start giving our partners the kind of power that our parents once had to make us feel shame or humiliation.

Knowing vs. Asking

Imagine going to a restaurant where the chef served you whatever he or she felt like fixing instead of giving you a choice. Imagine a gardener who never asked, "How do you like your bushes trimmed?" Yet when it comes to sex, many of us assume that we know what our partner wants, or we clam up instead of giving feedback. Worse yet is the kind of attitude that is reflected in the following advice that *Teen Magazine* gave to its millions of girl readers:

> "When you're French kissing, it helps to let the guy take the lead. Part your lips gently, and let him explore your mouth with his tongue."

Teen's smooch advice gives the impression that guys come out of the womb knowing how to French kiss. Don't the editors of *Teen* realize that the average American male's preparation for sex is jerking off to whatever comes up after hitting the "free tour" button on X-rated websites?

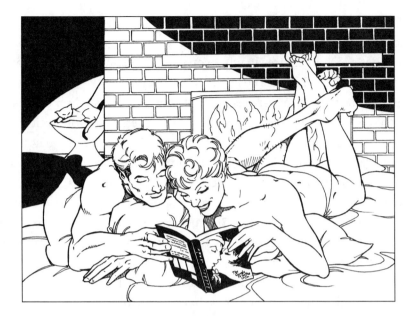

And why are guys always supposed to know what to do? Why aren't men and women encouraged to explore sex together, teaching each other what feels good along the way? One way to avoid being a *Teen* type of lover is by learning to talk to your partner about sex, about what feels good and what doesn't, and by exploring beyond what's familiar. Unfortunately, that's not always easy to do. That's why it sometimes helps to use props.

Learning to Speak

By discussing sex on a regular basis, if only once every couple of weeks, you may be helping your partner feel more receptive when you suggest that he or she try something new. Fortunately, there are "props" that can make sex discussions easier and more fun.

For instance, you might say to your partner, "Let's get a new book or magazine on sex every month." These don't need to be glossy jerk-off mags with the human crotch splayed wide, unless you are both into that. Why not try something that is a bit more upper-end? Consider explicit books from some of the better erotic photographers. Or you might pick up anthologies of erotic literature (smut with a college degree!); there are excellent collections out there. Browse through the erotica section of your local book store or visit an Internet bookstore and pump in author names like "Alison Tyler," "Susie Bright," "Marcy Sheiner," "Violet Blue," "Carol Queen" or "Rachel Kramer Bussel."

You can always highlight parts of this book that you find meaningful and would like your partner to know about. Or you can read parts of it to each other. Whatever your choice, do what you can to find humor. It helps any discussion that might otherwise be filled with anxiety.

Besides books and magazines, there are some really good sex videos and DVDs that range from informative to hot. When searching for erotic videos, you'll find some winners and plenty of yawners. Tristan Taormino has come up with a new series of videos for Vivid Entertainment where the porn stars script their own action and the female orgasms are actually real.

Some couples find it fun to play board games that promote discussion about sex or physical exploration. The nice thing about these games is that none of the players are losers. Games to consider range from *Enchanted Evening* and *Romantic Rendezvous* to *Cosmo's Steamy Sex Games*. (We list other board games on www.GuideToGettingItOn.com under "Dates.")

There are also Internet magazines that publish interesting articles on sex. These can be great discussion starters. For instance, consider the following from the excellent and erotic webzine www.Cleansheets.com:

> "Why is it that some men just can't deal with the idea that a smart, together, professional woman like me can actually deserve their respect and still want to be thrown down on the couch and pounded like a cheap steak now and then?" By Hanne Blank in *Clean Sheets Erotica Magazine* www.cleansheets.com.

Prevention

Of course, you might say, "Our sex life is fine right now. We don't need anything like that." Hopefully, your luck will hold, but therapists often see couples who had great sex lives two to ten years earlier. Things break down when we take them for granted, and the process of getting them right is not always pretty or fun.

Highly Recommended: For a wonderfully perceptive and well-written article on the elements that make for great sex, see *Building Blocks Toward Optimal Sexuality: Constructing a Conceptual Model* by Peggy Kleinplatz and A. Dana Menard, The Family Journal: Counseling and Therapy for Couples and Families, Vol 15 No 1, January 2007, 72-78.

11

Sex Lubes—A New Look

This has been one of the chapters in *The Guide* that kept swelling with each new edition. So it's probably significant that it's seriously changed its tune and was mostly rewritten for this edition.

Why People Use Lube

It seems that people use lube the most when they want to have intercourse but don't have as much time as they need for things to get all wet and sloppy, or when they have plenty of time but the vagina doesn't get as slick as they would like, as sometimes happens when a woman is taking the pill or other medications. Lube also provides a nice assist when using a condom makes for a dry time.

People use lube when they are giving each other hand-jobs, finger fucking, masturbating and for anal sex. Some couples like to incorporate lube into oral sex, and it helps with certain sex toys. Some women who are going through menopause find it to be really helpful. Other uses range from having sex in a hot tub to helping prevent UTIs or for sex during chemo for cancer.

Marketing Hype

Based on our sex-survey results, we've been surprised at how many young couples are using lube—highly amped couples who you'd think would be dripping wet and ready to go. Again, it could be due to the fact that people don't have the time for a woman to get seriously wet, however...

Companies that make sex lubes are dumping big dollars into some seriously slick marketing campaigns. These campaigns are suggesting that couples who coat their crotches with store-bought lubes will reach new levels of sexual bliss or will experience new dimensions of intimacy that the poor idiots who rely on nature's own lube are missing out on. Really? What about things like communication, fun, romance and respect? Does squirting chemicals up your crotch make up for a lack of that?

Don't Spit on Spit!

Given that people need lube, we contacted a professor of gynecology at a medical school and asked him, "What about the old standby of saliva? It seems to have gotten a bum rap these days. Is that because stores can't sell it by the ounce, or has science discovered something really bad about it?"

This professor checked in with one of the world's leading experts in vulvar pain, and both he and she shared the same opinion about saliva—*that it's an excellent sex lube!* She is also high on fresh olive oil.

Now, if you wonder why these experts might recommend saliva over the pricey stuff, let's look at the ingredients in a well-known lube that we have recommended in past editions of *The Guide*. This lube is described as water-based, hypo-allergenic and fragrance free. While that sounds good, here's a list of the chemicals that go inside of a user's love canal:

Highly purified water, Propylene Glycol, Isopropyl Palmitate, Dimethicone, Cellulose Polymer, Polysorbate 60, Sorbitan Stearate, Stearyl Alcohol, Glyceryl Stearate NSD. B.N.P.D, Di Sodium EDTA, Phenoxy Ethanol, Methyl Paraben, Butyl Paraben, Propyl Paraben, BHT

The good news is that only a couple of these ingredients are listed in the *Hazardous Chemicals Desk Reference.* And why they call it hypoallergenic is beyond us, when paraben and glycol are known allergens for some women. So we checked with a staff member of the FDA and asked what the criteria for hypoallergenic lube is. He couldn't find any criteria.

Worse yet, a company that distributes one of the most well-known personal lubricants recently petitioned the FDA claiming that vaginal moisturizers are actually cosmetics as opposed to drugs. It's a no-brainer why they are saying this. First, cosmetics don't require any more governmental scrutiny than hand creams or make-up remover. More importantly, if personal lubricants and vaginal moisturizers were classified as drugs, the manufacturers might have to do expensive clinical trials to show that these products are safe and effective.

Healthcare professionals often feel reassured about sex lubes because they assume that sex lubes have to be approved by the FDA. That's a nice fiction. As long as sex lubes are classified as cosmetics, they aren't evaluated for use in mucus membranes such as the vagina, rectum or urethra—where absorption of chemicals into your bloodstream can be quite high.

The fact is, no governmental agency is carefully watching over the things we buy in stores that go inside of our most private of parts.

According to FDA guidelines, Goofy Foot Press could easily set up its own sex-lube factory in a garage if it met the FDA's checklist, which isn't exactly rocket science. Because the FDA is so short-staffed they probably wouldn't visit but once every 3 to 4 years. So theoretically, we could go that long without washing our hands.

And there would be no problem if we had rodents or shedding cats in our little sex-lube factory. No agency checks to make sure that what's in the bottles of our Goofy Sex Lube is exactly what's on the label. A few years ago, researcher Bruce Voeller found something like mercury or arsenic in one of the brands of lube that he tested. Bruce suggested that if you buy lube, make sure it's made by a company that also manufactures pharmaceuticals because he felt the chances are greater that the factory is watched more closely by the FDA, although one such company has been selling a vaginal moisturizer whose main active ingredient was apparently turned down for use in cows. But maybe cow puss is more sensitive than people puss.

So, are we telling you that you shouldn't use store-bought lubes or vaginal moisturizers? No! But don't assume that the companies who make sex lube receive any more oversight than Wall Street did during the first decade of the century. Commercial lubes might be great for you, and a wonderful enhancement to your sex life, especially if your body is changing and you don't lubricate like the schoolgirl you once were.

What we are saying is why not try saliva first? If it doesn't work, by all means, go for something that's more slick. But if that's the case, why not consider what some of the medical-school urology departments are recommending—things like olive oil, almond oil and other vegetable oils for sex.

Oil in My Vagina?

You've probably heard, "I'm not supposed to put Vaseline inside my vagina." So why is it possible that olive, almond or other vegetable oils might be okay? The answer is that Vaseline is a petroleum-based product while olive oil, peanut oil, Crisco and the other vegetable oils are plant-based, and not thought to gunk up your junk. Unfortunately, we don't know of any science to back this up. The last thing the lube-making companies want to do is to fund a study that might show spit or vegetable oil being as good or better than what they're selling for $5 to $20 an ounce. And good luck finding a Congressperson who will spend tax dollars on research that's this useful when they can spend it on missiles-to-nowhere or abstinence only.

All things considered, the words "saliva" and "vegetable oil" sound lot better for a vagina than propylene glycol, hydroxymethylcellulose, sorbitol and polysorbate 60—harmless as they might be.

NOTE: Vegetable oils do go rancid, and you probably shouldn't use any with garlic cloves or hot peppers in them. Unless you are in charge of the party-room supplies for your local swingers club, it might be wise to buy your vegtable-oil sex lube in small containers and swap them out frequently. As for getting sex-lube olive oil that's virgin or pure—whatever put's a bigger smile on your face is probably the better choice.

What about Condoms & Sheets?

You should never use petroleum-based products like baby oil, mineral oil, hand lotions or Vaseline with latex condoms, as the latex in the condom dissolves in them. The same seems true for using vegetable oils with latex condoms, at least based on the experiment we tried here. As of presstime, the only condom that is safe for use with oil-based lubes is the Trojan Supra. The Durex Avanti has been discontinued, and the new non-latex Lifestyles Skyn is not supposed to be used with oil. So if saliva won't do the job with your latex condom, you'll need to use a store-bought lube.

As for oil stains on the sheets, it's not like you'll be using salad-dressing proportions. We're talking just a couple of drops of oil-based lube. And if it does stain, it will be easier to spray the spot with something like Shout while it's still on the mattress and then throw it in the wash. Or put an extra-large dedicated lovemaking towel under your rear before the banging begins. (Commercial lubes with silicone in them can stain sheets, too.)

Store-Bought or Commercial Lubes

Different lubes allow different amounts of sensation. The brand of lube to use will depend on the kind of sex you are having and the kind of feeling you and your partner enjoy.

Some lubes are thin, which allow you to feel more sensation, others are more cushioning. If you rub the lube between your fingers, see if you can still feel the ridges. If not, it's probably a more cushioning lube that might be better for weekend-warrior sex if your weekend warrior lasts for a long time.

There are also lubes that contain silicone. Some people love the feel, others don't. You might say, "I've heard that silicone is unsafe in breast implants. Why would I want to stick it in private places?" If you have ever been on the receiving end of a penis that's wearing a pre-lubricated condom, you've had silicone inside of you. Silicone molecules are supposedly too large to be absorbed into the body. The problem with leaky boob implants is that the silicone gets trapped inside the chest with no way to get out.

Most silicone lubes are water-based, which means you can use them with latex condoms. The silicone keeps the lube from drying out, but doesn't come off very easily. Another advantage of using silicone is if you are having sex in water. A possible problem with silicone lubes is their effect on silicone sex toys. It's not pretty. Also, if you are into electric sex—the serious kind with probes and electrodes—do not use silicone-based lubes. The silicone acts as an insulator. And silicone lubes can stain the heck out of your sheets, so make sure you don't use that particular set on the bed when your mom is visiting. **Note:** Silicone lubes become a sliping hazzard if they drip on the floor, especially if you use them in the shower.

The water in tubs washes away the body's natural lubrication, making intercourse difficult. Silicone-based lubes are slow to wash off and will help keep your piston pumping longer if you're doing it in hot tubs, bathtubs, lakes, rivers or oceans. Slop some on your genitals while they are still dry. You might also try a vegetable-oil lube for sex in water.

Glycerin in Lubes

Lubes that are glycerin-based tend to be slicker, which means if you rub them between your fingers you won't feel the ridges as much as with lubes like *Liquid Silk*. People who prefer lubes with glycerin say they feel "really fast." One problem that some women have with glycerin is that it's similar to glucose. In a woman's vagina, glucose is one of the things that yeast feeds on. Too much of it can encourage a robust yeast colony between the legs. So if you are prone to yeast infections, if you have diabetes, or if your are immunosuppressed, consider using a sex lube without glycerin.

Other Sex-Lube Woes

Believe it or not, women can get friction burns in the vagina when a lube is too gloppy or gets thick from drying out. So avoid gloppy lubes if you are experiencing discomfort. If you are having sex and your lube is getting gummy or is drying out, try adding a few drops of water or saliva to rehydrate it instead of more lube.

The propylene glycol that is in some lubes can be an irritant for some women. So can lubes with a high pH, such as Astroglide.

When a Woman Feels Too Wet

Some women on our sex survey say they naturally lubricate so much that they can't really feel the penis going in and out. If you are having this problem, have him pull out every now and then and dry the both of you off with a towel. Some people suggest trying an over-the-counter antihistamine to help dry up your natural lube if it's a problem. If you feel comfortable talking it over with your healthcare provider, by all means, do. If you are taking an antihistamine and are too dry as a result, be sure to try using some store-bought lube if you need to keep taking the antihistamine.

Lubes for Anal Play

Historically, the lube of choice for all things anal was a famous and well known brand of vegetable shortening. Then came the '80s, the plague, and the modern day sex-lube wars. Now just about everyone who is into anal sex has a "slippery top ten." Good luck finding a consensus on which is best.

Vegetable shortening remains the standard that today's anal-sex lubes are trying to copy, but without the downsides. [Vegetable shortening has no antibacterial properties, so dipping back into the can might contaminate it. While fine for your fries, vegetable shortening melts latex condoms, which are thought to be safer for anal intercourse than polyurethane condoms. It tends to leave rancid-smelling sheets with nasty stains, and there might be problems with a gnarly vegetable shortening/fecal ooze dripping from a woman's anus into her vagina if she is in an ass-over-tea kettle position.]

Fortunately, there are no warnings on the side of vegetable shortening cans that say, "Use only in your oven and not up your bum." There are no scientific studies on the safety of any lubes for anal sex, either. So while there are plenty of opinions, no one really knows. (Saying they use "FDA-approved ingredients" means absolutely nothing, as the FDA does not have a list of approved ingredients for anal intercourse.)

There are plenty of water-based lubes that will do the job without your butt dripping grease like the grill at McDonald's. Be careful with lubes that contain pain-killers, like *Anal-Eze, Anal Ease* or *Tushy Tamer*. These are like disabling the smoke alarms in your home because they bothered you when you burned the toast. Pain during anal sex is an important indicator that you are being too rough, aren't relaxed enough, turned on enough, etc. Plus, if something numbs your anus, it will numb your partner's penis, setting the stage for a marathon run in your rectum.

GNARLY WARNING Sorbitol and glycerin are used in a lot of sex lubes. They are also an active ingredient in laxatives and suppositories. Yikes!

Anal Fisting

The fisting world seems to be divided into your traditional vegetable-shortening fisters, your postmodern oil-based fisters who prefer *Elbow Grease, Boy Butter, ID Cream* and *Men's Cream*, and your reformed fisters who use thick water-based lubes like *Astroglide Gel, Probe Thick and Rich, Eros Silicone Gel* or *Eros Cream*.

Lubes for Hand-Jobs and Masturbation

Avoid hand creams for hand jobs and masturbation. Most hand creams and moisturizers are designed to be absorbed by the skin so people won't feel like greased pigs after they use them. The macro-molecules that make up moisturizers are designed to go flat fast. As a result, most hand moisturizers are poor performers for sex or massage, although you will occasionally find a good one.

Whether it is for giving your partner a super-dooper hand-job or just for jerking off, you'll want a lube that leaves a woody wet and slippery. One approach is to try an oil-based lubricant, such as canola, corn oil, coconut oil, vegetable oil, mineral oil, almond oil, baby oil, or massage oils. A popular and nearly legendary jerk-off lubricant is a facial cleanser called *Albolene*. Newer products that might feel similar are *Men's Cream* and *Boy Butter. Elbow Grease* has been a jerk-off standard since 1979. For those of you who like roasting your nuts but have no open fire, there's *Elbow Grease Hot* with menthol. Some wankers swear by *ID Cream*. **Note:** For those of you who use *J-Lube*, which is a powdered veterinary lube that you add water to, it only takes a tiny amount of *J-Lube* in the peritoneal cavity (gut) to quickly kill a horse or cow. We're talking maybe a few final moos before all four hooves are sticking straight up in the air. Do read the warning label before using.

If you've invested a major part of your stock portfolio in companies whose main product is men's masturbation lube, keep in mind that a whole generation of uncut males is entering puberty in the US. Uncut guys don't need lube for jerking off. Their factory-equipped foreskins work fine.

Women's Genitals (On the Outside)

Women have used saliva for masturbating since the beginning of time. *Vaseline* (petroleum jelly) or non-scented oils like mineral oil and olive oil work well for rubbing a clit during masturbation or vulva massage. Saliva, and the newer water-based lubes are excellent. Scented lubes should be avoided because they can cause irritation. Lubes that contain nonoxynol-9 cause irritation. Some women love old-fashioned *KY* in the tube for vulva massage. Add extra water if it starts to dry out.

Using *Vaseline*, baby oil or mineral oil may seem like a contradiction, because wisdom has it that petroleum-based lubes shouldn't go up your puss, but plenty of women seem to use them on the outside.

As for lubes to lick, some commercial lubes can taste awful. There are exceptions. Check with your favorite sex-toy store for their recommendation for lubes that taste good when mixed with vaginal juices. Some lubes come in a number of flavors including champagne cocktail, chocolate truffle, cinnamon toddy, egg nog, juicy fruit, lemon drops, orange and passionate pumpkin. Unfortunately for our readers in Tennessee, no Jack Daniel's.

12
Sex Legal

The legal realities have recently changed. Here are some strong words about relationship hygiene, or when it's okay to go for it and when it's not. Hopefully, you will make this your new mantra:

The Guide's Policy on
When to Call It Quits

An agreement to kiss is not an agreement to have intercourse. It never has been. Fucking requires a separate level of consent than making out. Likewise, feeling each other up and discovering that the woman's vagina is wet is not consent to put a penis in it.

If a potential partner doesn't want sex every bit as much as you do, go home and masturbate. If the relationship is worth it, phone the next day and talk things over.

If you need to convince someone to have sex with you, then it's the wrong person, time or place. If someone needs to convince you to have sex with them, then it's the wrong person, time or place.

Until the last twenty years, people thought of rape as something that was committed by a stranger who lurked in the shadows or pried a woman's bedroom window open. No one used to think of it as something your date did after you agreed to go upstairs to his bedroom and the two of you started making out. But as researchers interviewed more women, they started hearing accounts of when men would not stop, in spite of a woman's protests.

There are men who are adept at engaging women in kissing or petting, and then raping them in the same manner as "traditional" rapists who lurk in corners. Men like these can come from wealthy families who are on the social A-lists. They can be sports heroes. They can be divinity students at your local Bible college.

To help prevent date rape, the courts have had to push the limits of what consent is into a somewhat artificial and awkward place. Until we find a better solution, the new definition of consent will be the law of the land. The onus of stopping sexplay now rests on the male the moment a woman says, "Stop!" or "Maybe I should go" or "This doesn't feel good." She may have agreed to have intercourse, but if she changes her mind after 300 thrusts, the man had better pull out on thrust number 301 as opposed to number 306.

Males who do not take this seriously should read the recent decision for the State of California Supreme Court called *People v. John Z.* In that case, a woman had agreed to have intercourse, but at some point during the intercourse, she indicated that she might want to leave. She didn't say "Stop" or "I don't want to keep doing this." The court found that she was raped because the man did not stop the moment she indicated a change of heart. Interestingly, it was a female member of the court who dissented.

Making sure that a woman can legally consent to sex is now the job of the male, and it is very different from what you might think. For instance, even if a woman bought the first two rounds of drinks or brought the pot and rolled the joints, she is not legally able to consent to sex if she has been drinking or smoking. This can be true even if she is the one who went down on the man to help him get hard and put in the penis herself.

It doesn't matter if both of you were equally drunk or stoned: this does not excuse the male from the burden of realizing that a woman who has been drinking or smoking cannot legally consent to sex. Just the fact that she has been drinking before intercourse makes it sexual assault in some states. Also, it is not legal in many situations to have sex with a woman if you are her boss, her teacher, her minister, her physician or her coach.

Do not assume a woman is playing a game when she hesitates or says "No." And never, ever try to win her over with pressure or persuasiveness. The courts have made it clear that this will not be tolerated. In the absence of a woman making it completely clear that she wants sex, a man needs to assume that sex is neither desired nor is it legal. *Prison is no place where you want to be, and it's easy to find yourself there if you push sex on another person.*

If You Know You Have a Communicable Disease

If you know you have a communicable disease and do not inform a new partner, you can be sued. Not only is it morally right to inform someone you are about to have sex with that you have a contagious condition such as herpes, HPV or HIV, warning them will help you cover your legal bases as well.

Answers to Questions from Inquiring Minds

To Mark, formerly of the University of Georgia: When it comes to sex, we've all been misled (or led on) at one time or another. Some of us have even misled others. Even if it seemed like she wanted sex as much as you, the second she looked at her watch and said "Gotta go" you should have had your penis back in your pants faster than a tachyon through a crack in the cosmic egg. With good behavior, you should be out in ten to fifteen years. At that point, why not make sure that it's your date who makes the first move—she kisses you first, she takes off your shirt before you reach under hers, and she unbuttons or unzips your pants before you touch hers? And why not talk with her about the subject of sex when you both have your clothes on?

To LouAnne at Texas Women's University: You say that you and he had been slamming down Kamikazes in his bedroom and he was wearing blue jeans three sizes too small in all the right places and had on one of those little half-length T-shirts that was exposing each and every one of his washboard abs. LouAnne, it wouldn't matter if he were buck naked and had a red tassel on the end of his penis, when a person says "No more" you need to respect his wishes. None of us has a right to ignore another person's protests, no matter how hot, horny, hard, wet, willing, stoned, drunk, or sexually amped we might be. Even if a person has their tongue halfway down your throat for the better part of an hour, if they suddenly pull it out and wag it in a way that says "This is all you're gonna get," then you'd better stop. The same is true even if the two of you have been married for ten or twenty years.

To Randy at Fairleigh Dickinson University: The two of you had been flirting for weeks. She invited you to a party. Both of you had been drinking when she saw you from across the room. She threw her arms around you and said, "Let's go upstairs, find someplace private, and have the sex we've always dreamed about." The following Monday, you find yourself arrested for rape. How can this be? "Informed consent" implies that your partner was sober enough to make a rational decision. It doesn't matter if the two of you had been flirting for weeks and if she had been the one who initiated the sex. If she was not sober when she put the moves on you, it is you who can be charged with a crime in some states. And even if you win, which you very well might, it will cost you thousands of dollars to defend yourself and the personal toll will be immense.

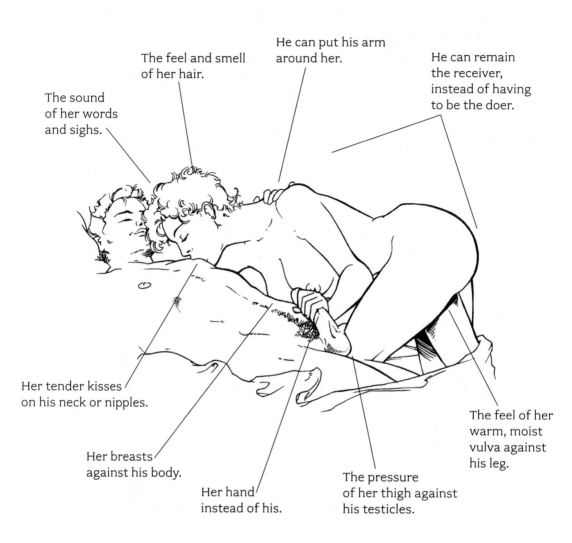

The sound
of her words
and sighs.

The feel and smell
of her hair.

He can put his arm
around her.

He can remain
the receiver,
instead of having
to be the doer.

Her tender kisses
on his neck or nipples.

Her breasts
against his body.

Her hand
instead of his.

The pressure
of her thigh against
his testicles.

The feel of her
warm, moist
vulva against
his leg.

**Things a woman brings to a handjob
that are missing when a man does himself.**

13

Handjobs
Different Strokes
For Different Blokes

Women often ask, "Why should I give him a handjob? I can't possibly compete with the hand that knows him SOOO well. Besides, there's nothing special about it. He can give himself a handjob any time he wants."

Talk about flawed thinking. This chapter describes ways of giving your man handjobs that will have his dizzy testicles saying to each other, "Holy Spermatogenis! She drained us dry and it felt SOOO good!" Hopefully, by the end of this chapter you will be thinking, "Any girl can give him a blow job, but I'm the only one who can give him a handjob that makes him want me more than he's ever wanted any woman."

Even if all you are doing is giving him a quick one to get him off and out the door, you and your hand have the tools to do things that he can only dream about when he's doing himself solo.

After all, let's think about this logically. Next time you are with him, grab his hand and smell it. How does it smell compared to you? Put it up next to your ear. Can you hear it whisper dirty nothings? Can it tell you how much it wants you, how good it feels to be stroking you, how cool it looks when his sperm shoots out? Nope. Chances are, his hand is as mute as it is hairy.

Now put that hand of his on your neck. Does it have hot wet lips that can kiss a neck from top to bottom? Does it have a hot wet tongue that can swirl around his nipples like yours can while you are jerking him off?

Feel the inside of his hand. Does it have soft, silky breasts and taut nipples? Does it have a head full of sweet-smelling hair that it can whip across his face and chest? Does it have a hot wet pussy that it can push up against his thigh? He gets none of this when he's choking his own chicken.

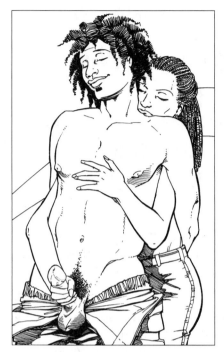

And what does he think about when he is jerking himself off? It's you! So when it is your hand that's doing the deed, you are there in person to flood his senses with what he can only fantasize about when he is jerking off alone.

That's just giving him a garden-variety handjob. Wait until you read about the luxurious handjobs that can turn his entire body into a giant sex receptor, with each stroke feeling like a little slice of heaven. But first, there's more to understand.

What You Bring To It

Before we get into technique, perhaps it might help to tell you about two very different reasons why guys jerk themselves off. There can be lots of other reasons—these are just two.

One reason is for alone-time fun. It's the jerking-off equivalent of jogging on a country road or walking though a park as the sun is coming up. He's alone, but it's nice in the way that reading the newspaper or going through the RSS feeds might be, or building a model airplane, or tricking out his car. Some women get all pissy when they discover that their boyfriend still jerks off; they don't understand the purpose of this kind of jerking off, and they view it as rejection. It is important for you to know about this form of jerking off, because if he lets you do it for him, then it's like he is inviting you to join him in his shop or private garden.

Then there's another reason why he jerks off. It has to do with misery. It's like heroin for the part of him that needs the sexual touch of a woman. It's comfort food for the crotch. It's when it feels like his inner horndog is going to eat him alive if he doesn't throw it a bone. This kind of jerking off is a cross between a Hank Williams ballad and calling an ambulance.

For a lot of us, this kind of jerking off helped us keep our sanity until someone like you came along. It was self-administered sexual life support.

So, depending on the mood and the situation, your handjob might be casual and fun—like the way he does himself when he's happy and it's a form of sport—or it might be to supply comfort and intimacy. You being the one who is doing it is like revisiting the scene of something that wasn't so great, and you are making it all better.

So even though it may look like your hand is doing the same thing as his, your mere presence gives a handjob a different dimension than when he does it himself. That's why it's important that you put more of yourself into it than just the muscles in your arm; why it matters that you make it a truly fun and intimate act. Cuddling close to him or giving him a tender kiss on the neck or nipple while you are doing him with your hand makes it special. Being genuinely into it on your part can be more emotionally comforting than you might know.

A handjob can be an opportunity for intimacy and closeness that a lot of women underestimate. And that's just an old-fashioned stroke-it-till-it-squirts handjob. Wait until you see what else you can do. But first, the basics.

Getting a Grip—Learning Boy Basics

"I could never move my fist that fast for so long. He really manhandles that sucker, and it doesn't seem to hurt!" *female age 55*

We usually don't think of the Hand of Mercy and the Vulcan Death Grip as being one in the same. But the two sometimes merge when you are giving a handjob. In fact, the usual complaint from guys about the way girls give handjobs is that women use too light of a touch. Remember, one of the major slang terms for masturbation is "beat your meat." It's not "tickle your meat" or "caress your meat." It's BEAT your meat. The technique that men use most when they masturbate can be summarized as: Grab it hard and give it a good workout. Mind you, there are plenty of exceptions, so as with all matters of sexual pleasure, be sure to ask.

To find the optimal hand position, lie parallel to your man and reach across his body as he does when he is masturbating. Ask him to form your fingers around his penis in the same way he does when he's alone and thinking about you. The way he holds the penis and where he puts his hand on the shaft are more significant factors than you might think. Try to imitate the exact place where he grips himself. There are reasons for this. One of the most sensitive areas of the penis is called the frenulum. It's just below the head on

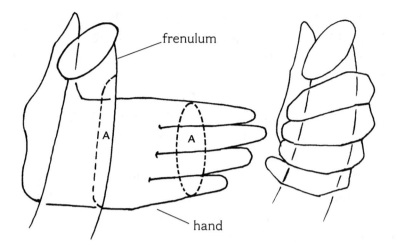

This is a rough approximation of where your hand should go when giving a hand job. Actual placement will depend on the size of your hand, the size of the object being grabbed, the amount of foreskin (tight circumcision, loose circumcision or no circumcision) and the preferences of the owner.

the side that's away from the man's belly when he has an erection. It shows good form to rub a finger—not fingertip—over this spot with each stroke, especially if you plan on getting this over with before next Christmas.

Wrap your entire hand around the penis so your thumb and index finger would touch if there weren't a big sausage in the way. Your hand should be in the same position as if it were holding a cup of tea. That's how we guys learn to masturbate, by drinking tea.

If your fingers were a belt, try to buckle them on the side of the penis rather than in front. Otherwise, your fingertips would go over the frenulum, which can be uncomfortable. It would not be hand-job cricket to have fingertips pressing into the frenulum.

Another reason to position your hand exactly where he does is because the foreskin is only so elastic—especially if he is circumcised. If your grip is too high or low on the shaft, the foreskin will be pulled beyond its stretching point. Much confusion can be avoided if you ask him to place your fingers where he likes them. Then have him guide your hand up and down so you can see how high and low to stroke.

Dry or Lubed?

While each man has his own unique spin, men masturbate wet or dry:

Dry The man wraps one or two fingers around the penis at a strategically placed point, slightly below the head. He then moves the entire foreskin up and down with each stroke. Because the foreskin glides easily over the shaft that it covers, most guys clasp it more tightly than might seem comfortable. Much of the sensation occurs as the fingers move over the highly sensitive part of the shaft called the frenulum.

Lubricated Using lubrication results in a handjob that feels more like intercourse. When giving himself a lubricated handjob, the man often wraps his whole hand around the penis. The lubrication allows the hand to glide over the shaft and the head of the penis. A man who is circumcised is more likely to use lube. If you've still got your foreskin, there's no need to use lube when masturbating, although some guys who aren't cut also like to use lube.

Dry vs. Lubricated Lube helps a man who is circumcised to get more sensation from the head of his penis; when he does it dry, he tends to focus finger pressure on the front of the penis below the head. The lubricated handjob can be a more sensuous experience. However, plenty of guys prefer doing it dry, and there are many times when masturbating dry is more practical. It is less of a production, and it is easier to clean up with a tissue or sock.

What Does a Penis Feel Like?

When a penis is soft it feels a little like human lips. The skin has a silky smooth, almost translucent texture that slides over the tissue beneath it. A soft penis is extremely flexible. It can be warm or cold to the touch and feels more like a squid than a hotdog.

To know what a hard penis feels like, find a fairly buff guy who lifts weights and ask him to flex his arms. A hard bicep feels similar to a hard penis, although a hard penis won't be nearly as big around except in guys' dreams. Poking a finger into a man's unflexed pecs will give you an approximate idea of what a semi-erect penis feels like. Here are some women's recollections about the first time they touched a penis:

> "It was sort of like 'Oh my God, what do you do with it?' I knew if you did something to it in the right way, that was good. I felt very, very careful, not sure what I was dealing with at all. It was like an alien

creature that you were supposed to automatically know how to please. As I listen to myself describing it, I must have considered it as separate from the individual who it belonged to!" *female age 34*

"It was not a pleasant experience then, but it sure is now."
female age 42

"I had intercourse a number of times but never touched it. I didn't get into that until much later." *female age 26*

"I didn't like the way it felt when flaccid. A couple of years later I finally got around to making friends with it, and it became exciting."
female age 21

"It took me a while to figure out that you could really handle it, that it wasn't fragile." *female age 27*

Your Touch vs. His

Men sometimes view their body and their penis as two unrelated entities, with the body merely being the chauffeur. They stroke the penis without caressing the other body parts that can help jerking off to feel more like a full-body experience. This is one of the ways that your giving him a handjob can be so special—not only will you be able to grip him like he does and manhandle his meat, but you will hopefully be adding your own special magic, perhaps by straddling some part of him and pushing your crotch into it, or by caressing him with your other hand, or by kissing him with your sweet soft lips, or by whispering into his ear...

Few women realize that they have the potential to control nearly every cell in a man's body with each stroke of their hand. Instead, they just jerk away until things get sticky.

Technical Points

Some women give handjobs that are jerky. After all, it is called "jerking off." And it might appear that when guys masturbate we use a single upstroke followed by a single downstroke, all in rapid succession. But that's not how we do it. We usually have a more fluid motion. The hand doesn't stop or even slow down as it changes direction from up to down. The motion is smooth rather than jerky—which means the term "jerking off" is a misnomer.

Another potential problem occurs when a woman slows down or stops pumping as the man begins to ejaculate. While some guys may want you to stop right away, most will greatly appreciate it if you keep stroking for a few minutes after they ejaculate ("stroking through"). Some might want you to proceed as though the penis were an udder, with you milking out each drop. As part of this process, some guys might push with their fingers into the hidden part of their penis that's between their balls, or into the perineum area between the balls and the bum.

As the handjob motion becomes familiar, you might want to caress your lover's testicles with one hand as you are jerking him off with the other. Your man might also enjoy being kissed while you are giving him a handjob, perhaps on the lips, neck, or nipples. Touchy-feely types claim that orgasmic rapture is enhanced if you stare into each other's eyes as he is coming.

Getting the handjob motion just right can also come in handy when you are trying to signal across a room to a friend what a bunch of bull someone is saying, or what a boring wanker some guy is.

Variation Consider doing your man when he is standing or kneeling as opposed to lying on his back. This could be nice for both of you.

Ball Trick When masturbating, some guys push the little finger of the stroking hand against the lower part of the shaft near the scrotum. This causes the testicles to jiggle or vibrate with each stroke, which can feel really nice. But it's always best to seek your man's input when first trying to do this, since your pinky might inadvertently poke him in the nuts.

Ultimately, it is unlikely you will get your sweetheart's hand motion exactly right unless you have him show you. That's because each guy varies in terms of grip, stroke, and rhythm—not to mention anatomy. Don't be surprised if it takes a number of tutorials before you get it right, especially if your hand is considerably smaller than his. If your own man is too uptight to teach you, it's likely that any number of his friends will be more than willing to let you learn the basics on them, or maybe one of your girlfriends can demonstrate on her boyfriend. Or she might use a banana. It can be both fun and helpful talking to your friends about their own special techniques for getting guys off, although you shouldn't assume they know better than you when it comes to the guy you are with.

In his wonderful books *Tricks: 125 Sex Tips to Make Good Sex Better, Vols. 1 & 2* (Greenery Press) author Jay Wiseman lists several tips to make a traditional handjob more fun. For instance, he suggests caressing the penis and balls for ten seconds with your fingertips, followed by one quick up-and-down hand stroke. Then caress for ten more seconds, followed by two quick up-and-down hand strokes. After every ten-second period of caressing, increase the stroke total by one.

Panty Play If he likes lingerie, take your panties off and drape them over his penis and testicles while you are giving him a handjob.

Thigh Sensation While facing him, have him straddle your thigh so it is touching or pushing up against his testicles as you are stroking his penis.

When a Man Helps a Partner Learn How to Please Him

A man can help both himself and his partner if he will turn the lights up, get naked, and let her learn about his genitals. The purpose is for her to tickle, squeeze, tug, and prod each part of the man's sexual anatomy so she can learn his comfort zones and become more confident in handling him "down there." She should gently, increase the pressure on each part until the man says something earthshaking such as "Ouch!" At that point, the woman eases up until he says, "Ah, that's good!" Here are a few specifics:

Penis Have her tug it, yank it, and squeeze it until she's able to distinguish your *Ouch!* zone from your *Good!* zone. Then help her learn how to grasp your penis to give you a handjob. Indicate how far up and down you like the strokes to go, as well as how fast to do them and how long you wish she would keep stroking after you come.

Testicles If the room is cold, and your cojones are in frostbite mode, turn up the heat and put something warm over them until you have coaxed them back down. Once they are hanging freely, have her tickle, caress, and play with them, letting her know what feels good and what doesn't. Then have her slowly squeeze each testicle, letting her know how far to go. Also, have her put a finger or two in the space between your testicles and push in until she is massaging the buried part of your penis.

Extreme Hand-job Techniques For an Extremely Good Time

Now it's time to consider special techniques for doing a boy with lube, even if he is uncut. The next couple of pages describe some of the strokes involved. Also, see the **Resources** section at the end of this chapter for a website that has excellent streaming videos of all of the strokes described here.

Lubricating your hands and his genitals is essential for this. Any number of oils will work nicely, as long as you're thinking peanut oil instead of Penzoil or coconut oil instead of Castrol. It's a penis you are massaging, not a piston.

Extreme Technique: Lube Him Up

The first thing to do is to get your man completely naked. This is usually not a difficult task.

The most civilized way of greasing a man's groin is to cup one hand over his genitals and drip massage oil over your hand. Gravity will pull the oil through your fingers and onto his genitals unless you are in outer space. Make sure that your man's testicles and penis are thoroughly basted with oil. To catch the excess oil, put a thick towel under him with a sheet of plastic under that. Plastic garbage bags work really well. If cleanup is going to pose problems, use less oil.

Different Massage Strokes

When doing him dry, it's best to be by your bronco's side so you can imitate his strokes. But when giving an extreme handjob, you will be using lube, so you can do a fine job from wherever you sit unless it's across the room.

These strokes make it possible for you to give a man extreme full-body sexual pleasure that he is not capable of giving himself—by massaging his genitals in specific ways. It is not necessary for him to have an erection for this to feel great. Many guys remain semi-erect when receiving penis massage. Some people think it feels best when the penis isn't erect. However, some guys will feel unmanly if their penis goes flat. Please reassure your man ahead of time that you don't expect him to stay hard.

Fists Going Up Be sure all skin surfaces are well lubed. Wrap one hand around the base of the penis, squeeze lightly and pull it up along the shaft, over the head and into the air. As this hand is making its upward stroke, grab the base of the penis with your free hand, squeeze and do the same thing. Create a fluid motion with one hand constantly following the other. Slow the pace if the man shows signs of impending orgasm. Some folks suggest giving a little extra squeeze or snap on the upward stroke just as your hand reaches the head of the penis.

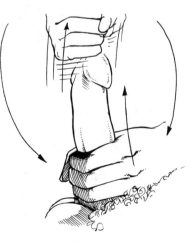

Fists Going Down Same technique as above, only in the reverse direction with your hands going from the tip of the penis to the base. Downward strokes such as these usually require an erection. Otherwise, the thing just flops there in your hand. Also, use a more open grip so you don't shove the penis into the body.

Thumbs Up While facing your man's crotch, clasp your fingers together as you might do when in deep prayer. The only difference here is that your hands are clasped around your man's penis. Use the pads of your thumbs to massage the front part of the penis where nature left the seam showing. Spend extra time rubbing the area where the head attaches to the shaft, or just below it (frenulum). Some people compare the sensitivity of this area to that of the clitoris, although they are probably overstating the case.

Open Palm Rubbing Head of Penis Some guys might like this; others won't. Hold the shaft of the penis in one hand so it is sticking straight out from the man's body. Open your other hand flat and rub it in a circular pattern over the head of the penis and down toward the frenulum, as though you were buffing it. Make sure that the palm of your hand is well-lubed.

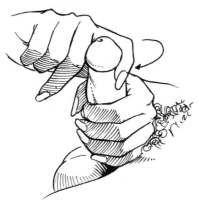

Twisting the Cap Off a Bottle of Beer Hold the shaft of a well-lubricated penis near the base. With your other hand, grasp the head of the penis as though it were the cap on a bottle of beer. Twist it as if you were opening a beer bottle, with your thumb and forefinger running along the groove under the ridge where the head attaches to the shaft.

Wringing a Towel Dry Grasp the lower part of a well-lubed penis with one hand and the upper part of the shaft with the other. There should be no gap between your hands unless nature endowed your man with an elephant trunk instead of a penis. Twist your hands back and forth in opposite directions.

How to Pull the Foreskin Taut

The penis can usually be made more sensitive by stretching the foreskin. In fact, guys who masturbate with lubrication often use one hand to pull the foreskin taut while stroking the shaft with the other. This also helps keep the baggy skin on the scrotum from rising up onto the shaft of the penis. There are a couple of ways to achieve this:

Clamp your thumb and forefinger around the shaft of the penis nearly an inch above where it joins the testicles (scrotum). Pull the skin down so your other fingers and palm rest on the testicles. This will make the foreskin taut. If the man is uncircumcised, reach higher up on the shaft to pull the extra skin down.

Or, when he's doing himself and trying to keep his foreskin taut, it is possible that your partner hooks his thumb around the shaft of his penis and uses the other four fingers to cup, squeeze or caress his testicles. There are many variations on this. Sometimes just the ring and pinky fingers lie over the top of the testicles; other times it's the index and bird fingers.

Strokes to Try When the Skin on the Penis Is Pulled Taut

Ouch Alert! Remember, only pull the foreskin taut when giving him genital massage if you are using lubrication.

Penis-Belly Rub The penis should be lubricated and resting flat against the man's belly. Pull the skin taut at the base of the penis. Open your other hand and lay it flat on top of the penis; then drag it toward the man's chest, as if you were trying to push or pull the good feelings out of his penis and onto the skin of his belly. Repeat.

The Corkscrew or Following the Stripe on the Barber's Pole Pull the skin taut at the base of your partner's well-lubricated penis. Wrap your other hand around the base, squeeze lightly and twist it upward as though you were following a corkscrew or the stripe on a barber's pole. If his penis is hard enough, do a reverse downstroke. This should return your hand to the same position where it started, or just do a series of upward strokes. Whether you are giving oral sex or a lubricated handjob, don't hesitate to use a twisting motion up and down the shaft of the penis, especially just beneath the head.

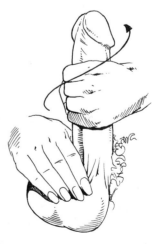

Thumbs Up — Thumbs Down There are two ways to grasp a penis that is lubricated. One is with your hand facing up, so the little finger is toward the base of the penis and the thumb is toward the head. The other is with your hand facing down, so the thumb is around the base and your little finger is around the head end of the penis. It can be quite impressive when a woman alternates hand orientation with her stroking hand, so he never knows if the next stroke will be thumbs up or thumbs down.

Octopussy Fingers Pull the foreskin taut with one hand. Lay the palm of your other hand over the head of the penis and drop your fingers down along the sides of the shaft. (Your hand will look like an open parachute or an octopus when it swims.) Your fingers will stimulate the sides of the penis as you move your hand up and down. You can also twist your hand sideways, or do a corkscrew stroke that combines both motions.

Massaging Under the Testicles

If his scrotum is tight, and his testicles are hiked-up closer to his shoulders than to his knees, heat the room and put a warm washcloth over his crotch.

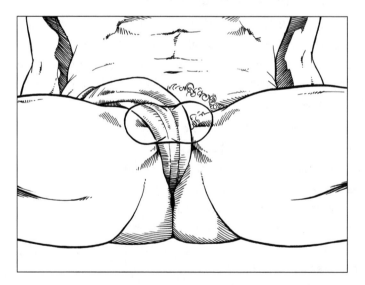

The Man with Invisible Balls

Women often assume that the penis is somehow glued or stapled to the front of a man's pelvic bone. In reality, it runs beneath his testicles and anchors inside his pelvis. Some men enjoy having the "invisible" part of the penis massaged. Push into the space between the testicles with your fingertips and gently rub. Also massage the flat space behind his testicles (aka "taint").

Let it warm up for a couple of minutes until the testicles hang freely. Press into the middle of the scrotum with your fingertips. You will be touching the part of the penis that is covered by the testicles. Massage this area all the way back to where the man's anus begins. There is often a single spot on this part of the penis where a number of ligaments, muscle fibers, and nerve endings seem to converge. Putting fingertip pressure on this spot while massaging the "regular" part of the penis with your other hand can make the entire shaft—from the base of the pelvis to the head of the penis—experience a subtle, warm feeling that some men will find enjoyable. This might be on one side of the shaft rather than in the middle. You might also try massaging this area when giving a blowjob.

A man's testicles will nearly cripple him with pain if they get hit, knocked or flicked, but not when a partner caresses and massages them. Being massaged in this area can feel like getting a really nice back rub, only it's between the legs. Be gentle at the start, and keep in mind that while some men find the sensation to be delightful, others don't like to be touched there.

Massage that Includes the Testicles

Here are a few techniques to try on the testicles, as well as some strokes that include the testicles and penis. None of these strokes should cause any pain or discomfort. If they do, stop. There is more information about your boy's balls in the chapter that follows.

Simple Testicle Massage Explore with your fingertips the space between and around the testicles. Be gentle at first, and seek plenty of feedback. Once you find a form of massage that pleases the man, do it often. For some men, the sensation feels like it's part back rub and part orgasm. They might even prefer this to stroking their penis.

Ball Rub With the thumb and forefinger of one hand, make a ring around the part of your man's scrotum where it attaches to his groin. Squeeze gently until his testicles are popping out a bit, but not enough to cause pain. Run the fingertips of your other hand up and down the sides of his scrotum with a light tickling touch.

Flat-Handed Doggy Dig Straddle your partner's chest while facing his feet. Lay his penis flat against his belly with the head pointing up toward his navel. Place one of your well-lubricated hands between his legs with your fingertips resting below his testicles. Pull the hand all the way up to his belly, dragging your fingers over his testicles and penis. Repeat with your other hand, rhythmically alternating strokes as a dog might when digging in the dirt. This same stroke is illustrated in the chapter: "The Zen of Finger Fucking," but as done on a woman.

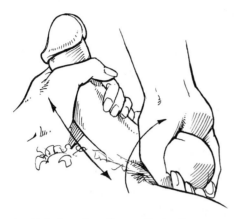

Penis Up, Balls Down Be sure that your hands are well-lubricated. Grasp the lower part of the penis with one hand. Clamp the fingers of your other hand around the base of the scrotum where it attaches to the groin. This should cause the testicles to pop out a bit, and the skin covering them should become taut. Squeeze both hands lightly, and then do an upward stroke with the penis hand while the testicle hand pulls gently in the opposite direction. Find a tempo that works for both of you, and keep repeating these strokes.

The Point of No Return

When doing an extreme handjob, you might want to keep your man highly aroused for long periods of time without letting him ejaculate. No, we haven't lost our minds, it is possible.

Think about a scale of 0 to 10 where 0 means no sexual arousal and 10 is an orgasm. Let's say your partner starts to ejaculate when he reaches a 9 on this imaginary scale. Past that, there's no turning back. Try to keep him between 7 and 8 for as long as possible before finally letting him squirt, an event that might be rather powerful when it finally occurs.

One way to keep your boy at such a high level of excitement is to learn his body language for when he is about to ejaculate. There are physical signs for when the wad is about to blow: the veins in his penis may start to bulge, or his penis might give a sudden throb, the color of the head might darken, his testicles may suck up into his groin, his muscles may suddenly tighten, his hips may thrust, and he might start to groan like a dying bull or invoke the names of the saints. Change the stroke, squeeze hard, or decrease the intensity when this starts to happen.

Some women find it very helpful if the man is able to report his levels of excitement by saying something like "6," "7," "8," or "9." Even the cues "more"

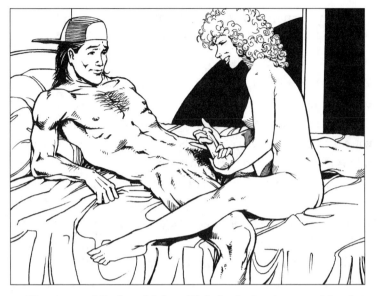

This position is great for hand jobs with lube, but not so good for doing it dry. Worse yet, her form is poor (fingertips on the frenulum), and his penis appears to be detachable. But he doesn't care, what with the washboard abs and cool cap.

or "less" are often enough. This will help you learn when to up the pace and when to back off. After a while you will become so familiar with his body language that you won't need him to tell you.

Ready, Set, Relax

It never hurts to begin genital massage by finding those parts of your partner's body where tension gathers. Who knows why, but the shoulders and back often become the body's collecting points for tension. There is no point in doing good work on a man's genitals when the weight of the world is parked between his shoulder blades. This is also true for women's bodies.

Some men believe that the only important part of sex is when a penis is being rubbed, sucked or fucked. They might not care about the tension in their shoulders. They will sometimes direct your hands straight to their crotch with the idea that an orgasm will help relax them. While this is true, think of how much more pleasure they could receive if they were relaxed to begin with.

If your partner is getting too penis-oriented for his own good, go ahead and fondle his testicles with one hand. At the same time, repeat your request that he close his eyes and relax. Inform him straightaway that you will do to his body what you like, when you like, and how you like. If he still objects, slap him upside the head and remind him what you are holding in your other hand!

Spreading the Excitement — Pavlov Between the Legs

Extreme handjobs can be used to help a man link the sensations in his crotch with other parts of his body. For instance, Hindu/Yoga types might have you stimulate the man's genitals with one hand while caressing various chakras (e.g. upper abdomen, heart, third eye, hair piece) with your other hand. It may help if he inhales deeply while you are doing this, as though he is sucking the warm glow from his genitals into the upper part of his body.

Western-psychology types might suggest kissing or caressing your partner's neck, shoulders, nipples, or chest while massaging his genitals. At various intervals, stop stroking the man's genitals but continue to kiss or caress the other designated body parts. If he were a dog and his name was Pavlov, he might eventually learn to have genital sensations when you caress these other body parts without reaching between his legs. Likewise, he might learn to have pleasant sensations in other parts of his body when his penis is stimulated. The goal is to help a man experience sensation over his entire body.

————————————

Dear Paul,

What if a guy is uncircumcised? Do you give him the same kind of handjob as a guy who is cut?

Helen from Troy

Dear Helen,

An uncut penis has lots of sensitive foreskin that slides up and down with each stroke. The foreskin also keeps the head of the penis moist. The skin on a cut penis is tighter and the head is dry. The skin doesn't glide up and down as smoothly. Doing a traditional handjob is easier on an uncircumcised penis, and it doesn't require lube.

With erotic massage, you will be using oil whether your boy's boner is circumcised or intact. On the strokes where you pull the foreskin taut, you will have more yardage to pull down, or ask him to hold the foreskin taut around the base of the penis while you use your hands on the shaft and head or shaft and scrotum. Also, if you pull the foreskin over the head of his penis, you can insert a well-lubed fingertip into the space between the head and the foreskin and swirl it around. For more tips, see Chapter 26: "Fun with Your Foreskin."

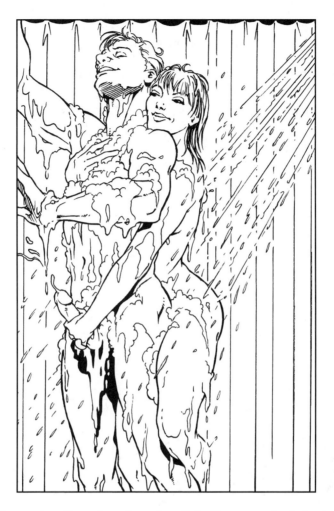

The shower is a fine place for a handjob. If you need a lube, try hair conditioner instead of soap, which can hurt if it gets into the urethra.

RESOURCES Highly Recommended: All of the strokes in this chapter are demonstrated on the website www.erospirit.org, or call (800) 432-3767. The website is dedicated to different ways of stimulating and massaging the genitals and rear end. It is not porn, but there is lots of full nudity. You'll need to get a month subscription for $10-$15, but it will be WELL worth it. Go to the "More Erotic Massage" section for streaming videos of a woman doing a guy as part of the *Expanded Orgasm for Him* series. There's also streaming content of guys giving guys erotic massage. Half of this site is men with men, but what does it matter? A gay penis looks just like a straight one, and if you turn us men upside down, we all pretty much look the same, give or take an inch

If you are in the mood for handjob instruction that has a much more upbeat tempo—something a couple can watch together but not with the rest of the family, consider *Penny Flame's Expert Guide to Hand Jobs for Men and Women.* This how-to DVD is porn-adjacent and partner friendly. It's part of the Vivid Ed series that Tristan Taormino created and directed, meant to help you learn at the same time that it helps you get hot.

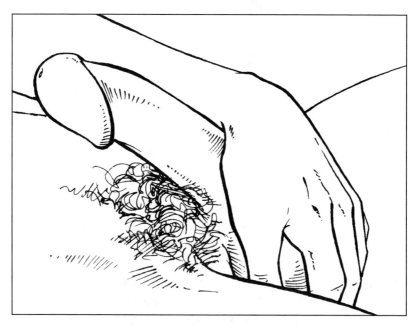

RU redE 4 balz, balz, balz?

14
Balls, Balls, Balls

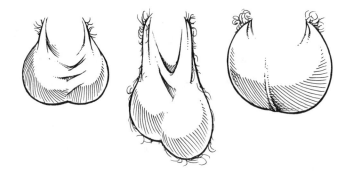

Balls usually take a back seat to the penis. One reason for this is the pleasure you get from your testicles is more subtle than the pleasure you get from your penis. But just because the pleasure is subtle doesn't mean it should be ignored. As one reader comments, "When my wife caresses my testicles, it's one part excitement, two parts relaxation, and six parts bliss. I didn't appreciate this when I was 20, but now I enjoy it as much oral sex. The sensation is different, but just as satisfying."

Ball Rules

Testicles are far more rugged than you might think. You can squeeze or pull them with no problem, and they can bang against a lover's thighs with impunity. But pop them with a simple flick of a finger and you might have to peel their owner off the ceiling. Heaven only knows why. They should feel a bit like hard-boiled eggs without the shell, but they won't be that big unless your lover is related to a racehorse.

As a man becomes aroused, his testicles tend to swell or become bigger. When he is highly aroused or just about to come, his scrotum and testicles will pull up to hug the shaft of the penis, some more than others. Another thing to know about testicles is that they can easily go from feeling soft to hard. It depends on the temperature and on the man's level of excitement.

Testicle Embryology

In the womb, males and females start off with similar-looking genitals. These appear to be female. However, the genitals of male and female fetuses may have different concentrations of hormonal receptors, so the idea that all fetuses start off with the same "female" genitals may be out the window. Still, our genitals sprout from similar fetal tissues.

For instance, the skin that makes up the male's scrotum starts from the same tissue as the lips of a woman's vulva. Have you ever noticed the seam along the center of the scrotum? If the guy with the scrotum had been born a female, that same tissue would have been used to make up the labia. So if a fetus is going to be a boy, nature glues the labia together to form the scrotum.

What's Inside a Ball?

Technically, the testicles are glands that produce testosterone and sperm. One ball is usually bigger than the other, and one hangs lower. Each testicle is a little factory. Sperm are produced in the tubules, stored and aged in the epididymis, and sent up into the abdomen through the vas deferens. Contrary to what you might think, sperm don't go straight from the testicles into the penis. Instead, they travel north, up into the pelvis to a place behind the bladder. That's where they make the connection with a tube that draws them in through the prostate gland. From there, they eventually shoot out through the penis. In the next chapter you can read what happens when you have an ejaculation and where the sperm go—before they leave your penis, anyway. The testicles are housed in a pouch called the scrotum. The reason the testicles hang away from the body is they need to run cooler than body temperature.

An Undescended Testicle

The medical term for undescended testicles is "cryptorchidism," which is Greek for "hidden gonad." One way to get a case of hidden gonads is to go surfing during the winter; another way is to be born with them.

Contrary to what seems logical, the testicles in the male fetus don't form between the legs. Instead, they develop inside the abdomen and do not descend into his scrotum until a month or two before he is born. They make the journey from the abdomen into the scrotum through the inguinal canal.

Almost 3.5% of males are born with an undescended testicle. This testicle often descends on its own without medical intervention, so that by one

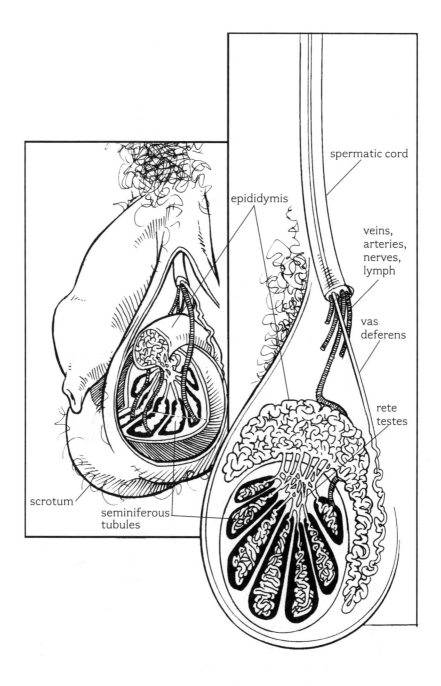

epididymis

spermatic cord

veins,
arteries,
nerves,
lymph

vas
deferens

rete
testes

scrotum

seminiferous
tubules

Ball Plumbing

year of age, only 1% of males (1 out of 100 or 150) still have an undescended testicle. In 90% of these cases, it's just one of the testicles that is undescended.

If the testicle remains undescended after the boy reaches one year of age, the current practice is to treat it surgically. This is often done as an outpatient operation. Attempts to coax the testicle down with hormone therapy have unacceptable side effects. Any gains are usually short-lived. The problem with a testicle remaining undescended past the first year of age is that it tends to become infertile.

If you are the parents of a child with an undescended testicle, be sure to get a second or even a third opinion from a pediatric urologist. As Dr. Joseph Dwoskin, a urologist from Texas Tech, says, "There are as many opinions about testes as there are physicians who examine them." It is also important to make sure that everything is well documented in the boy's medical records. This will be invaluable should there be any problems in ten or twenty years.

Late-Breaking News

Physicians are beginning to find that some guys who are sterile as adults got that way because they were playing sports without a cup and took a significant knock in the nuts. Any man or boy who is involved in a contact sport should wear a cup. Ditto if he is playing catcher

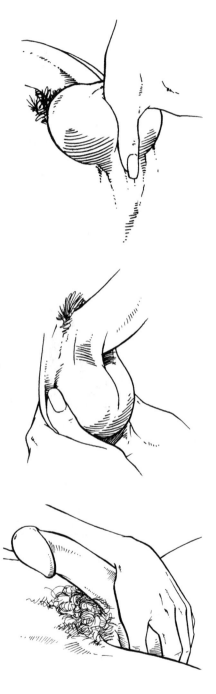

There are many ways to caress testicles. Here are three of them.

in baseball. Fortunately, they have soft cups these days which are a lot better than nothing for the weekend warrior, and they'll make you look like you are really well hung. See "Shock Doc" (page 970) for the latest in cup technology.

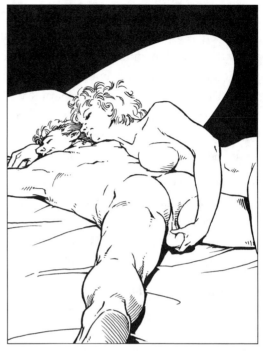

Ball Tending

If you are attempting give your sweetheart's testicles a good time, start by placing your fingertips on the sides of his scrotum and caressing lightly. Let his verbal feedback guide you. You might also try resting the palm of your hand over his penis with your fingertips pointing down. Experiment with lightly massaging the back part of the scrotum, where it attaches to his body. As your fingers move, the part of your wrist that's resting on his penis will move as well. This should give his penis pleasure, which might mix nicely with the more subtle sensations that your fingertips are providing his testicles.

Intercourse Extra

You can handle a man's testicles during intercourse from some positions, such as the reverse cowgirl where you are on top facing his feet. Different rear-entry positions may also allow you to reach between your legs and caress his testicles. Experiment and see what both of you and both of them like best.

The Exquisite Brush-Off

Have your cowboy spread his legs and gently brush his inner thighs, testicles, penis, and abdomen with a soft makeup brush or an artist's brush. Doing repeated circles around the scrotum can feel especially nice. The sensation is subtle, somewhere between a feather and a fingertip. It can feel relaxing and exciting at the same time. If you enjoy taking control, you can always tie him up first. Don't limit your strokes to just his genitals. If you're lucky, he'll grab the brush and return the favor.

Perineum

There is a patch of anatomical real estate between the testicles and rectum which is often ignored but has the potential for sensation. It is called the perineum. (Women have one, too.) Tantric and Hindu types get all excited about this particular area and regard it with the same kind of awe that we Westerners sometimes do the reset button on the computer. Place your fingertips on this area with just enough pressure so the skin moves over the tissue beneath it. Experiment and see what feels best.

Another Kind of Tenderness

Don't hesitate to reach between your man's legs and cup or cradle his genitals at nonsexual times, like when watching TV or while falling asleep. Some men will find this to be extremely thoughtful and caring. Others will find it too arousing, uncomfortable or intrusive.

Cancer of the Testicles

The term "cancer of the testicles" is a misnomer. It should be cancer of the testicle (singular), given how it's usually only one testicle that gets the cancer. The good news is we need only one testicle to be fertile and to have a perfectly normal sex drive. The reason for having the other ball is for playing pocket pool, and for back-up in case something happens to the other one.

Anyone with testicles can get testicular cancer, but it is more likely to affect younger men, particularly men between the ages of 15 and 35. It is curable 97% of the time if detected early enough. Considering that the testicles are hanging out and easily examined, you would think that it is almost always detected early. Unfortunately, the last thing a guy between the ages of 15 and 35 thinks about is the possibility of getting cancer. After all, cancer is something that happens to people your parents' age, so it is beyond the average male's consciousness to check his nuts every month for lumps or changes in texture.

Another problem is that a lot of men would rather sit naked on a fencepost than call the doctor's office and say, "I'm concerned about my testicle, and I'd like you to check it out." So they wait until the cancer has spread all over the place before getting care. This isn't good, since some forms of testicular cancer can double in size in fewer than thirty days, and you won't feel a bit of pain as it is happening. (If it hurt, he'd probably go to the doctor immediately, but cancer of the testicle usually doesn't hurt.)

A third roadblock in detecting cancer of the testicles is the extra meaning that we attach to testicles, as in the term "He's got balls!" Ever hear anyone say, "She's got ovaries!"? On a symbolic level, it's a big thing when a guy loses a ball, and we're not talking over the fence. Most of us would rather deny the possibility.

In spite of the way guys feel about their own testicles, women are not necessarily enamored by them. In fact, you don't want to know how some women describe the scrotum on our sex survey. Unless you've been caught cheating on them, most women would far more want to have you be healthy with one testicle than dead with two. In fact, we've heard that some guys who have lost a testicle due to cancer play the Lance-Armstrong card quite effectively. Far from being put off by the idea of scrotum with only one ball in it, women are sometimes quite curious.

It is often a partner who discovers the cancer. This can be a lifesaver. Hopefully, women readers will learn how to examine their man's balls in the name of health as well as pleasure, and hopefully they will insist that a partner see a healthcare provider if they find something that's worrisome.

The most common symptom to look for is a small lump or nodule on the side or sometimes the front of the testicle. It's usually not painful when you press on it. Another symptom is hardening of the testicle. Mind you, testicles swell and shrink, but it's time to get it checked when the entire testicle starts to lose its spongy texture. Less common symptoms include pain or discomfort in the testicles, back pain, swollen breasts (guy breasts), or a kind of heaviness or unusual discomfort deep in your pelvis.

There are a number of things that can look like cancer of the testicles. One of these is a spermatocele. This is a sperm-filled cyst in the epididymis that feels like a smaller third ball. These are pretty common and aren't usually a problem unless they get really big. Most of the things you will find in a scrotum besides balls aren't cancer and can often be treated with antibiotics. So don't assume that your doctor is going to present you with bad news.

It is very wise to do a routine ball exam once a month. The best time is when the scrotum is warm and saggy, like after a hot shower. Follow the instructions in the **Ball Check** chart on the next two pages. As for cancer of the testicles, the absolute mother of all websites is Doug Bank's incredible Testicular Cancer Resource Center: http://tcrc.acor.org

Also, please see Chapter 38: "Cancer of the Breast, Brain & Balls."

BALL CHECK!

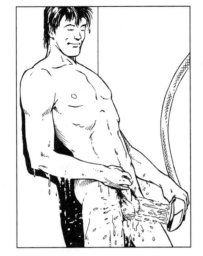

①

You need to do a ball check every 30 days or 3,000 strokes, whichever comes first.

The best time to check your testicles is after a warm shower.

One of the things you are looking for are changes, so it's important to know what your testicles usually feel like.

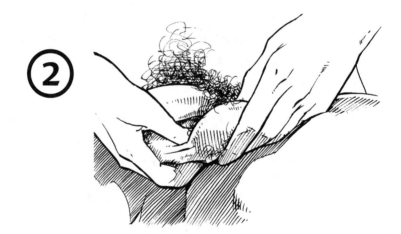

②

Use both hands. Grab a testicle. Roll it between your fingers. You are looking for any bumps or lumps. They can be smaller than a pea. Check the sides really well, and the top and bottom.

BALL NOTES If you ever get popped in the balls, and the pain lasts for more than ten minutes, have them checked by a physician. If not treated quickly, testicle trauma can cause your huevos to become sterile. Also, one ball is usually bigger than the other. Nature made them that way.

(3)

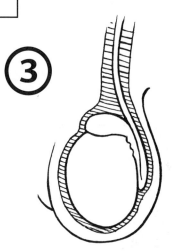

What You Are Feeling

When you feel your scrotum you may notice more in there than just two balls. There are a couple of spaghetti-like cords that attach to each testicle at the back, toward the top. They are called the epididymis. They form a structure that is shaped like a comma. These might be fuller if you haven't ejaculated in a while. It may feel a little weird, but check out your comma for any little nodes, lumps or changes since the last check.

(4)

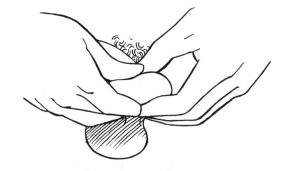

Squeeze that puppy. It should feel a bit spongy, although this varies depending on the weather and how horny you are. Be aware if a testicle becomes extra firm or tender or starts to lose its spongy texture. Also note if the testicle is larger or smaller or heavier than it used to be.

(5) Grab your other testicle, and have at it.

(6) If either testicle has any nodes, bumps or lumps, take it to a physician for a checkup. Chances are, it is only a cyst or infection, but that needs attention, too.

(7) **CONGRATULATIONS!** You are done. Now go grab your favorite lube and reading material, and liberate a few million sperm.

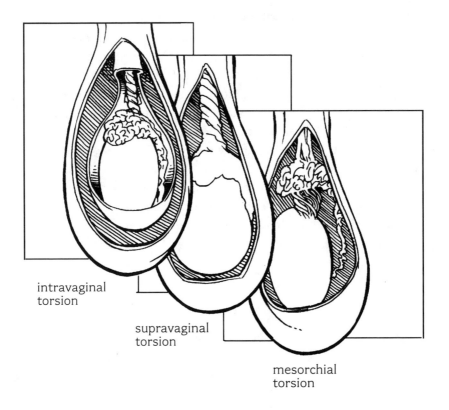

intravaginal
torsion

supravaginal
torsion

mesorchial
torsion

Testicular Torsion

Testicular torsion occurs when the testicle twists in the scrotum, causing the blood vessels in the spermatic cord to twist shut. It is very serious,
and if emergency surgery is not performed within four to six hours, it is
quite possible that the testicle will be lost. This is why any sudden or acute
pain in the testicles that lasts for more than ten minutes should result in an
immediate trip to the emergency room. The same is true for an excruciating
pain that appears for a few minutes and then suddenly stops. Don't take a
wait and see attitude, as it might be too late if you gambled wrong.

Torsion happens more often in teenagers, but adult males can get it as
well. The potential for torsion is created when the testicle is not properly
anchored in the scrotum. The three most common types of testicular torsion
are illustrated above.

Twisted testicles are modeled after the illustrations in the excellent book
Imaging of the Scrotum, by Hricak, Hamm & Kim, Raven Press, (1995).

15

The Zen of Finger Fucking

> **"** Rubbing lightly is what I do when I masturbate,
> so I like it even more when my boyfriend does it.
> I love it when he runs his fingers along my inner lips, up and
> down. I also love my genitals to be rubbed and tickled when
> I wear jeans or corduroy. I can come from that kind of stimu-
> lation." *female age 23*

Some men take the term "finger fucking" quite literally. They think that a woman's idea of a good time is having a man cram his fingers up her vagina. Or they attack a woman's clitoris as if it were a broken doorbell button, believing that the harder they push it the closer she gets to the big "O." The only "O" she is likely to experience is "OUCH!" rather than orgasm.

The truth is, finger fucking is not something a man does to a woman, but something he does with a woman. It's all of him–his smile, kiss, laughter, strength, and tenderness focused in the ends of his fingers.

Hopefully you will find this chapter to be helpful, especially if you are able to leave your bulldozer behind and are willing to try things with your fingers that maybe you've never felt before. However, none of it will make a lick of difference if she isn't turned-on, or if she won't give you feedback. In that case, there isn't much that you can do with your fingers that will put a smile between her legs.

And please, forgive us for choosing a clever title like "finger fucking" rather than one that makes sense, such as "Serenading Your Sweetheart's Clit." The last thing you'll want is for your fingers to be doing a bony imitation of a penis fucking a girl's vagina. If your fingers were supposed to do the job of a penis, something white and gooey would squirt out of the tips when you rubbed your knuckles.

Backseat Groping

There are several kinds of finger fucking. One encompasses the hot-and-heavy groping that's an extension of making out. It's when a guy gets his hand between a girl's legs because he can and because there's all kinds of passion and kissing and drooling going on. It's all about the moment. You don't need a chapter on that.

What follows is about learning how to please a woman with your fingertips. It's nothing you do in the dark or while you are stoned or drunk. The first dozen times, it requires lights, looking, and lots of feedback. And if all of the stars are lined up just right, and if she's finally forgotten how your eyes nearly popped out of your head when you met her seriously hot friend six weeks ago, you might just end up giving her incredible amounts of pleasure.

Altered Process, Altered Goals

The first thing to do is to banish the usual guy-goal of giving a girl an orgasm. She'll have one if she has one: maybe you'll be the medium, maybe not.

With the kind of finger fucking that's in this chapter, you'll try to help her walk along the edge of something intense and sweet for longer than she may have with a guy before. It's something she might do when she's masturbating, but not necessarily with a man. While the orgasm at the end of the rainbow is always a worthy goal, sometimes goals can get in the way.

This chapter asks you to stop trying to orchestrate an "Oh-my-God-I'm-Coming!" type of orgasm. The experience you are going for is different from the kind of fast blast that you get when you are jerking off, which is great for a guy, but sometimes doesn't reach the full spectrum for a girl.

The good news is, once you learn how to please a woman with your fingertips, it might make what you can do with your penis feel all the more satisfying for both of you.

NOTE: You might find inconsistencies in this chapter. Some of the top researchers in the world are still trying to make sense of the relationship between what's happening in a woman's crotch and the feelings in her mind. Please forgive *The Guide* if it trips up when it is trying to make mechanical that which has so many emotional components and variables.

Coaching, Patience & Practice

"I had to learn how to touch her clit... I can remember being clumsy about it early on. She'd have to stop me — I was going too fast, going too hard. I can remember her saying, 'You're in the wrong place.' 'Well, show me where. I mean physically, show me. Rub so I can see it. OK, now I understand.' Over time, I've learned where the places are. I can find them in the dark now. But early on I couldn't.... She would take my hand, or my finger, and she would put it right exactly where it was supposed to be, and she'd move it the way she wanted me to move it, and she would apply pressure to the back of my fingers, the amount of pressure she wanted, until I got the hang of it, and then she would take her hand away. If I got out of sync or something, she'd put her hand back and show me until I got it right. A few weeks later I might need some re-education, so she'd show me again." —From *Sex: An Oral History*, by Harry Maurer, Viking.

First, try to learn how to do your sweetheart in the same way that she does herself, assuming she does herself. Start by making an agreement with her that she will provide lots of coaching and patience, and you will provide an eager willingness to learn.

Also take heart in knowing that hands that are used to throwing a baseball, digging with a shovel, or torquing down engine bolts tend to get frustrated when it comes to finessing a woman's genitals; and that's only part of it. There's the additional matter of knowing when to speed up, slow down, push softer or harder, or stay your course. It will require patience and practice.

Differences in Attitude

"I've seen a couple of guys masturbate. I can't believe how rough they are with themselves!" *female age 26*

The reason why this woman can't believe how "rough" we guys are with ourselves is because she would never dream of finessing her genitals in that way. Think of how you squeeze or wag your penis when you are finished peeing. Try approaching a clitoris with that kind of careless abandon, and you are likely to be a dead man.

Try a Little Tenderness

"When women moan or gasp, it encourages me to press harder or faster on the clit. Always with poor results." *male age 41*

When it comes to touching a woman's clit, always err on the side of tenderness. Assume that softer is better. Push just hard enough to move the skin

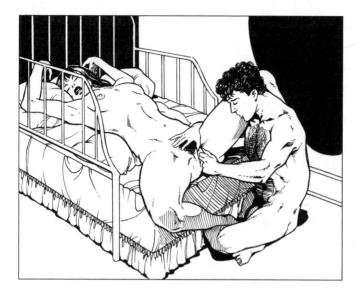

The Prince is finger fucking a very happy Snow White while the Dwarfs are away in the forest.

back and forth over the shaft of the clitoris, assuming you can find the shaft of the clitoris. And don't even get near the naked glans of the clitoris until you've paid your respects to her inner thighs, larger lips and mons pubis. A clitoris is best avoided until you see signs that the woman is sexually aroused.

If you put your fingertip under the hood of the clitoris and on its glans or tip, you will want to be sure that you have put lots of lube on it first. The tip of the clitoris is often more sensitive than any single part of the penis. You don't want the rough skin of your fingers rubbing across it. This is why you want to gently push and pull on the clitoral hood and labia (lips) rather than touching the glans directly. It depends on the woman and on how sexually aroused she is. (More on massaging the clit in the pages that follow.)

There are other kinds of genital massage where your lover may want you to be more vigorous. You'll learn as you go.

Showing Instead of Telling

Be aware that a woman's understanding of her own sexuality is sometimes on a body level and may have few words. Getting all frustrated and yelling "Just tell me" does absolutely no good. She probably would if she could, but it's like asking someone to tell you the meaning of life. She may simply have to show you by putting her own hands over yours and guiding your fingers as they go. Or she might say, "Keep trying different ways—I'll let you know when it feels right" or "Maybe my clit wouldn't be so shy if you didn't press quite so hard..." or "Try it here."

Also keep in mind that a woman might say "harder" when she actually means faster, or vice versa. And never make the mistake of thinking that if a little pressure feels good, a lot of pressure will send her through the ceiling. This is true, minus the metaphor. Guys also reason that if slow feels good, fast will feel even better. This kind of thinking does not work when you've got your fingers between your lover's legs. If faster is what she wants, work on establishing signals that will let you know.

Mix-ups will happen. You can get really frustrated. But it's not like anybody is going to die or lose their job because you confused harder with faster. After all, you have your hands between a woman's legs. Be happy.

Intrigue along the Inseam

In matters of love and sex, it never hurts for a guy to give his fingers a sense of humor. Fingertips that tease and dance will find an especially warm welcome. Gently running your fingertips up and down a woman's inner thigh is about a zillion times more enticing than shoving your middle finger up her crotch. When she's ready to have your fingers inside of her, she will let you know in no uncertain terms, and even then it's sometimes wise to hold back and tease and play some more.

Instruments of Pleasure or Weapons of Mass Destruction?

Make sure there are no rough edges on your fingernails. Get yourself a pair of nail clippers and a fingernail file. Keep your fingernails smooth and clean. Try to pry out any grease or dark gunk that's under them. And if your hands are rough, put hand lotion on them a couple of times a day.

Zen Boot Camp — Learning Her Style

> "It's not a dish of salted peanuts down there, don't just grab and hope for the best. It's very sensitive. Even the slightest movement can produce a reaction, good or bad." *female age 45*

OK, so you're going to learn how to masturbate her in the same way she masturbates herself. Grab a boddice-ripper novel with one hand, and have a big bowl of popcorn or chips close by. That's how some women do it sometimes. Read a few pages, rub a little clit, read a few pages... And if she doesn't masturbate, maybe you'll want to learn the fine art together.

When a woman masturbates, she often rests her wrist on her lower abdomen just above the pubic bone. Try to do the same, since it will influence the way your fingers feel on her vulva.

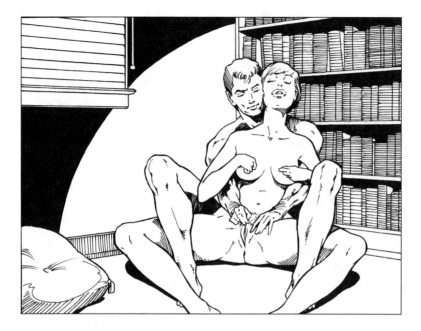

Lie next to her and reach your arm over her body until your fingers are touching her crotch. This allows your fingers to approach her vulva in the same way that her own fingers do. Or try sitting like the couple in the illustration above. Don't try to "masturbate" her while sitting between her legs and facing her vulva. This is a great position to use for the kind of genital massage that's discussed later, but it's not particularly effective if you are trying to imitate the way she touches herself. Here are some observations and tips for learning how to do a woman the way she does herself.

☂ Dry fingers on a dry clitoris do not make for the best of times. Don't start touching a woman's vulva near the tip of her clitoris. Try to bring lubrication up from bottom part of her vaginal opening, where the lips make a "U." Try dragging the fluid up your fingertips, or use saliva or lube. This assumes that you have spent the time and effort to arouse her in the first place.

☂ Ask if your partner uses extra lubrication when she masturbates, such as saliva, baby oil, Vaseline, KY, or Liquid Silk. If she's Italian or Greek, she might even use olive oil. (Vegetable oils are okay, honest.) Never be shy about using extra lubrication, especially if you'll be at it for long periods of time.

☂ When men try to masturbate women, they often use all finger and no wrist. When a woman does herself she might incorporate her wrist into the motion, even if only one finger is actually touching her vulva. This can be a subtle but significant detail, and it requires practice. (If you think your tongue wants to fall off during oral sex, wait until you try to do that giggling wrist-finger thing for 20 minutes. There are reasons why women use vibrators.)

🍄 Find out if your sweetheart has a favorite side of her clitoris or labia that she likes to stimulate. Be sure to follow her lead.

🍄 Some women will want you to pull back the hood of the clitoris. This will allow for much higher levels of stimulation. But if you do it before she's sufficiently aroused, or if she's got a super-sensitive clit, this can be a finger-fucking felony.

🍄 An excellent way to learn more about pleasing your partner is to rest your fingers over hers while she is masturbating. Then do the reverse, with her placing her fingers on top of yours, acting as guides. A woman shouldn't hesitate to take a man's fingers and put them exactly on those parts of her body where she likes to be touched. Most men will appreciate the assist, and after about the 500th time, they will probably remember how to do it in just the right way.

🍄 Another advantage of having your arm resting across your partner's body is that it allows you to feel how her body is responding. This is important, because as a woman becomes more aroused she may need you to stimulate her in a different way. Or it might be a cue to keep stimulating her in exactly the same way. Being able to read her body's signals is essential.

🍄 When they masturbate, some women direct the stimulation to just one spot. Others might stimulate themselves in a more global way, tugging and pulling on the surface of the entire vulva. Plenty of women use a circular motion when rubbing their clitoral area, while others move their finger side-to-side, or up and down like when plucking at a guitar string. If you live long enough, you might figure out exactly how to do it. She, of course, will assume it's all very simple and has no idea why you don't get it.

🍄 Novelty is not good. Try to achieve a steady tempo and rhythm with your fingers. That way if she says "faster" or "slower," you'll have a point of reference to work from. While one woman might want you to maintain the same rhythm and hand motion from start to stop, another might need an array of sensations because she quickly habituates to the same finger motion and it loses its effect.

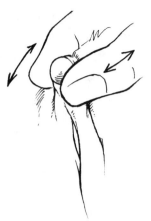

🍄 Ask if your partner puts something inside of her vagina when she masturbates. And some women like something in or on their anus. You're trying to duplicate everything she does, and it's not going to work if she forgets to tell you about that little vibrating butt plug that she can't get off without.

🍄 Try to use the fingers on your writing hand for working her clit, unless they are cramping and approaching paralysis. Finessing a clitoris usually requires a fair amount of fine motor skill.

It's Time for Genital Massage

Giving a woman the kind of genital massage that is described in the pages that follow differs from trying to "get her off by hand" in a number of ways. You will be working her into a high level of sensation and then trying to keep her there.

Whether you should roll the shaft of the clitoris depends on how long it is and if she wants you to.

By using specific finger movements on her clitoris, you might be able to help her stay near the peak for several minutes or more. But this will require finding the right spots around her clitoris to keep your fingertip on.

What's in It for a Partner: Gameboy for Grown-Ups?

Aside from the satisfaction of being able to truly delight your partner, you might be able to see her genitals open up, puff up, brighten, contract and pulse. In addition to the visual feedback, you'll be receiving sensory feedback from the tip of your finger that's on her clit. Eventually, you might be able to tell from the feeling in your finger where she needs it to be. Sometimes you can help her reach different levels of sensation as you change the length of your finger's stroke by just a hair, or by changing the speed, or pressure.

Getting Started with Genital Massage

The woman should be lying on her back. Her partner sits between her legs, facing her with her vulva in front of him, or he sits to one side of her, with one of her open legs across his lap. The point is for him to have good access to her vulva with both hands, and to have a good view so he can see the changes that are occurring in her vulva as she becomes more aroused.

You might start by caressing her inner thighs to help her relax and to build excitement. This seems like a contradiction, but the more relaxed a woman feels, the more sexually excited her body can become.

This is a good time to start talking to each other, because you will need a lot of that in order to learn where and how to touch. This simply won't work without the woman's input. Likewise, you will want to tell her exactly what you are going to do before you do it. So now is the time to tell her you are about to grease her groin—ah, put on the lube. Yes, lube—gobs of lube.

No matter how wet your partner is or gets, use and reuse lots of lube. The clit-massaging aficionados from *The Welcomed Consensus* who are referenced at the end of the chapter still recommend old-fashioned KY in the tube, and/or Vaseline on the clit itself. They haven't found anything better.

Put at least a tablespoon or two of lube on your fingers and start at her perineum. This is the area between her vulva and bum hole. Pull your fingers and the glob of lube up from there, through her labia, all the way up into the pubic hair area on her mons pubis. Relube and do this again. It's fine to not directly touch her clit just yet. Avoiding it can be part of the build-up.

Make sure she tells you how the lube feels as you are applying it. She should especially tell you about anything you are doing that feels good.

Clit Clocks—Finding Her Mark

Close your eyes and imagine a clock—the old-fashioned type that has a big hand, a little hand, and maybe even a cuckoo bird at the top. Mentally place the clockface over the tip of her clitoris. This will give you a map for how to find any special spot or spots, potential clitoral control centers.

Also, look at her entire vulva. Look at how the inner lips are sitting, their color, and observe the opening of her vagina. The landscape of her vulva will be changing as you find the right spots to massage. Visual cues will be both helpful and kind of amazing. People think nothing of a penis swelling when it is aroused, but we seldom think of a woman's vulva as changing. (Why not take before and after pictures? At least she won't have to worry about her hair or what she's wearing.)

Next, put a glob of lube on the tip of your index finger. Tell her you are going to lube her clit. Depending on your inclination and her anatomy, you

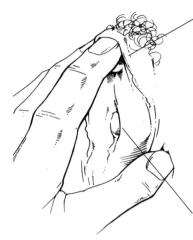

Reaching under the hood for the glans of her clitoris.

1. She needs to feel very aroused first.

2. Be sure there is a thick layer of lube between your finger and her clitoris.

3. Make very light, gentle movements.

4. Give each other lots of feedback, to find what spot feels best and how to move the finger tip over it.

5. Relube or add water to keep surface slick.

The opening of her vagina may become round if her vulva is engorged enough.

One form of stimulation that might work for some women. For others, it will be too much or too little.

might pull the hood on her clit back with the fingers of your other hand or you might simply push into the space between the hood and the glans. Gently circle the glans of her clit with the lube. Ask her to tell you what it feels like. Ask if she wants you to push harder or more lightly. Try gently rubbing each spot and see if it does anything for her. Make sure you notice what her clit feels like on your fingertip. How does it respond when you touch the spot? How does the rest of her vulva respond? This might sound strange, but does it make her anus contract? Observe as much as you can.

Her Johnny-on-the Puss Reporter

What you are trying to do is to find spots that generate nice feelings when you stroke your fingertip across them. For instance, you might try a linear motion, as if you are flicking a tiny light switch on and off. If you find any spots that she says feel good, experiment with the pressure and the length of the "on-off" motion.

Look at the rest of her vulva while you are doing this and describe for her what you are seeing. Have the inner lips gotten darker, fuller or brighter? Is the opening of her vagina getting wider or rounder? Has it started to open up? Are things contracting down there? She can't see what you can, so be sure to tell her if she would like to know.

Fist or Thumb on the Lower Part of Her Vaginal Opening

To help ground your lover's vulva, you might try pushing the thumb or the palm of your other hand against the lower part of her vaginal opening or on her perineum (see illustration below). This helps some women to feel a sense of solidness or comfort. Remember, you are providing comforting pressure to the outside of her genitals. You are not the little Dutch Boy sticking his finger in a dyke.

Anticipation vs. Dread

If it stops being fun for the two of you, or if it starts to feel uncomfortable or overwhelming, stop!

If you go beyond what feels good, her body will tense up the next time, and that's exactly what you don't want to have happen. If this is something the two of you try again, then she needs to look forward to it. Anticipation is an amazing thing. It can work for you, and it can work against you.

While the next part of this chapter describes techniques for stimulating the inside of a woman's vagina, it does so only in the name of exploration, and because some women find it enjoyable. Plenty of others don't like it.

Don't expect sexual pleasure to have rules and to be universal, which is what some of the women's magazines and the burgeoning home-sex-toy party circuit wants you to believe.

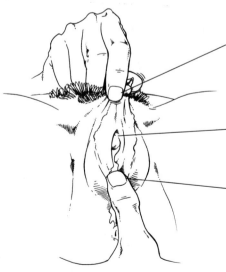

Clitoris stimulation by the hand above while the hand below puts pressure on the lower part of the vaginal opening and the perineum area.

The opening of her vagina.

Thumb pressure from below, or you might try using your entire hand against her perineum area at the same time that your are massaging her clitoris.

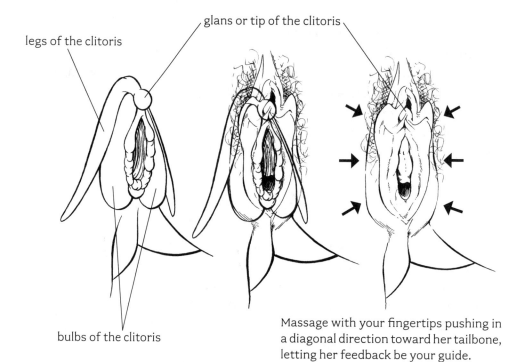

legs of the clitoris

glans or tip of the clitoris

bulbs of the clitoris

Massage with your fingertips pushing in a diagonal direction toward her tailbone, letting her feedback be your guide.

This was a challenging illustration! It helps show why finger pressure or deep tissue massage into the groin along the outer footing or base of the labia majora (bigger lips) can feel very pleasing to some women. You are not only massaging the labia, but the bulbs and legs of the clitoris which are buried beneath the labia. As with any deep massage, it is essential to get feedback from your partner. She will need to guide you on how deep your fingers should push into her groin. Some women enjoy it when you push your fingertips toward each other so your fingers make the sides of a "v" or a "u." You then massage the tissue that's between the tips of your fingers.

Fingers inside Her Vagina

You never want to surprise a woman's vagina by suddenly shoving an entire finger into it. A more satisfying approach is to ease your finger in, one joint at a time, and then only after she's spreading her legs and arching her hips into your caressing fingertips.

Once you get the signal that she wants your finger inside of her, slide it in as far as the first joint. Before you go any farther, make sensuous circles inside her vagina, gently pushing the tissue this way and that. After a while, if she gives you a cue to up the ante, glide your finger in a little farther until you reach the middle knuckle. Stop and play some more. At that point, she might want it to go all the way in, or maybe she'll prefer the added fullness of a second finger. She might want you to do an in-out motion with your fingers, or maybe she'll want you to stimulate the roof of her vagina. Maybe she will want you to jiggle your hand or pull upward, so the fingertip part stays inside her vagina and the inner knuckle part pulls up against the tip of her clitoris.

If you have been stimulating her clitoris with good results and her genitals are puffed up, you might want to keep pleasing her clitoris with one finger while exploring her vagina with a finger from your other hand. Think of using both hands as if you were playing a guitar. If the two of you give each other lots of feedback, you will soon discover what does and doesn't work.

Who knows where the fun spots will be, or if they will be. Think of it as a most excellent treasure hunt, one you will hopefully do time and again.

If Old-Fashioned Finger-Fucking Is What She Wants

In reviewing lesbian porn movies, author Jay Wiseman noticed that when lesbian performers feel each other up, they almost always use two fingers—not one or three. Wiseman asked a number of women about this, and most replied that two fingers simply feel better. Some of this Guide's women

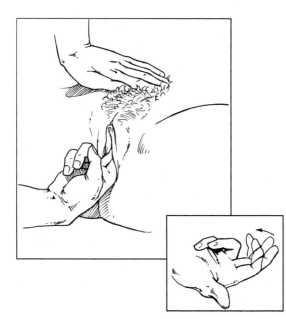

This is a common way to stimulate the "G-spot area."

For some women, it feels intense to stimulate the G-spot area along the roof of the vagina; some prefer a fingertip at 11:00 or 1:00.

Other women find that stimulating this area is uncomfortable and they enjoy other kinds of stimulation better.

readers said they enjoy one finger, three fingers, an entire fist or a big toe, but most agreed that two fingers is a fine number. The number of fingers a woman wants inside of her will also depend upon her level of arousal and sometimes upon her body's menstrual status.

You might consider wearing latex gloves when spending long periods of time with your fingers inside a woman's vagina. The smooth latex surface sometimes feels nice for the woman and helps to keep your fingers from stinging when they marinate in vaginal fluids, which are fairly acidic. Try putting a dab of water-based lube inside each fingertip of the glove and see if it makes any difference for you or her.

Finishing Off—Calling it Quits or Having Intercourse?

When the two of you have decided to call it a day, the man might try putting two fingers inside the vagina and applying pressure to help "wring out" some of the engorged blood. He might also put a towel over the woman's vulva and apply light pressure with his fist. Experiment with this to see if it is helpful. On the other hand, if you transition into intercourse, the extra engorgement might feel extra nice for both of you.

Isn't She Supposed To Scream with Delight?

Actually, no. Some women who are totally relaxed and receiving maximum sexual pleasure zone out and go into another world. While they certainly might moan or smile, hip-bucking and screaming aren't usually part of it. With other women, you might need to give the neighbors ear plugs. There is no correlation whatsoever between decimals and delight.

Other Kinds of Vulva and Vagina Massage

If what's been described in this chapter seems too involved or doesn't seem spontaneous enough, there are plenty of other things to try. Here are some things to consider:

☂ When massaging different parts of a woman's genitals, apply just enough pressure to move the skin back and forth over the tissue that's under it. Press harder if she asks.

☂ Finding a man's peehole is not a particularly taxing exercise; finding a woman's can take a bit of work. Why would you want to? Because there is a little dome of tissue that surrounds a woman's urinary opening. Some women might enjoy it if you stimulate this area. Ask.

☂ Think of the vagina as a tube that's about four inches long. Once a woman is sexually aroused, start at the rim (opening) of the vagina. Put pressure on each part of the tissue as your finger eventually makes a complete circle. She needs to give you feedback about any spots that she might want you to revisit. Then move your fingertip a little deeper inside and do the same thing all over again. Keep repeating this until you have done her whole vagina. It helps to be extra thorough about exploring the first third of the vagina, because that's a part that can be most sensitive to touch. Pay special attention to the upper half of her vagina between 9:00 and 3:00. A number of women report pleasurable responses in this part of the vagina.

☂ Some women feel a certain dull but enjoyable sensitivity around the base or deepest part of the vagina, a full finger deep. This part of the vagina might be more sensitive to pressure than touch.

☂ A woman's cervix can usually be found in the upper rear part of her vagina. It is easily felt if she is on all fours or brings her legs to her chest. The cervix feels like a little dome of tissue that's fun to run your fingers around. It may also have a small cleft in the middle, like your chin. Some women may enjoy it if you carefully stimulate the area surrounding the cervix. Others won't. Cervical sensitivity can vary with a woman's menstrual cycle; massaging it may release some blood if she is close to her period.

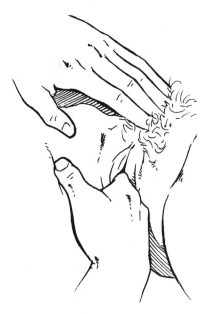

☂ Place your free hand over the lower part of your lover's abdomen. Experiment by applying different kinds of pressure with your top hand while you are exploring inside her vagina with the fingers from your other hand.

☂ The perineum is the groin's version of a demilitarized zone that separates the anus from the vagina. Push into the surface with your fingertips and see what she says.

☂ The ring of the anus contains a multitude of nerve endings. Women and men who don't have aesthetic problems with anal stimulation might enjoy an exploration of their rectal area. You may find that one part of the anus is more sensitive than others. Putting a finger on it might generate a deep sense of pleasure. But be careful about going from a woman's rectum to her vulva without washing your hands.

☂ Place a well-lubricated hand between the woman's legs with your fingertips resting below her vulva but not touching her anus. Pull the hand all the way up to her belly, with your fingertips gently separating her labia with each stroke. Then do the same thing with your other hand, alternating strokes.

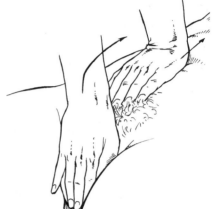

☂ While lying next to your partner, rest your arm across her body with your fingers on her vulva. Separate her labia with your first and third fingers and stroke between her inner lips with your middle finger, bringing lubrication up from the bottom of her vaginal opening. If she isn't already wet, lubricate your finger with saliva or store-bought lube. Also, some women like to have their vulvas tapped with fingers, and some even like to be lightly slapped on the genitals. Be sure to ask, first.

☂ Some women enjoy being touched from behind, when they are lying on their stomach or are on all fours or while they are leaning over something.

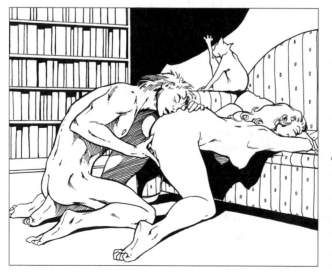

You can reach between your lover's legs from behind. This changes the angle that your hand and fingers make with her genitals.

☂ A woman's pubic bone can be a fine perch for a tired hand whose fingers are playing with the lips and folds below.

Massaging the Mons

The mons pubis is the fleshy mound at the top of the vulva just above where the lips begin to open. It usually has hair on it, or at least it did right after puberty. It's easy to ignore the mons and head straight for the clitoris, yet some women masturbate by putting moderate fingertip pressure on the mons and making a circular or back-and-forth motion with it. Some women enjoy it when a partner kneads the mons or taps on it with his fingertips.

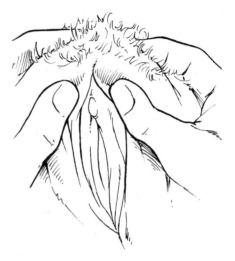

If you are looking for amplification of sensation, you might try pulling up on the mons with the fingers of one hand while gently tugging on the inner lips with the fingers of the other.

The Lip Part of Erotic Massage

Women's genitals have two sets of lips—the inner lips and outer lips. The inner lips attach to the glans of the clitoris. In erotic massage, much time is spent with the inner and outer lips.

After lubing the area up, you might begin with one of the larger outer lips. Put your thumb and forefinger around the lucky lip, clasping it at the base where it attaches to your partner's crotch. Then run your fingers or fingertip

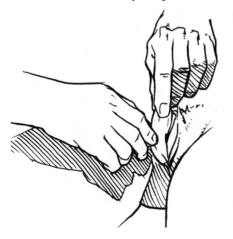

from the lower to upper part of the lip, as though you were tracing one side of a parenthesis. Repeat this as long as your partner finds it to be enjoyable.

Another form of genital massage is done by holding a lubricated lip between your thumb and forefinger. While squeezing just a little, pull your fingers straight away from the woman's body. Your fingers will end up in the air an inch or two above her body, as though you had pulled them off the edge of a sheet of paper.

Dry Humping vs. Finger Fucking

There's no reason why a woman shouldn't lube up a favorite part of her lover's body and rub against it with her vulva. This is known as dry humping. It was invented by Eve after she discovered that doing what the Devil taught her to do with Adam's penis resulted in unwanted pregnancies.

Some women like to do this on a man's back, thigh or hip. (There are women who think the penis would be more useful if it had been mounted on the front of man's thigh instead of between his legs. There is a special dildo harness that mounts a dildo on the thigh, achieving this very feat in an amusing way.)

Some women enjoy using the head of a sweetheart's penis for masturbating. This can be an invigorating experience for both partners. Even if the male doesn't ejaculate, unwanted sex germs can be passed on, or the woman can get pregnant from such activity. You can greatly diminish these risks if the man is wearing a rubber that is well-lubricated.

If getting pregnant or sex germs aren't a consideration, some women like to use a man's ejaculate as a lubricant to masturbate with. This might be fun to do when he comes first. She might add some saliva or her own lube.

The Extra-Sensitive Clit

Some women have a clitoris that is super-sensitive to touch. Even the most sensitive of lovers would feel at odds with it. This kind of clitoris is not

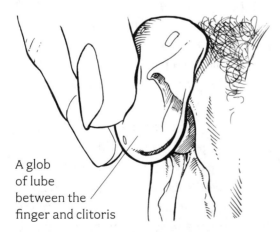

A glob of lube between the finger and clitoris

Never fear trying a glob of lube on the tip of the clitoris. This can be a helpful way to approach a clitoris that is hypersensitive. [Inspired by the "Illustrated Guide To Extended Massive Orgasm" by Steve and Vera Bodansky, Hunter House, (2002).]

particularly forgiving. Make sure the woman is highly aroused before your fingers go near her clit, and be mindful of how quickly it can go from being too sensitive to totally numbing out. Also, try to become a master of indirect stimulation, e.g. is it better if you caress her crotch when she's wearing blue jeans or underwear than when she's naked?

Agony vs. Ecstasy

We recently had to take a friend to the emergency room. From another part of the ER there was a young man who was moaning in excruciating pain. He would pepper his moans with an occasional "Oh God." If you had changed contexts and heard these exact moans coming from a bedroom window, you would have smiled in envy, sure the man was at the height of sexual ecstasy.

How is it that extreme pain and extreme sexual pleasure can sound identical? They certainly don't feel the same, not for most of us anyway. It seems that the sounds we make when our bodies are spinning out of control are similar, whether we are spinning toward ecstasy or agony. Keep in mind that it may be difficult for a partner to know when you are feeling pleasure as opposed to pain. It's up to you to help your partner learn the difference.

What Did You Discover?

It will take time to explore a woman's genitals. Maybe you will find one special place to focus on, or maybe ten. You might want to stimulate these spots while having intercourse or oral sex. Experiment with different positions that will help you take advantage of what you have discovered. Or try stimulating an outer spot with your tongue while using your fingers to reach a spot that's deeper inside. The sensations won't necessarily pack the kick of a mule, but the overall effect can be pleasing.

Contradiction—Aquatic Sex Is Dry Sex

Many couples find it sensual to grope each other in the shower, hot tub, or bath. However, water washes away natural lubrication. For a non-intercourse grope in a hot tub, keep a plastic squeeze bottle of vegetable oil or oil-based lube next to the tub. Stand and lube the outside of your dry genitals with oil, then ease your way into the water. This will help keep your genitals slick and slippery during aquatic hand play. For intercourse while submerged, try a silicone-based lube. Here are two advancements in hydrotechnology that have helped take the fingers out of aquatic fucking:

Hand-Held Shower Head If you don't have one of these gadgets, consider getting one. It shouldn't take more than fifteen minutes to install, unless your plumbing is really rusty. Hop in the shower with your sweetheart and try out the various settings. Keep in mind that when you hold the shower head point-blank against the skin it causes the water to bubble somewhat like the jet on a hot tub. This might feel good. Don't point a focused jet of water directly into a vagina, as it might force air inside the body, which can be dangerous.

Some men enjoy the feeling of the spray against the side of the scrotum. This might be one of those sexual experiences where the line between pleasure and pain is a fine but pleasant one.

Different brands of hand-held shower heads create different kinds of spray. You can find them for under $35. They often go on sale.

Powerjets in the Hot Tub Check with your hot-tub repair person about fitting an extension hose on one of the massage jets so you can direct the flow where you want. Tell him it is for your grandfather's hydrotherapy. Cut the air to the jets so it won't get into the vagina. Also, there are waterproof vibrators. These have only one conceivable purpose, yet the box shows a woman in a tub using the point of the vibrator against the side of her neck!

Winding Down

"The first time I felt a woman's vagina was with my first love. We were taking things very slowly, and when I would ask if I could go down her pants, the answer was no. I respected her wishes and we always did something else, usually making out. One day she finally told me I could proceed below the waistline. It was warm and wet and very soft. The wetness of her vagina was the most exciting feeling I'd ever had."

male age 25

For some men, putting their fingers between a woman's legs is a moment of magic. There's the woman's warmth, the start of her wetness, and how her body sometimes tenses and squirms.

While you are considering new ways to pleasure your partner's genitals, keep in mind that there are other parts of a woman's body where touch produces intense sensation. One reader reports that his lover has an area on the small of her back that is so erotically charged that her knees nearly buckle when he caresses it. He once nearly caused her to orgasm in the middle of

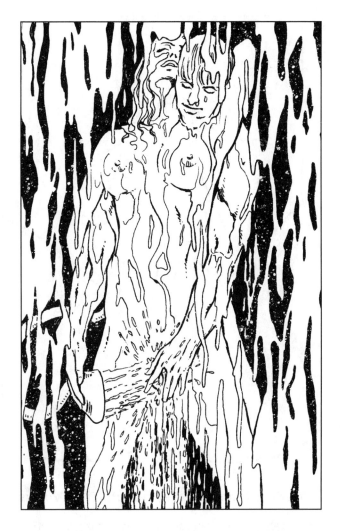

a busy hardware store by caressing this part of her back. Another reader is so sensitive to having her fingers touched that getting a manicure feels like a sexual experience. And sometimes, sensation happens purely by accident, like when you have been stroking those special spots on her body, playfully caressing her thighs and tugging on her inner lips, and suddenly, one just sneaks up on her. You weren't trying to give her an orgasm; you were just kicking back, letting your fingers play and enjoy themselves.

Some women readers have intimated that their lovers do the same thing each and every time they make love. It never hurts to experiment with new ways to touch your partner, both with your fingers and with your heart.

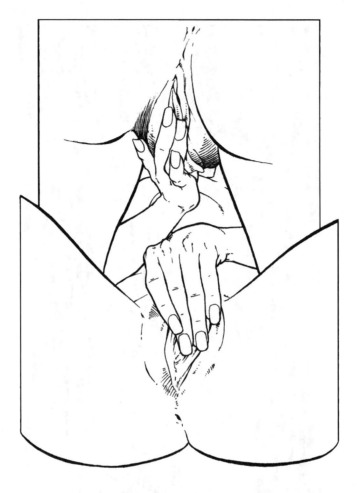

Reader's Advice on Playing with Their Vulvas

"I would first tell him to approach slowly. Having someone just dive straight towards where they think my clitoris is becomes overwhelming. I like to be teased, I like a slow and sensual working up to where they think my clitoris is. If they are totally in the wrong area (just because it's hard doesn't mean it's my clit!) I have no qualms about giving directions." *female age 22*

"Wait until I'm really turned on and I'm practically shoving your hand down my pants. Then, gently play around and see what I respond to. Once you've found my spot, start out slowly with only a little pressure. Don't focus exclusively on the spot, because that gets annoying, and it makes me less sensitive. As I get more turned on (which you can tell through body language like hip thrusting and my vocalizations), increase the speed but not the pressure." *female age 22*

"There's no point in approaching my vulva and clit unless I'm aroused. Touching me there is not the way to arouse me." *female age 23*

"Always get your fingers wet before touching where there isn't thick hair. Never, ever touch my clit dry. It hurts! Go ahead and play with my pubic hair. I keep it trimmed, but it means that every time you brush it, it sends a ripple of sensation through me. When I start arching up towards you, slip your finger just inside my outer lips and press gently, with a little circling motion. If I spread my legs more, please touch me! You should probably re-wet your fingers, either at my vagina (if I'm wet enough), or with some lube, or with your own saliva. I love being teased. Run your fingers along the edge of the inner lips, with just a little pressure. When I start moving against your fingers, caress my clit. Just barely touch me, that feels best. Again, that finger has to be very, very wet. In a very short while I'll be calling your name and God's!" *female age 20*

"The key word is GENTLE. At least in the beginning. Caress the pubic hair, then you could slightly penetrate with a finger near the vaginal opening. Gently move your hand forward till you find the clitoris. Never directly stimulate the clitoris, it's way too sensitive. Instead, position your finger(s) on top of the hood and gently manipulate it side to side. Be sure no matter what you are doing that there is plenty of lubrication, either from my natural supply or from a bottle."

female age 35

"Before you even think about coming near me with your fingers, please make sure that they are smooth. Long nails aren't fun, neither are sandpaper hands. I know that many men are very rough with their own members, but I do not need that. You'd be surprised what the lightest touch can accomplish. There is no need to "grind" your fingers into me. And please, when you find a pace that has me moaning, don't decide to switch to a different pace. That gets annoying."

female age 20

Reader's Advice on Fingers in Their Vaginas

"I like a finger in there, but please, don't dig for China." *female age 48*

"I like it if he inserts one finger until the opening relaxes, then adds a second finger. When I begin to breathe faster, he should start flexing his fingers." *female age 32*

"When I am sufficiently wet, I enjoy two fingers. I like it when he puts them in gradually and 'fucks' me with them gently. But no fingernails and no rushing!" *female age 35*

"Start with one finger, then go up from there. To find the G-spot, put your thumb over my clitoris, then insert your first finger into my vagina and feel for the rough spot on the upper wall. Rub this spot!!!"
female age 26

"I don't necessarily care for fingers in my vagina. I'd rather have a penis in there." *female age 43*

"I like him to rub the entrance of my vagina in a circular fashion, but don't like a finger all of the way inside." *female age 30*

"I like to wait until I can't stand it and beg him to put his fingers inside of me." *female age 25*

Resources

An excellent resource on erotic massage is www.erospirit.org. This site is dedicated to different ways of stimulating and massaging people's genitals and rear ends. It is not porn, but there is full nudity. You can get a month's sub-scription for $10-$15, and it is WELL worth it if you want to learn about erotic massage. It has many streaming videos on vulva and penis massage. It's not jerk-off material, but the information it shows will lead you and your partner to many happy and intense orgasmic experiences.

––––––––––––

Here's a finger-fucking resource that the author of *The Guide* found fasci-nating, but a female reviewer hated (to put it mildly).

This DVD series appears to have been made by a pod of mostly humor-less persons, consisting of five or six women and one man. Even their name is a bit unusual: "The Welcomed Consensus." They have devoted years to learning how to stimulate the clitoris, seemingly with the one man's finger. Their website is www.Welcomed.com. In the first DVD of their *Deliberate Orgasm Collection*, the members appear to be wearing uniforms from the original *Star Trek*. The fourth tape has the stiffest, slowest, and perhaps most awkward introduction of any how-to video in history. And if a bikini shaver ever got close to these womens' abundant mountains of *au natural* crotch hair, its bearings would cease in horror. When one of the women said, "Can you move your finger up just a hair?" the possibilities boggled the mind.

What Paul found fascinating was purely anatomical—how these women's vulvas changed with arousal, and how they pulsed for twenty minutes at a time. He thought it showed something that might be highly instructive. The finger-under-the-clitoral-hood illustration from earlier in this chapter shows what The Welcomed Consensus does.

The female reviewer, who is a Ph.D. in all things sexual, said there was nothing here that a woman who masturbates wouldn't know, and that the woman who is on the screen looks like a display object. She felt it was judgmental and it implied that this was the only way to have a truly good orgasm. She believed that some women would find the stimulation to be way too much, while others wouldn't find it to be enough. She feared that men who watched it would think this was the only way to touch a woman's genitals, and if they did, she feared their wives or girlfriends would be awfully bored.

———————————

See also *Penny Flame's Expert Guide to Hand Jobs for Men & Women*,
which is listed as a resource on page 166.

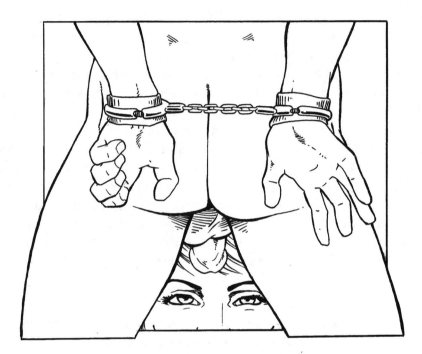

Sam had been reluctant to get a prostate exam.
Nurse Helga responded, "We have our ways..."

16
The Prostate &
The Male Pelvic Underground

One of the truly cool things about the prostate is that it is completely hidden. It is the one sex organ a guy doesn't have to worry about the size of when he's naked at the gym or when he is with a new lover. Prostates are measured in grams instead of inches, and a man has to be pretty neurotic before he'd worry about how his prostate stacks up against another guy's. In fact, you would have to be chewing on some seriously strong mushrooms before you would ever hear one young woman say to another, "You won't believe the size of Bobby's prostate!"

Like the prostate, the seminal vesicles are important sex glands that are tucked inside a man's pelvis, but you don't hear as much about them because they rarely give a guy a hard time. The seminal vesicles sit on top of the prostate like a pair of rabbit ears on a 1960s television. Without seminal vesicles and a prostate, ejaculation would be a non-event. The wad would be a no-show.

In this chapter, we will discuss a range of prostate and seminal-vesicle matters, like why a woman's vagina drips after intercourse and what happens when a man gets his prostate examined. We'll also talk about prostate problems, including infections and cancer. So here's the skinny on the two sex glands that allow a guy to launch his load—and they are not his testicles.

The Prostate in Ancient Greek Mythology

You've probably heard how Zeus was the head of the Gods on Mount Olympus, and how he was a jealous man with paranoid tendencies. What you probably don't know is how the prostate gland came to be. To make a long story short, there was a rather peculiar god by the name of Prostateus whose saliva smelled like chlorine bleach. Zeus feared that Prostateus was scheming to overthrow him, so he asked his wife Hera to land Prostateus in the underworld near the River Styx. Hera didn't get the message quite right. She thought Zeus said to make Prostateus a gland by the river of shit.

To this day, you can still find Prostateus, who the Romans called Prostate, by sticking a finger about two inches up the male rectum. He'll be sitting just below the bladder, right where Hera put him. If you reach up a little farther, you will find the two bota bags that Prostateus used to carry his wine in. They are now called the seminal vesicles.

From Marbles to Golf

If you take any fourth-grade boy, you can be pretty sure that his prostate is the size of a marble. If you take his dad, you're dealing with a prostate the size of a walnut or a golf ball.

If a fourth-grade boy jerks off, he'll produce only a drop or two of clear sticky fluid. While he can still enjoy the nice feeling of an orgasm, he won't start to ejaculate until puberty begins. Until then, his small prostate and sleepy seminal vesicles are just a twinkle in the eye of his older, semen-producing self. It will take a jolt of juice from the teenage testicles to make his little marble morph into a man-sized gland.

Geography of the Glands

The prostate is located between the bottom of the bladder and the start of the penis. The urethra (tube you pee through) runs through the prostate like the Mississippi runs through the heartland. If you are thinking in three dimensions, the prostate wraps around the urethra like a donut around a straw, or your hand around your penis when your partner says, "Not tonight, dear."

The prostate is made up of smooth muscle fibers, connective tissue, small tubes, and clusters of glands that produce a clear fluid. If you find fruit metaphors helpful, the prostate is like an orange, with a tough skin and pulpy insides. The fluid from the prostate makes up around 30% of each ejaculation. As a guy is starting to ejaculate, the muscle fibers in the prostate squeeze the fluid from the tiny glands into the urethra.

The seminal vesicles are about two inches long. They sit above the prostate on the side of the bladder where the foul winds blow. They are long and

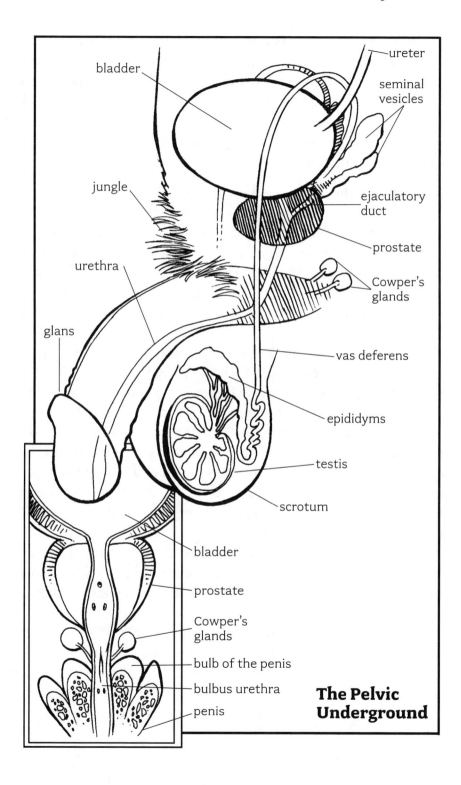

bladder

ureter

seminal vesicles

jungle

ejaculatory duct

prostate

urethra

Cowper's glands

glans

vas deferens

epididyms

testis

scrotum

bladder

prostate

Cowper's glands

bulb of the penis

bulbus urethra

penis

The Pelvic Underground

narrow like a pair of puffy rabbit ears. The seminal vesicles have special cells that make a gelatin-type of juice that puts the "thick" in semen. The seminal vesicles manufacture about 70% of the volume that's in each and every wad.

Note While the testicles are the master glands of the male pelvis, they contribute less than 1% of each ejaculation. The testicles are hugely important when it comes to keeping a male looking like a man, but they don't produce much of his ejaculate.

Why Girls Drip after Intercourse without a Condom

Did you ever wonder why ejaculate shoots out of the penis thick, but ends up dripping out of a woman's vagina as she tears out of bed and tries to get to work or class on time? The easiest way to find out why is to have a guy come in a glass. Then sit around and watch. In a few minutes, the thick whitish cum in the glass will start changing into a thin watery fluid. If a woman who's had intercourse stands up when the ejaculate is in its thin-as-water state, it will drip. And drip.

How come? To find the answer, we'll need to explore what happens when a guy has an ejaculation. When a man is about to come and he reaches the point of no return, a couple of different things happen in his pelvis. It's like when you pour lime juice, tequila and triple sec into a blender.

There's a collector part of the urethra that's located at the very base of the penis. It is called the bulbus urethra. When a man is about to have an orgasm, the ingredients that make up semen collect in the bulbus urethra. These ingredients include a tiny squirt of sperm, a big squirt of gelatin juice from the seminal vesicles, and a medium-sized squirt of prostate fluid that contains an enzyme called PSA. (All in all, semen has more than 300 ingredients.)

When the bulbus urethra fills with the different ingredients that make up semen, the pressure seems to trigger the muscles around it to convulse. This sends the wad flying through the penis and out the end: "Houston, we have an ejaculation."

As for explaining the trick in the glass, the key is the PSA from the prostate: when it mixes with the thick gelatin juice from the seminal vesicles it causes the gelatin juice to change its state from thick to thin. This makes the semen get watery. Scientists think this happens so the semen can more easily be sucked up into the woman's cervix. Evolutionists will say it's so other males will smell her dripping and will realize that their sperm has been out-competed. Socialists will complain that it's a capitalist plot to sell more tissue.

Prostate Has the Right Name, But Not the Seminal Vesicles

The prostate was named around 300 B.C. by Herophilus, the father of anatomy. The word prostate supposedly means "guard of the bladder." The prostate glands that Herophilus studied were apparently fresh and in working order, as he was allowed to do his dissections on criminals who were being put to death. Herophilus deserves credit for disseminating correct information about the prostate. This was not the case for those who eventually found and named the seminal vesicles.

The name "seminal vesicles" implies that they are containers that hold the semen. But the seminal vesicles aren't containers. They manufacture several ingredients that go into semen, but the seminal vesicles never see fully-mixed semen any more than an ice-cream machine sees a hot-fudge sundae.

Curiosity Will Not Kill the Prostate

Some people can read about the prostate and be perfectly content leaving well enough alone. Others will want to reach out and touch one. It probably depends on whether you view the prostate as a lump in a landfill or a diamond in the rough.

If you are interested in finding out more about the prostate and there's a guy around who is willing, get yourself some fingernail clippers, latex exam gloves (without powder), and KY Jelly or something like it. Have the guy bend over, like in the illustration of the DRE (digital rectal exam) that you'll see after you turn the page.

Use the clippers to eliminate any claw on your finger. Put on a latex glove, and lube up your index finger and the guy's anus. Chapter 23: "Up Your Bum" describes how you can give the anus a lubricated finger massage, which isn't a bad way to begin. It will help your finger to go in easier and might make the man feel grateful.

Some books on the prostate say to have him push out like he's trying to pass gas, since this will help him to relax his anal sphincter. But the methane nozzle that you are about to stick your finger into is a lot closer to your face than it is to his, so think long and hard before offering advice like this. Instead, you might use your free hand to pull one of his butt cheeks out a little.

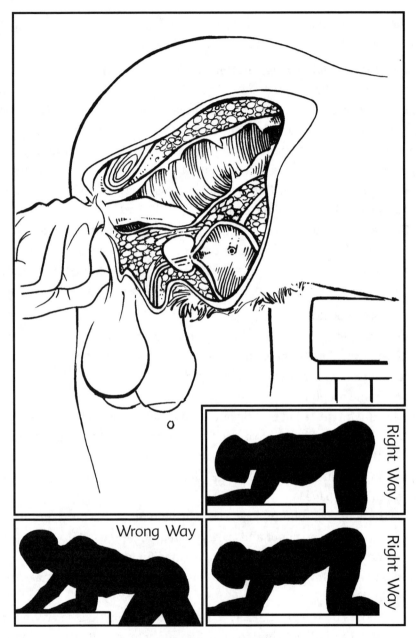

Right Way

Right Way

Wrong Way

DRE—Digital Rectal Exam

The examiner can reach only about a third of the entire prostate. The rest remains a mystery. So she tries to check for symmetry in the lobes of the gland. The only way to determine this accurately is if you are standing or squatting square, with your butt sticking up and out.

For a good way to approach, let's begin by looking at what you don't want to do. You don't want your finger to enter his anus at the same angle that an arrow does when you've shot it at a bull's eye. Instead, you want the pad of your finger laying flat against his anus and your wrist downward and against his balls, or in that general area between his thighs. You want your finger to be against his anus like it is when your are putting it against your lips and going "Shhhhh!

Eventually, as you are pushing the pad of your finger against his anus, it is going to blink or momentarily relax. This is your opportunity to ease the pad of your well-lubed finger farther into the opening. Simply flick the tip around and in. In the flicking process, your finger will suddenly go from the "Shhhhh" direction to the arrow in the bull's eye. The quick flick can't really be seen because it happens as your finger is pushing into the anal opening. As long as you are gentle but firm there shouldn't be any need to peel the man off the ceiling or call an ambulance.

Slowly push your finger in a couple of inches and start to explore the neighborhood. The illustration on the opposite page should be an adequate guide. While the prostate will be a lot bigger than the tip of your nose, the surface will probably feel a bit like it or like the padded part of your thumb as it meets your wrist.

If you explore the entire surface of the prostate from side to side, you might discover that it has an indentation running down the center. Also, experiment with different levels of pressure. Be sure to get lots of feedback.

For men who want to stimulate their own prostates, an S-shaped lucite sex toy (Crystal Wand) or a special butt plug might help. If you are able to sufficiently contort yourself, you should be able to feel it with your own finger. But the notion of a man being able to do an accurate exam on his own prostate is kind of silly.

Prostate Play for Lovers vs. Prostate Massage

It's one thing when you are exploring a friend or lover's prostate. It's quite another when a guy is having prostate problems and a health care professional tries to do a prostate massage or milks fluid from it to study under a microscope. Looking at what causes prostate problems might help explain why.

One theory says that some types of prostate problems are caused by small pockets of infection that get trapped inside the gland. These pockets become surrounded with a hard material that encapsulates the infection. The purpose of a prostate massage is to push hard enough to burst these pockets of infection open. This requires a good deal of pressure that's not any more sexually arousing than getting your breasts squeezed during a mammogram.

However, when you are stimulating a guy's prostate in a sexually exciting way, you are pushing only as firmly as he tells you to. There is no agenda, and the motions are based on your mutual pleasure.

Stimulating a prostate isn't going to get most guys off, so if that's your goal, one of you will need to be playing with his penis. When he does start to come, his prostate might feel like it's starting to dome or swell. At this point, you might rub your finger around his prostate or push down on it. In the gay community, putting finger pressure on a man's prostate when he's coming results in an ejaculation that they call a "gusher."

Getting a Good Prostate Exam

Feeling a guy's prostate will help you appreciate what an art it is to do a good prostate exam. A lot of physicians who are too embarrassed to do a good exam tend to stick a finger up a guy's rear with lightning speed, touch it long enough to say, "Tag, you're it," and yank their finger out. It's a wonder why they even bother; they aren't doing the patient any good. This is the same thing as waving a wand over a woman's crotch and telling her she's had a pap smear.

One of the reasons why a "Tag, you're it" type of exam is useless is because on a really good day, the examiner is able to feel along the surface of only one-third of the entire prostate gland. He or she is trying to get a lot of information without being able to put a finger on most of it. Some of the things they are trying to determine are the size and symmetry of the gland, if there are lumps in it that might raise suspicions about cancer, and if it is spongy or hard.

Our medical consultant on this chapter estimates he has done more than 35,000 prostate exams during his career in urology. He says a thorough prostate exam takes time and concentration. He tends to close his eyes once his finger reaches gland zero so he can focus better on the limited amount of information he is receiving. For him to feel like he's done a good job, he has the man stand or kneel square with his butt pointing up in the air.

So here you've got two grown ups, one with his finger up the other's butt, both have their eyes closed, and each is hoping that when it's over, the one with the finger can give the one with the prostate a big thumbs-up.

Why Healthcare Professionals Will Grope Your Gland

When a health care professional examines your prostate, it's called a DRE or digital rectal exam. There can be a number of reasons for this to happen. One is if you are a younger guy who is having pain or discomfort in his pelvis, or you are having trouble peeing and the doc is trying to rule out an infected gland as the possible cause. Another reason for having this done is called middle age. A white guy who is 45 or older will usually receive a prostate exam during every routine physical. Black men get prostate cancer at a significantly higher rate, so they often begin to receive prostate exams at a younger age. They will also do prostate exams on any man whose father or brother has had prostate cancer.

While a DRE isn't going to provide any answers by itself, it is one piece of information that might be helpful in ruling out conditions like BPH, prostatitis, and cancer. Yikes, did we say BPH, prostatitis and cancer?

Trouble in the Pelvic Underground

Did you really think that a gland that has to spend its entire life inside a guy's rectum isn't going to get uppity now and then? We're talking life without parole inside a human porta-potty. So if the gland is going to revolt, what are its options? Its most immediate targets are the bladder and the urethra. With a little enlargement here and there, the prostate can nearly cripple a man's ability to do everything from peeing in a straight stream to making him drip for a long time afterward. It can cause such an urgency to urinate that he can't hold it for more than a couple of minutes and it can make him wake up three times a night. It can also interfere with his ability to ejaculate without pain or to even walk or sit without discomfort.

Most prostates get bigger as a man gets older, yet there's no room for expansion. As you can see from the illustration on the next page, if the gland grows one way it's into your bladder, the other way it's up your rectum. Or the prostate might not feel enlarged, but the growth is on the inside of the gland in the central zone, where it can push against the urethra and clamp it shut.

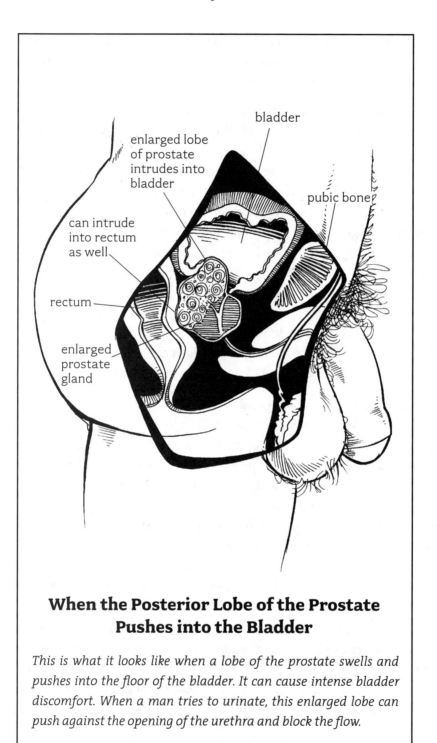

enlarged lobe
of prostate
intrudes into
bladder

bladder

can intrude
into rectum
as well

pubic bone

rectum

enlarged
prostate
gland

When the Posterior Lobe of the Prostate Pushes into the Bladder

This is what it looks like when a lobe of the prostate swells and pushes into the floor of the bladder. It can cause intense bladder discomfort. When a man tries to urinate, this enlarged lobe can push against the opening of the urethra and block the flow.

If this weren't bad enough, the prostate is one of the most understudied parts of the human body. Scientifically valid studies on the prostate are few and far between. Although prostate cancer is the third-most-common kind of cancer that men get, there is little good science to guide physicians. Half of all men will at sometime have BPH or prostatitis, yet treatment remains more of an art than a science. While studies are now being done, it will be years before there is a decent body of findings to help health care practitioners make quick and accurate decisions.

Prostatitis—A Young Man's Disease

Prostatitis is a syndrome that can include pain in the pelvis, painful ejaculation, pain with erections, an array of urination problems, and pain with life in general. Some men say it feels like they've got a golf ball up their butt, and it's not because they were bending over and someone forgot to yell "fore!"

Prostatitis is often described as a young man's disease, yet it can pummel the pelvis of any man at any age. It can be caused by anything from an infection to chronic tension in the pelvis, although infection is found in less than 10% of all cases of prostatitis. To quote a recent article in the *Journal of Urology*, prostatitis is a syndrome that is "poorly defined, poorly understood, poorly treated, and bothersome." Or to quote our own prostate expert, "Prostatitis is a young guy's disease that is not diagnosed properly and is not treated properly."

If you've got a sudden, acute attack of pain in your pelvis, get yourself to a physician as soon as possible. This kind of prostatitis can usually be treated successfully.

If you have chronic prostate problems, educate yourself about prostatitis. A good source of information is www.prostatitis.org. Then, after you have an idea of just how many theories there are and how complex the problem can be, find a good urologist. The prostatitis.org website usually keeps a list of urologists with whom people have had positive experiences.

Since chronic prostatitis tends to wax and wane, a lot of men take course after course of antibiotics, thinking that the antibiotics helped it improve the last time around. This is not a good idea. You need to approach chronic prostatitis with patience and intelligence.

Regarding sexual practices and prostate health, there aren't any studies to offer guidance. Having anal sex without a condom (barebacking) makes the man who inserts vulnerable to prostatitis because E. coli can cause prostatitis, and there are abundant legions of E. coli in our rectums. There are also concerns that couples who are having vaginal intercourse can be passing some prostate infections back and forth, so if you have prostate problems, discuss this with your urologist.

BPH (Benign Prostatic Hyperplasia)—Middle-Age or Older

Let's say you are getting close to 50 and you notice that the wall doesn't shake anymore when you are peeing at a urinal. Or maybe you don't make it through the night like you used to. This could be due to a prostate that is getting larger as you are getting older.

It is called BPH when your prostate gland is enlarged and physicians don't think you have cancer. The symptoms can range from mild to severe. One of the fascinating things about BPH is that the prostate can be greatly enlarged in a man who experiences no troubling symptoms, or it can be completely normal in size but the man is going through hell. In the latter case, the swelling might be on the inside of the prostate, clamping the urethra shut.

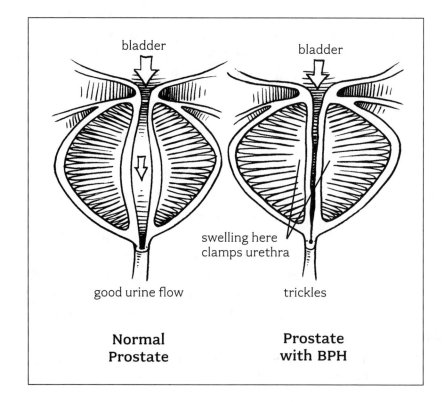

bladder

bladder

swelling here
clamps urethra

good urine flow

trickles

**Normal
Prostate**

**Prostate
with BPH**

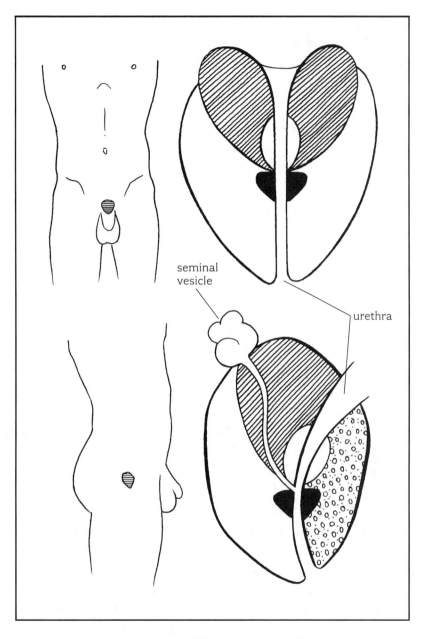

Prostate Cut in Half—Front and Side Views

Some people think of the prostate as a lump. However, as you can see from this diagram, the prostate is a complex organ that has a number of different parts to it.

Although BPH and prostatitis are supposed to be two different things, a man who is under 40 is likely to be given the diagnosis of prostatitis while a man who is over 50 is likely to be given the diagnosis of BPH, even if they have the exact same symptoms.

Prostate Cancer

It has been estimated that half of all grown men have an early form of prostate cancer called microcarcinoma. It usually stays where it is and you never know it is there. When this kind of cancer does grow, it often remains inside the prostate and is not aggressive. However, some forms of prostate cancer can be very aggressive. The challenge is in knowing which is which.

Prostate cancer is sometimes diagnosed on a wing and a prayer. One of the big challenges with prostate cancer is deciding when to treat it aggressively and when to take a "wait and watch" attitude.

One test that can possibly indicate the presence of prostate cancer is called the PSA test. PSA is the enzyme that makes a guy's ejaculate go from thick to watery. When the level of PSA in the bloodstream starts to rise, it might be due to cancer of the prostate. On the other hand, BPH can also cause the PSA level to rise, and some men who have prostate cancer show no rise in their PSA level at all.

At this point, scientists wonder if doing routine PSA tests are helpful, as they sometimes result in a wild goose chase. If you have reason for concern, check with your doctor on a regular basis. Long-term studies are being done that will offer more guidance.

If you are concerned about prostate cancer, educate yourself and check out numerous resources like some of the following:

The Prostate Health Workbook by Newton Malerman, Hunter House Press, Alameda, California, 2002. The title is misleading. This is a book for men who have prostate cancer, and it's a good one. The author had prostate cancer and he's tried to provide answers to questions that others have been too embarrassed to ask or answer, such as "What Do I Tell My Grandkids?," "Do I Have to Shave?" and "What Is That Strange Thing Between My Legs?" The author has excellent suggestions such as the following:

> "If you are diagnosed with prostate cancer or any other serious illness, take someone with you to your doctor's appointments. My wife was able to ask much clearer and tougher questions than I was.

If you are single, or your spouse or partner is too emotional about what's happening, take a trusted friend or family member."

"If you are treated to a rough digital exam, find another urologist. The procedure is not too unpleasant if the doctor has a gentle touch."

💡 Explore several websites. Some of your best help will come from other men who have been through it before you, and they often post. However, be aware of which companies contribute funding to the websites you are searching. It is unlikely that companies will be supporting websites that question the wisdom of taking their products.

💡 If you have cancer or BPH and if surgery or radiation is being suggested, ask if it will cause incontinence, impotence, a shorter penis, dry ejaculations or if you will squirt urine when you ejaculate. Also inquire about vacuum pumping your penis after surgery. Some urologists recommend it.

A Healthy Prostate Diet?

Long-term studies on diet, prostate irritation and prostate cancer are just starting to come in. Check with your healthcare professional about what foods might help and which to avoid. Smoking definitely causes bladder cancer, and it causes men with prostatitis to have worse symptoms.

RECOMMENDED: for chronic prostatitis, one of the most highly-regarded books is *A Headache in the Pelvis: A New Understanding and Treatment for Prostatitis and Chronic Pelvic Pain Syndromes,* 4th Edition by David Wise and Rodney Anderson (2007).

Also visit the extremely thorough and competent www.prostatitis.org.

THANKS: A very special thanks to Dr. Joe Marzucco, formerly of the Portland Kaiser Urology Department and now a sex therapist in private practice in Portland, Oregon. Thanks also to John Schulman, a sex educator in Corvallis, Oregon, who helps students learn how to do prostate exams.

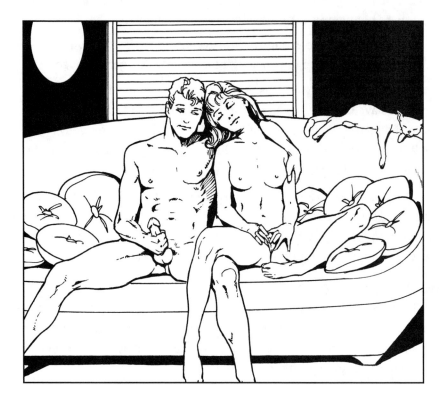

17
Doing Yourself In Your Partner's Presence

Some women have never seen a man masturbate, and some men have never seen a woman masturbate. Yet plenty of us would find it erotic to watch a partner do it. That's what this chapter is about.

Many of us have the fantasy that once we get into a relationship, we won't be playing with ourselves anymore. In some cases, that's how it is for the first couple of months or years. You either don't have the urge to masturbate, or can't remember why you used to do it so often. In other relationships, which can be just as satisfying, you don't really stop masturbating. And some women report that they actually start masturbating more once they are in a satisfying sexual relationship.

While there are plenty of times when masturbation is something you will prefer to do alone, there are other times that doing it with or in front of a partner can be extremely satisfying.

For straight people, masturbating in front of a partner can sometimes take a lot of trust. That's because masturbation tends to be more self-disclosing than other types of sex. It can also leave you feeling vulnerable if your partner finds you doing it: "Oh, hi, honey, I was just sitting here in front of the computer jerking off."

Being open about it can help expand sexual enjoyment for both partners. Here are nine reasons why:

There is often something erotic and even forbidden about seeing your partner masturbate. This is just as true for women watching men as for men watching women.

If your partner can see how you please yourself, it might help him or her understand more about pleasing you.

Orgasms from masturbation can be more intense than other kinds of orgasm. It might increase the level of intimacy in your relationship if you can ask your partner to hold you while you get yourself off.

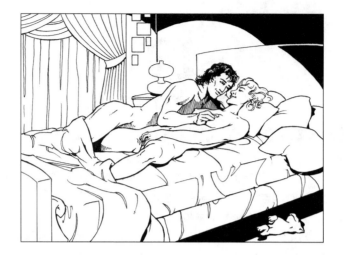

🔆 Masturbating together is an excellent way to share intense sexual feelings without the risk of unwanted pregnancy or STIs.

🔆 People often have unreal expectations that a partner can satisfy all of their sexual urges. There will be plenty of times when one of you is in the mood and the other isn't. There may also be times when your partner is so pleasantly drained by what you have just done (oral sex, genital massage, etc.) that he or she curls up and falls asleep on the spot. If the two of you are comfortable about it, then the spent one can hold the horny one while he or she masturbates, or you can masturbate while your partner conks out.

🔆 There are times when people feel like doing it solo. If this is an accepted part of your relationship, you won't have to hide or feel like a weirdo when you want to control your own orgasmic destiny.

🔆 Although the sex you have with your partner can be really satisfying, masturbating is the only way some people can have an orgasm.

🔆 When you do masturbate in each other's presence, don't forget that a partner's pleasure might be greatly enhanced with a special assist on your part. For instance, a man might enjoy it if his partner caresses or massages his testicles while he masturbates, and a woman might find it delightful if her partner licks her nipples or whispers sweet but nasty things into her ears while she masturbates. The possibilities abound.

🔆 Summers in the East, South, and Midwest are sometimes so miserably hot and muggy that the last thing you'll want to do is hug an equally hot and sweaty partner. Masturbating together is one way you can share sexual pleasure without full-body contact.

When It Is Difficult to Talk About

Perhaps you would like to talk to your partner about masturbation, but aren't sure how to bring it up. Or maybe you discovered him or her doing it, and you feel jealous or worried that your partner isn't satisfied with you.

One way of approaching it might be to ask your partner if he or she would hold you while you gave yourself an orgasm. A lot of lovers would find this to be a turn-on, and it would help make the subject of masturbation safe for conversation. Eventually, you might ask your partner if he or she does it in addition to the sex that the two of you have together.

Readers' Comments

"I wish he would do it in front of me more often. I've even named his penis Squeegy Loueegy." *female age 37*

"I never realized it was possible for a guy to be turned on by seeing a woman touching herself. Needless to say, once I figured this out about him, I put on a good show." *female age 45*

"It took a while for us to get comfortable with it, but I like to watch my husband stroke his penis. He enjoys watching me, too. I often masturbate as part of our loveplay because I like stimulation in more places at once than two hands are capable of doing." *female age 47*

"During intercourse one of us always has to touch me so I can have an orgasm, so in that respect, he's seen me do it. And we both chat about how we masturbate when we are alone sometimes." *female age 30*

"Masturbation is the act in my life that keeps me sane. My wife even helps me sometimes." *male age 38*

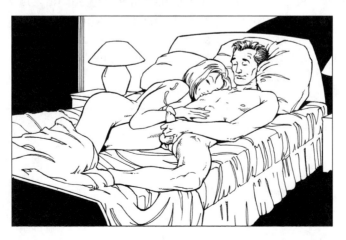

"I masturbate in front of my husband, mostly with a vibrator. I still find it a bit embarrassing." *female age 35*

"I masturbate at least once a day. My lover loves it when I masturbate with him or beside him. He thinks it's one of life's great mysteries. I like to watch him masturbate, though sometimes it makes me jealous. I'd like him to take the time and attention he spends on himself and use it on me." *female age 24*

"I masturbate regularly because in the fourteen years that I have been sexually active I have never received an orgasm from intercourse. The only way I can come is from a vibrator or by my husband performing oral sex on me. Sometimes I masturbate privately, other times in front of my husband right after intercourse." *female age 35*

"I masturbate several times a week, and if she doesn't know after twenty-five years, well, I'd be surprised." *male age 48*

"Sometimes, you just want to come and not have intercourse with your partner. It makes sense because you know how to make yourself get off better and faster than anybody else. You might also get to know yourself and discover new techniques." *female age 26*

Virgin Birth Alert

Be sure to wash male ejaculate off your fingers before touching female genitals. While the risk is low, a reader actually became pregnant from masturbating after giving her high-school sweetheart a handjob.

18

Nipples, Nipples, Nipples

While the title of this chapter is fun, it should have been "breasts, breasts, breasts," or "nipples/breasts, nipples/breasts, nipples/breasts." That's because for many women, the part of their breast that they prefer having kissed and caressed is between the neck and nipples as opposed to just the nipples themselves. Plastic surgeons discovered this when they were doing studies of sensation in women's breasts.

There's also the implication that nipple stimulation is only for women. However, a 2006 study on nipple/breast stimulation found that 52% of males enjoy tender kisses and caresses of their nipples. There was probably another 25% of the males who were too manly to admit they enjoyed it, or unable to allow themselves to ask a partner to do it. Men seem to have similar variations in nipple and chest sensitivity as women do. Some men get an erection and nearly come when their nipples are caressed. Some find it enhances their orgasm if a partner sucks on or caresses a nipple at the same time that they are coming.

Plenty of women and men have mega nerve endings in their nipples, chests and breasts. The sensations can be both pleasant and annoying.

One woman might find it heavenly when a lover barely breathes on her nipples, but convulses in pain if he is the slightest bit rough. So her partner learns to traverse her tender nipples like a butterfly and becomes a master at the art of subtle stimulation. Another woman wants her lover to handle her nipples with authority and doesn't find it erotic until his lips latch on like an industrial vacuum cleaner. Also, some women's breasts become more sensitive during certain stages of their menstrual cycle, especially if they are taking birth-control pills. Know your lover's body and be sensitive to the ebb and flow of what feels good and when. And don't assume it's the nipple that does the trick when it might be the area a couple of inches above or to the side of the nipple.

A Fascinating Take on Breasts

Here are some women's perspectives on their breasts as reported to Meema Spadola in her wonderful book, *Breasts—Our Most Public Private Parts,* Wildcat Canyon Press:

From Elaine: "My preferences vary constantly. What feels pleasurable one moment can feel annoying the next. Sometimes I hit sensory overload and can barely stand to have my breasts touched."

Cecilia says, "My nipples are very sensitive and I could be aroused almost to the point of orgasm just by touching them, but only very gently, almost not at all." At the other end of the spectrum is Heather, who prefers a firm touch that includes clothespins and biting.

Then there is Carrie, who was known as the girl with the big boobs. "Guys were sometimes more attracted to my boobs than to me." One day when Carrie was wearing a large rain slicker which hid her breasts behind a wall of thick yellow plastic, she met a man from out of town, and they seemed to hit it off. They talked on the phone and wrote letters for the first year of their relationship, with him never knowing that her bras were the size of saddlebags. Assured that he liked all of her and not just her mammaries, Carrie eventually married the man.

One woman reports, "When a man touches my breasts, I feel a little removed from the whole experience—as if he's on a date with my breasts." Another woman says, "My boyfriend loves to suck on my nipples, but sometimes I get this sense that he is focusing on them and tuning me out, and I can feel a wave of resentment, almost jealousy, when he latches onto my breasts." A third woman says, "I would feel like I had this 180-pound baby in my arms, and occasionally he'd fall asleep there sucking my breasts. I'm sure he thought he was giving me great pleasure, but it just didn't do it for me."

On the other hand, there are women who describe their breasts as being "a place of warmth and love," and "without breast stimulation, sex is purely physical with no emotional component." Another perspective comes from Scarlet, with 38DD breasts, who says, "I can't wait to take my clothes off in bed because I know that men will get excited; they always want to suck on my breasts. They think that I get incredibly turned on by it, but my breasts aren't as sensitive as men expect. Honestly, I could be balancing my checkbook while they're doing it. It's really not a big deal. But I do get turned on seeing them getting very turned on."

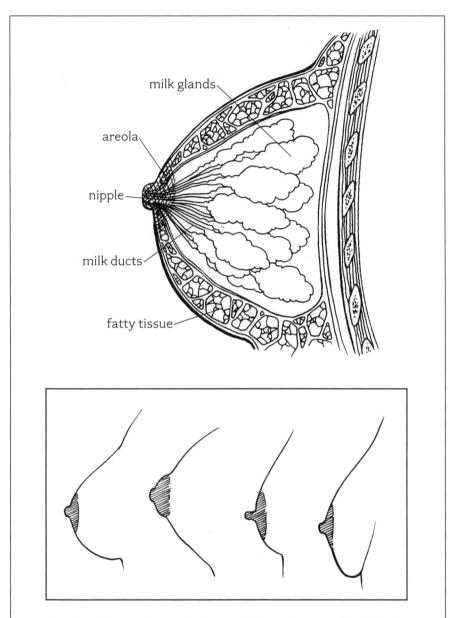

milk glands

areola

nipple

milk ducts

fatty tissue

The breast is made up of glands, ducts, and surrounding fat. In younger women, the proportion of fat in the breast is usually lower, and it tends to increase with age. It is the fat that gives the breast its unique size and shape. Because there is fat in the breast, it is completely normal for breasts to feel lumpy.

Finally, Ms. Spadola quotes a woman who has had sex with both men and women: "The men didn't seem to grasp that twisting them like radio dials does not work. They treated my breasts as something separate from my body. Women seem to know instinctively what to do with breasts. Women sense that there are times when you want your breasts to be touched, and times you don't. It didn't seem to occur to the men I was with that there might be mental and cultural baggage wrapped up there."

A Suggestion for Female Readers

Even if your guy has a big hairy chest, tell him you are going to touch and kiss his "breasts" the same way you like to have yours kissed, and then do it. If there are times when you like it to be gentle, tell him, "This is what I like when I say *gentle*." If there are times when you like it extra-rough, grab a pair of vice grips, and let him know what you mean when you say *rough*. If you like your nipples tugged, show him exactly how and for how long. And please, don't get all bent out of shape if he requires refresher lessons. The learning process is not nearly as straightforward as you might think.

Techniques for Happy Breasts

There is no "one-size-fits-all" bra, and there are no sets of breast-stimulation tips and techniques that will work for everyone. Here are a few to pick and choose from. Please be aware that many of these techniques focus on the nipples. If this doesn't work for your partner, find out what parts of her neck and chest do bring her pleasure when you kiss and caress them.

Size vs. Performance As with a clitoris or penis, the sensitivity of a breast has nothing to do with its size. Small ones can be like lightning rods, while big ones might not be sensitive at all.

Making the Nipple Taut Place your fingers on each side of the nipple, not quite touching the nipple but around the perimeter of it. Push down lightly and slide your fingers apart. This will make the nipple taut. Some people find that taut nipples are more sensitive.

In and Out Pucker up your lips and use them to make a gasket around the nipple. Then suck in and out without breaking the seal—so the nipple feels alternating currents of vacuum and pressure. This method is described in more detail in Ray Stubbs's book *The Clitoral Kiss*. It also works well on earlobes and the clitoris. However, if you are sucking earlobes in this way, be sure that earrings are removed first. As for jewelry in the nipples or clitoris, be sure to discuss suction limits with their owner lest one of their favorite good loops or bars ends up in the bottom of your stomach.

Five-Finger Breast Grab This works best if the breast and your hand are lubricated with massage oil. Rest the palm of your hand over the breast with your fingertips around its circumference. As you lift your hand, let your fingertips caress their way up the sides of the breasts until they are clasping the tip of the nipple. Pull on the nipple just a little or a lot, depending on what your partner likes and her level of arousal.

Nipple Between Your Index & Middle Fingers The ability to do this will depend upon the size and shape of the nipple. Cup your hand over the breast in such a way that the tip of the nipple rests in the space between your middle finger and index (or other) finger. Squeeze the fingers together so that when you lift your hand the nipple follows, pulling the rest of the breast up with it.

Nipple and Penis Some women find it highly arousing when a man caresses their nipples with the head of his penis or by pulling his foreskin up around the nipple. If he pulls apart the opening of his penis, he can sometimes stick the tip of an erect nipple into it.

The Whole Enchilada Women Find out if your partner wants you to lick or suck on the entire breast and not just the nipple, and remember to alternate breasts every once in a while.

Hand and Mouth Chances are, your partner has two breasts, and you have only one mouth. Perhaps she might like it if your fingers are caressing one breast while your lips are tending to the other, or perhaps she would prefer your hand to be caressing some other part of her body. Ask.

Variations in Sensitivity & Menstrual Effects Sometimes one breast or nipple is more sensitive than the other. Find out if your partner would like you to spend more time on the sensitive side. Also, breast sensitivity can change with a woman's monthly cycle or if she's taking the pill.

Different Temperatures An ice cube in the mouth can be a rousing way to greet a partner's breasts. Or for nipples that are already cold, drinking something warm just before licking or sucking them can feel quite exquisite.

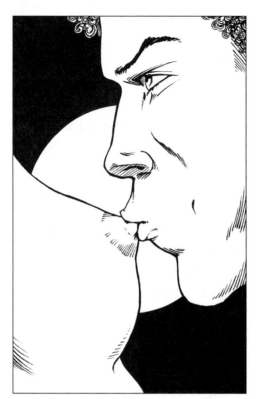

Playful Plate Fruit salad, all kinds of fruits, dessert foods, and certain liquors can be served on chests, abdomens, backs, and other body parts with extremely pleasing results. Do what you can to keep sugars out of the vagina.

Getting to Watch Some people find it highly erotic to watch while a partner plays with her (or his) own nipples and breasts. So if you enjoy playing with your own nipples, there's no point in keeping it a secret.

Hard-Nipple Alert

Let's say you are playing with your partner's nipples and they get hard. Is this a good sign? Sometimes yes, sometimes no. Until you learn more about your partner's body, don't assume that hard nipples mean happy nipples. Nipples can get hard from unpleasant stimuli such as roughness, abrasion, and cold—so be sure to ask your partner if he or she likes what you are doing. Also be aware that what a person wants in terms of nipple play can vary with their state of sexual arousal.

Dads and Their Daughters' Growing Breasts

Growing breasts come between some dads and their teenage daughters. For instance, some of a daughter's fondest childhood memories can be of wrestling and rough-housing with her dad. But suddenly, it all stops when her chest develops, and he becomes uncomfortable. Hopefully, dads will understand the huge loss to their daughters. They can gradually transform the physical closeness into involvement of other ways—with everything from playing catch to taking their daughter some place special each week like a museum or out to lunch. The important thing is to maintain the intimacy which is so important to most daughters and dads while moving the physical relationship into something that's more age-appropriate.

Readers' Comments

"Kissing my breast depends upon my mood. Sometimes I like being touched gently with fingertips and then gentle circles of a tongue followed by a very light sucking on the nipples." *female age 27*

"Most of the sensitivity is in the nipple, but there are good feelings from having the whole breast caressed and sucked. Swirling your tongue around the nipple is good. Sucking the nipple is great! Biting the nipple is a MAJOR no-no." *female age 34*

"Depending on how aroused I am, I like to be sucked hard and even gently bitten on the nipple." *female age 45*

"There doesn't seem to be any logical pattern or reason behind it, but sometimes even touching the breast area can hurt. Other times, pretty much anything is okay." *female age 32*

"I had to have a breast biopsy last year for a lump. I had not thought of my breasts as pretty before. They have always seemed too small compared to what all the boys were paying attention to. With a gain in self-esteem and self-respect and with the help of my current boyfriend, I've found that I really do think of my breasts in a whole new way, especially after going through the experience of surgery. My lump was benign, but it made me think about myself in a new way and what I really have to appreciate." *female age 20*

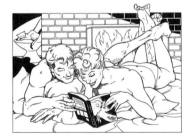

Dear Paul,

My boyfriend wants me to lactate for him. I am not pregnant nor have I ever been and I don't know how to lactate. I don't know if it's safe or if it is going to turn me into a hormonal wreck. If you have any advice or know any books I would be really grateful.

Madonna in Montana

Dear Madonna,

For starters, what you are asking about is different from the breast play that couples often enjoy during lovemaking. You are talking about a situation where your breasts would be lactating and your boyfriend would be nursing on them two to four times a day, seven days a week. If he missed a nursing, you would need to pump or express the milk from your breasts. This wouldn't be a problem if you were also donating breast milk to infants. This is actually becoming a cottage industry in America.

Adult couples who nurse refer to it as an "Adult Nursing Relationship." It usually begins after the woman has had a baby. The father may have started nursing alongside junior, or maybe mom encouraged him to take over once the baby was weaned. There are adult couples who keep nursing for years. Junior could be graduating from high school, and dad might still be sucking milk from mom's breasts.

The notion of having to nurse so often might cause even the most eager of couples to abandon the concept. However, couples who continue this kind of nursing seem to cherish the added closeness and shared dependency. Not only is one partner dependent on the other for milk, but she is dependent on him to relieve her swollen mammaries. In fact, the woman's milk will often let down at the sight or sound of her partner's presence, just as a nursing mother's breasts will let down when she sees or hears her hungry infant cry.

There are two ways that someone who hasn't been pregnant can try to jump-start her non-nursing breasts. These methods have been pioneered by adoptive moms who are trying to breast feed their adopted infants. One method involves the use of drugs to trick your body into thinking you were pregnant and have given birth. The other involves seriously intense sucking on the part of your boyfriend, several times a day for several weeks. Even then there is no guarantee he'll be sporting a milk mustache when all is done.

If this did work, your breasts would probably get bigger, so you would need to get new bras and blouses. As for the potential of getting stretch marks, I don't think it would be any different than with mothers who nurse infants.

Also, you would need to supplement your intake of calories and calcium just as a nursing mother does. Otherwise, your body might start robbing your bones of the extra calcium that your breasts need to produce milk. And if your boyfriend didn't cut calories in other ways, he'd probably start to get fat. As for the safety and impact of all this on your body—women have been nursing babies since the beginning of time, but does that have the same impact on your body as what you would be doing? I honestly don't know of any studies.

We keep links to adult-nursing websites on our totally weaned website at www.GuideToGettingItOn.com.

19
Oral Sex
Popsicles & Penises

Some women enjoy giving oral sex to a man. It provides them with feelings of intimacy and closeness that can be both soothing and erotic. It also provides a feeling of power and control. Other women don't find anything special about doing oral sex, but will go down on a guy if he enjoys it. And some women would rather suck on a rusty old pipe than let their lips stray south of a man's beltline.

Whatever your preference, this chapter offers tips and techniques about giving oral sex to the male of the species. It starts with a candid discussion about male ejaculate and then offers techniques for giving splendid blowjobs. It also includes suggestions for the man who is receiving oral sex—things he can do to help make it a neat experience for both partners.

When Gay Guys Blow

Straight women often get the feeling that they need to swallow a guy's ejaculate in order to give a truly fine blowjob. If this were true, you'd think it would apply just as much in the gay community, where the giver of the blowjob knows exactly what it feels like to receive a blowjob. But that's not true. Gay guys don't always swallow when giving blowjobs. As one gay male reader says, "No way am I going to do all that work getting a partner to come and not watch him ejaculate. Besides, I don't exactly love the taste."

Of course, you might love swallowing your man's gonad glue. But do it only because you want to and not because there's some *Emily Post of Blowjobs* who says it has to be.

To Swallow or Not to Swallow—That Is the Question

Considering what happens if you suck on a penis for long enough, a woman who gives oral sex eventually has to decide if she wants to swallow ejaculate. While some women don't mind swallowing, others find it weird.

For some women the salient factors are how they feel about the guy and how they feel within the relationship. For others, it's the taste and texture.

Different guys come in different flavors. As a female reader states: "My current lover tastes great, I like swallowing his ejaculate. But when my former boyfriend came, it felt like battery acid in the back of my mouth." Another reader comments that she has no problem with the taste or texture of male ejaculate, but that it sometimes upsets her stomach. A British sex expert with a Margaret Thatcher-like voice says that male ejaculate is an acquired taste, like swallowing raw oysters. She says it's nothing to get worked up over. We're not so sure, given how nobody around here likes swallowing raw oysters. As for the smell of male ejaculate, it's like a weak solution of Clorox—original scent rather than Lemon Fresh or Spring Rain. It also smells like alfalfa sprouts. (For more on taste, texture, smell and volume, see Chapter 6: "Semen Confidential.")

Who knows what to advise about swallowing male ejaculate, except that a man shouldn't push the issue unless he is willing to swallow a mouthful of his own, although the actual amount is closer to a teaspoonful. Suggestions for how to give a really good blowjob without swallowing are listed later in this chapter.

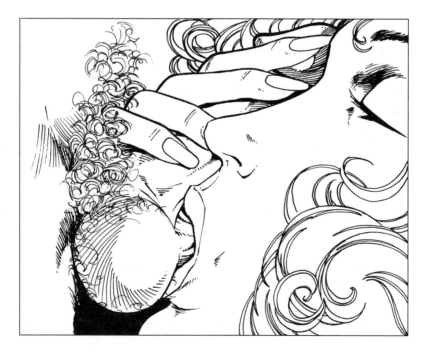

To Swallow or Not to Swallow: Hormonal Considerations

Women sometimes wonder if they are going to get a dose of male hormones when they swallow male ejaculate. While the testicles produce the lion's share of male hormone, most are dumped directly into the bloodstream. Those in his cum are already being absorbed into your body when you have intercourse. If you haven't sprouted a beard or grown a big Adam's apple from intercourse, you won't from swallowing your partner's cum. And the only way you will gain weight from male ejaculate is if it makes you pregnant.

Regarding the issue of health, ejaculate from a healthy guy has fewer germs than saliva. It seldom causes an allergic reaction. The main health concern about male sex fluids is whether the man has a sexually transmitted infection. For more on STIs, see chapter "Gnarly Sex Germs."

Have an Understanding

The important thing to remember about giving a blowjob is that no matter what you are doing down there, it is going to feel pretty wonderful to him. So lighten up, loosen up, stare that one-eyed squid in the scrotum and say, "Listen here, you floppy little strange thing, you might be able to spit, but this lady's the one with the teeth!" Blowing a boy is about being in charge. Enjoy it and have fun calling the shots.

Quick & Easy

Going down on a man isn't as much a mystery as going down on a woman, given how the penis is pretty much in your face from start to finish. The childhood experience of sucking on popsicles will give you an idea of how to begin. However, popsicle-sucking does not make for an excellent blowjob unless your man keeps his penis in the freezer.

There are many different kinds of blowjobs. Some women like to include lots of kissing and licking; others mainly suck on the thing. Using your hands while giving oral sex adds an extra dimension.

It never hurts to ask your partner what he likes.

Gag Prevention

Some women complain that they gag when giving blowjobs. When asked if they ever bothered to tell their partners about this, the gagging girls usually reply no. What follows are four suggestions to help keep yourself from being gagged while giving a blowjob, but the most important and intelligent suggestion is clearly the first:

Tell Him! If he thrusts and it gags you, let him know. Tell him that the two of you need to work on it, because you enjoy giving him blowjobs except for that part. Be specific! If a little thrusting is OK, help him recognize the difference between good and painful thrusting.

Fist on Shaft Make a fist around the shaft of your lover's penis, with your little finger resting on his pubic bone. This will give you four knuckles' worth of washer or buffer. If your man has an average-sized penis, there should be less than three remaining inches to go into your mouth. If your man is luckier than most, use two hands instead of one, as you would if swinging a baseball bat. As an added benefit, keeping your fingers around the shaft can be nice for him if you use them to pump the foreskin or pull it taut. More on the pleasure aspects later.

On His Back Some guys thrust involuntarily when they come. To deal with this, keep your bronco on his back and position your body between his legs. When he is close to coming, keep both of your hands around the base of his penis and your forearms flat against his pelvis. The weight of your body distributed against his pelvic region will help discourage any unwanted thrusting, and if he does thrust, it will pull you up with him.

Get Him By the Balls Clamp your thumb and forefinger together around the upper part of the man's scrotum where it attaches to his groin. This will place the testicles in the palm of your hand. Some men find this pleasurable, especially if the woman gently pulls downward. If he thrusts more than you want, increase the downward pull, as though you were pulling back on a horse's reins.

Positions for Penis Sucking

A highly effective position for doing oral sex is to place yourself between your partner's legs, facing his body. This gives your tongue direct access to the most sensitive parts of his penis and scrotum, and the angle minimizes the tendency of the head of the penis to bang against your molars. It's a comfortable position for most women, and it lets a man watch you giving him head, which some men find to be reassuring and a turn-on. Another variation is to sit, kneel or crouch in front of your partner while he is standing or sitting.

Some couples like the woman to straddle the guy's chest. She faces southward as she would if the couple were doing 69. This can be particularly nice for the guy if staring at his sweetheart's crotch and rear end provides

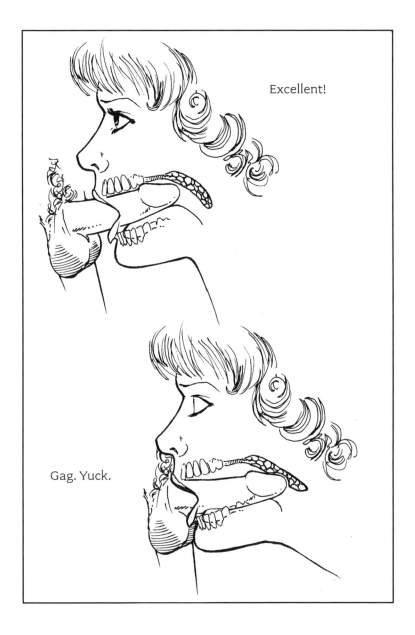

Don't Gag the Girl!

an extra turn-on. But it places her mouth in a poor position to give his penis maximum stimulation. It puts her tongue in contact with the back side of the penis, which isn't as sensitive as the front.

In the positions mentioned so far, the guy lies still, and the woman provides the up-and-down motion. Another way of doing a blowjob is where the woman keeps her head still, and the guy moves his penis in and out of her mouth. The fancy term for this that nobody but the Pope ever uses is "irrumation," which is Latin for "altar boy, hold still!"

The position the woman sometimes takes in irrumation or "face-fucking" is on her back with her head propped up on a pillow. The man sits astride her upper body and gently thrusts his penis in her mouth. The woman lets the guy do some of the work and she has good access to his testicles and rear end, or she can easily masturbate while she's blowing him. The couple can also alternate penis thrusting with French kissing. On the other hand, some women become bored or feel claustrophobic giving a blowjob with the guy on top, or they fear that the man might be rough or thrust too deep. Putting your hand around the shaft of his penis while he thrusts will greatly decrease any chance that he might thrust too deep.

A final position that some couples enjoy is where they lie side by side, with the woman's mouth in front of the man's genitals. She can lay her head on a pillow.

Deep-Throat Myth

You wouldn't stick an entire popsicle down your throat, so why try it with a guy's dick? Truly great blowjobs have nothing to do with deep-throating a man. Deep-throating is more of a novelty than something that makes a penis feel great. If your man insists that you deep-throat him, go to the market and buy a vegetable that's the same size as his erect penis, hand it to him and say, "Okay, let's see you shove this thing down your throat!"

Also, don't confuse a penis with a clitoris and think that every square centimeter is packed with thousands of nerve endings. As was said in the porn film *How to Perform Fellatio:* "The most sensitive part of the penis is the top part, so stop wasting your time on the bottom," and the male actor who uttered this profound statement had a penis with a great deal of bottom part to suck.

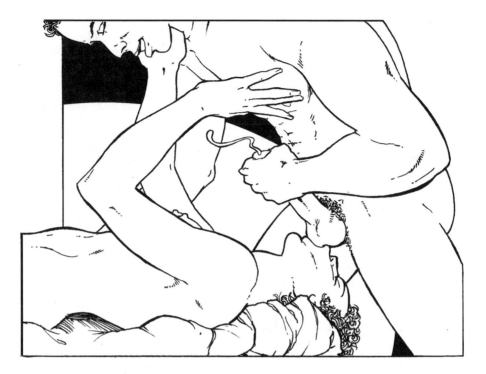

**This is a position that is also used by couples
for deep-throating.**

The average penis has certain parts that are sensitive and other parts that are mostly for show. For some guys, especially those who are uncircumcised, the head might be really sensitive. Find out how he likes you to suck or lick the head. Also, there is a sensitive nickel-sized area just below the head on the side of the penis that's away from his body when he has an erection. It's called the frenulum, and some guys can be brought to orgasm from stimulating this area alone. The seam of the penis that runs from the scrotum to the head usually responds to tender kisses, as does the entire scrotum.

If you still insist on deep-throating your partner, it might help if you position your body so you are either on top of the man in a 69-type position or are lying on your back with your head over the edge of the bed. These positions will help to straighten the pathway down your throat. They are better for deep-throating but not nearly as good for regular blowjobs.

Blow-Job Basics

Several tips and techniques are listed in this section for giving a really good blowjob.

Slobber People who are neat freaks often try to swallow all of their own drool when giving blowjobs. Such people have been known to nearly drown. Smart women let gravity carry their saliva down a lover's penis. They can also use it as a lubricant for pumping the bottom part of the penis with one hand while doing the upper part by mouth. Don't hesitate to toss a towel under the man's rear or to wedge one beneath his testicles; that way there won't be a big wet spot or stain on the mattress, couch or seat of the Greyhound Bus.

If It's Still Soft Some women enjoy sucking on a soft penis and feeling it grow inside their mouth. Just because it's soft, don't think for a moment that each kiss, lick and suck doesn't feel exquisite. One of the few times when a man can be totally passive and feel no need to perform sexually is while he is receiving a blowjob. Don't assume it's a negative sign if it takes a while to get hard or if it doesn't get hard at all. A man can still have a lovely time with his soft penis when it is in your mouth.

Lubrication for Licking When you first lick a man's genitals, coat your lips and tongue with extra saliva. This will make it feel better. Honest. If you suffer from the dreaded pre-blow-job dry mouth, try sucking on a mint beforehand to help kickstart your salivary glands. The mint might also help take the edge off the taste when the wad hits your buds. And never hesitate to keep a glass of water nearby, or a bottle of your favorite designer water.

Teeth Some women wrap their lips over their teeth when giving a blow-job, given how the mere hint of teeth on the penis scares the tar out of some men. However, a set of sexy choppers can sometimes feel erotic, assuming the girl's not in a pit-bull mood. Some women make a ring around the penis with their thumb and forefinger. They then push their lips against their fingers which are making a gasket around the shaft of the penis. Experiment and see what you come up with.

Little Kisses & Flickering Tongues Never hesitate to lavish your man's genitals or any other part of his body with little flicks of the tongue or sweet little kisses. The kisses not only feel nice, but allow you to rest your jaw without having to yell "Intermission!" It usually works better if the area you are flicking your tongue over is already lubricated with saliva or massage oil, so get it good and wet first.

Twisting Your Head Twisting your head when going up and down the penis (in a corkscrew pattern) provides the penis with a higher level of stimulation, especially when focused on the upper half of it.

Twisting-Corkscrew Action (for the experienced) While on the upstroke, wait until you are halfway up the shaft and put the tip of your tongue under the ridge of the penis head. Not only does your tongue press against the sensitive frenulum while your head is twisting, but the tip of your tongue adds extra stimulation to the sensitive ridge below the glans.

A Shirley Temple You can lick the penis with the pointed end of your tongue, or you can soften your tongue and give it a long flat lick that covers more real estate. The latter is called a "Shirley Temple" because it's similar to the way a person licks a big lollipop.

Partners Who Aren't Circumcised #1 Without retracting his foreskin, stick the tip of your tongue inside his foreskin and run it in a circle around the head of his penis. You can hold the foreskin up with your fingertips as your tongue does circles between it and the glans.

Partners Who Aren't Circumcised #2 By varying the level of vacuum in your mouth, see if you can make the foreskin come up and down as you bob your head.

Partners Who Aren't Circumcised #3 A most excellent conversation to have with a boy about his foreskin is at what point he wants you to retract it (pull the extra yardage down the shaft so the head is bare).

The Long Lick Mother nature left a seam on the penis that runs from just below the head to halfway down the scrotum. Never hesitate to take a long, wet lick from beneath your partner's testicles all the way to the tip of his penis, along the length of the seam.

Making the Foreskin Taut This applies as much to men who are circumcised as for those who aren't: using your hand to pull the skin taut over the shaft of the penis can sometimes enhance the pleasure of a blowjob. It might also encourage the man to come sooner if that is what you want. Wrap your thumb and forefinger around the shaft of the penis an inch or so above the base. Then pull it down to the base. This makes the skin tighter on the penis and usually increases the sensitivity in the upper part of the penis. If he isn't circumcised, you may need to start higher up the shaft before pulling the foreskin down.

Pumping the Shaft While your lips are focusing on the upper part of the penis, there's no reason why you can't be pumping the bottom part of the shaft with your hand or fingers. Let your saliva flow down the shaft, lubricating both it and your hand, and start pumping. Some women synchronize the shaft pumping with their head bobbing, so their hand follows just beneath their lips at all times.

The Vacuum (Hoover Fellatis) Some men will like it if you draw a light vacuum with your mouth. One way to draw a vacuum is to take as much of the penis in your mouth as feels comfortable, make a seal around the shaft with your lips and suck some of the air out of your mouth. Then, as you pull your head back, a vacuum is created.

Na-Na-Na-Nipples Some guys have nipples that are highly sensitive. Caressing them with your finger while doing oral sex might add to the man's pleasure. The best way to find out is to experiment and seek feedback.

Inner Thighs and Other Places The inner thighs of both men and women can be extremely sensitive. There's no reason why you can't alternate a blowjob with licking and sucking on your man's inner thighs, or caress them with a free hand.

Fingers in His Mouth When you are blowing him, you might try sticking your fingers in his mouth. Some guys will find this to be very erotic.

Perineum (between the Testicles and Rear End) There is an area behind the testicles called the perineum that is often overlooked but has the potential for good feelings. Licking this area can light some men up. A gentle finger massage down here can also add an extra dimension to oral sex.

The Blow Hole You know the little slit in the head of the penis where the semen comes out? It might be fun to explore it with the tip of your tongue.

Rear End Some men find that a finger on or up the anus when receiving a blowjob can be enough to make the cannon fire. Some men claim that the most intense orgasms they have ever had occurred when a woman was giving them oral sex while putting a little pressure on their prostate. Other men hate this sort of thing. Also, a small vibrator up the rear might catch some men's attention, and some couples enjoy rimming (oral-anal contact).

Visual Assist There are plenty of men who enjoy watching a woman give them head. Some women might be offended by the notion, thinking that this has something to do with submission. The chances are that the man is way too appreciative to be thinking about gender-power issues when you are giving him a blowjob. In her video on how to give blowjobs, porn star Nina Hartley comments, "It took me a long time to be able to do a blowjob in the light and not get embarrassed." She apparently got over it.

Oral Intermission If your mouth gets tired, do him by hand for a while, or run your hair over his genitals. Or if you feel like playing with yourself, let him watch you do that. Some women say that they give their best blowjobs when they are just as turned on as their partners. Don't be afraid to let him know about it if you are. It may help speed things up.

Tap & Hum It might enhance the feeling of a blowjob if you occasionally hum or tap the shaft of the penis when the head and frenulum are in your mouth.

Hot, Cold, Etc. Don't hesitate to suck on ice cubes to make your mouth cold, or drink hot liquids to make it extra-warm before and during oral sex.

Going Down after Intercourse Some women enjoy giving blowjobs after intercourse. They find it highly erotic to suck on a penis after it has been inside of them.

A Little Help from Your Friends If you have a friend who is more experienced at giving blowjobs, consider asking her (or him) for pointers, but keep in mind that you will soon be evolving your own personal style. What you do will also vary depending on the guy you are doing it with and whether the friend you are asking used to sleep with him.

Oral Sex with Men of Size

Oral sex may be problematic if your man's salami is on the enormous side. Never fear. The illustration on page 243 shows how you can still lick and kiss it into submission. Use your hands to pump the shaft while focusing your efforts on the frenulum and head.

Cojones with Hands

Using your hands is as important to blowjobs as it is in doing sign language. Be sure to include lots of finger and hand work. For instance, at the same time that your mouth is on his penis, consider caressing your partner's testicles. There might be places along the lower shaft of the penis — the part that is covered by the testicles—that respond nicely to fingertip massage. Massaging this area with your free hand can substantially increase the sensation. If you make hand play an active part of the blowjob, he's not as likely to notice when your mouth needs a rest.

Cojones by Mouth

"I love my boyfriend's testicles. I like taking them into my mouth one at a time and sucking on them. The skin on the sack is really soft and feels great in my mouth." *female age 23*

Some men will be highly appreciative if you take one or both of their testicles in your mouth. Don't fear doing this. Just go slowly the first couple of times until you get the hang of it. The skin around the testicles (scrotum) also loves being licked and kissed. The sensitivity of the scrotum has been compared to the lips of a woman's genitals. If he doesn't have an erection, you might be able to fit his testicles in your mouth as well as his penis.

Right before He Comes

There might be certain things that you can do just before a man starts to come that will increase his pleasure. Some women wrap a hand around the bottom part of the penis so the entire shaft feels like it's inside a vagina. Others place their fingertips along the seam on the front side of the penis and apply a bit of pressure. They might be able to feel the ejaculate surge through the penis when they do this. Some men appreciate it if you increase the vacuum in your mouth as they are about to come, but be careful about sucking the surge of ejaculate into your sinuses. Some men enjoy it if you hold or caress their testicles or massage the part of the shaft that's beneath them. Since this is a highly individual matter, let him know that you would like to experiment with a couple of new things and seek his feedback.

An experienced prostitute who consulted on this chapter said she finds that many men like to have their nipples pinched as they are about to come.

Learn When He's Coming

If you know the right signs to look for, you can often learn when your man is about to come. This will give you options if you don't want to swallow.

Until you learn his body's signs, ask him to tell you when he's about to ejaculate. You might notice that his penis starts to swell and contort just before it spurts. You can feel this in your mouth. A hand over the testicles may be a good source of information, as testicle tend to draw closer to the body when a man is about to ejaculate. Also, his buns or abs might tighten up or his hips might give a thrust when coming is inevitable.

If You Don't Like the Way He Tastes

If you know you're not going to swallow, keep a hand around the base of his penis while you are sucking on the upper half. As the signs of ejaculation

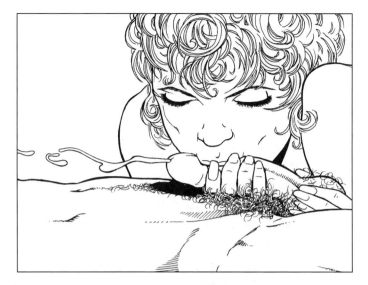

An Effective Way To Get Him Off Orally Without Swallowing

This feels so good that a lot of guys won't be able to tell that you aren't swallowing unless they are actually looking. The trick is to focus your lip action on the sensitive frenulum area while cradling the penis with your hand. This area is just beneath the head of the penis. Use lots of saliva and put plenty of tongue into it—almost like you are French kissing this part of his penis. Occasionally fill your hand with your hot steamy breath. This also works well if your lover's penis is a little on the huge side and you'd more easily fit a zeppelin in a one-car garage than get it in your mouth.

present themselves, free your mouth from the line of fire, slide your hand up the shaft, to just below the head, and start pumping for Old Glory. Be sure your grip is firm and pump fast and furious. This is no time for a gentle touch. And don't stop pumping just because he starts to ejaculate. This would be like the cable or satellite signal going dead during the last two minutes of your favorite show. Keep stroking until you have milked out the lasts drops of ooze.

Here are some other suggestions that you might find helpful:

Toothpaste, Mints, or Sweet Liquor Sticking a dab of toothpaste in your mouth before inserting a penis can improve the taste greatly. Or try sucking on a mint beforehand. The flavor of blowjobs can also be enhanced by sipping on your favorite sherry or liquor, unless you are a confirmed whiskey or Scotch drinker. Most of these will drown out any flavors from your man's wild turkey. Or you might try glazing his yam with things like honey, jam or whipped cream. Champagne blowjobs can be fun, although they can result in nasty hangovers. If you enjoy experimenting with minty liquors such as creme de menthe, do a small test patch on the side of the penis beforehand. While a little menthol on the skin can feel great, especially when you blow on it, too much can burn. It takes a few minutes for the full intensity of the burn to peak, so wait before declaring your test a success.

Slobber and Punt When Old Faithful is about ready to blow, start to mobilize a pool of slobber in your mouth. When he comes, let the floodgates loose. The saliva will help thin the ejaculate, making it run out of your mouth faster. And don't worry about the mess. The more goo and slime running down the shaft, the better.

To the Rear If you are going to swallow but want to decrease the taste, place his penis as far back in your mouth as you can while still being comfortable. Then start swallowing fast. Unless he comes in buckets, it should decrease the amount of ejaculate that hits your taste buds.

Sublingual Ejaculation This tip is in the excellent book *Tricks — 125 Ways to Make Good Sex Better* by Jay Wiseman. When it feels like a man is close to coming, put your tongue over the head of his penis. He won't know the difference, but the first splash will hit the underside of your tongue where there aren't any taste buds.

Let Him Help Some guys won't mind finishing themselves off with their own hand if you have taken the time and energy to give them a really good blowjob. It might be a special treat if you kiss or suck on their testicles while they pump themselves to orgasm, or push a finger against their anus.

Bag It Not only will putting a condom on a penis before a blowjob protect you from getting sexually-transmitted infections, but they allow you to bring him off without swallowing a drop.

Putting a Condom on with Your Lips

A competent prostitute can slip a condom over a man's penis with her mouth and he will never know it is there. This suggests that the problems some guys have with wearing condoms might be psychological. (So what else is new?)

In her book *The Ultimate Guide To Fellatio*, Cleis, Violet Blue suggests that you wet your lips and put the unrolled condom up to your mouth. Pull just enough vacuum to suck the reservoir tip of the condom into your mouth a bit. This should hold the rest of the condom, which is still rolled up, against your lips. Bend over the penis and pop the unrolled part over the head. Then walk the unrolled part down the shaft either with your lips or fingers. You might want to practice alone once or twice on your favorite banana.

A key to all of this is getting non-lubricated condoms. Condom lube tastes absolutely awful, as do spermicides. Some condom brands to consider for oral sex include the Durex Natural Feeling Non-Lubricated, the Trojan Regular Non Lube (no reservoir tip, either!) and the Trustex Flavored Condom. As of press time, the word on flavored condoms is that they were pretty dreadful except for the Trustex, although some people will beg to differ. Either way, the flavor is just coated on and goes away fairly soon.

Also, if you don't mind the taste of the lubricant, the condoms made of polyurethane might transmit the warmth of your mouth better, and the warmth is one of the things that feels extra nice about receiving a blowjob.

Dealing with Condom Balkers

Contrary to what we used to think, people can most certainly give and get sexually transmitted infections when giving and receiving a blowjob. Here are two approaches to consider if you want a man to use a condom while blowing him but he balks.

1. In a loud and clear voice, say, "Forget it, Charlie! If you think it tastes THAT great, suck on it yourself." Actually, he probably would if he could, and has maybe even tried a couple of times.

2. Try making the whole process of oral sex more fun and pleasurable for both of you. If he knows that the blowjob is going to be lots of fun, putting a condom on won't be such a big deal. You might hawk a small wad of spit on the head of a man's penis right before bagging it with a condom. This will help the sensations translate through the condom betters. Or if you are really prepared, use a drop or two of water-based lube on his penis or put it in the condom before rolling it on. Once you have rolled the condom over his penis, squish the lube around the entire head.

While He's Coming, and Afterward

At the end of a blowjob, there are two micro-epochs that happen in rapid sequence: the time when he is coming and the time after he comes. If you keep his penis in your mouth while he is coming, find out what he wants you to do while he's in the process of ejaculating. Does he want you to suck harder, suck less, pump his shaft with his other hand?

Then try to get a sense of how soon after he ejaculates the head of his penis starts to get extra sensitive. For some guys, the head of the penis can become painfully sensitive. What you were doing before he came might have felt great, but actually hurts after. Does he want you to keep his penis in your mouth, but to slow the action way down? Or maybe he's got callouses on the thing and wants you to keep going as if nothing happened. Another option is to keep the penis in your mouth, but to stop the sucking action and instead pump the shaft with your hand. Pumping by hand usually is no problem for a sensitive head, as the foreskin acts as an insulator. The only way to learn this is from experience and plenty of helpful feedback on his part.

Clearing the Pipes After He Comes

When a guy is masturbating, right after he comes he might reach into the perineum area (between his balls and butt) with his fingers to sort of push out any cum that's still in the pipes. Or he might push into the hidden part of the penis that's between his testicles to do the same thing. It's the post-jerk-off equivalent of wagging your penis after you pee.

While this would certainly be an advanced oral-sex technique that he wouldn't expect of most women, you might ask him about it and see if he can show you how to do it, assuming it's what he does.

What If He Doesn't Come?

This is a situation where one woman's blessing is another woman's curse. Some guys don't come from oral sex no matter how great your blowjob. If that's the case, you and he will need to settle on how long the blowjob should last. You will also need lots of reassurance from him about just how good the blowjob feels, and that he's just wired in such a way mentally or physically that this is not one of the ways he can ejaculate.

Pre-Cum Jitters

Some people who are giving oral sex experience a brief paralysis or mini-dread right before the penis ejaculates. If this keeps happening, try to talk to your partner about it. Maybe he can give you plenty of warning before he's going to come so you can stop sucking and start pumping by hand. Or maybe it will help to put a condom on his penis while giving blowjobs, or perhaps you can switch into the position we illustrated where you bring him off with your lips but the wad doesn't go in your mouth. With time and experience, it's likely any dread will go away.

Hands on Your Head

Men will often put their hands on a woman's head when she is giving oral sex. For most guys, this is a loving gesture which can also be used to let a partner know what feels good and what doesn't. However, some men will put their hands on a woman's head in an attempt to forcibly push it down onto the penis. This is rude, and you need to tell him to stop.

Counterpoint: One woman says, "It can be particularly exciting, when a man pushes my head down on his penis. But I would never have sex with a man who I didn't love going down on. Also, you make a joke out of it when a woman grabs a man's head and pulls it into her crotch in the prior chapter, but call it assault when a man does this to a woman. You present a double standard that says we women are either more fragile than men or more easily offended when it comes to sex."

Research Findings

One of the more interesting research findings of all time is in an article about the hazards of oral sex. It was written by a group of dentists and published in a medical journal (Bellizi, Krakow and Plack, *Military Medicine* 145 (1980):787—honest, his name is Dr. Plack and he's a dentist). The article is titled "Soft Palate Trauma Associated with Fellatio."

The article tells about the daughter of an officer who was taken to the base hospital because she discovered a black-and-blue blotch in the back of her mouth. Several dentists eventually converged on the mystery blotch, trying to discover its origin. After eliminating all other possibilities, the dentists finally asked the officer dad to leave the room and then popped the big question: "Gotta boyfriend?"

In the back of the mouth near where the tonsils hang is a highly vascularized mass of tissue (highly vascularized means lots of small blood vessels). An erect penis hitting against this sensitive tissue can cause a bruise.

This isn't a common injury. It goes away like any other bruise, but it is a reminder that the woman, and not the man, should control the level of movement during a blowjob. It's fine if she wants a lover to thrust in and out of her mouth, but the choice needs to be hers.

Ejaculate-Related Sinus Infections

When some women give blowjobs, they like to create a slight to moderate vacuum around their lover's penis. Men who enjoy this kind of sensation find it to be heavenly. However, a problem can occur when a man comes with the head of his penis in the back part of a woman's vacuum-pulling mouth. The vacuum can sometimes draw ejaculate up into the woman's sinus cavities, creating what might be a cum-related sinus infection. If this is the case, the woman and her partner need to work on keeping the head of his penis in the middle part of her mouth when he is coming. Another solution is for him to wear a condom.

Lasting Shorter (as Opposed to Lasting Longer)

"Why is it when you are giving men head, they take forever to come, but are so much faster when having intercourse?" *female age 29*

During vaginal intercourse, most guys make an effort to last as long as their partners want, sometimes successfully. While this might be a noble gesture during intercourse, it is not appreciated nearly as much during oral sex. That's because oral sex tends to tucker out the mouth of the giver. So if the purpose of the blowjob is to get the man off, he shouldn't try to hold back his climax just to show what a stud he is. On the other hand, some guys love oral sex but can't come from it. The best course of action is to discuss this matter with each other. If the male is one of those lucky guys who can pretty much orgasm at will, he and his partner might devise a signal for when she'd like him to come. For the rest of us, the woman can ease up if we are approaching orgasm too fast, or she can try some of the measures listed on pages 60-61 to speed us up if her jaw is about to drop off.

Do Men Blow Men Better Than Women Blow Men?

In researching different sexual techniques, we have reviewed many videos on sex. Videotapes made by women, many of whom are bisexual or lesbian, are often (although not always) a good source of information. The absolute worst source of information is traditional straight pornography.

It wasn't until this book was nearly finished that we took stock of the fact that no gay-male videos had been reviewed—except those on male genital massage. With this in mind, the following question about oral sex was posed:

"Is it possible that gay men give better blowjobs than straight women?"

Armed with several gay videos and lots of buttered popcorn, this question was examined by a small group of straight men and women, with the men being somewhat uncomfortable and the women being highly curious. The videos themselves caused a few unanticipated comments.

Most of the actors in the gay videos were exceptionally good-looking and appeared totally straight. At the very least, these men were more buff, attractive, and likable than some of the actors in traditional straight-porn movies. Upon making these discoveries, one female reviewer exclaimed, "It's a straight woman's nightmare: five naked men who are physical gods, and I couldn't get one of them to look at me if his life depended on it!" Another woman viewer stated: "It's one of the few times in my life when I wish I had a penis. I'd let that cute blond guy with the dimples suck on it all night long."

As for conclusions, it seemed that these men handled each other's bodies with a kind of skill and effectiveness that some straight women might do well to imitate. The one technical difference was that the gay men used their hands more than most women do when giving blowjobs. However, the real difference wasn't so much in technique but in intensity. It's difficult to put into words, but viewers had the feeling that the gay male actors seemed to form an intense relationship with the penis itself. No matter how much they might enjoy doing oral sex, few women make an emotional connection with a man's genitals in quite the same way as these gay men appeared to.

Granted, few people who have ever worked with actors consider them to be representative of average people. And this Guide's methodology is lacking in scientific rigor, but the conclusion is, yes, it's quite possible that gay men blow men better than women blow men, at least in porn movies.

In turning the question around, it can be asked if women do a better job of giving oral sex to women. The answer? Who knows, although one female reader who is bisexual was kind enough to offer the following comment:

"Having received oral sex from many men and women, I believe women's superiority at this activity is mostly myth."

An Oral-Sex Postscript over at the Beta House

Let's say a very straight, homophobic college fraternity man who prides himself on his conquests of women has just volunteered to take part in an experiment on sexual response. The researchers put EKG leads on his chest, blindfold him, restrain his hands and inform him that he is going to receive a blowjob from "a very sexy blond." After receiving the blowjob, he responds that she seemed to know more about how to please him orally than any sorority girl he's ever dated, and pleads for "her" phone number. The researchers then inform him that the sexy blond is a male who starred in one of the previously mentioned gay videos. As they show him a tape of this sexy blond giving him his blowjob, the identity meltdown begins. Suddenly, our fraternity brother's enthusiasm isn't quite the same and he's not sure if the blowjob was all that exceptional. More importantly, if this subject had been told the true identity of the sexy blond ringer before receiving the blowjob, it is likely that he wouldn't have been able to get an erection or ejaculate.

In this hypothetical experiment, our subject's pleasure was determined as much by his fantasy of who was giving the blowjob as the reality of it, assuming the blowjob was competently done. MORAL: Never underestimate the role of the human mind in determining what does and doesn't influence sexual outcomes and perceptions.

Things a Guy Can Do to Help a Woman Who Is Trying to Give Him Oral Sex

To help a partner give you the best blowjobs, you might start by re-reading earlier parts of this chapter about bruising in the back of a woman's throat, how she can prevent gagging, and how it can be nice when a guy doesn't last quite so long. Also try reading this chapter with your partner. The key to really good blowjobs is being willing to explore and give each other feedback.

Also, keep in mind that most women won't go down on guys who smell rank. Whether you are going out on a first date or have been married for twenty years, here are a few things to remember: #1: Shower at least once a day, unless you are seriously into grunge or are a holdover from the court of Louis XIII, in which case bathing is irrelevant. #2: Don't wear the same socks or underwear for more than one day without washing them. If everyone including the dog and cat runs out of the room when you take your shoes off, use foot powder or spray. #3: While not particularly popular with the organic crowd, deodorant can be a wonderful thing. #4: Brush and floss your teeth often, as kissing often precedes and follows a blowjob. #5: If you wear cologne, ask your partner or a woman friend how she likes the smell of it, as well as how much you should use. Some guys smell great from just bathing alone. On the other hand, she might like you marinated with a bit of citrus or spice.

Uncut? If you haven't noticed by now, this Guide abhors circumcision. However, all good things have their downsides, and smegma is one of the downsides of having a healthy, intact penis. So if you haven't taken a shower in a couple of hours, why not establish a pre-blowjob routine where you go to the bathroom, retract your foreskin, and tidy up a bit around it? And if you buy the sometimes silly theories of evolutionary biologists, anything they write about male smells being important in attracting females, they are referring to intercourse, and not when she has your penis in her face.

Pube Tug Tug on your pubic hair ahead of time so you'll pull out the strays that might end up in her mouth. It's now the height of straight male fashion to trim pubic hair as well. A few years ago this would have been considered weird.

Arrogance Don't assume that a woman automatically wants to suck on your penis just because it's there. (How would you like to suck some guy's dick?) Never take blowjobs for granted, and be thankful whenever you get one, even if your partner loves doing it. Tell her how good it feels. Also, it never hurts to ask yourself, "What have I done lately to deserve a blowjob?" Did you give your partner a long lingering body massage? Did you help her with a project she's been struggling with? Did you do more than your share of the housework? Did you respond kindly in a situation where most men would have been jerks? Are you a loving partner and good friend?

Talk Is Not Cheap Oral sex requires a doer who is willing to accept helpful feedback and a receiver who is willing to give it. If words don't come easily, pick up a book like Violet Blue's *Ultimate Guide To Fellatio* or Saddie Allison's *Tickle His Pickle* and go through it together.

Mutuality Never, ever cop an attitude such as "My last girlfriend blew me really well. Why can't you?" There are reasons why you aren't with your last girlfriend. With enough mutual caring, love and experimentation, the chances are good that you will soon be receiving oral sex, but don't expect it to happen magically.

The Deep-Throat Fantasy A throat is not a vagina. Any extra thrills you might get from this are mostly psychological. Besides, why would you encourage your partner to do something that might trigger a natural gagging reflex? If she gags on your penis, do you really think she's going to be excited about putting it in her mouth again?

He Who Gives, Gets A fine way to get great oral sex is to give great oral sex. This assumes that the rest of your relationship is in good shape. Do not expect that being a great lover will make up for being a selfish person. Some women will overlook bad manners and social lunacy for a good lay, but women who are so inclined tend to have their own emotional problems and will find other ways to make your life a living hell.

Asking vs. Not Asking

Every once in a while you might have a horrible day and are totally frazzled and in desperate need of a blowjob lest you further decompensate and have to be hauled off to the loony bin. If you don't abuse the privilege and have a loving partner who hasn't had an equally hideous day, she will usually do the mercy blowjob even if she's not particularly into it. For this type of situation, it is fine to ask or beg for a blowjob. However, in the course of normal lovemaking, it might not be such a good idea to routinely ask for oral sex. That's because some women don't take well to being pestered for blowjobs. Granted, they might love blowing you and will do so often, but only if it's on their own initiative. Of course, there are other women who are just fine with being asked. Why not ask about asking?

Improving the Way Your Ejaculate Tastes

Some people claim that vegetarians, both male and female, taste better than their carnivore brethren. However, it is likely that this is just propaganda from the cows and chickens. It has also been said that dairy products make ejaculate taste bad, but not nearly as bad as asparagus. Smoking and/ or drinking coffee might cause a guy's ejaculate to taste strong or bitter. Perhaps Starbucks can formulate a new blend of beans and call it "Sweet Tasting Wad." Regardless of their impact on semen, the combination of smoking and drinking coffee makes for bad-smelling breath. (Ejaculate, like cow's milk, can definitely take on flavors of what the beast eats, including its favorite vices.)

One woman said that her partner's ejaculate tasted good unless he was under a lot of stress at work. Then it would start tasting bad. This makes sense, and is reason to take long semen-rejuvenating vacations.

One common suggestion for improving the taste of male ejaculate is to eat celery or fruit each day, especially pineapple and apples. The sugar in the fruit is supposed to give a guy's ejaculate a sweet edge. Perhaps this is useless folklore. However, if this is what a partner requested before doing more blow-jobs, most guys would go to work each morning munching on stalks of celery and finishing their lunches with slices of fruit. Either way, if your partner is willing to be the taster, why not experiment with different combinations of food? Does ingesting a little cinnamon make a difference in the way you taste? What happens if you drink less coffee or eat less broccoli or garlic?

If your partner says that your ejaculate is really bitter, consider seeing a urologist to screen out the possibility of an infection in your prostate or other glands of sex. Although you might not be feeling any pain, it's still possible to have an infection. Unfortunately, in this day of HMOs, you will probably need to see a family physician or internist first, and it might be embarrassing to say, "Heather claims my cum tastes bitter. Can I see a doctor?" Urologists, on the other hand, see genitals all day long, and it's usually easier to say something like that to them. In either case, rather than telling the receptionist or nurse the exact reason for the appointment, you might say that you'd like to rule out a prostate or urinary-tract infection. Then tell the physician the real reason once you see him or her in private. And under no circumstances should you take antibiotics unless tests have been done and they show a problem. Antibiotics are not breath mints for the prostate gland.

Readers' Comments

"I am certain that women would give more blowjobs if they didn't feel like they had to swallow." *female age 43*

"Cum is not a gourmet treat, but not unpleasant. I'd rather be eating mocha-chip ice cream, but getting there isn't half as much fun. My partner's orgasm is often a total turn-on for me, and occasionally just a relief that the blowjob is now over with." *female age 47*

"If he smells bad down there, it's a turn-off for me." *female age 34*

"If I'm in the mood it's really sensual. If I'm not it's like a job." *fem, 43*

"It is a major power trip for me if he comes in my mouth. I like knowing I have the ability to take this big strong man and turn him into a sack of Jello." *female age 37*

"I used to tell my partner that I was semen-intolerant." *female age 26*

"I like running my tongue around the head and sliding it in and out of my mouth. I like to take his penis in my mouth as far as possible and rub my tongue on the underside of it, pushing the head into the roof of my mouth. It seems to drive him crazy." *female age 37*

"More than anything it feels so good because I am in control." *fem, 43*

"When it comes to blowjobs, let the lucky son of a bitch treat you like a queen, honey, because you are." *female age 48*

"I never was very good at blowjobs until I had a lover who had a small penis. Then I felt comfortable with him in my mouth." *female age 43*

"I like to give head, so I don't need much persuasion. I get really wet from giving someone that kind of pleasure, and I always feel so powerful when I do it." *female age 23*

"It feels very sensual if he lets me take it at my own pace. I think the penis has the most wonderful velvety skin." *female age 38*

"I only like it if I can keep the hair out of my mouth. I enjoy it only because I know he enjoys it so much." *female age 35*

"I like it. I especially like the little leaks before he comes. I think cum has an interesting taste, sort of fizzy." *female age 38*

"I have discovered that we both find it erotic to have him come on my face or on my breasts when I give him head. I don't care for the taste of his semen." *female age 22*

"I really don't like it when he comes in my mouth. I kind of gag on it."
female age 26

"It's fun to suck on a limp penis until it hardens." *female age 37*

"One thing that's really neat about sucking on a guy's cock is watching it change shape and color and get harder. You're right up there in the front row. You don't get that with intercourse." *female age 42*

"I've observed that not all guys come as much; some have very little, and others lots and lots." *female age 27*

"Never forget to caress and tickle the balls." *female age 44*

"My mouth and hand work as a team. As I pull away with my mouth, I twist my hand almost like a corkscrew." *female age 26*

"I love to give head, but I hate to feel pressured into doing it. Also, remember what goes around comes around. If I'm the only one going down, I'll be less likely to do so again." *female age 26*

"Please don't do it like they do in the porno flicks, where the girl just about bobs her head off. Not a turn-on." *male age 46*

"Don't be fooled by the name. Blowing has nothing to do with it."
male age 26

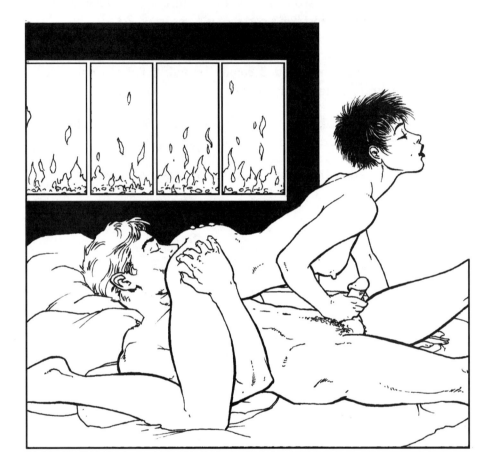

20
Oral Sex
Vulvas & Honeypots

Having powerful feelings for a woman can leave some men with an insatiable need to kiss and lick her genitals. It's hard to explain why, but it's a primal need that can be triggered by a mere wink of her eye. Other men are happy to give a woman oral sex because it pleases her sexually, but they aren't really into it. And some men would rather lick a cat.

Whatever your preference, this chapter is loaded with tips and techniques for giving a woman all of the oral pleasure her heart and thighs could possibly desire.

Talking to Elvis from between Your Sweetheart's Thighs

It's a funny thing about oral sex, at least when you are a guy on the giving end. The woman whom you are giving oral sex to, a person whom you know and often love, sometimes just disappears. All that's left is a strange, twitching, moaning protoplasm which only partially resembles the person who was there just minutes ago. You are left virtually alone, with your tongue feeling like it's running the Boston Marathon. You might as well be talking to Elvis. After it's over, you might want to ask, "Hey, where did you go?" but you learn not to because she'll usually just give you a big smile and want to curl up in your arms.

A female reader offers a possible explanation. She says that when she is receiving oral sex, she isn't as aware of her partner's presence, so it's easier to let her fantasies run wild. She wouldn't necessarily want to tell him "where she went," since her fantasy might have been with someone else. Little does she know, guys who are sexually secure might get off on hearing about her fantasy escapades, no matter who they are with.

Does She Want His Penis or His Mouth?

We have been asking women survey takers on *The Guide's* website if they had to choose between receiving oral sex and intercourse, which would it be. We assumed it would be an even split. No one anticipated that close to

95 out of every 100 women would say intercourse, hand's down. The deciding factor was intimacy over orgasms.

Of course, we also posed the question "Sex or chocolate?" and expected a 50-50 split, so what do we know? It turned out 97% for sex. Fortunately, when we have asked women specific questions about receiving oral sex, it has been abundantly clear that many love to be on the receiving end. And of those who don't, about half were concerned about the way they might taste, smell, or the way their labia look. So before this chapter starts to yodel at your sweetheart's yoni, it looks at her labia.

The Way Women Taste

Most carpet munchers know that some vulvas taste great, while others don't leave fond memories. Beyond that, men are fairly useless when it comes to discussing genital taste. Lesbian and bisexual women, however, will talk your ear off about the subject of how women taste:

> "One woman who I loved going down on suddenly began tasting different—not nearly as good. As it turned out, she had started taking vitamin pills. It was never a problem if she took herbs, but vitamin pills would ruin the way she tasted."

> "A former girlfriend was a tennis pro. Sometimes she would play tennis for a few hours and I could go down on her without her taking a shower and she would still taste sweet. There are other women whom I have gone down on right after we showered, and they still didn't taste good. In making my own inquiries, I found that the sweeter tasting women didn't eat red meat."

> "I watch my diet carefully, but I have to admit, the sweetest, best-tasting lover I ever had was a meat-eating, beer-drinking dietary disaster."

So much for consensus. Finally, a thought from the cleanest lesbian in all of Hackensack, New Jersey:

> "Some women spend more time filing their toenails than they do taking care of their pussies. When I'm in the shower, I always separate the lips of my vulva and wash between them. I'm also careful about little bad-tasting pieces of gunk that collect under my clitoral hood. These are what uncircumcised males get under their foreskin if they don't pull it back and clean it."

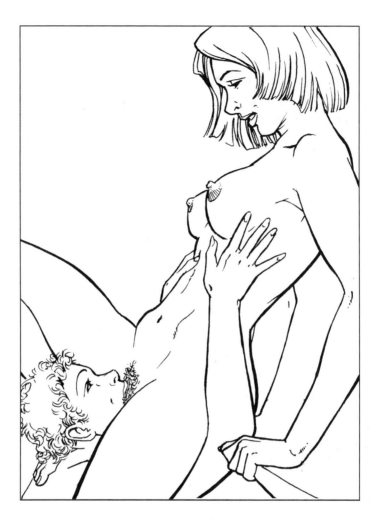

A Q-tip dipped in mineral oil works well to get rid of any "little pieces of gunk" that stick under the clitoral hood. When it comes to keeping your kitty happy (besides making sure it gets lots of oral sex), please see Chapter 51: "Vulva Care–Keeping Your Kitty Happy."

Lips in Photoshop

If you've been watching a lot of porn, keep in mind that pussy lips in porn are touched up with computer software. And women in porn tend to have funky surgical things done to their labia almost as often as they have them done to their breasts. Plastic surgeons would be smart to offer porn stars a two-for-the-price-of-one special, even if it's really four for the price of two. As Diana Cage, author of the excellent *Box Lunch: The Layperson's Guide to Cunnilingus*, says:

> "Lesbians are at an advantage in the vaginal knowledge department because we see our lovers' pussies all the time. We get up close and personal with real cunts in all of their real imperfection. But most straight women don't have the kind of access to vaginas that you get from licking box all the time. Many of my straight female friends have told me that the majority of up-close-and-personal views they've had of various vulvas have come from porn. And worse than that, some women feel insecure about their own coochies when they don't look like the ones in *Playboy.*

> "Well, let me just set the record straight: Cunts don't really look like that. Trust me. I'm a pornographer."

> —From Diana Cage's *Box Lunch: The Layperson's Guide To Cunnilingus,* Alyson Books, (2004).

So whether you are the lickee or the licker, you won't any more find perfection between a person's legs than you will find it between their ears. A lack of symmetry is one of the wonderful things about being human. So is going down on your girl.

Talking With Tongues—Suggestions for Pleasing a Woman with Your Mouth

According to some women, a smart and loving tongue between their legs can offer feelings of pleasure that fingers or a penis simply can't. Yet many a male merely pushes his face into a woman's crotch, sticks his tongue out like when the doctor asks you to say "ahhh" and wags away. What follows are suggestions to help cure a chronic case of tongue wagging.

On the Tip of Your Tongue

The human tongue, like the penis, can be made hard or soft. To understand the difference between a soft and a hard tongue, spend a few minutes licking the palm of your hand. This may not be as much fun as when LuLu sits on your face, but a moment's practice on the palm of your hand can be a good way to learn about subtle variations in oral-sex technique.

First, if you've just been installing a new head gasket or fertilizing the lawn, it might be a good idea to wash your hands. Then, pretend your palm is a woman's vulva and give it a good licking.

Notice how quickly the end of your tongue goes dry. So much for the fantasy that the human tongue is always wet. A dry tongue creates drag or friction. Nature did not create the clitoris with a high tolerance for friction. In fact, nature did not create the clitoris with very much tolerance for friction at all.

This is why you'll need to coat your tongue with saliva before licking a woman's private parts. After a few minutes, saliva from your mouth will automatically run down your tongue and keep everything well-lubricated, but not at the start. (There's nothing wrong with keeping a bottle of water or good-tasting lube by your side when you are giving your lover a licking.)

Try licking your hand again. You may find that your tongue is somewhat taut with the tip hard and pointed. Try to let it go soft, in a way that would cause you to slur your words if you were attempting to speak. You may need to push your hand closer to your face, since a soft tongue is not as long as a hard tongue. Some women will prefer a softer, more rounded tongue when you are licking the underbelly of the clitoris, given how it isn't insulated by the clitoral hood. On the other hand, if she's highly aroused, she might want the tip of your tongue to feel like an arrowhead.

This may all sound like French if you have yet to go down on a woman. Not to worry; no matter how experienced you might be, she will still need to teach you where and how she wants you to lick. This can take a while. Also, it's normal to feel clumsy when you are with a new lover or if you haven't performed oral sex in a while.

The Mood Is Much More Important Than the Method

While there is much in this chapter about different things you can do with your mouth and fingers once you get them between your lover's thighs, equally important is taking your time getting there. In fact, if your put your lips on a woman's crotch before she's nearly begging for it, you are working against yourself and particularly against your poor jaw.

A wet tongue is not an antidote for an unaroused clitoris—fantasy, romance, teasing, kissing, caressing and the early stages of sexplay are. Your tongue can only amplify what you've already got going on down there through other means. Your tongue is totally useless if the anticipation and desire for it aren't there.

The Initial Approach — Getting There

"Gentle teasing brings me to an orgasm. I like him to start off gently, with light licks and kisses all over my vulva. I can't take too much pressure on my clitoris, though, and sometimes that ruins it for me."

female age 23

The best approach to a woman's genitals is anything but direct, especially if you are hooking up or it's a new relationship and you don't know what she likes. Once you've been with a woman for a while, you will discover what body parts she likes to have licked. One woman might love it when you kiss her inner thighs or rear end, but hate it if you kiss her abdomen. Another woman might want the opposite. Find the body parts that she likes having kissed and caressed, and spend plenty of time on them. Work your way down slowly, planting occasional kisses on her vulva, but only as a preview of what's to come. An indirect approach helps assure a warm welcome when your face finally drops into your lover's saddle.

Kansas Or the Yellow Brick Road?

Think about it, what was more exciting, the journey down the Yellow Brick Road, or the balloon trip back to Kansas? Some men think they haven't pleased a woman unless they have given her an orgasm. That would be fine if sex were football and orgasms were touchdowns, but this kind of philosophy can spoil your love life. It means that instead of trying to delight your lover's senses, you'll always be playing to her clitoris. This can get tedious.

Of course, there are times when it's important to be single-minded about a woman's orgasm, but not as a rule. You will do better if you let yourself have fun, be close and want her dearly. If your lips convey this when they are working their way toward her thighs, you'll have a leg up on most other men.

Avoiding Beard Burn

When it comes to receiving oral sex, one thing that women often complain about is men's beards. Their advice: grow a full beard or keep your face clean-shaven. Grunge is not good on a woman's thighs. Five o'clock shadow is even worse on a shaven or bare vulva. It doesn't have the pillow of pubic hair to protect it.

If you are the kind of guy who grows a five o'clock shadow ten minutes after shaving, find a favorite set of towels and drape one over each of her legs, like mechanics do on the fenders of cars when they are working on the engine. Talk to your partner about this and see if it would help.

Three Oral Sex Caveats

#1 Until shown otherwise, don't assume there are similarities between the way you like your penis sucked and the way your partner likes having her genitals licked (a corollary from the chapter "The Zen of Finger Fucking").

#2 If your main exposure to oral sex has been through watching porn videos, forget all you have seen. So you, the viewer, can see what's going on, the porn industry has invented its own version of oral sex. In porn oral sex, a woman sits with her legs six miles apart while a guy tries to lick her vulva without blocking the camera shot. While this is good for the cameraman, it's not going to please a woman.

#3 A mediocre lover always knows what his or her partner wants without having to ask. An accomplished lover implores a partner to provide copious amounts of advice.

Body Positions

There are some oral-sex positions that might look great, but don't work as well as others. What follows is a description of oral-sex positions where your bodies are both pointing in the same direction. These provide the best face-to-vulva alignment, where your tongue has clear access to the tip and shaft of the clitoris. In this alignment, you will be licking in an upward direction. This gives you the most options, especially if she likes you to retract her clitoral hood and lick the underbelly of her clitoris.

To start with, imagine that you are standing in a swimming pool and the lucky lady is sitting on your shoulders. Only she is turned around so you are staring into her stomach and her feet are dangling over your shoulders. You are getting a mouthful of bathing-suit-crotch material, but this beats the heck out of anything you ever learned in Red Cross swimming lessons. Envision yourself falling forward, so she lands on her back and you are on your stomach. You will be staring up at her navel. One disadvantage of this position is that your head is looking up and this causes your neck to bend backward. This can be uncomfortable after awhile, and it is not a position you want to be in if she's on Prozac and takes an hour to come.

For the second oral-sex position, which might be more comfortable than the first, go back to the swimming pool and imagine the two of you falling to one side or the other. You land on your sides, except for your head which is between her legs. Your mouth is on her crotch, and her inner thigh becomes a pillow for your head. Your neck doesn't have to bend backward as it does in the first position, since you can move your entire body to form more of a right angle to hers. One disadvantage of this "sides" position is that you don't have the full access and degree of control that you do when her legs are spread apart. So some guys will start off in the first position, when her clit is more sensitive and mouth and tongue control are more critical. Then they ask the woman to roll on her side so they can get into a more comfortable position and keep at it for as long as she likes. Another disadvantage of this position is if she's got really strong thigh muscles and clamps her thighs together when she comes. Big Time Wrestling is not what you were bargaining for.

In another oral-sex position, she is "sitting on your face." Go back to the swimming pool and imagine you fell straight backward. You end up on your back and she's above you on all fours. The term "sitting on your face" is rife with deception. While it might look as if she is sitting on your face, she shouldn't be. It might feel good to have her in this position over your face, but the human face isn't the most comfortable object to sit on. As an alternative, she might want to stay on all fours, with you propping your head and upper body on a bunch of pillows to give your lips the necessary altitude.

Another good position for giving a girl oral sex is when she is sitting in a chair or on a stool, with you sitting or kneeling between her legs. She'll need to slouch so you don't get a mouthful of chair cushion, oak or leatherette.

There are other positions, like if you were doing 69. In these positions, your head is pointing in the opposite direction from hers and the alignment is not optimal. With time, you may evolve your own variations, but these are excellent no matter how experienced you are.

Protect Your Neck

Whenever you fly on a plane, the attendants instruct the passengers that in the event of an emergency, they are to first put the airmasks on themselves and then on their children. A similar philosophy should be employed regarding your neck during oral sex. If your neck is in a strange position or making a strange angle, you won't have the stamina to do a good job. First and foremost, make sure your neck is comfortable. Always assume that you may be in this position for longer than anticipated. Sometimes much longer.

Pillows to the Rescue

As with any kind of sexual activity, a strategically placed pillow under your partner's bum can provide better access to her genitals. Also, don't hesitate to put a pillow under your head if it makes you more comfortable.

Some vendors such as Libida.com sell a special cushion wedge for help with oral sex called The Liberator (www.liberator.com). It is not cheap, but you might want to check it out. If you can't afford it, it is possible you've got something around that might work as well.

Ground Zero

Perhaps you are a total pro at giving oral sex, or maybe you know more about the dark side of the moon than licking a woman's genitals. Regardless of your experience, what follows is a blueprint for giving really good oral sex—as long as you get reliable feedback from the woman you are doing it with.

💡 The tongue can be an abrasive little organ unless it is lubricated. Coat your lips and tongue with extra saliva as you approach your lover's vulva.

💡 Oral sex tends to make your salivary glands sing. Instead of swallowing or letting it pool in your mouth, let your slobber flow wherever gravity wants to take it. That way, you won't have to worry as much about pubic hairs wrapping themselves around your tonsils each time you try to swallow. Putting a towel under your sweetheart's rear will help to keep the mattress from turning into a lovemaking lagoon. Some women will appreciate it if you push an edge of the towel against the area that's just below their vulva so the saliva doesn't trickle down their butt crack.

💡 When a woman flexes her legs, her pelvis arches forward. This will provide access to give good oral sex. A lot of women will do this themselves by putting their legs over your shoulders, or by planting one or both feet on your shoulders. Some pull their legs up to their chest. The guy can also wrap his arms around the back of the woman's thighs and push them forward.

💡 As a woman becomes more aroused, she might want to change leg position or flex her thighs to help get her off. This could limit your access to her vulva, but if it's what does the trick, so be it.

💡 Some women provide all the oral access a man needs by simply spreading their legs. On the other hand, you may want to separate the outer labia with your fingers. This gives your mouth better access to the inner lips, and can sometimes feel like the difference between kissing a woman whose mouth is open versus one whose lips are closed. Some women will offer a helping hand by separating the lips themselves.

🔆 Lavish the outer lips with licks and kisses. Then try running the tip of your tongue up and down the furrows between the outer and inner lips of your lover's vulva.

🔆 The mons pubis is the little mound of flesh that sits directly above the labia. It is where the bulk of the pubic hair grows. Some women enjoy it if you rub the mons in a circular pattern. Also, pushing or pulling up the mons while doing oral sex can heighten the intensity for some women.

🔆 Some women will enjoy it if you run your fingertips through their pubic hair, and some will particularly enjoy it if you tug lightly on it or nibble gently on the mons.

🔆 The inner lips of women's genitals tend to be longer around the vaginal opening. Some are prominent enough to clasp between your fingers and tug upon gently. When a woman is highly aroused, she may enjoy this tremendously. Be sure to ask!

Her Clitoris

"Don't immediately dive into the clitoris and stay there. Warm up by licking all of the vaginal area. Suck on the labia. Then turn your attention to the clitoris. I like my clitoris to be licked, flicked and sucked. Sometimes I get off faster if my partner licks lower on the clitoris, rather than at the top of the hood. It makes for a different kind of orgasm." *female age 25*

No matter how small your penis is, nobody's going to have trouble finding it. However, nature designed the average clitoris to play a mean game of hide 'n' seek.

After you kiss and caress the other parts of the vulva, some women will appreciate it if you focus your oral efforts in the vicinity of the clitoris. "Vicinity" might mean simply in the neighborhood, or it might mean knocking on the front door. Sometimes all it takes to expose the tip of the clitoris is a single finger to pull the hood up. Sometimes it takes both hands and a litany of prayer.

To find the tip with your tongue, separate the outer lips with your fingers. Make sure your tongue has plenty of saliva on it for lubrication. Take a long slow lick from the bottom to the top of the vulva where the big lips meet. Somewhere along the way you will most likely feel a small knob or slight protuberance. Find out from your partner if this is the tip of her clitoris. Have her explain to you exactly how she likes it licked.

As your sweetheart becomes aroused, it is likely that the tip of her clitoris will swell. Some swell predictably; others don't. This process can be challenging until you become more familiar with the way her clitoris changes. With some women, you learn to lick on a specific spot rather than relying on finding her clitoris with your tongue. You simply go on faith and past experience.

You might think that the surest way to arouse a woman would be to start at the tip of the clitoris, since that's where so much of the action seems to be. But this is not the way it usually works. For most women, you don't even approach the clitoris until you have planted plenty of kisses in the surrounding area. With some women, you never touch the tip at all. Of course, if your lover wants you to start by throwing a liplock on the tip of her clitoris, far be it from this Guide to suggest anything different.

Some women enjoy it if you kiss their vulva in the same way that you do their mouth. Some crave a gentle nursing action on the clitoris. Some like it if you flick the tip of your tongue over the clitoris in a sideways direction; others prefer an up-and-down motion as though you were rapidly turning a light switch on and off, and some enjoy a circular motion. These different motions may seem awkward at first, but you will eventually learn to flick your tongue back and forth (or is it hither and yon?) with enough grace to humiliate a hummingbird. Also, some women will want you to speed up or change locations as their arousal grows, while others prefer a constant motion.

Your partner might have a favorite side of her clitoris where she wants you to lick. To help improve access to the favored side, she might try flexing one leg while the other lies flat and a bit to the side.

The clitoris sometimes disappears right before orgasm. Who knows why, but it is almost always good news. With helpful input from your partner you will eventually learn how to respond; in the meantime, let The Force guide you. (When a clitoris disappears on you, you might try giving a little suck to pull it back out.)

After learning more about your partner's responses, you might experiment by puckering your lips around her clitoris and making a light vacuum.

You can then push the clitoris in and out of your mouth either with your tongue or by reversing the suction every couple of seconds. Tricks like this can be found in Ray Stubbs's book *The Clitoral Kiss*, Secret Garden Press.

Your partner's clitoris or the area around may begin to pulse once she is highly aroused. This is probably an indication to stay your course without any variation in speed, tempo or rhythm. Problems start when you assume that if she's pulsing at this speed, she'll love it even more if you double the tempo or do it harder. This is a mistake. These pulses happen every second or so and seem to be in direct response to the stimulus of your tongue. If you speed up, you will quickly lose them.

The contractions of orgasm are said to happen every seven-tenths of a second. Some men say the best way to stimulate a woman's clitoris either by mouth or by hand is to use strokes that last seven-tenths of a second. Good luck making that one work.

Some women prefer to receive different kinds of stimulation depending on the time of the month. For instance, at one point in her menstrual cycle you avoid the tip or glans, but two weeks later you lick the tip silly. It's nothing you're going to learn in a one-night stand, and these changes don't apply for a lot of women.

Body Language Rather than Words

Some women reach a certain threshold of arousal where they can't tell which direction your tongue is moving. All they know is if it feels good or not. Be sure to pay close attention to your partner's body language as your tongue touches her exposed clitoris. If her body suddenly convulses or jolts, you have probably hit the right area but too early or with too much force. It never hurts to retreat and find a safe spot that's protected by plenty of hood. She will usually let you know when she wants more. The ways she might do this include telling you, pulling your head into her body with her hands, or grinding her crotch into your face. Hopefully she won't grab you by the ears, although men's ears make fine rudders for oral sex.

Unless she is in the throes of orgasms, if she is moving her hips, squirming or trying to move your head, the chances are good you aren't getting your tongue where she needs it to be, or how she wants it to be. It is also very possible that you are licking too hard. The only way you will ever find out is by asking her.

Her Vagina and Beyond

Using terms like "urinary meatus" or "the area around her peehole" can cause an aesthetic flat tire. However, the part of a woman's vulva between her clitoris and vagina which contains the urinary meatus is definitely worth exploring with the tip of your tongue. For some women its stimulation might be the difference between good oral sex and great oral sex. If you have aesthetic problems with this notion, think about what your lover dips the tip of her tongue into when she is sucking on the head of your penis. Also keep in mind that urine and the urinary passageway are more sanitary than the human mouth and that kissing her down here is more hygienic than kissing her on the mouth.

The opening of the vagina is in the lower half of a woman's vulva. A man might occasionally be swept away by an urge to stick his tongue far into his lover's vagina. This, of course, is ridiculous unless he has the same gene pool as Lassie. Still, it's a nice thing to do, or want to do. Realistically, your tongue will be able to stimulate the outer edges of your partner's vagina and maybe an inch or two inside of it. This is good, because it's the part of the vagina that responds best to touch. Reaching too far inside a woman's vagina can cause your tongue to get a nasty cramp.

Some women may treasure a finger or two inside the vagina during oral sex, but usually not until they have reached higher levels of arousal. As for what to do with your fingers once they are inside, you will need to ask. Some women like them to stay perfectly still, while others will enjoy it if you twist, jiggle or thrust your fingers in and out. Also, there might be special spots in her vagina that your partner enjoys having stimulated.

The inner part of a woman's vagina often balloons open when sexually aroused. A number of women enjoy having this filled up. While a man's fingers will usually do the job, some women find that a silicone dildo works better. For some couples, inserting a dildo during oral sex can be a turn-on. Also, a woman might fantasize about having one man's penis inside her vagina at the same time that another man is licking her clitoris. Using a dildo while receiving oral sex can help satisfy this fantasy unless you are actually into threesomes. (There are actually oral sex dildos that strap on a guy's chin!)

One highly-athletic advisor to this Guide so loved doing oral sex on his women friends in school that he was considered an important resource off the court as well as on. His secret? When a woman was about to have an orgasm, he would gently insert a fingertip into her rectum. He says this would invariably launch a cascade of pleasure. There is no need to stick your finger in very far; just putting pressure on the rim around a lover's anus might light up thousands of nerve endings whose sole experience to that point has been to endure storms of methane and toilet-paper abuse. A variation is to insert a well-lubricated butt plug or vibrator in the woman's rear while doing oral sex. Just don't put this or your fingers in her vagina afterward.

You can always go for a triple play: lips on her clitoris, one finger in her vagina and one up her rear.

Some women push a man's head away from their vulva after they begin to come. Others pull it in tighter. Don't fret if she pushes it away. This will give your tongue a well-earned rest. Also, some women are extremely sensitive after orgasm, when barely breathing on their genitals can hurt.

If She Starts Bucking

It's not unusual for some women who are receiving oral sex to start bucking their hips with pleasure when they are having an orgasm. This kind of motion can knock a guy off her mound.

While it is important to discuss this with your partner, a response that some women appreciate is as follows: Wrap your arms around her thighs from behind, as in the illustration. Put your hands firmly on her hip bones. The female hip bones provide a perfect handle and were clearly put there for this very purpose. Flex your arms so that she has to lift the weight of your upper body in order to buck. This shouldn't hurt her at all and will keep her pelvis still enough so you can give her more of what's causing her to buck in the first place.

Fun at The Y

🔅 Find out if your sweetheart likes you to play with her breasts or other body parts while you are going down on her. One reader loves her partner to squeeze her toes when she is receiving oral sex—it can be the difference between coming or not for her.

🔅 Here's a game suggested in *Ultimate Kiss* by Jacqueline and Steven Franklin. Bring your lover to the edge of orgasm with oral sex and then pull your mouth away for a count of fifty. Then bring her to the edge again and

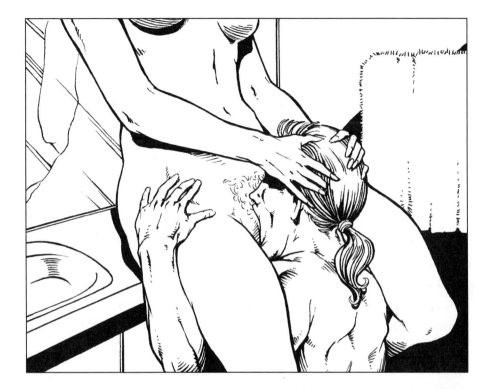

pull your mouth away for twenty-five seconds. Then bring her to the edge and pull your mouth away for ten seconds. Do this once more, pausing for just a few seconds. Be sure to explain this game beforehand so she doesn't become seriously annoyed when you stop for the first fifty-second pause. One female reader suggests that this game can work equally well when masturbating a woman.

Sometimes it is fun to give a woman oral sex when she is still wearing her panties or bikini bottom. Start with your lips on her inner thighs, work them up to her crotch, and then sneak your tongue under the material. Eventually push the material to one side with your tongue, teeth or fingers. This will provide more working room. Some women might like it if you blow warm moist air through the front panel of their underwear. But never blow air directly into a woman's vagina.

Consider pulling your lover's panties off with your teeth. But be careful not to leave any holes or rip the material, given how lingerie can often cost an arm and a leg; it's best that she not remember you as the one who destroyed her favorite undies. Then again, the memory might bring quite a smile!

💡 It is difficult to do oral sex when a woman is standing. The access is too limited. Think nothing of crawling under her dress when she is standing to plant tender kisses in places where other guys only dream of touching, but she'll need to sit or lie down to receive your oral finest.

💡 After she is highly aroused, place the tip of your tongue on the side or bottom of her clitoris. Then push the tip of a small vibrator on the other side of your tongue.

💡 Separate the outer lips with your fingers and lay your tongue flat against her vaginal opening at the lowest part of her vulva. Take a slow, long, wet lick that lasts for about 60 seconds. This way, her clit gets a slow protracted licking as your tongue creeps up her vulva.

💡 Some women like so many pillows under their rear end that their entire body is on an incline with their crotch angled up in the air. This provides great access plus an intriguing view. And your neck doesn't cramp.

💡 A more subtle way of making your tongue vibrate is to hum while placing it on your partner's clitoris. A well-hummed aria can push some women into orbit. Others will start laughing hysterically.

💡 On a hot muggy day, ice cubes can always spice up any kind of sex play. Some women enjoy an occasional ice cube in the vagina. If you try this, use small cubes that won't cause frost burn. During the cold of winter, sipping a warm drink before kissing a woman's vulva can leave her with warm and sensual feelings.

💡 Some couples enjoy placing a slice of banana, mango or papaya inside a woman's vagina for the man to retrieve with his tongue, as long as she is not prone to fruit-induced infections. You may need to douche to get out any remaining fruit if your man is a sloppy eater. Honey and syrup should be used with caution. While they are fine on nipples and other parts of the body, residual sugar in the vagina might inspire its resident yeast cells to procreate with painful delight. This may not be a problem for most women, but is worth noting.

💡 There are special swings that are great for doing oral sex. They can be hung from a door jamb or ceiling rafter. The swing spreads the woman's legs and places her at the perfect height for a man to give her oral sex while he is sitting upright. Beware: many swings are poorly made and uncomfortable. You'll need to shell out a lot for a good one.

🔆 Some couples occasionally pour champagne into a woman's vagina when her legs are elevated. (Vamosa?) Her partner then licks out the champagne, although this is not recommended for men in twelve-step programs or for women whose vaginal tissue might become irritated. (The sugar in the champagne can cause a yeast infection.) An extremely dry champagne with low residual sugar might be preferable. Avoid putting cold duck in a woman's crotch, although a loving goose on her rear is usually welcome.

🔆 Some women have a problem with being kissed on the face after being kissed on the crotch. If that's the case in your household, consider keeping a wet washcloth handy. Run it across your face before kissing above after kissing below.

Safety Note: It can be very sexy to blow warm moist air over your lover's vulva, but very dangerous for her to blow air into her vagina. Never lock your lips on your partner's vulva and blow air into it, unless your partner is made of plastic and is inflated that way.

Female Fluid Flow

Some women who are highly aroused expel fluid from their vulva around the same time that they have an orgasm. One female reader who gushes says that her male partner finds it exciting. Guys who are fluid-shy should discuss it with their partners and explore ways of ducking when the tsunami begins.

If your partner gushes and you have a problem with it, take solace in knowing that you've done something incredibly right to get her there.

Feeling Like a Crash-Test Dummy

Some women are not particularly subtle when it comes to signaling their oral sex wants and desires. In fact, it is not unheard of for a woman in the heat of oral passion to grab a man's skull and yank it one way or another with enough force to cause whiplash.

If she grinds your face into her crotch with a nose-flattening swoosh, she probably wants you to up the tempo or pressure a bit. But don't be silly and let your tongue go full throttle, because this might cause her to whip your head in the opposite direction. Learning to shift tongue-gears gradually can add years to the life of your neck.

Neck Pain, Lock Jaw & Tongue Cramping

Tongue cramping and jaw paralysis are common side effects of giving oral sex. These usually occur just moments before the woman blurts out, "There, that's perfect, don't stop!" Being able to continue when every ligament and muscle fiber from your neck up is screaming for mercy is what separates the oral-sex men from the oral-sex boys.

With experience, you will discover which positions land you in traction. Do not suffer in silence. Discuss this with your partner so you can find positions that are mutually pleasing. That way you'll be able to give her more of what she likes. And don't hesitate to give your mouth a breather by gently replacing the tip of your tongue with the tip of your wet finger.

Damn Those Dental Dams & Latex Beaver Tarps

Several years ago, some bozo decided that the way to safely go down on a woman was to spread a dental dam over her crotch. Why not just use neoprene or Naugahyde?

Lately, they've come up with an alternative that's supposedly thinner and more lick-friendly. It may be made for vulvas instead of molars, but good luck. First of all, you have no clue what you're licking. It might as well be the president's face under there. And then there's the texture problem. Try whipping your tongue back and forth over latex. No matter how much slobber you throw on it, your tongue drags and your RPM rating goes to hell. A more satisfactory barrier is Saran Wrap. You can see through it, it doesn't slow your tongue action, and you can always re-use it afterward to cover the Peach Melba or Apple Brown Betty.

When a Woman Doesn't Like Her Own Body

"I have a lot of hang-ups about oral sex because I think the guy wants to get out of there as soon as possible. So I need to be reassured you really enjoy it. The orgasm I have with oral sex is the most wonderful, but it often takes a long time and would try the patience of anyone." *female age 38*

Some women don't like their bodies and are uncomfortable when a man has a close-up view. If this is the case in your relationship, it might help ease your partner's mind to do oral sex with the lights out. On the other hand, if your partner is looking for an excuse to feel bad about herself, she will assume that you turned the lights out because you find her body ugly. Either way, it never hurts to talk about this. One possible solution is to start doing oral sex when the two of you are in the shower. She might feel more comfortable with this, reassured that she is clean enough for you to enjoy.

Maintaining a Hard-On While Giving Oral Sex

If a guy is giving his sweetheart oral sex, it might be nice if he kept doing it long enough to get her off. But once he feels his hard-on starting to go, a man will sometimes surface from between a woman's legs and try to have intercourse before it's "too late." Otherwise he feels unmanly about his penis going soft.

So why does a man sometimes lose his erection while going down on a woman? First of all, doing oral sex requires the kind of concentration that isn't always conducive to maintaining an erection. It's a little like playing catch or strumming a guitar, things that can be immensely enjoyable but don't necessarily make a guy hard. Also, for some men, doing oral sex on a woman can bring up all sorts of primal feelings that aren't fully in sync with getting a hard-on. These can be pleasant and even deeply moving feelings, but they might not be the stuff that erections are made of. For other guys, it's instant wood when tongue touches thigh.

There is also the matter of mouth fatigue. It's not easy to keep a hard-on when your tongue and jaw start cramping. On the other hand, it's kind of fun to see how far you can lick a lover into an altered state of consciousness even if you can't talk too well afterward.

Whatever the cause, it's not unusual for a man to lose his erection when he is going down on a woman, but not because he is unhappy or a wimp. Women might consider what a drag it would be if they had to stay hard while doing oral sex. Nobody ever gets on their case for losing an erection.

Things a Woman Can Do to Help a Partner Who Is Going Down on Her

Here are suggestions for women who like to receive oral sex:

Tugging on Your Bush Take a moment to tug on your bush before your man goes down. You'll pull out the loose hairs that would otherwise end up sticking to the back of his throat.

Trimming Your Triangle While some women feel that trimming the triangle defiles the natural appearance of the female body, others take pride in showing off more of their genitals. A woman so inclined shouldn't hesitate to put her lover in charge of muff maintenance and coiffure. Many men find this a joyful duty.

Labia Laundering Separating the labia and washing between them once a day will help to keep your genitals clean and tasty. Douching usually isn't necessary nor advisable, and avoid soap that is scented or is alkaline.

Not Helpful Women who think that their own genitals are dirty or not likable seldom do themselves any favors when it comes to oral sex. For instance, a guy might be having a wonderful time kissing and caressing his partner's genitals when she suddenly pulls him up because she's decided that he surely can't be enjoying something "as gross as that." If a woman fears that her genitals don't taste good, she should ask her partner. And if she feels there is something bad about her genitals, she should tell her partner lest he feel hurt by her rejecting behavior. Perhaps his reassurance will be helpful. On the other hand, if it's something that genuinely makes her feel uncomfortable, then he shouldn't keep trying to do it.

Information As long as it's done with sensitivity, most men will appreciate any input or suggestions that a woman has about giving her oral pleasure. If you feel shy, hand your lover a copy of this chapter or Violet Blue's *Ultimate Guide to Cunnilingus* or Diana Cage's *Box Lunch* and ask if he'll read it with you. And if your man's ego is so fragile that he can't handle your input, perhaps he would do better with a mindless partner who has no input to give. If you aren't equal partners in sex, you aren't equal partners, period. Is that what you want?

Masturbating Don't hesitate to reach down and masturbate while your partner is doing oral sex. Of course, this may be more easily said than done, so be sure to let him know that you want him to keep licking. While this can be fun, it may require some interesting tongue-finger logistics.

Attitude Issues There is a section at the end of the preceding chapter on blow jobs that is similar to this, only it is addressed to men. You might look over the parts titled "Attitude Issues." If the shoe fits...

Humor Next to bathing, humor is the most important sex aid there is. Try not to forget this.

Oral Sex during Her Period

Some couples are fine with oral sex while the woman is having her period; others wait a few days until the flow has stopped. Here are some solutions if you want the action but not the extra nutrition:

Instead, The Keeper, Diva Cup These are tampon alternatives that collect menstrual flow inside the vagina. They work well for oral sex during your period. Pop one in before oral sex and it will catch most if not all of the bloody flow. These are not for birth control.

Tampons A woman who is menstruating can insert a tampon before a man goes down on her. The tampon will usually catch most of the flow, assuming that you don't attempt to tickle the woman's cervix with the tip of your tongue. If you douche before putting the tampon in, which might do more harm than good, consider using a gentle solution with a lower pH.

Diaphragm Some women get a diaphragm for the sole purpose of having sex during their periods. The diaphragm becomes a barrier that traps the menstrual flow. Some couples use the diaphragm for oral sex but not for intercourse, since period flow can help make intercourse feel extra nice.

Plastic Wrap A simple way of dodging menstrual flow is by putting plastic wrap over the woman's vulva before going down on her.

NOTE Little if anything is known about the risks of AIDS transmission when doing oral sex on a woman who having her period, but it is a way to give and get hepatitis. A conservative approach is in order if the woman has any sexually transmitted infections. You should never do unprotected oral sex on a partner if you have a canker sore or active oral herpes in your mouth, or if your partner has a herpes outbreak on his or her genitals.

Sixty-Nine

69 is when a man does oral sex on a woman at the same time that she does oral sex on him.

There are plenty of couples who enjoy oral sex but don't necessarily like doing 69. That's because when a person is on the receiving end of oral sex, he or she might want to kick back and not have to worry about getting the other person off. On the other hand, some couples enjoy 69 as their favorite way of having sex. 69 might also be good for people who can't tolerate receiving pleasure without giving it at the same time, or vice versa. 69 should also be avoided if either partner involuntarily clenches his or her jaw when having an orgasm.

Readers' Comments

"Get a good rhythm going. Don't suck or lick too hard on the head of the clit. Also, either be smooth-shaved or have a beard, but no in-between. Beard burn really kills down there!" *female age 45*

"Stubble on the face is not welcome in tender areas down below."
female age 48

"Please quit when I say so; it gets really tender and ticklish after I come." *female age 43*

"Lick around the area of the clitoris, not directly on it, until I am more aroused and then only part of the time." *female age 35*

"Start out slowly, working around the outer area with your tongue. Don't just push in. Do a lot of gentle rubbing and caressing on the insides of the leg. Gradually probe the vulva with your tongue. Develop a rhythm and keep going until I come." *female age 32*

"If my partner's tongue gets tired, he uses his finger and sometimes it feels the same." *female age 25*

"I like a man to first shave me smooth, then gently kiss and finger me." *female age 34*

"It's great when he puts a finger into my rear while giving me oral sex. It makes for quite the explosion!" *female age 38*

21
Body Massage
The Ultimate Tenderness

I n doing research for this book, almost every way that humans give each other sexual pleasure was considered. Attempts were made to view sex through the eyes of mate-swappers, Tantric-sex masters, gays, lesbians, conservative born-again Christians, bondage enthusiasts, and those whose sex lives are really boring. Having left no sexual stone unturned, one and only one universal truth about human sexuality emerged:

No matter what your sexual beliefs, fantasies, kink, or persuasion, nothing beats a good back rub.

Nobody, absolutely nobody, had a single bad thing to say about a good back rub. Ditto for foot massage.

Hard vs. Soft? Male vs. Female?

Just about every book ever written on sex loves to state that men touch women too hard, and that women touch men too soft. Baloney, says a straw poll taken by the Goofy Foot Press. There are two types of touch that both men and women like a great deal:

Feather-light to Light This is where the fingertips lightly dance across the surface of the skin, resulting in a delightful tingling sensation that may or may not raise goosebumps. It can also be done with the flat of the hand doing light, long, gentle strokes.

Deep & Hard This is when muscles are kneaded with a strength and authority that chases away stress and tension. The men commented that they often fear they are doing this too hard, but their female partners almost always say it's just right or to do it harder.

Fortunately, numerous books on touch and massage have been published in the last twenty years. There are also several nicely done videos on the subject. An hour spent reading one of these books or watching a tape will probably do more for your relationship than a lifetime of looking at *Cosmo* or *Playboy*. Pay special attention to the chapters on foot rubs, hand rubs, and scalp and facial massages. These body parts are often ignored because they aren't considered blue-chip erogenous zones.

Spectators vs. Participants

Some people struggle to get fully into their bodies. Some have trouble relaxing enough to enjoy what is being shared with them sexually. They need to be hypervigilant about what is going on around them. The same thing happens when a person always needs to perform and has difficulty becoming passive enough to allow sexual things to happen to his or her body.

Learning to massage and be massaged is one way that might help you to relax your body's armor. This might be anxiety-producing at the start, so go slowly and try to enjoy the gains you are able to make.

Combining Sex & Massage

One reader comments: "My husband often massages my shoulders while I'm giving him head. It feels wonderful and serves to relax me so I can become more easily aroused." Another reader ties her naked partner's hands together above his head, lets him watch as she slowly removes her satin panties and then caresses his entire body with them. A third reader drags her long hair across her lover's naked body and eventually wraps it around his genitals. One man reports that the best way to drive his partner into total ecstasy is by brushing her hair or massaging her scalp with his fingertips. Another couple takes long, candlelit showers together, shampooing each other's hair and soaping each other's body.

Perhaps you have your own favorite ways of combining massage with sex play. Whatever your inclination, if there is only one thing you take from this book, make the resolve to make massage an integral part of your sexual relationships. Touch and massage might be the most important aspects of human sexuality, outside of the occasional need to replenish the species.

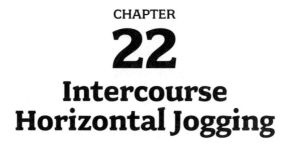

CHAPTER

22

Intercourse
Horizontal Jogging

Intercourse can mean different things. As presented in this chapter, it is an intensely private and delicious act. You can use it to honor and expand your relationship at the same time that you are doing satisfying things with your body. It is also what couples do when they want to create new life. We try to present it with a level of feeling and intelligence not normally found in popular books on sex that mostly focus on positions.

Dick, Laura & Craig

To learn more about the role of intercourse in sex, this book has invaded the privacy of three young adults, Dick, Craig, and Laura. Laura used to go out with Dick, and now she's involved with Craig. Here are their stories:

DICK

Dick is a very nice-looking guy who won his fraternity's "Mr. All-America" title two years in a row. Dick has a nice job, a nice social manner, drives a nice sports car, wears nice clothes, has nice biceps, triceps, and pecs, and goes out with nice women. Since this is a book about sex, you might as well know that Dick has a tree trunk of a penis that stays rock hard from dusk to dawn. A former girlfriend referred to it as "the sentry."

CRAIG

Craig is the same age as Dick. Craig is a sports writer. Craig is no longer eligible for the Mr. All-America contest. During a football game a few years ago, Craig went airborne to catch an overthrown pass. On the way down he got sandwiched between two spearing linebackers. Craig's spinal cord snapped, and he hasn't been able to walk or have an erection since.

LAURA

Laura is a fine young woman who just left a big corporation to form her own company that makes sporting gear. Laura's had sex with both Dick and Craig. Let's see what Laura has to say about these two different men.

"Dick's the kind of guy that many American women have been raised to worship. Parading him around your friends or taking him home to your parents would win you the female equivalent of the Breeder's Cup. I've always really enjoyed sex, and until recently I could never understand why a woman would want to fake an orgasm. But it didn't take too many nights with Dick before I started faking orgasms. There was Dick, Mr. Right Stuff, making picture-perfect love. I didn't want him to think there was something wrong with me since I couldn't get into it like he was, so I started faking orgasms."

"Craig is nowhere near as perfect as Dick, but he has a great sense of humor and he is genuine. Craig is able to laugh at himself, which Dick never could. Craig has taken the time to learn exactly how to kiss, touch, and caress me, and the sex I have with him is great. When I'm with Craig I don't need to fake a thing."

"This may not seem relevant to your question about sex, but I work in a totally male-dominated business. I have to think like a guy from morning to night. Sometimes it leaves me feeling alien from my femininity. With Craig it's easy to find it back again. Craig never wakes me up at 3 a.m. with a hard-on poking in my back, but he feels just as masculine as Dick. With a lot of guys there's a huge difference between how they treat you in bed and how they treat you the rest of time; with Craig that's not the case. Maybe that's another reason why sex is so nice with him, even if it's not intercourse."

Okay, so here we have Dick, more functional than a Sidewinder missile. He fulfills everybody's definition of what a sexual athlete should be. Then we have Craig, who redefines the term *sexually dysfunctional.* If Craig had the same erection failure but no spinal-cord injury, psychologists and sex therapists would collect a small fortune trying to make him "normal." At the very least, they would have him munching down blue boner pills as if they were M&Ms. And probably Prozac, too.

And finally, there is Laura, a woman who enjoys sex a great deal. She is telling us that the man who can't get it up is a more satisfying lover than Mr. Erectus Perfectus.

In telling you about Laura, Dick and Craig, the intent was not to dump on intercourse. Intercourse, when it's good, can be one of the sweetest things there is. What this book is dumping on is the assumption that intercourse is good just because it's intercourse and that a man is a man because he can get

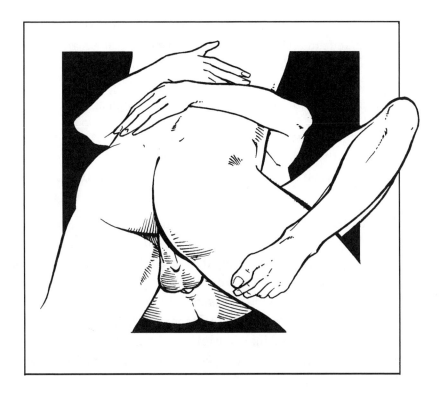

hard and fuck, or that a woman is a woman because she can get wet and fuck him back.

What Does It Feel Like When You Have Intercourse?

"Oh God—It's like describing the universe. It feels like I might explode and can't wait to but at same time want it to last forever. Breathless, hot, turned on in the extreme. I want to engulf and squeeze his penis, get it in me as much as possible. I love the connection of it."

female age 48

"When his penis first enters me I want to feel every inch of it because it is exquisite. I feel like I need it inside me and I don't know if I can describe that. The actual sensations of his penis sliding in and out of me are sometimes over-powered by the pleasure I feel all over my body, so I don't necessarily concentrate on the intercourse."

female age 23

"As he enters me I feel myself spreading open to accommodate him. Emotionally it feels right that he is inside of me. I have a feeling of fullness when he is inside me. I can feel the head of the penis as it slides in and out and can feel my vagina collapse or expand around him. If he plunges deep I can feel the head of the penis bump my cervix, a not altogether unpleasant feeling. From rear entry I can feel the penis more acutely rubbing the top of my vagina." *female age 37*

"It feels different every time. Sometimes it is very satisfying. Sometimes it hurts inside my vagina if I'm not lubricated enough. And sometimes when his penis hits my G-spot it takes my breath away!" *female age 34*

"At first I feel the light pressure of my partner's penis against my unopened vagina. It is often deeply pleasurable to feel the head penetrate, and then a slow, smooth slide all the way in, and a jolt of excitement when my lover's penis is completely inside me. The most sensation is around the outer part of the vagina, but there is also a pleasurable feeling of fullness when he is fully inside me. My hips want to move and match his strokes, or create my own rhythm for him to match. Different types of strokes and rhythms create different sensations." *female age 47*

"The first thrust is the most vivid for me. I like to slowly slide down his cock and feel it go up me. I love it when he is trying to hold back from coming; I can feel him get more swollen and hard and I get very excited when I feel that. It actually is the time when my vagina gets the most pleasure from intercourse." *female age 23*

"It depends on how sexually excited I am and whether I'm in the mood or if I'm just doing it because he wants to. If I'm into it, it's like ecstasy!" *female age 43*

"I enjoy the pumping and grinding a great deal. I love it when we are rubbing our pelvic bones together and when the penis is in deep." *female age 21*

"My favorite part of intercourse is when he comes; his entire body stiffens." *female age 55*

"I'm strictly a clit person. I love having sex with men, but I don't like intercourse." *female age 36*

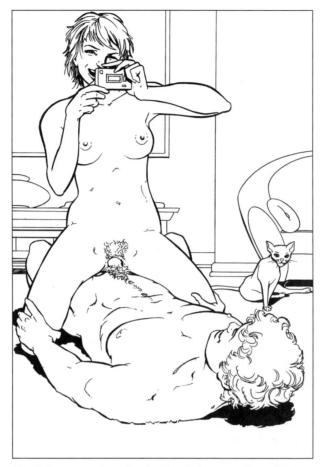

This Kodak moment was inspired by photographer Trevor Watson.

At the Start — New Relationship or New to Intercourse

For a lot of couples it takes time and familiarity for intercourse to get that kind of sloppy-intimate-erotic edge that makes it so much fun. This means that intercourse won't necessarily knock your socks off at the start. It may not even feel as good as masturbation.

Also, each partner brings his or her own hopes and expectations, as well as physical anatomy and body rhythms. Patience can be a virtue. For instance, some couples who are having dynamite intercourse during the fifth year of their relationship had lousy intercourse during the first year. And even if the sex is great at the start, chances are there will be periods in any relationship when sexual desire falls flat. Hopefully you continue to grow as a couple during those times.

Your First Intercourse

The Guide is happy to have a separate chapter for people who are about to have intercourse for the first time. Here's why:

In their study on first intercourse that included 659 college students, researchers Schwartz, Sprecher, Barbee, and Orbuch found that while 79% of the men reported that they had an orgasm during their first intercourse, only 7% of the women reported having an orgasm. Males had far more overall pleasure than females.

The mean age for first intercourse was 16½ years, although those who waited until they were 17 or older reported having a better experience than those who were younger. A year or two of added life experience can go a long way when you are only 16.

Both males and females reported more pleasure if they had intercourse for the first time in a more serious or long-term relationship than in a casual or brief one. People who used alcohol during their first intercourse (about 30% of the total) reported significantly less pleasure and more guilt than those who did it sober. Those who used contraception reported more pleasure than those who didn't.

On our own sex survey, we've asked hundreds of women to compare how their first intercourse felt with how it feels now. While most of these women say it feels great now, it is an unusual woman who says she cherished her first intercourse, even if it was in a loving relationship. If this will be your first time, please see Chapter 28: "Goodbye V-Card—Your First Intercourse."

Intercourse Orgasms vs. Masturbation Orgasms

While masturbation orgasms sometimes feel more intense than intercourse orgasms, a group of researchers in the UK have found that after an intercourse orgasm, the amount of prolactin released into the body is 400% more than the amount that is released after a masturbation orgasm. (One learns to take such findings with a grain of salt until they are replicated in other labs, which they seldom are. But let's run with it anyway.)

Theory has it that the hormone prolactin helps mellow us out following the rush of dopamine that accompanies sexual excitement. It has also been suggested that the prolactin after orgasm is what helps make some men want to snooze after coming, as well as what keeps most guys from being able to get a quick rebound erection.

We would also want to know about the number and sensitivity of pro-lactin receptors in the male body versus the female body. It could be that the same rush of prolactin does a bigger number on men than on women. This makes sense given that some women enjoy intercourse more if they have an orgasm before the penis goes in, while a penis often wants to pack it up and go home after having an orgasm. Clearly, there is still much to learn.

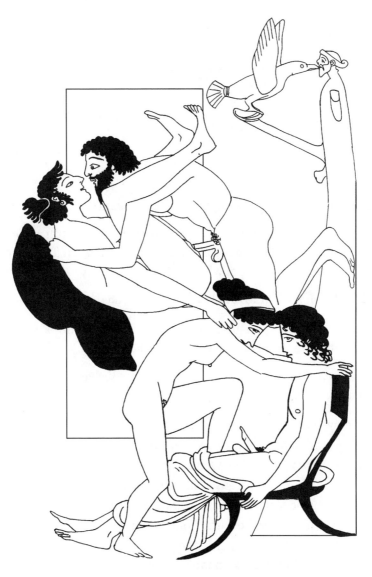

Intercourse in the old days.

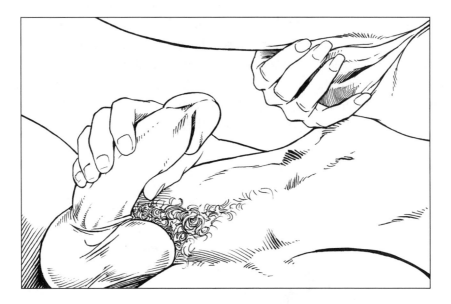

One in the Hand. Who Sticks It In?

"I generally prefer to put it in; otherwise we seem to miss a lot." *fem, 32*

"I like to put his penis in me because it seems no matter how many times we have had sex, he still misses a little bit when aiming. Also, I find it exciting to hold him while he thrusts into my vagina." *female 23*

"It's really whoever grabs ahold first." *female age 36*

"He prefers to put it in, because if I do, he thinks I think he doesn't know where in the heck that hole is." *female age 38*

"She always does. No matter how many years we've been doing this, I still manage to miss!" *male age 43*

This may seem like a dumb thing to talk about, but the issue of who sticks the penis into the vagina can sometimes be significant. A rule of thumb is that either the woman, or the woman and man together, should stick it in the first few times. That's because only a woman knows when she is ready to have a penis inside, and all those years of inserting tampons have taught her exactly where the head of little Tonto needs to go. Some women might be shy about grabbing a guy's penis and guiding it in for a landing. This kind of reticence is silly, but understandable. Once your penis-to-pussy GSM is up and running, it's catch-as-catch-can regarding who puts it in.

Note: Whoever puts it in needs to make sure the woman wants it and that her vagina is wet enough to take it. If not, a bit of spit or water-based lube is in order. See the chapter "Sex Lubes—A New Look." If you are using water-based lube and it starts to dry out, a drop or two of water or saliva will give it new life, while more lube will just gum things up. The women at Good Vibrations suggest keeping a water pistol handy for just this purpose, although women without humor will find this offensive, and wives of NRA members should be careful not to grab the Glock by mistake.

The First Thrust

As we were reading the questionnaires of our women readers, an amazing pattern emerged. A large number of women said that the part of intercourse they liked best was the first stroke. For a lot women, it seems like the first stroke is a nearly religious happening, assuming they're primed and eager for the thrusting to begin.

Do not hesitate to ask your sweetheart how she likes you to do your first stroke. Does she like you to start by teasing her with a series of short little thrusts, going in only an inch or two? Or does she like one big straightforward glide for the gold?

Legs Bent or Straight, Open or Closed

The biggest variable in the physics of intercourse is often the position of the woman's legs—whether they are straight or bent, open or closed, over your shoulders or in your face. When the woman's legs are straight, penetration is not as deep, but the tip of the clitoris might receive more stimulation. When a woman bends her legs and brings her knees closer to her chest, the penetration is deeper. This can be nice if she likes more pressure in the back part of her vagina.

If the woman's legs are together, the penis is hugged more snugly. This might offer better clitoral stimulation, because the extra snugness may push the inner labia more tightly against the shaft of the penis as it goes in and out. If the woman's legs are open, there is greater skin-to-skin contact between her vulva and the man's genitals. This can also result in more bouncing-testicle action if the man is on top.

Some couples enjoy intercourse with one leg straight and the other flexed. And some women like to reach between their legs and push on the

Rear Entry

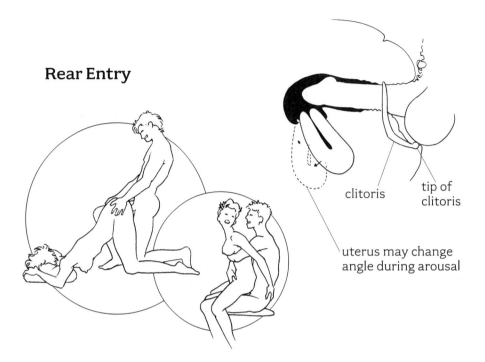

clitoris

tip of clitoris

uterus may change angle during arousal

tip of their clitoris with their fingers. Depending on the mutual anatomies, it might push it against the penis.

If this isn't confusing enough, some women keep their legs straight and together while flexing their thighs to help push themselves over the top.

Legs Bent or Straight, Anatomical Consideration

A woman's decision to keep her legs straight or bent might vary with the length and thickness of the man's penis. A woman whose partner has a really long penis may find that she gets poked in the cervix if she opens and bends her legs during intercourse, while a woman whose man has a short penis might prefer the feeling of deeper penetration that bent knees allow.

Porn star Nina Hartley has a shallow vagina and can't take guys who are really long. Mind you, "shallow" and "long" are defined differently in the world of pornography than in the average bedroom. Ms. Hartley suggests that women can add another inch or two of thrusting room by using positions that allow the penis to move into the space behind the cervix that is called the fornix. You will need to experiment on your own: Nina doesn't say what these space-enhancing positions might be.

Missionary

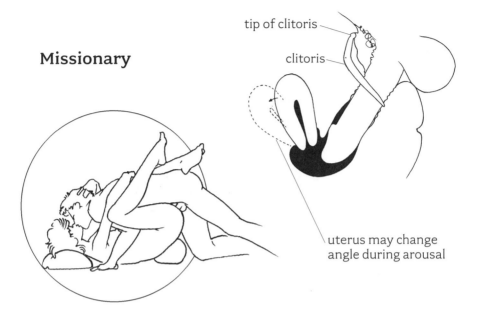

tip of clitoris

clitoris

uterus may change
angle during arousal

Apologies Sex books these days don't use the term "short penis." Instead, they say a penis that isn't overly long. The latter phrasing is meant to protect the allegedly fragile male ego, yet this Guide hates to think that today's male is so fragile that he can't say "I've got a short one" without experiencing a crisis of character. As for the sentiment expressed by the 20 Fingers song *(Don't Want No) Short Dick Man*, making peace with body parts is discussed in a latter chapter entitled "Techno Breasts & Weenie Angst." For now, keep in mind that when a woman is highly aroused, her genitals usually puff, which can make for a tighter fit. So one way a man with a smaller penis can even the playing field is by being better at the things that come before intercourse.

Thrusting—Shallow vs. Deep

The walls of a woman's vagina change shape with each thrust of intercourse. This means that with each stroke, thousands of nerve endings are being pulled and tugged, which, neurologically speaking, can feel quite nice. (This doesn't feel half-bad for guys, either.) The most sensitive part of the vagina is usually at the opening, up to an inch or two deep. This can also become the snuggest part of the vagina when it is aroused.

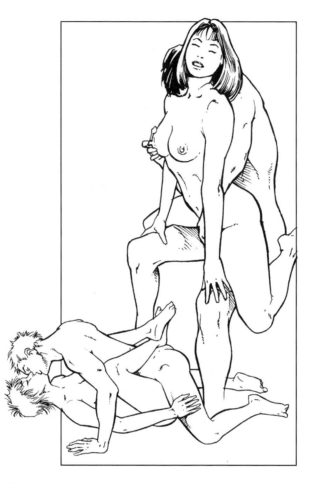

Shallow thrusting encourages the snuggest part of the vagina to wrap around the most sensitive part of his penis, which is just below the head. Shallow thrusting also allows the ridge around the head of the penis to stimulate this sensitive part of the vagina. An exception might be if the man's penis has a compact head and is thicker around the middle of the shaft. In that case the woman may prefer the thick part to be in the vaginal opening.

Deeper thrusting offers its own advantages: 1. Unless the man's penis is really long or the woman's vagina is shallow, deep thrusting can help to position his pubic bone in direct contact with more of her clitoral area. Rubbing against a man's pubic bone helps some women have orgasms during intercourse. 2. Deeper thrusting may allow the penis to pull on the labia minora (inner lips) for a longer period of time, providing more stimulation to the clitoral area. 3. The deeper part of the vagina is often sensitive to pressure.

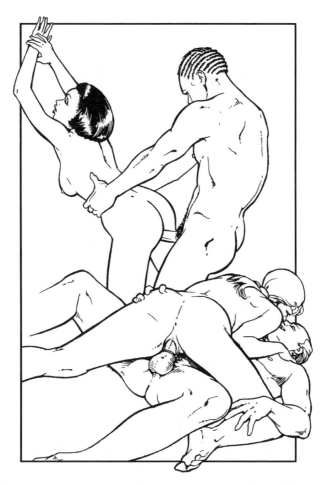

As some women approach orgasm, they find it pleasurable if there is a penis or penis-like object in the back part of the vagina that it can contract around.

The Tantric Police Talk Thrust

Some Tantric and Oriental sex masters caution against constant deep thrusting during intercourse. They believe that the vagina does best with a ratio of five to nine shallow thrusts to every deep thrust. This is an interesting observation, given how they don't allow women to be monks or masters and they don't even allow them to enter business meetings unless it's to bring tea. But they have no shortage of suggestions for pleasing them sexually.

If you are following the nine-shallow-for-every-one-deep thrust dictum, increase the ratio to two deep for every four shallow as she becomes more aroused, or live dangerously and go for one shallow to one deep.

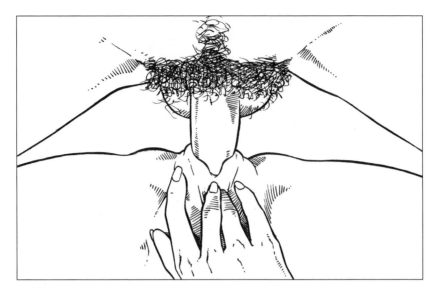

*Some women use their fingers to give themselves
extra stimulation during intercourse.*

Mixing up the trusting between shallow and deep is definitely something to experiment with. But if your partner starts threatening you with serious grief if you don't knock off the shallow stuff, you can safely assume she wasn't an Asian princess in a past life.

Battering Ram or Pleasure Wand? Mosh Pit or Symphony?

Some men use a penis as a battering ram, believing that women always enjoy being slammed during intercourse. Other men, perhaps a bit more sensitive or experienced, realize that there are different thrusting rhythms that can help make intercourse feel more symphonic than metallic. Maybe she will like it slow at the start but strong at the end.

An excellent way to find out what works best during intercourse is when the woman is on top. That way a man can feel how she moves up and down on his penis and what parts of her vagina she focuses the head on. For instance, is she up and down on it repeatedly, or does she keep the penis deep inside of her and rub her clitoris on the his pubic bone? Does she like to rub her clitoris or breasts while a penis is inside of her, or would this be an unwelcome distraction? Where does she like to look, and what does she do with her mouth? How does she help to orchestrate the rhythm and speed? Sometimes a hand pushing on a man's hip or rear end can speak volumes.

Eager for Beaver — Intercourse as Two Separate Acts

If you are feeling terminally reflective and have nothing else to do, it might be helpful to think of intercourse as two separate acts—the thrusting part and the orgasm part. If the sole purpose of the former is to achieve the latter, then the intercourse might not have much emotional depth to it. That's because it is during the thrusting part of intercourse (before orgasm) when feelings of love, friendship and gratitude are often shared.

Most couples have a variety of thrusting modes—hot and furious, fun and playful, giggly, tearful, passionate, powerful, passive, and maybe even angry at times. This becomes part of the private language that lovers share.

Using Your Head

The first inch or so of a woman's vagina is sensitive to touch. That's why a bit of gentle finger or penis-head action around the rim can be a nice way to begin. The art, of course, is in making those shallow little thrusts without pulling out too far and having your dick fall out. If it falls out enough times, she'll start thinking your middle name is "Goober," or maybe she does already and she loves you still.

Beyond the first inch or so, you need to start thinking pressure. That's because the back part of the vagina feels stretching and pressure more than it does light touches. This is when it's wise to learn which parts of her vagina respond best to pressure when the head of your penis pushes against them. You'll find that you can combine certain positions with certain angles to put pressure on the different parts of her vagina.

A good way to learn about a woman's genitals is with your fingers as well as with your penis. This will give you a better understanding of what needs to be done with your penis. (As one female reader says, "It wouldn't hurt for women to know this about themselves.")

Popping Out

During some orgasms, the vagina contracts enough to expel a penis. When asked about this, most women advise, "Push It Back In!"

Thrustless in Seattle

Some couples don't thrust at all during intercourse, but move their entire bodies in sync. Or the man might do a circular motion with his penis or pelvic bone grinding against the woman's vulva. Some couples occasionally

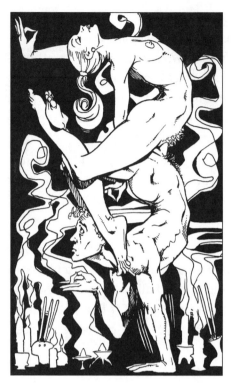

stay really still during intercourse and try to coordinate their breathing. One partner breathes in at the moment that the other breathes out.

You don't have to be a yoga master to achieve peak experiences with breathing instead of thrusting. You don't even need to meditate or stand on your head while chanting mysterious incantations. All you need to do is be in sync with each other.

Another way of enjoying intercourse without thrusting is to play "squeezing genitals." This is based upon the anatomical fact that when the male squeezes or contracts his erect penis it momentarily changes diameter, and when the woman squeezes her vagina it hugs the penis—sometimes rather snugly and with memorable results. To play "squeezing genitals," partners alternate squeezing their genitals. This can be quite interesting, and it doesn't require a particularly high I.Q. or a daring sense of adventure.

Riding High—Tom Landry Remembered

Each year a new book comes out that promises to reinvent the wheel sexually. One book talked about a radical "new" way of having intercourse. The couple starts by assuming the missionary position with the man on top. Right before the thrusting begins, he makes a quick shift toward the head of the bed, like the Cowboys used to do at the line of scrimmage before the set call, back when they were America's team and Tom Landry was coach.

During this quick shift, the male pushes his entire body a couple of inches forward over the head of the woman. This puts him in the position of being able to say, "Honey, your roots are showing something awful, time for a new weave job." This new position is supposed to bring the man's penis in more direct contact with the woman's clitoris, assuming his weenie doesn't snap off between the down-and-set-calls.

There is no in-out thrusting in this new form of intercourse. The couple simply move their hips back and forth in synchronized form, like those women swimmers with the ugly caps at the Summer Olympics.

This intercourse position does attempt to maximize clitoral stimulation by making the man "ride high." Guys who are sensitive lovers figured this one out long ago, although an occasional man may have had the knowledge forced upon him by a rambunctious lover who rode so low that she made him wonder if his penis would survive the night. Her riding low is the equivalent of his riding high. Again, a good way for a man to learn what angles his partner prefers is to pay close attention when she's on top. Or ask.

Nasty Reflections

Watching your genitals at work or play during intercourse can be an awesome way to pass time. There are several positions that allow one or both partners to watch the vagina swallowing up the penis and then spitting it out again, or passionately enveloping it, if you prefer. A good-sized hand mirror can offer a nice view of genital play until one of you accidentally kicks it over. Also, try using the magnifying side of the mirror. It will make you look huge! A woman reader comments: "That's a frightening thought."

Some couples also like to pull out the camcorder and tape themselves when having intercourse. Entire books have been written on this subject. Precautions for making home movies are mentioned in the fantasy chapter, such as putting a big X on the cassette and keeping it in a separate place from the movies that go back to Blockbuster. There are also special video locks that can be put on tapes of mom and dad having sex so the kids don't watch and suddenly have the ammo to blackmail you out of every last dollar in your retirement fund.

Kissing When Thrusting—Size vs. Intent

Sometimes there's nothing nicer in the world than kissing passionately when your genitals are locked in a loving embrace, but this simply isn't possible for some couples. For instance, if a woman is 5'1" and her partner is 6'4", there is no way her tongue is going to play inside his mouth when they are having intercourse.

One reason why it is impossible to make recommendations regarding intercourse positions is because different couples come in different sizes. Some positions will feel better for couples who are relatively the same height and weight, while those positions might be a disaster for a union between someone who is really tall and someone who is really tall. Likewise, certain positions will feel better or worse depending on the size and angle of your respective genitals. And some positions that feel best during the first part of a woman's menstrual cycle might give way to other positions during the later part of her cycle. And that's just physical differences. It really gets complicated when you factor in each partner's emotional desires and needs.

Signaling

Sex seldom works well when a partner is too passive or inhibited to let the other know what feels good and what doesn't. Fortunately, signaling during intercourse doesn't need to include words, because hands on a partner's hips or rear end can be great rudders—as long as the partner with the hips is hip to the hands.

To Come or Not to Come...

People have this silly notion that women are supposed to come during intercourse and by thrusting alone. Some do, some don't. As you will see from the following comments, many women who do come during intercourse need a little help from either their own or their partner's fingers.

> "I rarely have orgasms with intercourse, unless I'm playing with myself at the time. The best way for me is oral sex or using a vibrator."
> *female age 36*

> "I don't usually have orgasms during intercourse. In a very open relationship, I can have an orgasm after intercourse by manually stimulating my clitoris or by rubbing myself on his flaccid penis."
> *female age 26*

> "I usually have them with intercourse if my husband is rubbing my clitoris or using a vibrator while he is thrusting. Sometimes when I am really excited, I can have one just with thrusting." *female age 35*

> "I come faster sometimes when he's inside me, but I always have to rub my clit to climax." *female age 25*

A woman can love the feelings she gets from intercourse, both emotional and physical, but still not have orgasms from it.

When Is Intercourse a Success?

Most books imply that intercourse is a success if you give each other orgasms and a failure if you don't. Hardly. This Guide takes the position that intercourse needs to convey certain feelings between partners that are too primal for words alone. These feelings rest on the boundary between body and soul and are transmitted from one person to another in many different ways. If orgasm is part of that process, fine, but having an orgasm is no guarantee that anything special has taken place. On the other hand, it's possible to have intercourse with no orgasm and experience it as wonderful or enchanting.

When is intercourse a success? Intercourse seems successful when it leaves you feeling more solid, less grumpy, more able to face the day, and less afraid of the world when it's an overwhelming place. Intercourse is successful when it allows you to give and get something from your partner that makes you feel more whole or wholesome and secure.

When is intercourse a failure? This book's criterion for failure is waking up at three or four in the morning, looking at the person who's sleeping next to you and thinking "I wish I were home in my own bed, ALONE." This can be a particularly nasty dilemma if you are married or living together. And intercourse that conveys less pleasure than when someone leaves you a free hour on a parking meter is not necessarily worth having.

After Intercourse — The Drip Factor

Unless a guy is wearing a rubber or pulls out and squirts to the side, he usually leaves ejaculate inside a woman's vagina during intercourse. OK, so where does the ejaculate go?

"Runs down your leg," says one female reader. "It usually drips out," replies another. "Like water in a cup that's turned upside down," says a third. This might not be a problem if you are going to sleep, except for the wet spot on the mattress, but what if you had intercourse in the morning or at lunchtime? "You can usually get it out in the shower" was one response, while another woman says, "Not true. It tends to drain out at its own pace, and all the showering in the world isn't going to hasten it along." Either way, what if you already took a shower or don't want to take one just then? "Sometimes I'll wear a panty liner," said one woman, "but it's not worth a tampon." All of the women said they know of other women who douche right after intercourse even when they have it at bedtime. Most thought this was silly and unnecessary. As one woman said, "It's not dirty; I put the stuff in my mouth!" Another woman said, "I don't have sex with a man unless I really care about him. I find the occasional dripping to be a sweet and sometimes exciting reminder that he's been here."

As for why the ejaculate goes in thick but drips out thin, you can find the answer in Chapter 6, "Semen Confidential."

Top Dog

It has been said that people who always need to be on top during intercourse are insecure, while people who have it more together are happy to switch off. If this is true, then intercourse is no different from life in general. What's probably more true is that the couple has tried it both ways and likes it better with the top on top.

Also, feminists claim that intercourse usually follows a prostitute model of sex—once the male comes, the sex is over. If that's true in your relationship, a workaround is in order. Perhaps you can work on ways to help the woman get her share of pleasure before the man comes.

On Not Pulling Out

Staying inside your sweetheart after the thrusting is done can sometimes feel magical. Since most men lose their erections after coming, the two of you need to keep the fading member in while getting comfortable enough to stay in each other's arms. Some couples like to fall asleep this way.

The desire to stay inside your sweetheart after ejaculation is one of the downsides of using a rubber. A man who is wearing a rubber needs to pull out soon after he's come. Otherwise he might leave the rubber inside his partner.

Missed the Train Again

Men who have trouble coming tend to pump faster during intercourse, hoping this will provide extra stimulation to help them ejaculate. This is a bad idea. The rapid thrusting desensitizes the penis, and it's possible the female partner won't be able to walk right for a few days afterward. For more information, see Chapter 57: "Delayed Ejaculation."

Passive Intercourse vs. Masturbation

Let's say a woman wakes up at 5:00 a.m., horny as can be, and would like to have intercourse. Her partner, on the other hand, is not a morning person and is pretty much comatose until noon. Assuming he's just slow to rise and not an early-morning grouch, he might allow her to stimulate his penis to a point of erection, or maybe he's already got an early-morning (REM-state) hard-on. They then have intercourse in a position where he can be passive while she is active, or she massages her clitoris while his penis is inside of her. In a sense, she is using his penis as a dildo.

Or let's say it's nearly midnight and this woman's partner is feeling sexually amped, but she is pretty much dead to the world. She doesn't mind his using her vagina for intercourse, but doesn't want to have to be into it either. So she rolls on her side and allows him to have rear-entry intercourse.

Ah, you might say, why didn't the horny partner just masturbate instead of bothering the one who is zoned out? Sometimes a partner honestly doesn't mind being "used" for sex as long as he or she isn't expected to get all turned on. He or she might even enjoy the other's pleasure. However, it is essential that the passive partner feels comfortable saying, "Naw, not now," and the horny partner should be willing to masturbate. And it requires a sex life that is fairly rich at other times, given how an entire diet of passive sex might leave the active partner feeling unvalued or the passive partner feeling used.

What's the Frequency, Dan?

When it comes to frequency of intercourse, people who ask, "What's normal?" usually aren't asking the right question. If you are in a relationship, good questions to be asking are, "Do we have intercourse as often as each of us likes?" "Do we have intercourse more often than one or both of us likes?" The reason these questions are more important than, "What's normal?" is because the only thing that matters about sex is what feels best for you— whether it's three times a day or three times a decade.

Nookie Noise

Some vaginas make fartlike noises during intercourse. This is due to air that has been pushed into the back of the vagina. If you get embarrassed about these sounds, it might be helpful to remember that the silly sounds are the result of the pleasure you were giving each other. If it really bothers you, you might experiment with different positions, or perhaps ear plugs.

Pillows under Your Parade

Don't underestimate the power of a pillow under the rear to enhance intercourse. Changing the angle of the hips can dramatically change a person's experience of intercourse, sometimes for the better. Experiment to find what placement might be good for you. If you like intercourse from the rear, keep a lookout for the right big pillow that will provide support and raise the woman's rear end to an angle that is comfortable and inviting. The more humongous the pillow, the more fun. Experiment with bolsters and different kinds of cushions.

Environment

If intercourse is seeming a bit stale, it might help to scout out some new locations. It never hurts if that new location is a four-star hotel in Europe, but most of us will need to consider other possibilities:

The Kitchen Always a fine place for intercourse until you have kids. Once the kids reach school age, the kitchen is game for an occasional nooner.

In Front of the Fireplace There's nothing quite like doing it in front of the fireplace, until they deliver wet pine instead of seasoned oak and a slew of hissing, burning embers showers your naked back and rear end.

The Yard It's a shame to spend all that time and money making the grass grow and never have sex on it.

In Water Hot tubs, bathtubs, pools, and other large bodies of water can be great places for people to do all sorts of nasty things. But intercourse in water provides its own unique hazard because water washes away natural lubrication. One solution is a silicone-based lubricant. Why hot-tub manufacturers don't include samples of silicone-based lubes is beyond us. Another solution is to bury the penis inside the vagina while both sets of organs are outside the water. To help facilitate underwater hand play and sexual groping, coat your genitals with something oily while they are still dry-docked.

Sex at the Office Sex at the office often has the right elements of risk and mischievous fun. One reader is a commercial-real-estate agent who has keys to some of the finest offices in all of Los Angeles. When he and his girlfriend want a dramatic change of scenery, they check out the upper floors.

Candlelight An old standby for erotic ambiance is candlelight. Make sure that the candle wax doesn't drip on your carpet, because it will cost you a fortune to have it commercially removed. (A reader kindly comments: fold up a paper towel a few times and place it over the cooled wax on the carpet. Then put a warm to hot iron on top of the towel. It will melt the wax into the towel and the carpet is wax-free! Another reader cautions that some types of candleholders get hot enough to scorch furniture.)

Extra Odds'N'Ends

🔆 Some couples enjoy it greatly when the woman uses a vibrator during intercourse. The sensations can be very pleasing for both partners. This can work in any number of the usual positions, or you can get all artsy and try doing it like the couple in the illustration in the sex-toys chapter.

🔆 A woman who is on top and facing a man's feet can watch his penis go in and out of her vagina, especially with a mirror. She can reach forward and play with his toes or testicles.

🔆 Rear-entry positions allow the head of the penis to focus on different parts of the vagina than missionary positions do. Rear entry also provides extra padding, which can be welcome if one or both of you is really bony.

🔆 Rather than thrusting, some couples find that rocking back and forth with a penis inside feels pleasant.

🔆 Some couples take an intercourse break to have oral sex; some do oral sex afterward.

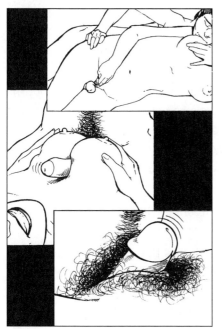

Intercourse between the thighs, breasts, and femoral intercourse—where the penis slides between the lips of the vulva without going into the vagina.

🔆 In Veronica Monet's DVD of women masturbating, some used dildos. However, it was not unusual for the woman to run the dildo between her labia rather than pushing it into her vagina. Some couples enjoy a lubricated penis moving between her labia, like a hot dog going back and forth through a bun. The ridge around the head of the penis can feel especially nice as it glides back and forth over the clitoris. The woman can increase the pressure by pulling the penis tighter against her vulva with her fingertips, aka femoral intercourse.

🔆 In the highly recommended book *Tricks - More Than 125 Ways to Make Good Sex Better*, author Jay Wiseman suggests having the man lie on his back and the woman places a pair of her panties over his penis. The penis sticks through a leg hole, with the panties draping down over his testicles and between his legs. The couple has intercourse with the woman on top. If the panties are silky or rayon-like, the material might stimulate him with each stroke.

Some couples find a well-trimmed and freshly bathed big toe to be a fun penis substitute, especially those who work at Dr. Scholl's. Also, a heel that's jiggled back and forth can be used to stimulate a woman's genitals.

There are couples who like to gently bite each other's shoulders or run their teeth along each other's skin while having intercourse. This works best when the skin is well-lubricated and the lovers are good with feedback.

Some men and women particularly enjoy the feeling of intercourse after a woman has had an orgasm rather than before.

If for some reason a vagina doesn't get as wet as a couple might want, keep some water-based lube handy, or pick up glycerin suppositories from the drug store that can be put into the vagina ahead of time. If vaginal infections are a problem, you might experiment with water-based lubricants that have no glycerin. As the former baby-boom generation hot flashes its way through the new century, a plethora of pricey new "personal moisturizers" have been flooding the market. Whether they have anything on saliva is still unknown.

Women might not lubricate very well for the first couple of months following pregnancy. Extra lubrication can also help if the woman is taking drugs such as antihistamines, alcohol, or pot, and if the man is wearing a condom or the couple is playing with sex toys.

Why not try feeding each other while having intercourse? That's what nature created papaya for.

Some couples enjoy a finger, thumb, small vibrator, or butt plug on or in each other's anus during intercourse.

Most sex stores sell little plastic thingies that fit over a man's penis and provide extra stimulation to the woman's clitoris when she rubs up against his pubic bone. There is also a plastic vibrating cock ring that some couples enjoy, and a special vibrator in a harness can be strapped in place over the clitoris for use during intercourse.

Positions where you are sitting up might allow more blood to pool in the pelvic region, which could, theoretically, help some men get better erections and women get more vaginal engorgement. For instance, there is

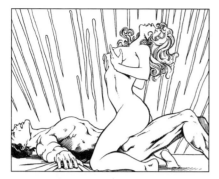

Warning! This can hurt you. Really.

Intercourse injuries can cause a penis to forever bend in a strange way. Most of these injuries occur when the woman is on top. Urologists strongly suggest that when using this position, the woman be well-lubricated and that she restrict her up-and-down motion. This helps decrease those instances where she sits down on a penis, but at a funny angle, or when it comes out on the upstroke and gets crunched on the downstroke instead of sliding in the way it's supposed to. A good way to compensate for the decreased thrusting is to put a pillow under the man's rear end. This can help make his pelvic bone more accessible, and his partner might enjoy pushing down against it (grinding). That way she has the penis deep inside and gets her clitoral area worked too. She might also try squeezing, as if she is peeing and trying to stop the flow.

one position where the man sits on a chair and the woman sits in his lap, wrapping her legs around his waist. While this doesn't work for heavy-duty thrusting, the penetration can be really deep. You might try a similar position where the man sits in the chair and the woman sits on his lap but facing away from him (sitting spoons position?).

Betty On Intercourse

What better way to wind down a chapter on intercourse than with a few passages from Betty Dodson's book *Sex for One?* These refer to things that transpired during Ms. Dodson's sex groups for women.

On Pretending You're a Guy during Intercourse "One amusing and informative exercise was called "Running a Sexual Encounter." It involved reversing sex roles with the women on top. We made believe that our clitorises were penetrating imaginary lovers, and we had to do all the thrusting. I would set the egg timer for three minutes, a little longer than the Kinsey national average. As the fucking began, I would participate and at the same time comment on everyone's technique. 'Keep your arms straight; don't crush your lover. You're too high up; your clitoris just fell out. Don't stop moving, you'll lose your erection. Don't move so fast; you'll come too

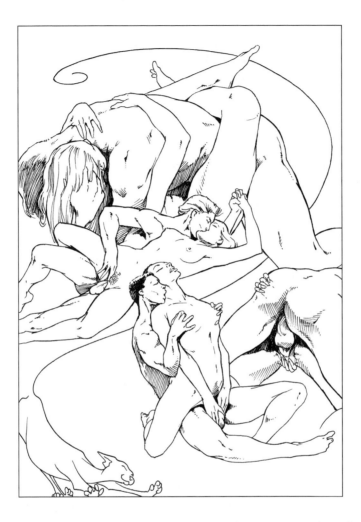

soon. And don't forget to whisper sweet things in your lover's ear between all those passionate kisses.

"Watching the egg timer, I coordinated my theatrical orgasm with the ding of the bell, frantically thrusting for the last ten seconds. Then, falling flat on my imaginary lover, I muttered, 'Was it good for you?' and promptly began snoring loudly. It was always hysterically funny. Panting and exhausted, the women all exclaimed, 'How do men do it?' Complaints included tired arms, lower-back pain, and stiff hip joints. Most of the women had fallen out long before the bell went off. After that, there was always more empathy for men, and the women showed an increased interest in other positions for lovemaking."

Odds & Ends "Some of the women talked about experiencing pain with deep thrusting intercourse, while others claimed to want a hard fuck. In my youth, I'd confused hard pounding intercourse with passion, and experienced internal soreness afterward.... While I enjoyed a strong fuck when we were two equal energies in sync, I also loved the slow intense fuck.

"Another problem the women complained of was lack of lubrication and the pain of dry intercourse. Some women felt inadequate if they weren't wet with passion. My experience varied; sometimes I lubricated when I wasn't even thinking about sex. Other times I could be dry even though I felt sexually aroused..."

On Orgasms "Some women had good orgasms with oral sex but not with intercourse. Others could come with intercourse but couldn't get off alone. Still others were having orgasms with themselves but not with a partner. All of the orgasmic women agreed on one thing: Their experiences of orgasm varied greatly from one orgasm to the next."   —From *Sex for One* by Betty Dodson, Harmony Books.

Readers' Comments

Some of your favorite intercourse positions?

"My favorite position is doggy style, with me on my hands and knees, and him behind me. I like this best for two reasons: my vagina is tighter this way, and I can easily rub my clitoris and have an orgasm. I also love to sit on a guy while he is sitting up. This just feels wonderful. Our bodies are so close." *female age 26*

"Good old missionary, with me on the bottom and him on top!"
female age 32

"One of my favorite positions is sitting in his lap in a chair. He can kiss my neck or armpits, which drives me nuts, and I can move freely. If we are on the bed, I can also lie back and touch my clit if I want."
female age 38

"My favorite position is sitting on top of him. That way I can stroke my clitoris or I can watch him do it." *female age 43*

"I like it best when we're doing it doggy style and I hold the vibrator and rub my clit with it. The sensation is wonderful!" *female age 25*

"I enjoy having him on top but recently discovered that if we lie on our sides with me in front and I throw my upper leg over his, he can enter me from behind and it's very exciting." *female age 45*

"I like to bend over a table and have my partner insert his penis from behind. We get great penetration this way, and he is also able to hit something in there that makes me feel really good!" *female age 34*

"I like to be on my back with my legs up while he is on his knees entering me and rubbing my clitoris. We started using this position when I was pregnant and I still like it best." *female age 35*

What do you like the most, and least, about intercourse?

"Worst part—the big wet spot. Best part—making the big wet spot."
female age 27

"It is wonderful when we first start having intercourse and I love the cuddling after. I don't like how, if you don't clean up afterward, the ejaculate runs out of you (sometimes cold) and drips down your butt onto the sheets." *female age 30*

"I like it when he first inserts his penis into my vagina the best. The thing I like least about sex is having to really work for a long time to get him to orgasm when he's had too much to drink." *female age 34*

"I like the beginning the most and orgasm, of course. If somebody takes too long, the middle gets dull." *female age 25*

"The first moments of penetration are the best. The wet spot on the bed, the worst." *female age 44*

"The part I like best is when my man spends a long time getting me hot until I want him so badly I can't wait and he finally sinks his penis into me. It's such a relief to finally be joined together. I like it least when he enters too soon and comes too fast and says, 'I'm sorry' when I had my hopes up for more." *female age 38*

"I love feeling him on top of me, kissing and caressing, and I love the feeling of his penis inside me. The part I don't like is the mess." *fem 35*

For Exploring Different Intercourse Positions: You can't beat Sadie Allison's *Ride 'Em Cowgirl! Sex Position Secrets For Better Bucking*, Tickle Kitty (2007). Explains the how and why in addition to showing what.

23
Anal Sex
Up Your Bum

66 I grew up in the country. We had neighbors, Amos Wheatley and his wife. One night while washing dishes, Mrs. Wheatley told my mother that she let Amos 'use the other hole.' Then they had a baby girl, and I heard my father comment that Amos must have got it right at least once. Sometime later, Amos, who was uneasy about the expense of having a new baby, told my father he'd rather have had a team of horses. My father said, 'Isn't that expecting rather a lot of Mrs. Wheatley?' "

—The recollections of a 71-year-old woman, as told to Julia Hutton in her *Good Sex: Real Stories from Real People,* Cleis Press.

Some couples would rather drink goat sweat than try anal sex; others enjoy an occasional rear-end soiree. You will be hard-pressed to find too many parts of the body that have more nervereceptors than the anus, plus a lot of the nerves that light up during vaginal intercourse also light up during anal-sex play. This, rather than the perverse thrill of it all, is why some men and women enjoy anal massage or anal intercourse. It is an enjoyment that cuts across all orientations.

Whether you are straight, gay or somewhere in between, the chances are good that at some point in your life you might try anal sex. That is why the topic is covered in this book. Please be aware that this Guide couldn't care less whether you do or don't practice anal sex, but it does have a few suggestions in case curiosity nips you in the rear.

Anal Massage

Although sex includes much more than intercourse, if someone says they had sex last night, we assume they had vaginal intercourse. When you add the modifier "anal" in front of the word sex, we assume that it was the same penis going into the same pelvis, only using the back door.

Yet one of the nicest forms of anal pleasure comes from anal massage, where nothing is inserted into the anus. As anyone who has ever had a hemorrhoid will tell you, the anus is alive with nerve endings. A well-lubed finger or thumb massaging the outside of the anal opening can bring subtle but wonderful waves of pleasure to any partner who can allow him- or herself to receive it.

"I hate admitting this, but I like it when Dave wets one of his fingers and slides it into my anus. It is a huge turn-on, and there are times when it makes me orgasm. The only problem is pulling out. It always hurts coming out and usually throws off my bowel movements for the next few hours. It feels like I have to go...." *female age 26*

"When Erica is all worked up, she sometimes really likes me to massage her anus. When I slip a lubricated finger inside her, it is often the thing that puts her over the edge. If I have a finger inside her vagina and one in her anus, she reacts very well to the sandwiching of the wall when I press the two together. Other times, she really hates it when I touch her there. I can never quite guess when it's going to be a green light." *male age 25*

Rimming

Rimming is a slang word for kissing ass, literally. It means sticking your tongue up or around your partner's anus. Keep in mind that it's probably not a good idea to rim just anyone, as it can be an effective way of getting hepatitis and intestinal parasites. In a one-night stand or brief encounter, cut a condom lengthwise and lay it over the person's anus before licking.

One gastroenterologist has said that by the time a couple has been together for a couple of years, they pretty much share the same anal flora. This means you probably won't get anything more from licking your partner's anus than you would from licking your own.

Penis, Plug or Dildo into Rectum

Anal sex—Penis into Rectus—is often associated with homosexuality. However, it appears that 30% to 40% of all heterosexual couples in this country have tried anal intercourse, and that's just intercourse. While 2 to 5 million straight American couples are said to practice anal intercourse with regularity, only about 50% of gay males bury the weenie in the wazoo.

The remainder of this chapter is about the kind of anal sex that includes something going in the anal opening, be it a penis, finger, butt plug, or dildo.

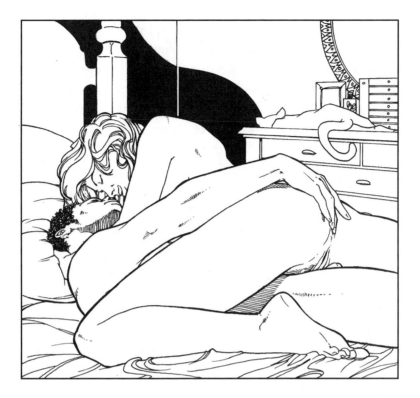

What Can Brown Do For You?

Some couples like anal sex because it's forbidden. Some women have anal sex who would like a partner's penis inside of their vagina but can't because of chronic pain. Some men have anal sex as a way of getting work in the entertainment industry. But the most obvious reason why people have anal sex is because they enjoy the experience.

> "Anal sex helps me feel a whole different part of my vagina and vulva. The fact that it is so tight and kind of nasty is a turn-on to me too."
>
> *female age 23*

> "My wife asks for anal intercourse on occasion, usually late at night when she is very aroused and her inhibitions are down." *male age 41*

> "I can come from anal intercourse, but not from vaginal intercourse."
>
> *female age 32*

> "Both of us like it. I will sometimes put a finger in her anus while we are having intercourse. It's very exciting for her, and I can feel my penis through the wall, which I find to be very erotic." *male age 39*

Most people have the notion that the only reason women do anal sex is to please a male partner. Not a single woman in our survey who does anal sex mentioned anything about pleasing a partner. Each one said she did it because she liked the way it feels. Some women report getting an extra-intense orgasm when they stimulate their clitoris at the same time that they are having anal sex. Some find anal sex to be emotionally intense, as well.

As for men's pleasure, some enjoy having their anus massaged or penetrated, and some report having memorable orgasms when their prostate gland is being pressed. Seldom do men have an orgasm from anal stimulation alone. Usually it includes penis stimulation.

A final reason that some couples do anal sex is for birth control. It is possible that anal sex is practiced as birth control in countries that take seriously the Catholic Church's opposition to contraception. Perhaps this isn't what the Vatican had in mind. Or maybe anal sex would be a hot concept in these countries regardless of where they pray. Is anal sex an effective means of preventing pregnancy, or can ejaculate run out of the anus and into the vagina? Pregnancies from anal sex are common enough that the term "splash conception" is used to describe them. Perhaps this is how people with anal-retentive personalities are conceived.

Big Mama Nature & The Human Backside

When Big Mama Nature designed the female body she gave it a vagina that's rough, tough and durable. She made the walls of the vagina so they would stretch, swell, lubricate and straighten out at times of sexual excitement. This allows objects of desire to slide in and out with a fair amount of ease and enjoyment.

Mother Nature was working from a different set of blueprints when she built the human rectum. That's because the rectum's main purpose is for elimination rather than romance. As a result, the walls of the rectum don't stretch and lubricate, although they comfortably fit objects that are even larger than a penis on a nearly daily basis. Think about it. Reports that anal sex will damage your rectum are not backed up by medical fact as long as you use lots of lube and leave your crowbar in the toolshed.

The rectum includes a pair of pugnacious sphincter muscles that guard the gates of your anus. These muscular rings were designed to facilitate outgoing rather than incoming objects, although they can be taught to yield in either direction. The anal sphincters are two of the most important muscles in the human body if you plan on living and working in the vicinity of other human beings.

A Brief Summary of the Structure & Function of the Human Rectum from the Time of Cro-Magnon Man Until the Founding of Ancient Greece

If you consider the history of the human rectum, say from the time of Cro-Magnon man until the founding of ancient Greece, its sole purpose was to hold things in. It wasn't until the ancient Greeks invented sodomy that our bums became multipurpose. (In giving credit where credit is due, the Old Testament may have had an interest in the subject of anal sex that possibly predated the Greeks. At the very least, one of the early Biblical plagues visited upon the Egyptians apparently included hemorrhoids.)

Thanks to the inventiveness of the ancient Greeks, we now have things in our lives like politicians, lawyers, doctors and anal sex. The only one of these that should never cause you any pain is anal sex. If it does, you are doing it wrong, says psychologist Jack Morin, who has written the bible on the subject, called *Anal Pleasure and Health, 3rd ed.*, Down There Press (1998).

The key to pleasurable anal sex is training the anal sphincter muscles to open for incoming objects. One set of these muscles is under conscious control. It's what people use to maintain their dignity when waiting to use the bathroom. The second set of sphincters is a total free agent that automatically closes whenever something pushes against it. To have comfortable anal sex, the second set of sphincters must be taught how to relax when you ask.

Popular Culture Historical Note When Jack Morin published the first edition of his *Anal Pleasure* book, it was such a taboo subject that few bookstores stocked it. Now, a little more than two decades later, Jack's book has been joined by Tristan Taormino's *Ultimate Guide to Anal Sex for Women,* and it is not unusual to see both on bookstore shelves. And if you look at today's porn, you might think that couples have anal sex as often as vaginal sex, when the reality is that most couples prefer vaginal intercourse way more.

The Three Key Elements

The next sections have been written as if the male is doing the inserting and the female is receiving. Far be it from this Guide to say how it is in your own relationship. (*Pegging,* or the insertion of penis-like objects into the straight male butt might not be as popular as blogging, but it's not totally uncommon, either.)

There are at least three keys to anal insertion: relaxation, feedback and lube. The difference between anal pleasure and pain is having generous amounts of each. Interestingly, one of the new safesex guidelines for anal sex includes trust or relaxation. It seems that even the toughest of condoms can tear if the anus isn't relaxed. So if you are highly turned on and relaxed, the sensations will be very different than if you aren't.

Consider the following question that one female reader had for us about her experience with anal sex:

> "I truly hated anal sex the two times I had tried it before. But I agreed to do it with my new boyfriend, and it feels incredible with him! Am I weird, or are there any other women who enjoy anal sex?"
>
> *female age 28*

We posted this reader's question on our sex survey and found a surprising number of women who said they'd had a similar experience. Many said the two key elements were being able to feel totally relaxed with the guy and feeling exceptionally horny. Few mentioned anything about penis size. Even a finger can be annoying if the key elements of trust and arousal are missing, while a good-sized penis can feel fine if a woman is relaxed and ready.

If you have had a painful anal experience in the past, it will make the relaxation part more difficult to achieve.

Strange vs. Pain

When you are first experimenting with anal play, you will need to appreciate the difference between physical sensations that are unusual or strange, versus those that are painful. When you or your partner first start groping inside your anus, it might feel quite strange. With time and experience, the initial strange feeling can evolve into a new kind of sexual pleasure. Or, it might just remain strange. You never know how your brain will translate the sensations until you are in the throes of sexual passion and desire.

If the sensations are painful as opposed to strange, back way off and try to figure out what's causing the pain. Don't explore again until you have come up with theories about the pain and possible fixes.

Practice Makes Perfect

When it comes to the rectum, jagged finger nails are weapons of mass destruction. Make sure that your fingernails are trimmed and your hands are washed. The best way to prepare for anal sex is in the shower, for a couple of weeks before you do it with a partner. Try inserting your finger up your bum. Think of it as a rectal rover. Its job is to provide you with valuable information about the geology of your anus. As you do this with each ensuing shower, you will learn more, and you will be teaching your anal sphincters to relax.

Another thing that some people might find helpful is to try masturbating with an anal toy or finger in your rear. This will help you get used to the new sensations.

Psychologist Jack Morin suggests the following technique for teaching your rectum to relax: Each night for a week or so the one partner lubes up a clean finger and gently inserts it in the other partner's rear, pushing very softly and slowly. This should encourage trust and relaxation.

Rectal expert Erik Mainard—known as the Avatar of Ass—encourages a gentle massage of the anus and suggests angling the finger slightly upward toward the tailbone, since that is how the rectum curves. He says to push in slowly and only as the resistance eases. This should feel good for the receiver; otherwise the person who is inserting the finger is either rushing it or violating your comfort zone. (That's not the only thing he or she is violating.)

One way to help relax the anal area is for the receiver to push down as though she were trying to move her bowels. In addition to relaxing the sphincters, this adds a bit of suspense to the exercise. However, anal purists say that with the help of a patient, caring partner, one needn't trick the sphincters into relaxing. It also seems that even though only one partner might be inserting a penis, each should experiment with fingering the other's rear. This will help build knowledge and trust—bum-bonding with your sweetheart.

The receiver needs to feel comfortable with finger penetration before trying any further unnatural acts. It is not until the second sphincter learns to relax that anal sex will feel comfortable, and if it doesn't feel comfortable, you shouldn't be doing it. If there is any discomfort other than a feeling of fullness, which shouldn't be painful, spend an extra week doing the finger exercises or give up the concept of anal intercourse entirely.

Simultaneous Clit Play

Women frequently find that clitoral stimulation helps take anal sex from being nothing to write home about to something that feels really good. The two of you need to talk about ways of making sure that her clitoris gets plenty of attention at the same time that her rear end is. This can range from fingerplay to a vibrator, and just about everything in between.

Swabbing the Decks of the Hershey Highway

Some people prefer to give themselves a quick enema ("short shot") with a bulb syringe or a prepared store-bought solution before having anal sex. Others will equate this with removing the patina from the Statue of Liberty.

Keep in mind that the rectum is not usually a storage space for poop. It is merely the toll booth between the colon and the toilet. A good soaping in the shower should make most anuses sparkle. They should be more than ready for the tongue of a partner who is so inclined.

If you decide to give yourself an enema, do it a couple of hours before sex. A bulb syringe with water should do the trick. Follow the instructions on the box. Do not use a Fleet or Fleet-like enema for sex, as it contains a laxative. Empty it and fill it with clean tap water. Make sure it's not too cold, unless you enjoy giving yourself cramps. For more cleaning options, see Tristan Taormino's *The Ultimate Guide to Anal Sex for Women,* 2nd ed. Cleis Press, (2006).

Anal Play Combined with Other Kinds of Sex Play

"I like to have my anus stimulated when I'm receiving oral sex. I like to have one finger inserted, but it doesn't have to be very far, just past the sphincter will do. And rather than sliding all the way in and out, it is better if there is just a slight tugging movement. It adds one more sensation to the myriad of sensations involved in oral sex." *female age 37*

"My boyfriend likes me to rub a finger on his anus while I give him oral sex. Gentle pressure and a rotating finger add a lot to his pleasure." *female age 23*

Plenty of couples enjoy adding a finger or toy in the rear when doing sex that isn't anal focused, such as handjobs, oral sex and vaginal intercourse. You will need to ponder whether you want the anal accessory to move in and out, or to stay put once it is where the person wants it. And remember, brown and pink don't mix—keep anything that has touched an anus out of a vagina.

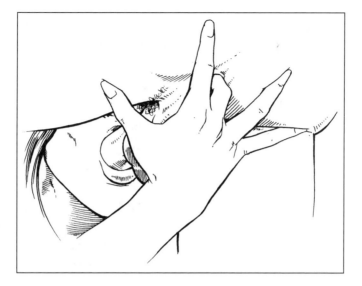

Playin' the Back Nine? Bag It

Straight or gay, single or married, monogamous or slut, you are always wise to use a condom when having anal intercourse. The reasons extend beyond concern about AIDS. It is just as much to keep the male from getting a possible prostate infection as it is for protecting the woman.

Fluids deposited in the rectum are absorbed more easily into the body than fluids deposited in the vagina. In other words, deposit a wad of male ejaculate up a partner's rear, and chances are her hungry colon is going to slurp it up. Heaven only knows how her immune system is going to respond, and science won't be helping straight couples answer this question any time soon. If you bag the penis before it goes up her bum, you've eliminated a potential source of concern.

Also, *men can get prostate infections from having anal sex without wearing a condom.* Both of our prostate consultants, who are nobody's prudes when it comes to matters of sex, nearly come unglued at the thought of sticking an unbagged penis up a rectum, even if it's with a wife of twenty years. That's because the same bacteria that are prevalent in the rectum can also cause a difficult case of prostatitis. He feels that the reason more men don't get bladder infections from doing anal sex is because the infection settles in the prostate. Also, no matter how hard you wash your penis after a rectal rendezvous, bacteria-laden chunks can still remain inside the urinary opening if you haven't used a condom. This is not good for either of you, and at the very least can give her an infection if you then have vaginal intercourse. If you are

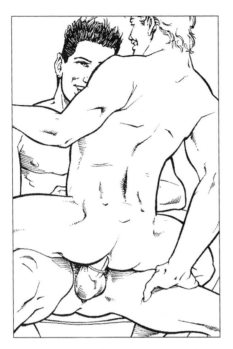

These young lads want to remind you to use condoms with anal sex, even if you are married and straight as a road through Kansas. Condoms help protect the prostate from infections.

going from anal intercourse to vaginal intercourse, not only should you wash your penis, but try to take a leak as well. When it comes to condoms and anal sex, polyurethane condoms should be a butt pirate's dream, however, they have not been approved for anal-sex usage by the FDA. They are made thinner than traditional latex condoms and can be used with oil-based lubricants, but they seem to have a higher rate of breakage than the old latex war horses.

Using latex condoms with silicone/ water-based lube Silicone lube is the lube of choice for some anal enthusiasts. It won't harm latex condoms and it seems to give good bang for your buck. It won't dry out as fast as most water-based lubes. Also see Chapter 11: "Sex Lubes—A New Look"

Female Condoms You hear more and more anal sex aficionados trumpeting the value of the female condom for anal sex play. Why not see if it works for you? Plus, you can leave it in if you want to take an anal intermission, or maybe go shopping or something. However, these kinds of uses have not received FDA sanction, so buyer beware.

Don't used ribbed or studded condoms for anal sex; you don't need the extra resistance. It's best to put a new condom on any sex toys that go into the rectum and to wash the toy afterward. If you have favorite toys for butt play, dedicate them for that purpose only so they never see the inside of a vagina.

Beware the Buttman

If the thought anal intercourse intrigues you, you might like to watch some anal-sex DVDs. In her book, *The Ultimate Guide to Anal Sex for Women*, Tristan Taormino warns that anal-sex videos leave out the most important

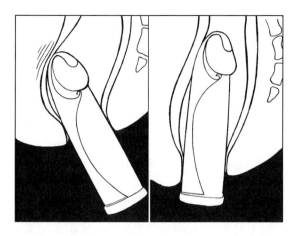

Positions

Unlike the vagina, the rectum curves. So you will want to experiment with different positions that will help straighten out the rectal curves. Otherwise, an incoming penis or dildo might have a rear-ender with the wall of the rectum.

parts. Even when they are making X-rated movies, the actors don't just go plowing each other's rear ends without lots of preparation and anal foreplay, none of which the viewer actually sees in the video. So while it's fine to enjoy Gonzo anal releases such as *Bongwater Butt Babes*, don't for a moment try to replicate it in real life with a real partner, unless she's inflatable.

In Slow—Out Slow

No matter what you are putting inside a rectum, it needs to go in very slowly and come out very slowly.

Most people have no difficulty grasping the former, but they don't realize that anything being pulled out of a rectum, whether it's a finger, penis or butt plug, needs to be pulled out slowly. Otherwise, extreme discomfort and even physical damage might result.

Anal-Intercourse Alternatives

One of the most sensitive parts of the human body is the skin that surrounds the outer rim of your anus. It's easy to stimulate this area with a thumb, finger, tongue or butt plug without sticking a penis all the way up it. For instance, some women who are receiving vaginal stimulation enjoy it when a partner puts pressure on their anus with a thumb or finger. Just be sure to avoid putting something that's been up an anus into a vagina.

All's Fair in Anal Play

It's only fair that if a guy wants to stick his penis up a partner's rectum, she should be able to stick something of comparable size up his. Plus, it will help him become a more sensitive anal lover. Vegetables aren't a good idea.

You don't want a vegetable breaking off and taking up permanent residence inside your man's rectum. Use a dedicated anal toy or butt plug.

Butt Plugs Galore

Butt plugs are dildo-like objects made specifically for the rear end. They have flared bases to keep them from getting lost on the Hershey Highway. Butt plugs come in many different sizes, and some even vibrate. People use butt plugs to give their rear ends a feeling of fullness. They are much better suited for this purpose than a dildo, which is made for thrusting.

Dildo Deluxe

If you are considering a dildo or butt plug, be sure to check out places like Good Vibrations, Toys in Babeland, JTs Stockroom, and Blowfish to find which dildos are best for anal penetration. They will also be able to tell you which dildo will fit into which harness, if you are so inclined.

If you plan to use a dildo for both vaginal and anal recreation, it is a very good idea to get a separate one for each port of entry. Having dedicated dildos helps decrease the chance that fecal matter will get into the vagina.

You will find that sex toys vary greatly in price. If all you are doing is experimenting, a jelly butt toy or even a cheapo latex one might be OK. But be sure to put a condom on them before each use. That's because the surfaces are porous and might collect fecal matter that won't wash out.

Pegging or "Bend Over Boyfriend"

> "My boyfriend of five years actually made the suggestion that I penetrate him anally. I lubricated the finger with the shortest nail on it and slowly slid it into his anus. He enjoyed it so much that he asked for two fingers and then three. While doing this, I also alternated sucking and manually pumping his cock with my other hand. He had a mind-blowing orgasm. He tells me it's the kind you feel deep down to your toes…. I'm now looking for a strap-on that stimulates me as well as him!" *female age 40*

Some people feel that only gay guys like things up their rears. Yet straight men have rectums that are every bit as sensitive as those of gay men. While plenty of straight guys would just as soon be boiled in oil as have a dildo or butt plug put up their rear, other manly guys enjoy the feeling tremendously. In fact, there are popular series of straight adult videos titled *Bend Over Boyfriend* and *Babes Ballin' Boys*.

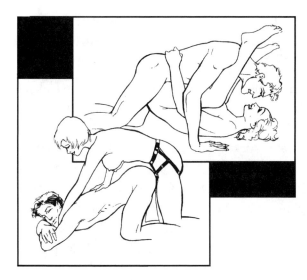

Positions for anal intercourse are the same as with vaginal intercourse. Some are more intimate and allow for the couple to kiss, while others provide better access to the clitoris or penis of the receiver.

As for penetrating their men anally, some women hold a dildo with their fingers; others put it in a dildo harness and propel it with their hips. A dildo harness looks somewhat like a jock strap and holds the dildo in the same position as a man's erect penis. This allows the woman to thrust in and out, more or less. Learning how to use a dildo in a harness is an acquired art that takes time and patience. Also, keep in mind that a man's anal sphincters need just as much rectal foreplay as a woman's.

Consider trying a harness that straps to your thigh. It might be easier to control than the model that goes over your crotch.

Toy Precautions

Rectums are hungry orifices. Make sure that anything going up them is firmly anchored on the outside of the body so it can't get sucked up inside. Dildos or butt plugs with flared bases are best for anal play, as it is unlikely you will need the assistance of an emergency-room crew to get them out.

Be sure that anything inserted into the rectum is smooth with no points or ridges.

Anal beads consist of five large beads on a string. They resemble worry beads, but each bead is held in place on the string so it doesn't slide. While anal beads can be used to count your worries on, people usually stick them up their butt. They are slowly pulled out, often at the point of orgasm, which can make for a super-charged orgasm. Anal beads can be as small as mothballs or as big as golf balls. If the beads are plastic and have sharp blow-mold edges, file them down first. Also, it is wise to encase them in a condom before inserting. That's because they are very difficult to fully clean.

Prostate Stimulation

The only time most straight men get anal stimulation is during a physical exam. Then and at tax time.

Men who are curious about feeling their own prostate can do so by reaching between their legs and sticking a well-lubricated finger up their own anus. Pressing on the prostate will probably cause a dull, subtle sensation in the penis. Some men find that the physical contortions necessary to reach their own prostate can result in unanticipated trips to the chiropractor. To avoid this, you can purchase specially curved sex toys that help a guy to stimulate his prostate. For more on sex play with the prostate, see Chapter 16: "The Prostate & The Male Pelvic Underground."

Double Penetration

"I have had anal sex intermittently. It's OK. I was double penetrated twice and *THAT* was the most incredible thing, but it was a dangerous science to get the positioning just right." *female age 28*

The Guide has a separate chapter titled "Double Penetration" (pp. 557-560). Please give it a look if you are planning to party with two penises.

Anal Fisting

Yes, Martha, there is such a thing. It can be very dangerous if done by the inexperienced. The best book on the subject is said to be Bert Herrman's *Trust: The Hand Book—A Guide to the Sensual and Spiritual Art of Handballing*, Alamo Square Press (1991). The subject is also covered well in Tristan Taormino's *Ultimate Guide to Anal Sex, 2nd edition*, Cleis Press (2006). It never hurts to check with a physician first, perhaps one who is recommended by your local gay and lesbian health center. Even if you are not gay, they are more likely to know about the practice and will send you to a more fisting-friendly practitioner. There are also organized groups of fisters in large cities who sometimes offer talks and demonstrations.

Lost Condom in the Dungeon of Doom?

According to the excellent book *Sex Disasters*, a condom lost up your rectum can go farther up than your partner can reach with his or her fingers.

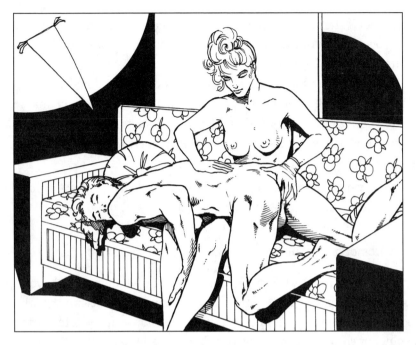

*Using the forefinger instead of the middle finger allows for a deeper probe,
as the knuckles on both sides of the bird finger act as governors.*

Not to worry, it will most likely come out the next time you have a BM. However, if you are worried you will die from the condom up your crapper, call your healthcare provider or visit an ER. As for a sex toy lost up your bum, this is a different story. Do not try to reach up and grab it, as you are likely to shove it farther up. If you can't squat and push it out, seek medical attention. Depending on the object, this can be a very serious situation.

Precautions for Anal Sex—A Recap

💡 Straight or gay, married or in transition—if you are doing anal intercourse, use a condom and LOTS of condom-friendly lube.

💡 Make sure that anything about to go up your rectum is both clean and well-lubricated. Re-apply the lube often.

💡 You will need to discuss which positions and angles feel best. Positions are similar to those used with vaginal intercourse.

💡 Remove anything you have placed in the rectum very slowly. This includes a penis.

Don't stick a finger, penis or other object directly into a vagina when it's just been up an anus. Wash it first with soap and water. Make sure that your nails are well-trimmed.

People who have anal intercourse should occasionally get a rectal swab done to check for VD, yet few individuals own up to doing anal sex, so they don't tell their doctors. It might be easier if doctors simply asked, "Have you ever tried anal sex?" but it seems unlikely that the answers given would become a barometer of truth.

Never, ever have anal sex unless your rectum is in 100% good health. Do not do anal sex if it is painful. Unless you are sure of what you are doing, check with a physician or qualified expert first.

Do not hold your breath. Breathing deeply will help you relax.

Once your get your finger, penis, dildo or whatever inside your partner's rear end, don't start thrusting with it. Leave it in place and gently start making circular motions. If and when your partner wants you to start thrusting, pull out slowly and as far as possible, and add more lube. Then you can start thrusting slowly.

Using a latex glove helps fingers slide in more smoothly, using a condom helps a penis slide in more smoothly. They also protect both partners from getting and giving sexually transmitted infections.

Don't have anal sex when you are drugged or drunk. Your rear end is more easily damaged by sloppy sex than other body parts. Anal sex requires that the driver as well as the passenger be alert and sober. Likewise, don't use a lube like *Anal Ease* that numbs your butt.

The author of this book went to a university with a top reputation in the sciences. Many of his classmates became medical doctors. A number of them did not seem like they would be comfortable dealing with questions about sex, anal or otherwise. Or, it is possible that you won't be comfortable asking a physician who you know if you have questions about sex. An alternative is to call your local free clinic or a national sex hot line. And as mentioned earlier, while you may not be homosexual, a friendly place to call with questions about anal sex might be the nearest gay and lesbian health center.

Resources

If you are into anal recreation, consider the following:

Jack Morin's *Anal Pleasure and Health*, Down There Press, (1999). Morin's book is not shy with the "love your anus" mantra, but anyone who is having anal problems of any kind will find it to be helpful. He really does get you thinking about your anus in a different way, and if you have any kind of stress-related anal problem (especially hemorrhoids), this book will be more than worthwhile. It's also a highly-regarded book to read if you are thinking about trying anal sex.

Tristan Taormino's Ultimate Guide to Anal Sex for Women, 2nd edition, Cleis Press, (2006). This book is just as informative for men as for women. Tristan Taormino's infectious zeal and zest for life and sex provide a welcome backdrop to all things anal. An excellent resource, well-organized and easy to read. Definitely a book to own if you are into anal. Get the 2nd edition.

Tristan Taormino's Expert Guide To Anal Sex DVD (Vivid Ed/Vivid Entertainmen). Ms. Taormino's sex-ed series will do for your screen what her books have done for your library.

For a DVD on anal massage, try *Anal Massage for Relaxation and Pleasure* from www.erospirit.org. Expect to see couples of all ages and all orientations massaging each other's butt cheeks and anuses. If your goal is to be a pro at anal massage and finger penetration, you will definitely learn a thing or three from this quietly-paced DVD. Better yet, get a membership on the Erospirit.org website. You can watch all sorts of streaming videos by the calm, thoughtful and kind anal massage expert Chester Mainard.

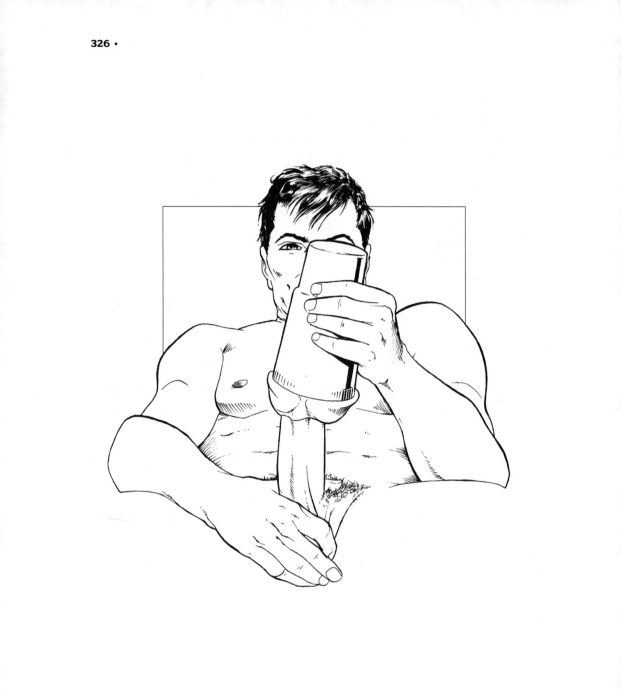

24
Playing with Yourself

Before the 1960s, people who wrote books on sex stated with an almost religious fervor that playing with yourself (masturbation) was a very bad thing to do. Today, people who write books on sex speak with the same kind of religious fervor, only now they say that playing with yourself is a very good thing to do.

It doesn't seem as though anything has changed. That's because none of the experts are asking you what you want to do. When it comes to the question of whether you should or shouldn't be masturbating, this book doesn't have any answers. It's your hand and your pants; if you want to stick one into the other, that's totally up to you.

What we can tell you is that as teenagers we felt certain that masturbation was an adolescent thing, something people get over when they become adults. That never happened.

There are times when people do it a lot, and times when they hardly do it at all; times when it feels great, and times when it's a letdown. But during those times when the world doesn't seem like such a nice place, masturbation can usually be counted on to help take off some of the edge. It also helps ease the transition between wakefulness and sleep, and contrary to what you might think, it will sometimes play an important role in relationships even when the sex between you and your partner is totally satisfying.

Some people find that their bodies simply work better if they have an orgasm every day or two, with masturbation being a natural way to help this happen. Sometimes, you might find that you get into a certain state of mind where you need to masturbate just to relax enough so you can get the rest of your work done.

Whatever the motivation, if you are going to get yourself off by hand, why not try to get the most out of it? That is the focus of this chapter.

Wanking Protocol—When You Have Roommate

Even if they're not particularly horny, a lot of people masturbate in bed at night to help turn their brains off. This can be especially necessary when you've had a full or stressful day and you need as much sleep as possible. Lying there awake just makes you feel more stressed.

Firing up a 30-amp vibrator or humping your teddy bear until his stuffing starts to explode is usually not a problem when you have your own room. But tender moments with yourself can be few and far between when you have a roommate. Add to this the fact that most of us would find it less embarrassing to be walked in on while we are having sex with a partner than when we've got our hands in our own pants.

The usual solution is to wait quietly until your roommate is making sleeping noises. This is not as easy as it sounds, since your roommate is probably waiting for you to make sleeping noises as well. Fortunately, there are common-sense solutions that they usually don't tell you about at your college orientation.

First, is to pull out your trusty copy of *The Guide*, point to this page, and say to your roommate, "Hmm. I wonder if we should talk about this?"

Of course, there are those roommate situations where you'd rather be anally penetrated by a herd of buffaloes before talking about masturbation, but let's say your current roommate is reasonable and probably has some of the same needs that you do. So here are some solutions that roommates in the past have found to be helpful. Some roommates are most comfortable only adopting the first solution, others more. It depends on your situation and your comfort level:

- You agree to share with each other your class and work schedules, and if there is a change, you will notify your roommate, especially if a class was cancelled and you're returning early. A quick call or a long, loud series of knocks on the door accompanied by a thoughtful, "I can come back in ten minutes" shows consideration.

- You agree that if you are leaving and won't be right back, to tell your roommate, "I'll be gone for at least ??? minutes," and don't come back before then unless it's totally necessary, in which case you'll knock loudly and wait to hear "Come on in" before coming on in.

- You agree that after the lights are out, it's fine to masturbate as long as you are reasonable about it. While it's usually impossible to be totally silent, one doesn't need to sound like porn star or a Mr. America-wannabe at the gym who can't unrack a dumbbell without grunting loudly.

You agree that it's okay to rub one out first thing in the morning while you are still in bed to help to tame a raging A.M. erection or to relieve a crippling case of sunrise horniness.

You agree that if one of you has a significant other at a different school or on a another part of the planet, you will try to work out specific times when that person can be alone on the phone with his or her lover. That way, if they want to get themselves off while aided by the sound of their lover's voice, or if they want to share some kinky webcam moments, there's no problem. However, this is one of those things that a less-than-sensitive roommate can easily abuse, so the one doing the phoning needs to be fair, reasonable and not overdue it.

You agree that if one of you is dating a person who is abstinence-only to the fullest degree or not interested in having sex—that upon returning from a date or evening with this person, at least fifteen or twenty minutes of alone time will be provided.

Two things to avoid:

Masturbating with earphones or plugs in your ears, as you won't be able to hear your roommate's warning knock;

Never, ever masturbate in a bathroom stall unless it's in your own dorm and it's pretty well understood that everyone does it. The problem with relieving yourself in a public rest room is that it could be against the law and you could get busted if there's a sting operation going on. It doesn't matter if you have the stall door locked and are being discreet.

And finally:

Tissues and toilet paper remain the usual standbys for guys to masturbate into, although socks and dark-colored underwear are strong contenders.

For guys who are wanking in the shower, it's better to use hair conditioner for lube than soap, although when the conditioner claims that it adds volume or thickness, your penis is not what they had in mind.

Vital Statistics

The following was told to Harry Maurer by a young woman for his book *Sex: An Oral History,* Viking Press:

"My mother has a vibrator that my father gave her one year. When I used to come home from college, I knew where she kept the vibrator, and I knew they never used it, so I would put it into my room and use it for the vacation. One summer I came home and it wasn't there. I was going crazy, I'm really a vibrator addict. Finally I was just so horny I said, 'OK, Mom, sit down. Where's the vibrator?' She's like, 'What!' I said 'Look, here's the deal. I've been stealing your vibrator for three years, and I need it now.' She was blown away, but she goes into her room, comes back with the vibrator, and says, 'By the way, have you ever used the jet in the hot tub?'"

According to just about everyone who has ever researched the subject, somewhere between 80% and 95% of guys eventually masturbate. Depending on whose statistics you look at, between 50% and 85% of women do it.

Contrary to what you might think, people don't masturbate any less as they get older. In fact, many people who are married or deeply involved in a sexual relationship still get themselves off by hand. Masturbation doesn't decrease a person's desire for shared sex. For some people, it increases it. And some people report that they masturbate more when they are in a relationship rather than less.

How often do people masturbate? It varies from a couple of times a day to sometimes never. As for the number of orgasms per effort, researcher Thore Langfeldt interviewed children in Norway from kindergarten through high school. Langfeldt found that the younger boys and girls could give themselves multiple orgasms when they masturbated. But as they got older, the boys started reporting fewer orgasms per attempt, while the girls reported more. This is a trend that continued with increased age and experience.

Also, while intercourse remains the most popular sex act for couples, far more men than women have orgasms during intercourse. A woman is much more likely to have an orgasm when she masturbates than when a penis is in the picture.

What the Sandman Knows about Masturbation

"In my younger years, it usually took an hour or so before I had an orgasm. Now, if I'm especially hot, five minutes with a vibrator can do it, or about fifteen to twenty minutes by hand. Sometimes I like to keep things slow; I prolong it by starting and stopping. Other times, I just want to get off as fast as I can. Sometimes I masturbate, but not to orgasm. It feels good and relaxes me without wanting to come." *female age 47*

According to the Sandman, the most common time when people masturbate is at night before they go to sleep or before taking a nap. People get themselves off at other times, too. For instance, it sometimes feels good to masturbate after a workout, since workouts can be sexually arousing. Plenty of people masturbate as a study break or when they have to spend long hours doing a paper or a project. It helps them refocus and return to the work at hand. Some people masturbate before a date so they will be more intellectually present. Women sometimes masturbate during their periods to help relieve cramping, or before intercourse to help it feel better. Some people wake up feeling really horny. They sometimes masturbate early in the morning, when the cock crows, before having their Wheaties®.

Some Seriously Twisted Lunacy from Kellogg's of Battle Creek

That should have read "Corn Flakes" instead of Wheaties, since Kellogg's Corn Flakes were created to give children more stamina so they wouldn't want to do horrible things like masturbate. John Harvey Kellogg, M.D., founderof the flake, told anyone who would listen that masturbation was a worse sin and "more immoral" than adultery. He called it the "most heinous, revolting, and unnatural vice."

Kellogg proposed a six-point program for every American male that included taking cold enemas every day and wearing a wet girdle to bed every night to help prevent masturbation.

His advice for parents whose children were caught masturbating included bandaging the genitals and covering them with cages, tying the child's hands together, and circumcision without anesthesia. He felt that the pain would be a helpful punishment for the act that had been committed. Whatever foreskin was left should be sewn shut over the glans of the penis to keep the young man from having erections. Kellogg was an interesting guy.

Kellogg's cereal is still known as "Kellogg's of Battle Creek." Battle Creek was the name of his mental asylum, where he served his special cold cereals to help keep the inmates from masturbating. Of course, the finest medical minds of the day couldn't quite agree on the specific horrors that masturbation would cause. Some claimed it caused a man to become feeble, lackluster, feminized, impotent and to have underdeveloped genitals. Others claimed it had the opposite effect, turning the young men into sex fiends who would have uncontrolled eruptions of lust and blow the family fortune on prostitutes. Ads in popular papers promised to cure "the excesses of youth" and "underdeveloped genitals," which were what happened if you masturbated.

To keep Dr. Kellogg spinning in his grave, this book encourages its readers to occasionally masturbate while eating a bowl of Kellogg's Corn Flakes.

How Guys Learn

> "When I was ten, an older friend showed me how to masturbate. He had a full ejaculation; nothing came out of my penis. Astronauts were first orbiting the earth, and I believed that technology could fix anything. So I decided to create a jack-off machine. Planning and building it kept me busy for days. But it didn't make anything more come out of my penis than my hand did. Time, rather than technology, was the answer to that problem." *male age 45*

A lot of guys learn to masturbate from other guys, often friends or a big brother. Guys who don't learn about jerking off from other guys eventually learn on their own. That's because a teenager has to be pretty numb to himself to miss the connection between soaping the thing up in the shower and the nice feelings that result. Also, when lying face down on a mattress with a hard-on, most guys are eventually compelled to hump or rub. More than other human organs, the penis pleads to be yanked, stroked and squeezed. (Anyone who has raised daughter in a non-repressive environment might disagree, saying that clitoral hoods get a pretty good working out, as well.)

If they haven't heard about ejaculation before having their first one, some guys will experience anything from concern to terror when they have their first ones, e.g., "Oh no, I broke something," to "Please God, I'll never ever do it again! I promise, just make it OK." And then they do it again the next day. Today's porn-saavy pre-pubescent junior high males might have the opposite concern, "Mine doesn't squirt worth squat; where's the wad?"

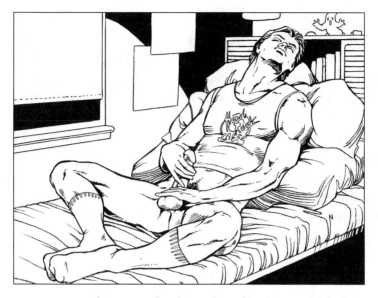

This young buck is taking his time.

The Group Thing

"I can understand all sorts of things about guys' sexuality, except
why they jerk off together. It seems so gay. Why do they do it?"

female age 23

Good question. First of all, the majority of men will tell you that they
have never jerked off with another male. And for those who have, it may have
to do with the maturation process. Most young guys need little encouragement to take their pants off and explore. Getting naked can be so exciting for
some boys that they get hard-ons from that alone. It's also natural for boys
to share experiences, whether it's checking out an abandoned house or cave
or showing each other the things you do with your dick. After all, you would
want to show your best friend the model you just built or take turns doing
the latest skateboard trick, so why wouldn't you want to jerk off together
and see what happens when you get hard or come?

"When we became teens, some of us boys would get together for a
masturbation meeting in the treehouse, but it was more the thrill
of something exciting and forbidden than anything else. *male, 26*

Plenty of men will say, "No way. You'd never catch me jerking off with
another guy when I was a kid." Others will say, "Sure, that's how we did it."
Some even might say, "It was neat back then, simpler, and fun."

As for masturbatory etiquette, some males have guy-like tea parties called circle jerks where they stand around and masturbate. There might be games connected with this, like who shoots the farthest or who comes the fastest (it's interesting how priorities change as you get older!). It's even been said that some young men feel excluded until they have been allowed to beat off with members of the local gang. The urge to beat off together seems to peak before high-school age and drops off significantly after that. However, there are some adult males who appear to be straight who enjoy masturbating together. Perhaps this isn't as much of a contradiction in terms as it seems. Straight men sure enjoy watching other men ejaculate in porn movies. Perhaps it's acceptable to be curious about another guy's ejaculation if he's just had his penis in a woman's body, but not acceptable if it's just two guys together.

The following answers to a survey in the newsletter *Sex & Health* help to summarize some of what's involved:

"While partying with fraternity brothers, someone suggested a contest to see who could ejaculate the farthest. Each of the five of us took our turn in a tiled shower room. Surprisingly, the least endowed among us won!"

"Sometimes when I'm camping with a couple of my buddies and our girlfriends are otherwise occupied, we get to joking about sex. We soon get so aroused that when one of us whips it out to pee, we start joking and the others whip theirs out, too. Then we just start stroking ourselves and talking about our favorite techniques. We don't touch each other, but we do comment on each other's members and may cheer one another on to climax. We're all good friends and have become much closer sharing our sexuality this way."

Sex & Health had a large male readership. 95% of the men characterized themselves as strictly heterosexual; most were married and many had children. Still, a number reported fantasizing about masturbating with other men, e.g., 'Although I'm happily married with two children, I do sometimes fantasize about masturbating with friends. I've thought about asking one friend in particular, but I haven't had the nerve.' "

How Girls Learn

"When I was young, climbing a flagpole always brought on such intense tingling feelings that I was only able to hold on tight and my legs would clamp around the pole. When the feelings subsided enough, I would resume climbing." *female age 37*

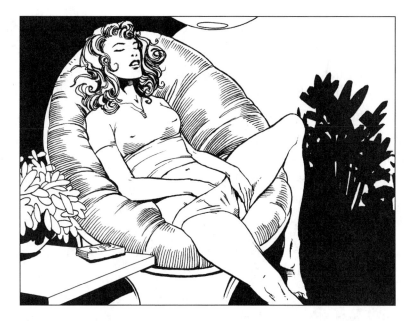

"It was my freshman year of high school. I was kissing this guy and was getting really turned on. He put his hand on my inner thigh and I was going crazy! This was my first heavy petting session. I didn't quite know what to make of it. When I got home, I went to the bathroom. My underwear was very wet. I went to touch myself and BAM!—instant orgasm! My very first. I've never had it that easy since." *female age 27*

"When I had my first orgasm I kept saying, 'Oh my God!' over and over. I was really shocked because I didn't know I could do that to myself!" *female age 25*

When it comes to masturbation, girls don't do "show and tell" nearly as often as boys. They tend to learn about masturbation on their own or by reading about it or seeing a woman do it in porn. Some women learn how to masturbate from the sensation they experience while cleaning their genitals, from climbing trees, poles, or ropes, while on swings or when riding bicycles. Some learn by putting a pillow between their legs or by leaning up against the washing machine when it's on the spin cycle. It might also happen when they have a sex dream and wake up before it's over—the sensation is still alive in their genitals and all they need to do is reach down and rub. One woman learned to masturbate by pushing a sanitary napkin against her vulva; another by stroking the shaft of her clitoris with a pencil. The possibilities for discovering how to masturbate are too numerous to name, but here are some of the ways women readers say they do it now:

> "Bathtub, vibrator, boyfriend's fingers (my own don't work). Electric toothbrush handle, my ex-husband's hammer (the handle), even celery once." *female age 26*

> "I get the most intense orgasm by leaning on a hard surface like a counter and wiggling around till I come. I also use a dildo, and I use my fingers to massage my labia and clit, occasionally fingering my vagina." *female age 37*

> "I use a finger, then fingers." *female age 49*

> "Occasionally I use my hands, but usually I use a running faucet before I take my bath." *female age 19*

> "I rub my clit in a circular motion with my fingers or use a trusty old Prelude 3 [vibrator]. I've tried putting things inside my vagina, but so far that's been a very neutral experience — I need my lover's hand or torso to be attached to what's going inside. Sometimes I gently rub my chest as I masturbate, or run a soft piece of cloth over my nipples." *female age 47*

> "I do it while reading a book or having a fantasy. Usually I stimulate my clit directly with one or more fingers. Only rarely do I put anything inside my vagina, although I do like the feel of a tampon. I also like anal stimulation. That will make an orgasm more intense and more diffused." *female age 36*

It is impossible to list all of the different ways that women masturbate. A lot of women use their fingers while lying on their backs or sitting in chairs. Some do it on their sides, or while lying face down so nobody can see what they are doing. Some women may even occasionally prefer to squat.

Men sometimes have the fantasy that a woman who is masturbating sticks her fingers inside her vagina. Some women do, but many don't. Instead, they might squeeze the lips of their vulva together or push against it in ways that create pressure rather than penetration. A woman who has responsive nipples may make nipple stimulation an enjoyable part of her masturbation.

Plenty of women use lubrication when they masturbate, either their own (vaginal or saliva) or store-bought. Lots like to use vibrators for masturbating, and some use dildos. Some like to masturbate by using the faucet in the bath-tub. After they get the water temperature just right, they lie down in the tub and push their bum against the wall of the tub where the faucet comes out. It might help to have an inflatable pillow to put under their rear to get the angle just right. Some women say it works better if they spread their labia open with their fingers so the water cascades onto their awaiting clitoris.

Water Safety When masturbating with a water jet in a hot tub, sit back at a distance. The current might be stronger than you think, so approach slowly. Some women like to pull their labia apart; others don't. Do not get extremely close to the jet, and don't aim it up your vagina or rectum.

Thigh High

The woman writer who contributes to the female part of JackinWorld.com suggests that some women can teach themselves to come by squeezing their thighs together. She suggests that you start by masturbating in the nor-mal way, but press your thighs together when you start to have an orgasm. After a few weeks of doing this, masturbate yourself to the point where you almost have an orgasm, but pull your fingers (or whatever) away at the last minute and try to finesse yourself into orgasm by squeezing your thighs together. Once you are able to do this successfully, start with the thigh-squeezing action a little earlier each time. Some might prefer doing this with tight jeans on so they get an assist from the seam in the crotch.

Additional Ways

One woman says she can have an orgasm by doing stomach crunches (mini sit-ups). What an incentive for keeping your abs in shape!

Other women get off by humping pillows or water bottles, swinging on swings, tugging on underwear, rubbing up against things, using peeled cucumbers, and riding a bike down bumpy roads. Some like to stimulate their anus, either by putting pressure on it or by sticking a finger or butt plug inside it. Some like to look in mirrors, some get turned on by wearing their boyfriend's shirt or underwear. Heck—fill in your own blanks.

Say It Ain't So!

Tennis elbow is a form of tendonitis. One reader, a female physician, suspects that some of her patients with tennis elbow got their tendonitis from—gulp—the number-one repetitive finger motion that many women do. So if you are having tendonitis or repetitive-stress syndrome on the arm that you masturbate with, try using a vibrator for masturbating and see if the problem doesn't improve. Ditto for lovers who routinely masturbate their female partners. This physician adds that guys with unexplained tendonitis might try masturbating differently, too. If you do it dry, you might try using lube. The hand motion can be quite different.

Rubbing the Nub? Beating the Bush? Giving Girl-Masturbation a Name

There are numerous slang terms for male masturbation. This is not the case with female masturbation (Diddle? Jill off? She Bop? These are not exactly universal terms). Since women don't usually masturbate together, they haven't needed to establish slang to convey what they are doing. In fact, it has only been during the last couple of decades that our society has openly acknowledged the existence of women's masturbation. Maybe it's time that women adopted a universal slang term for masturbation. Perhaps one of the women's magazines could have a contest, or maybe the First Lady could announce what she calls it.

Women, Masturbation & Intercourse

Some women give themselves orgasms during intercourse by pushing against a partner's pubic bone or by reaching down with their fingers and playing with themselves while the penis is inside of them. Is this masturbation, intercourse, or both? It happens often and is totally normal.

It's not unusual for a woman to masturbate before intercourse to help her genitals be more into it, or after intercourse because she wants more stimulation or enjoys the feeling. It is unfortunate that women often hide this and think that their partners might not want to know about it. It seems like a sign of a good relationship when a woman feels free to finish what we couldn't, or when we help her get started and she takes it from there.

It's also nice when a partner feels free to masturbate on his or her own. Far from being a sign of deficit, this might be an indication there is a great deal of love and understanding in the relationship.

Girls, Their Horses & the Fifty-Minute Hour

"My first orgasm? I was riding my horse and I felt a strange sort of pleasure between my legs. I felt like I wanted it to stop so I could concentrate on my riding, but it felt so good." *female age 18*

"I was standing in the barn with my horse when I had a spontane-ous orgasm. I gushed and everyone laughed at me for peeing in my pants. I was fourteen or so. I didn't discover masturbation until I was twenty, and then I thought orgasm was so incredible, I wanted one every day." *female age 37*

"My first orgasm ever was when I was riding a horse. I thought I was perverted and never told anyone. Then at a slumber party one of my close friends who also horseback rides admitted that she'd had a similar experience." *female age 18*

Having grown up close to livestock, your author knew from a young age that it was unwise for any man to come between a woman and her horse. But can you imagine his amazement years later when an occasional female patient would describe the euphoria she gleaned from the back of her favor-ite gelding? It's information that's usually relayed in hushed tones of revelry and delight—warm, pleasing, primal sensations with one of nature's most magnificent creatures between her legs. Women rarely speak about their husbands or boyfriends with the kind of knowing sensitivity that is reserved for their favorite horse.

From Trigger to Hitachi

After having an orgasm, women's genitals often stay primed. Some women experience waves of orgasm that can be finessed for the better part of an hour. Other women find a single orgasm to be very satisfying.

Because of the different possibilities, one woman might masturbate on and off for an entire evening, reaching between her legs every page or two while reading a book. Another woman might masturbate with the sole purpose of reaching a single, discrete orgasm, going from beginning to end without pause.

There are plenty of women who don't like to masturbate. Some never feel the urge. For others, touching themselves implies an uncomfortable investment in their own sexuality. Sex with a man makes it OK to be a sexual rocket ship, but masturbation might feel dirty. This might be true even if their body badly needs an orgasm to help it unwind. There are also women who like to masturbate but don't like to touch their genitals. They might use a vibrator or masturbate with their fingers on the outside of their underwear.

The Limitations of a One-Grip Rhythm (for Both Sexes)

If you always use the exact same touch and rhythm when you mastur-bate, you might be teaching your body to expect that and only that. Given how it's difficult for someone else to do you in precisely the same way that you do yourself, you might consider occasionally mixing it up. For instance, if you usually get yourself off dry, you might try it with lotion. If you use your right hand, experiment with your left or try it with a vibrator one time and another time in the bathtub, but not with a vibrator in the bathtub unless the vibra-tor is waterproof.

On Sucking Air (for Both Sexes)

Learning to breathe right is an essential part of being an athlete, unless maybe your sport is billiards. It's no different with sex.

When you are having sex, be it solo or with a partner, you might occa-sionally pay attention to your breathing. Tantric types encourage taking long, slow, deep breaths where you imagine pulling the air all the way into your groin. This may help some people have a more intense experience. From this book's more geriatric perspective, the extra O_2 helps keep us from having a coronary.

Guy Tricks—"First, Nuke a Jar of Miracle Whip, Then..."

> "I made a false pussy out of bicycle tire inner tubes, and it worked quite well. I have also used banana peels, watermelons, and a hole in a piece of wood." *male age 42*

A lot of guys use their hands to jerk off with. Some do it dry and some add lubrication which includes saliva, soap, hair conditioner, Vaseline, vegetable oil, coconut oil, baby oil, baby oil gel, and anything else under the sun that can make their pecker slick. Guys do better using an oil-based lubricant, and some even use a special type of facial cleanser called Albolene which is greatly admired for its jerk-off properties. The trouble with standard moisturizers is that they dry up quickly, as do water-based lubes when exposed to air. If you use a water-based lube, try adding a few drops of water or saliva as it dries instead of adding more lube. Otherwise, you might end up with two sticky messes instead of one.

A lot of guys masturbate in the shower using soap as a lubricant, but that's kind of iffy because the soap can get up your peehole and irritate the living daylights out of you. A fine substitute is hair conditioner, or, if you must use soap, you might start each stroke by grabbing your penis around the base and pulling outward only.

Another way that guys sometimes masturbate is by lubricating the inside of a condom with a water-based lube like KY. They slide a condom on their erect penis, wrap their fingers around it and pump away. A variation of this is to lube up the inside of a Baggie or plastic bag and put it between your pillows or mattress and box springs. You then get on your knees and hump the bag, being careful not to get your mattress pregnant.

Banana peels can come in handy. If you are having trouble with the peel falling apart and condoms are plentiful, try putting a condom over the peel.

If you make an artificial vagina and heat it in a microwave, be cautious. It could feel nice and warm around the outside, but could sizzle your little pecker when you stick it in the center.

Foreskin Tricks for Men Who Are Uncut

Fill a turkey baster or syringe with warm water. Pull your foreskin over the head of your penis and crimp it with your fingers over the end of the turkey baster. As you squeeze the end of the turkey baster, the warm water fills your foreskin and causes it to balloon out. Then let go of the bulb and the baster sucks up the water. Keep repeating until you come.

Another unusual method is to keep the foreskin retracted. Tug the foreskin lightly by pulling it down toward your scrotum. This will cause it to become taut. Keep repeating this until you come. It will take a while, but might be pretty intense. (Thanks to JackinWorld.com for these suggestions.)

Rushin' Roulette (for Men)

Guys tend to rush themselves when they are masturbating. There are a couple of reasons for this. First, a man often wants to get to the heavy-duty pleasure part as soon as possible. Second is the matter of privacy, or lack of it, when you are growing up. (The same privacy challenge repeats itself when you have your own children.) The last thing most guys want is for someone to walk in on them when they are stroking themselves, so they teach themselves to come quickly and quietly. Also, if they are doing it in the shower, the extra speed helps them finish before the hot water runs out. And if you take a really long shower, most everybody knows what you are doing.

In employing the basic theorem of jack-off relativity, $M = Q^2$ (masturbation = quick x quiet—Betty Dodson), the body becomes numb to anything but the rush of coming. This might desensitize a man to some of the more subtle sensations that can feel so wonderful when he is sharing sex with a partner.

Learning to Live in the Zone of Subtle Sensation

Taking extra time when masturbating might help a man learn about subtle sensations that he won't notice if he's red-lining it. For instance, if he slows down as ejaculation approaches, he might discover a rush of feelings in his stomach, bladder, or rectum. Instead of going for the big squirt, he might try to back off a bit, teaching himself how to live in the zone of subtle sensation. If allowed to emerge slowly, pre-squirt feelings can be quite intense and last for long periods of time without becoming an actual ejaculation. Learning to stay with these feelings might help a man experience deeper levels of intimacy when he is with a partner.

Also, instead of reaching for his crotch each time he masturbates, a man might start by touching or massaging other parts of his body: scalp, face, neck, shoulders, chest, hands, feet, etc. This can be a way of reminding himself that sex is a full-body activity rather than something that just happens between his legs. (One female reader says that this section should have been written for women as well as men.) For new ways of stroking yourself that you might not have thought about before, check out the "Extreme Handjob" part of the chapter on handjobs.

Reader Comment "This is just as true for women when they masturbate as for men!"

Intercourse Spoilers

Grip of Death Guys tend to grip themselves tightly when masturbating. Yet few vaginas can come close to generating that kind of squeezing action. This might be one reason why some men have more intense orgasms when they masturbate than during intercourse. You might try masturbating with a lighter grip, at least occasionally.

Face Down The last thing we want to do is amplify anecdotal science, but it seems that some men who always masturbate face down have erection and/or orgasm problems when trying to have sex with a woman. So, if you are having erection problems or delayed orgasm and masturbate face down, try to limit your jerking off to sunnyside up. And if you masturbate face down and have erections of steel each and can come on a dime, have a good laugh over this paragraph of caution.

Warnings

URETHRA SAFETY See "sounds" in the glossary at the end of this book. Some people, both men and women, are tempted to stick things up their urethra (pee hole) when they play with themselves. This is known as *urethral play* or *sounding*. If you don't know what you are doing, this can be a dangerous thing. It may end up requiring an embarrassing visit to a hospital emergency room and maybe even surgery if the object gets lost in your bladder.

BUTTHOLE SAFETY Some men and women enjoy sticking things up their buttholes when they play. Be sure it the object is well-washed and has no sharp edges. The advantage of using a finger is that it's not likely to get lost up there. Always wash your hands ahead of time and make sure that your fingernails don't look like Elvira's. A good alternative is to use a butt plug.

BAGGING and REALLY TWISTED STUFF Over the years, people have tried some seriously dangerous and life-threatening ways of getting themselves off. If you are into that sort of thing, there are two ways to go. If you need to act out scenes or levels of kink that are risky, search out a community of caring, thoughtful people who are into similar things and can help you to do it as safely as possible. The other way is to get yourself some therapy from a sex-positive psychotherapist or sex therapist. Bagging or erotic asphyxiation is discussed in Chapter 50: "Kinky Corner."

Chapter Notes Dr. Tom Szasz made a presentation which was similar in content to this chapter's introduction. This similarity was discovered after this book was already written and is a pleasant coincidence

Readers' Comment Quiz

Guess which answers are men's and which are women's.

Have you ever needed to masturbate while away from home?

a. "I have done so occasionally in the car, while driving. Tricky, but doable."
age 37

b. "I would pretty much masturbate anywhere if I could. I know it sounds silly, but when I am on the beach or catching a killer wave I get kind of horny." *age 23*

c. "Yes. Although never at my current job, I have masturbated at work."
age 26

d. "Yes. I've masturbated driving in my car; the urge was just too great and I had to deal with it right then." *age 36*

e. "It has happened. I feel pressure like I'll go nuts if I don't get relief, and I'll sneak off." *age 38*

f. "Except for when I was on a long vacation, I've always been able to wait until I got home." *age 26*

g. "One time I was driving and I had a terrible urge, so I brought myself to orgasm. I've also done it at work once." *age 43*

h. "I was once on a long-distance bus trip and a teenage boy was next to me. I don't remember why, but I got very aroused, so I put my coat over me and masturbated while he slept." *age 45*

i. "While my partner lived in a different city, I used to all the time. I would lock myself in the bathroom and put my feet on the wall while sitting on the toilet, with my legs bent and above my head. It was most satisfying this way." *age 37*

j. "I was using the computer at my brother's house when no one was home. While on the net, I was talking to someone who was so hot that I had to masturbate to release enough tension so I could keep talking online."
age 27

Darned stereotypes...

a. female b. female c. female d. female e. female f. male g. male h. female i. female j. female

25

Oscillator, Generator Vibrator & Dildo

It used to be "sex toy" meant getting yourself a vibrator or dildo. Vibrators were one of the first electric machines created back in the 1800s, and they have been a hit ever since. Other useful toys include bondage devices for people who are into BDSM, good old-fashioned butt plugs, and some of the really cool double dildos. Additional spicer-uppers include adult literature and DVDs.

In recent years, sex toys have become the new Tupperware, with people selling them at parties, on the Internet, and anywhere else you can think of. So rather than being a fluff piece on the joys of sex toys, this chapter takes a more balanced view. It hopes to broaden your notion of what a sex toy is in a relationship, and it looks at what makes a toy sexy. It has suggestions for how to size a dildo, and it considers when a partner might feel threatened by your vibrator or dildo. Also, while sex-toy aficionados will call this blasphemy, keep in mind that there are lots of people who don't use sex toys and still have wonderfully fun sex lives.

Sex Toy Strategy, Part 1

Before investing money in the latest sex toy or getting your hopes up that the hype is real, why not think about what it is you want a sex toy to do for you? If you are trying to get a sex toy for a partner, think about the things that turn him or her on. If your gift doesn't resonate with a lover's fantasies, it will end up being just another buzzing piece of plastic or a suggestive *whatever* without any sexual oomph.

Another thing to ask yourself is, "Would my partner prefer flowers and the latest book by her favorite author?" "Would he like it better if I got him a new computer gizmo or brake cable for his mountain bike rather than this strange looking sex toy that he's supposed to stick up his ass?"

As for haphazard sex-toy shopping, let's say you are a woman who is trying to rev up her partner's interest. You could always buy him a thick sleeve-like vagina-device that he sticks his penis into. Forget that it might feel like the vagina of a woman who's been dead for two weeks—the websites that are selling it claim it's even better than blow-up dolls!

Or you could take a smarter approach.

NOTE: Over the years we have tried a $1200 sex-toy device that had nothing on a $20 vibrator. We also tried a $600 male masturbating device that made you appreciate just how good your own hand feels. Just because it's supposed to be great doesn't mean it's great for you or your partner.

Sex Toy Strategy, Part 2

You might find that the perfect sex toy for your lover is one that you use on yourself. Perhaps he'll be turned on by watching you use it. Or make a deal with your partner: she selects a toy for you to use on her, and you select a toy for her to use on you. Then go shopping together. The neat thing about using toys in this way is they help you reveal new things about yourself to your partner, and vice versa. Sex can get boring when you think you know all there is to know about the person you are sleeping with.

Beware the Phthalates

Not long ago, Greenpeace issued a warning that sex toys put off a dangerous class of chemicals known as "phthalates." Were schools of dildo-using dolphins in danger? Unfortunately, it's much worse than that.

Phthalates have been linked to liver damage, kidney damage, lung damage, and damage to the developing testes in the fetus. Phthalates are added to plastics to increase their flexibility. They are used to create favorite sex-toy materials such as Cyberskin, Softskin and Futurotic. Phathalates put the jelly in jelly rubber sex toys.

Flat out—do not buy plastic sex toys from dealers who are not highly reputable, and only buy toys that these dealers will certify do not contain phthalate residues. Hard plastic toys usually do not contain phthalates, nor do 100% silicone toys or dildos made of glass. The trouble with silicone is that it doesn't need to be 100% silicone to be called silicone.

As for the supposed quick fix of putting a condom between you and your phthalate-containing sex toy, keep in mind that the amount of phthalates in a number of sex toys has been described by researchers as being so high that they are "off the charts."

Books, DVDs & Websites

If you are going to get something sexy, why not search out some cool DVDs that the two of you could watch? Check out sites that only carry titles they think you will enjoy, e.g.: *ComeAsYouAre.com Goodvibes.com, Blowfish. com, Babeland.com,* and *Stockroom.com.* These people work really hard to screen X-rated movies so you don't have to. Read their reviews. Even if you aren't a girl, you might start with Violet Blue's *The Smart Girl's Guide To Porn.*

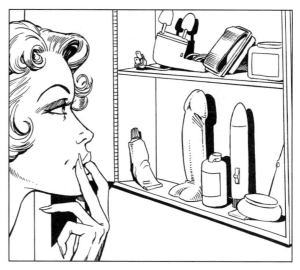

There's a new world of erotic books and literature that you and your partner can read together or to each other. Collections of short stories by competent writers abound. The quality is leagues above the typical letter to Penthouse. Some will get you going, others will fall short, but it's nowhere near as bleak as it used to be. A collection of erotic short stories might be the best sex toy you ever gave or got.

And if you want to visit sexy websites with a partner, there are a dozen or so sites that do nothing but review other sites. Try JanesGuide.com, where their motto is "We waste our time so you don't have to!" Fleshbot.com, TinyNibbles.com, and PuckerUp.com are some of dozens of sites to visit.

Creative & Low Cost

There are plenty of great sex toys that cost hardly anything. For instance, you can make a series of coupons that you give your partner. Each lists a special thing you are willing to do, from giving her a bath and full-body massage to things we can't print even in *The Guide.* Your partner gives you the coupon when she wants you to do what it describes. (Author Laura Corn's *101 Nights of Great Sex* is built around this concept.)

Another idea is for each of you to describe a scene that is a personal turn-on. Then go shopping for props to make the scene happen. For instance, if one of you has the fantasy of being stopped and frisked by an officer in uniform, you can go to a used-clothing store and buy the perfect uniform for acting out the scene, perhaps including handcuffs. If the fantasy concerns a visit to the doctor, do your shopping at a medical-supply house.

If you don't like that idea, try surprising your partner with a sex toy that's found at your local pet store. When your lover comes home, you can be standing there in your underwear with your new dog collar around your neck; hand her the leash and say, "I'm yours for the night!" But don't forget to attach a bow to the collar, as they do at the fancy pet groomers, and pray that she isn't bringing her parents home for a surprise visit.

A Moldy Penis

If your partner feels his penis is adequate, consider getting a kit from your local art-supply store that allows you to make a mold of his little soldier. Best to tell the clerk that you want to make a mold of your son's foot or hand. It's the same kit and won't cause you unnecessary embarrassment. You and your lover will be laughing yourselves silly as you make the mold and the whole thing becomes an adventure. He might even be paralyzed with excitement when you use the finished casting of his penis on yourself or place it proudly on your bookshelf. You can make it out of different materials.

You can find a kit that's specially designed to mold your man's penis at www.artmolds.com. Put the words "intimate" or "penis" into their search engine once you reach their site.

Oscillators, Generators, Vibrators and Dildos

Some people claim that the light bulb is the most important electrical invention of the last 130 years; others say it's the vibrator. The rest of this chapter is about vibrators and dildos. Its emphasis is on the use of these devices by couples as opposed to individuals, although many people use them for solo sex. If what you want is a vibrator, dildo or butt plug, the people who work at reputable stores try them out themselves and are pretty conscientious about what they will and won't sell.

Confusing Vibrators with Dildos

People often confuse the vibrator with the dildo, which is like confusing a rhino with a giraffe. Both are native to the bush, but that's where the similarities end.

Vibrators are valued for their buzzing properties and are usually rested on the surface of the genitals rather than placed inside them. Dildos are penis-shaped and are used as such. Most don't vibrate like a vibrator, but are made to be kept inside the vagina to give a feeling of fullness or to be thrust in and out. They can also slide up and down between the lips of the vulva.

The common battery-operated plastic vibrator is sometimes thought of as a dildo. While some women use them as such, the vibrating part of these little devices is usually located on the tip, which means a woman can't insert it deeply inside her vagina and expect it to keep her clitoris happy. These are also made of hard plastic, and some of them don't pack much of a wallop compared to the more adequately appointed AC models. Most of these novelty devices aren't in the same league as a well-made dildo or vibrator, although some highly devoted users will disagree.

Vibrators, Dildos & Couples

Most guys have no problem with a partner who uses sex toys; many find the situation a total turn-on. However, some males worry that their sweetheart will start preferring the vibrator or dildo to them. Some believe that a sex toy means they aren't hung well enough or can't deliver the goods.

On the surface, these are not irrational fears. First of all, the vibrator keeps running long after most men have delivered the mail, and nobody's ever heard of a dildo that needed Viagra. Also, women can put the vibrator or dildo anywhere they want and totally control the proceedings.

But strangely enough, if he is a considerate, caring, real flesh-and-blood guy, most women will still want him regardless of how often they fire up the old magic wand. In fact, it's hard to have a meaningful conversation with a vibrator, and no dildo has ever played catch with the kids or gotten up in the middle of the night to feed the baby. Also, sex toys aren't the sort of thing that you can cuddle up next to and feel safe with—not that you can with all men.

In purchasing a new vibrator or dildo, a woman who is in a relationship should consider making her partner a part of the selection process. This way, her partner won't feel left in the dust, resentful or inadequate. On the other hand, good luck getting a guy to attend an all-woman's sex-toy party.

Perhaps it might not hurt to show your partner this chapter, which encourages men to take pride in a woman's sex toys. It might also help to let him know that women who buy vibrators and dildos are often extremely happy with their sex partners.

Making Friends with Your Lover's Toys

There's no point in feeling at odds with your lover's vibrator or dildo. If you are a man and you partner orders up a new sex toy, ask her to show you how she uses it. Hold her tight while she's getting herself off with it. If she has a vibrator, why not let her use it on you? And for heaven's sake, be sure to have her use it during intercourse. Some couples find the sensations to be sensational. It's even possible to combine vibrator play with oral sex. The man pushes a small battery-operated vibrator against the bottom of his tongue while the tip of his tongue is touching his partner's clitoris. Or you can gently push a dildo in and out of her vagina while planting wet kisses on her clit.

Vibrator Bits & Pieces

Here are a few vibrating facts that might be helpful if you have never used a vibrator. (People with medical conditions such as phlebitis should check with a physician before using a vibrator.)

Coil vs. Wand When it comes to vibrators that plug into the wall, there are two different types of vibrator design: wandlike vibrators with longer bodies and large heads, and coil vibrators with compact heads. Each type delivers a unique sensation. Coil vibrators are smaller and nearly silent. The sensations they produce tend to be more localized. The more popular wand vibrators are bigger and make a distinct humming noise. Newer models are rechargeable and will hum for up to an hour per charge. Some come with two heads which can be used for a variety of purposes, including on your genitals and bum at the same time, as well as for up and down your spinal column. Try to compare the feel of different coil vibrators, as some pack a serious vibe.

Be a Brand-Name Snob While some people swear by the little battery-operated vibrators, plenty of other people swear at them. The beefier AC-powered vibrators, such as those crafted by Hitachi, Oster, Wahl, and Panasonic, deliver more bang for the buck and won't let you down at critical moments. They are also well-made and have warranties.

First-Time Users If you are new to a vibrator, be sure to use it on the lowest possible speed at first while you learn to navigate the head around your pubic bone. Some new users have actually bruised their pubic bones by plopping the head of a vibrator on a bony pelvis.

Geography Some women move a vibrator around the entire vulva rather than park it in one particular place; others find a favorite spot and leave it there as though it were welded.

Sensation Levels Some users like the sensations full blast; others like to muffle the vibrator with a towel or even a pillow, and some hold the vibrator in a way that allows their fingers to transfer the vibrations. Some vibrators have variable-speed controls.

Hands Some vibrators strap on the back of your hand. Your fingers deliver the vibrations. These can be great fun to use, but they do tend to numb out the fingers temporarily.

Fingers The Fukuoko vibrators fit on your finger. They are incredibly small and almost unnoticeable.

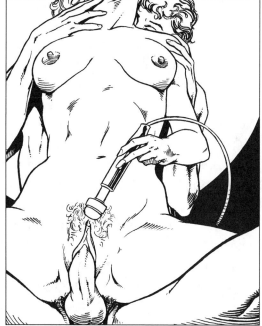

No Hands Some women rest a vibrator between their legs so they can use their hands for other things such as holding a book, playing with their nipples, touching a partner's body or channel surfing. There are special harnesses which hold the head of a vibrator snugly between your legs. There is even a small vibrator with built-in straps that is sometimes called *Joni's Butterfly*. It can be worn during intercourse, in public, at work, on a date or wherever a woman might want to get a private buzz in a public place. However, this type of vibrator can sometimes be heard in super-quiet places like elevators or libraries, so plan accordingly.

Positions Unlike most men, vibrators are meant to be abused. Be sure to try different positions with it on top of you, with you on top of it, with it between your legs and as you lie on your side.

Vibrator Vacations People sometimes worry that a woman will become used to the vibrator and want only that. If you are concerned, consider taking vibrator vacations for one week every month.

Attachments There are a number of vibrator attachments for both coil and wand vibrators. They can deliver a finger of vibration to any location a man or woman wants.

Vibrators and Boys Women aren't the only ones who appreciate an occasional mechanical assist. Some boys learn to wrap a towel around their dad's hand-held vibrating sander and hold it against their genitals for a quick and easy orgasm. Just about anything around the house that vibrates will eventually find a young man leaning against it to see how it feels. Likewise, some girls first learn about good vibrations by leaning against the strangest things. The vibrating handles of some vacuum cleaners can also be enlightening. Be careful if the device grabs or kicks.

Vibrators and Men Given how many times the average male masturbates during his lifetime, it makes a certain amount of sense to try out a couple of gadgets that are made for that purpose. Some are interesting, most are disappointing. Many are nowhere near as convenient as using your own hand. For instance, there is a special attachment for certain types of vibrators called a come cup which fits over the head of the penis. (Be sure to lube up the cup first.) To make a come cup of your own, push the head of a vibrator against your hand as it is holding your penis. Some men wrap a vibrator with a towel and lean into it. The towel helps to muffle the sensation, since some vibrations can be too much and you're left with a numb dick and no orgasm. There are even vibrating sleeves that a penis can fit into. Of those we've tested, none came close to using your hand and five-cents-worth of lotion. We also tried a vagina substitute that's shaped like a big flashlight. Sticking your penis into cold mud would have been more fun. Perhaps the problem was not being able to get a fantasy going.

Battery-Operated Personal Massagers There are different vibrators crafted in every possible shape known to woman, from interesting contours and cute little lady bugs to vibrating silver bullets and even vinyl hummingbirds. Some of these hold up well and are made by reputable companies.

Flying High When viewed through X-ray, vibrators can resemble detonating devices on bombs. Airport security will make you open up purses, briefcases and suitcases that have vibrators in them. Resist informing them about what your vibrator does and doesn't detonate.

Dildo Logic

Vibrators have become so socially acceptable that most department and drug stores display them. Few manufacturers mention why people buy vibrators, although most of the boxes show scantily clad women using them on their calves. With dildos, there are fewer options for subterfuge and denial. Big stores would be hard-pressed to advertise that dildos help relax tense muscles, although they clearly do. And if people hear a woman say the word "dildo" in a public place, they are more likely to think that she is referring to a man she used to date than to something that gives her pleasure.

The next couple of pages offer enough information about dildos so you won't be in the dark even if you use them in the dark.

Dildo vs. Penis

It is a biological fact that the human penis, when fully anchored to the human crotch, imposes certain limitations upon a woman's sexual pleasure that the silicone dildo does not. A real penis can't be radically flipped upside down without necessitating a trip to the hospital for the man whose body it is or was attached to. There is also the matter of hardness: the male penis isn't always hard when a woman wants it hard, nor for as long as she might desire. And finally, a penis is not like a car that you can trade in every couple of years. Even if her spouse's penis might not be the best size and shape to fit her psyche or anatomy, a married woman is pretty well glued to it till death or divorce do they part. Fortunately a woman needn't ditch the man she loves just because she prefers a Chevy-type penis when nature gave him a Ford or, gulp, a Yugo. She can purchase a dildo instead.

In Search of the Perfect Dildo

Dildos are made from a large variety of materials, including jade, acrylic, alabaster, latex, leather, glass, brass and wood. However, the most highly regarded dildo material is usually silicone. Silicone has a soft but firm texture with a smooth surface that is durable and easy to clean, although it doesn't stand up to cuts too well. The silicone material also warms up rather nicely, which is an added plus unless you like cold things in your vagina.

Since there is a fair amount of craftsmanship involved in producing a high-quality dildo, be sure to purchase dildos from places that carry only proven products and take pride in pleasing their customers. Check how long they've been in business and how well they support their products. As for dildo particulars, here are a few to consider:

Price Expect to pay from $50 to $120 for a good-quality silicone dildo. For instance, rubber dildos have little divots in the surface which make them next to impossible to keep clean. You should always use a condom over them.

Size The most important consideration in sizing a dildo is girth. One strategy for determining which width is best for you is suggested by the women at Good Vibrations. They say to buy different-sized zucchinis, carrots or cucumbers that have an inviting girth. Steam or nuke them for just a few seconds so they won't be cold, wash them, and put condoms over them. Add lubricant and try them in your vagina. Don't hesitate to use a vegetable peeler to fine tune the girth. When you find one that feels just right, cut it in two and measure the diameter, which will most likely be somewhere between one and two inches. If you are the one who will be inserting the dildo, order one that's sized just right. However, if a friend will be doing the inserting, consider getting a dildo with a slightly smaller diameter. As for length, a four- to five-inch-long dildo should be just right if you plan to keep it stationary inside your vagina, while a six- to eight-inch length might be easier to handle if you like thrusting.

Shape When it comes to dildos, there are plenty of variations within a basic theme. Some dildos are made to look like penises, complete with veins and testicles, some look like dolphins or bears, and some have ridges. Dildos also have different-sized heads. With a small amount of effort, you are likely to find the dildo of your dreams.

Lubrication No matter how wet you might be, it's best to lubricate the dildo and yourself before inserting, but don't lose track of where you put the tube of lube. You may need to add more as you go. If it's a silicone dildo, don't use silicone-based lube. It can melt the silicone toy.

What to Do With It Women don't necessarily use dildos for thrusting in and out. A woman might like a dildo to be stationary inside her vagina while she uses her fingers or a vibrator, or while a partner provides her with oral or anal attention. Or she might enjoy running the dildo up and down between her labia.

Numbers Some women have one favorite dildo; others have dildos of different shapes and sizes for every day of the week.

Clean Dildos should be washed and dried after each use. If not properly cleaned, the porous surface of some dildos will grow microorganisms that are best not introduced or reintroduced into your body. If you are sharing sex toys, sterilize your dildo with hydrogen peroxide, rubbing alcohol or a light bleach solution (nine parts water to one part bleach).

Anal Play If you use the dildo in your arse, be sure to wash it with soap and water before putting it into a vagina. Better yet, slap a condom on it before it goes up anyone's rear. Also, limit your anal play to dildos with a flanged end or use a butt plug which won't get lost up your rear end (bum bummer). People who enjoy both anal and vaginal penetration are wise to have dedicated dildos for each orifice.

Dildo Harnesses Dildos with a flared base can be worn in harnesses which make them appear like erect penises. With a moderate amount of skill and effort, the person wearing the harness can use the dildo to penetrate a partner. This can be disappointing, though, because the dildo isn't connected to the wearer's nervous system like a real flesh-and-blood penis and she can't feel what the dildo is feeling. (Talk about an existential crisis!) Nonetheless, there are plenty of couples, both straight and lesbian, who enjoy using a dildo in a harness. The best harnesses are made of leather or nylon webbing. The actual geometry of harness construction and fastener application can be tricky; call or e-mail the sex-toy store for advice about the do's and don'ts of dildo-harness buying and wearing. Also, there are other kinds of dildo harnesses such as those that fit on the thigh. Users of these marvel at the versatility of such an arrangement and claim that the human penis should have been attached to the thigh of the male rather than between his legs. There is even a dildo mounted on a beach ball that a person can bounce up and down on.

Dildo Harnesses for Inner Wear Let's say you're shopping at the supermarket or have a hot date and want to spice things up a bit. Now you can do it with your favorite dildo inside your vagina and no one will ever know unless you want them to. That's because they now make dildo harnesses that hold the dildo inside a vagina so it won't pop out when you are seeing patients or when making a special presentation to that hugely important client who just flew in from Algiers.

Doubles? A double dildo is worn in a harness, with one end going up the wearer's vagina and the other end sticking out in front like a penis. There are a couple of highly rated double dildos on the market. The old champ used to be the Nexus, but the new kid on the double-dildo block is the Feeldo.

Full-Court Press Some women like to be penetrated in both the front and the rear at the same time. In lieu of doing a double penetration with a threesome, the dildo can penetrate one gate while her partner fills the other.

Techno Dildo Some dildos are motorized and move in circles. Some have vibrating appendages that can be parked over the clitoris.

Beware Of Gumby-Like Dildos Some dildos are embedded with wire rods to help keep whatever shape the person bends them into. Be aware that if the wire separates from the dildo material, it will become embedded in the wall of your vagina or rectum.

Menopause Masturbating with a dildo fully inserted might help some menopausal women without partners to keep their vaginas in good shape.

Suction Cups There are even dildos with suction cups on the bottom so the woman can stick them on a wall or the floor while she moves her entire body up and down or forward and back while the dildo remains stationary. These can also be planted on the wall as decorations for your dorm room.

Backdoor Men & Women Good Vibrations reports that about half of the dildo harnesses they sell are to heterosexual couples in which the woman wears the dildo to do her man in the rear.

Sex-Toy Layering—Dildos & Vibrators

Some women who have never enjoyed masturbating with their fingers or a vibrator go to town once they get the right dildo. The dildo provides an internal fullness that might make it more satisfying when they stimulate the vulva with their fingers or a vibrator.

SEX-TOY LEGAL UPDATE

In 2007, the federal courts declared it is legal for Alabama to ban the sale of devices that are designed or marketed primarily for the stimulation of human genitals (Williams v. Morgan, Eleventh Circuit, February 14, 2007). While sodomy in the privacy of your home is now protected, you can't buy a sex toy in Alabama to save your soul.

HOWEVER, our gynecology consultant offers a solution that won't get a Belle busted: "My new favorite item is a vibrating toothbrush. The vibration is a perfect frequency for clitoral stimulation. I remind my patients not to use the bristle side but the back side of the bristles. Travels great, is inexpensive, doesn't threaten a man's masculinity..." [This disposable, battery-powered toothbrush is from a well-known oral hygiene company, has bright, multi-colored bristles that pulsate, and is pretty cheap. Where ever toothbrushes are sold!]

CHAPTER

26
Fun with Your Foreskin

66

Cut to the chase: I am an RN and have seen hundreds of uncircumcised males. No turn on. But when my most recent lover happened to be such it was so totally unexpected that my sexual arousal rate went up 200%. I am very turned on by stroking him to expose the head, kissing and licking it and then covering it again by pulling the foreskin back up. Sucking ever so gently with the skin covering the head gives him pleasure, but pulling it down near the base of his penis completely exposes him and his reaction is amazing. All it takes is tender gentle swirls to drive him crazy.... The wanton horny bitch that resides within myself has now been released and owes you all at the Goofy Foot Press gratitude and the author the best blow job ever!"   *female age 27*

Drive south on I-5 until you reach the Corvallis exit, go west...

Medically speaking, routine circumcision makes about as much sense as removing a kid's eyelids or cutting out the labia of a baby girl. So why are so many American boys routinely circumcised?

During the 1880s, a few influential men like John Harvey Kellogg, physician and founder of a famous American cereal company, started preaching that boys masturbate because the foreskin rubs on the head of the penis. Until that time, most American men were not circumcised. As a leading anti-masturbation fanatic, Dr. Kellogg believed that boys who were circumcised at birth would be less likely to play with themselves. His influence helped circumcision to become a routine operation in America. Swell guy that he was, Dr. Kellogg also recommended that girls who masturbate have their clitorises burned out with acid.

There is No Medical Need for Circumcision

America's medical establishment has tried to justify its hand in circumcision by saying that it prevents cancer of the penis, cancer of the cervix and now AIDS.

Cancer of the penis is extremely rare—more men get breast cancer. In Sweden, where few men are circumcised, cancer of the penis is just as rare as in the circumcision-happy United States. In fact, when circumcised men get cancer of the penis, it tends to break out on the circumcision scar. It would be interesting to compare the number of penises lost to cancer with the number of penises mutilated through botched circumcisions.

As for cancer of the cervix, the HPV virus is the main culprit. Women who live in countries where men aren't circumcised have no higher rate of cervical cancer than women in America.

The idea that circumcision is protective against HIV is the brainchild of pro-circumcision advocates in America. These advocates fail to mention that although the vast majority of adult males in America are circumcised, America has one of the highest rates of HIV infection in the industrialized world—higher than a number of European countries where the vast majority of men are not circumcised.

Studies from Africa that show a higher rate of HIV among uncircumcised men are preposterous. None of the three studies were carried out to completion and none of the studies showed that male circumcision would protect women from being infected. In fact, a report done in 2007 suggests the opposite. Once a penis is in a vagina, an intact foreskin allows it to thrust without causing as much abrasion to the vagina as a circumcised penis. This would help decrease, rather than increase, a woman's chances of being infected.

Any competent analysis of the HIV data from Africa reaffirms the fact that circumcision is not an effective means of preventing the spread of HIV:

> "Given what is known at the individual level, one would have expected HIV incidence or prevalence in circumcised groups of men to be consistently about 20% lower than in uncircumcised groups. This was not the case according to the results of this study. Until this discrepancy between demographic evidence and expectations from epidemiological evidence is resolved, is it wise to recommend mass circumcision? Also, the implementation of mass circumcision raises serious ethical concerns, well documented elsewhere."

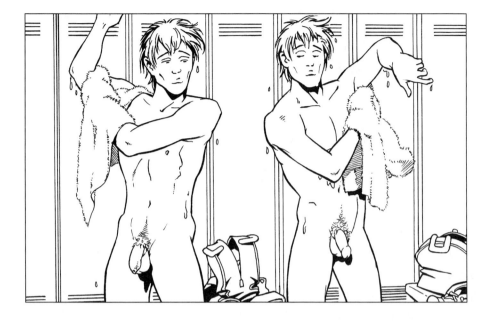

"Once more, the dynamics of generalized HIV epidemics in Africa appear more complex than originally thought. Male circumcision appears only as a minor factor amid many others contributing to the spread of HIV, such as the complex web of social, cultural and economic interactions surrounding sexual behaviour, especially among adolescents and young adults. These complex relationships merit further field studies, as well as investigations through mathematical modelling." —*"Long-term population effect of male circumcision in generalized HIV epidemics in sub-Saharan Africa," African Journal of AIDS Research [2008, 7(1): 1–8]*

The only thing that is clear about the African studies is when strong proponents of circumcision get funding to carry out circumcision research, science takes a backseat to politics. Their recommendation for circumcision was clearly an ideological one. It's what they appear to have wanted and expected to find from the start. Questionable data and poor research design wasn't going to get in their way. John Harvey Kellogg would be proud.

What is particularly disturbing is that the proponents of circumcision would have us spending millions of dollars coercing African men to have needless circumcisions, while ignoring more effective solutions like the use of condoms. In Uganda, HIV infection rates decreased by 49% following a

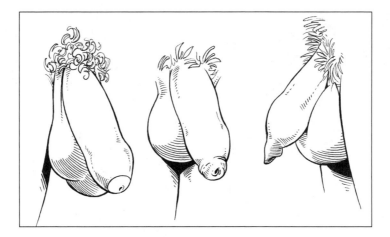

highly effective condom use campaign to educate people about HIV. On the other hand, assuming the decreases reported in the three circumcision studies were correct, circumcising every male in Africa would result in only an 8% decrease in the number of HIV cases, with only a 1% reduction in the number of deaths. Could the money be more effectively spent on education and condom distribution?

Why are we willing to expend sizeable resources on the dubious practice of circumcising African men when we could use that money to install badly-needed sewer systems and water purification plants that would save countless African lives?

The Risks of Circumcising

For those of you who genuinely care about your infant son's health, why not consider a danger that is a wee bit more immediate than dubious studies from Africa? It is called Methicillin-resistant Staphylococcus aureus (MRSA). This infection has at times reached near epidemic levels in the United States, and it can be a serious problem in newborn nurseries. Its most frequent infant victims are circumcised boys, although more research on this is needed. The infection gets into the body through the circumcision wound, and it can cause impetigo, staphylococcal scalded skin syndrome, bacteremia, cellulitis, pneumonia, arthritis, osteomyelitis, pustolosis, pyoderma, empyema, and sometimes death.

There also exists a myth that large percentages of uncircumcised babies will have foreskins that don't retract (phimosis), and that these males will need surgery when they grow older to correct this condition. In reality, fewer than 1 out of every 100 uncircumcised men have this condition, and a foreskin-friendly urologist can almost always help to resolve the problem without having to cut the kid.

So Why Do They Keep Doing It?

A physician in the US makes between $150 and $300 per circumcision. Doing one circumcision per day, five days per week, at a fee of $150 each minus time out for a six-week vacation nets a physician an extra $34,500 per year for a procedure that takes less than ten minutes. And that's only one a day at the lower rate. No wonder pediatricians and obstetricians used to fight over who got to do the circumcision!

Another reason for doing circumcisions is medical bias. Until recently, physicians in this country have had a long-standing bias that hysterectomies are good for women and circumcisions are good for men.

In short, there appears to be no medical reason besides possible income enhancement for doing routine circumcision. There does, however, appear to be a very good reason why nature equipped the penis with a foreskin. Not only is the foreskin rich in pleasure-producing nerve endings, but it also keeps the head of the penis moist and the extra skin provides added sliding pleasure during intercourse and masturbation. The foreskin is extremely elastic and is said to be as sensitive to touch as the human lips. Far from being unnecessary, a foreskin is usually a nice thing to have.

How They Do It

During male circumcision, physicians stick a prodding instrument into the foreskin to tear it away from the head of the penis. One-third to one-half of the skin on the penis is then cut off. Traditionally, male circumcisions have not been done with anesthesia, but even when anesthesia is used, there is still pain from the raw scar on the penis.

Religious Considerations

Some people will say, "But circumcision is done for important religious and cultural reasons." The same is true for female circumcision, which we refer to as genital mutilation.

Some people say this is being disrespectful of an important ritual in the Jewish faith. This is true. We are also disrespectful of the Catholic Church's ban on birth control and masturbation. If Jewish men want to be circumcised as an expression of their faith, why not let them wait until they are 18 years old and able to call the Mohel themselves? That would be a far greater expression of faith than having the end of your penis chopped off when you are only a few days old and can't tell the Torah from a phone book.

According to psychologist Ronald Goldman, not all Jewish men are circumcised. Theodore Herzl, the founder of modern Zionism, did not allow his own son to be circumcised. Even Moses did not circumcise his son, and circumcision was not done during the forty-year period in the wilderness. It is quite possible that this custom arose out of the Egyptian practice to circumcise their Jewish slaves. Over time, this became a ritual or custom, and eventually became associated with the Covenant.

The ultimate goal of circumcision, according to ancient rabbis and Jewish scholars from Philo to Maimonides, was to decrease sexual pleasure for both men and women. This would give men more time to study the Torah, and result in women receiving less sexual pleasure from a man who was circumcised.

In 1843, Reform-Movement leaders in Frankfurt, Germany started a mini-house revolt against circumcision. This group argued that 1) Circumcision had not always been practiced among Jews; 2) It was not commanded to Moses; 3) It's not unique among Jews, given how Muslims do it as well; 4) It is only discussed once in the Mosaic law and not repeated in Deuteronomy; and 5) There was no comparable practice for females.

Perhaps one of the most interesting elements of circumcision in the Jewish religion is that for the first 2,000 years of the practice, only the tip of the foreskin was cut. This was called Milah. It was only after the first 2,000 years of Milah that they started whacking off the entire foreskin.

Resource: *Questioning Circumcision—A Jewish Perspective* by Ronald Goldman, Ph.D., Vanguard.

For Parents—Foreskin Care

Do not try to retract the foreskin of a young boy unless there is a specific medical reason. During infancy and childhood, the inner surface of the foreskin is physically attached to the skin on the head of the penis. This protects the opening of the penis from irritation, infection and ulceration. Over time, the cells that attach these two surfaces together will start to dissolve on their own. By trying to retract the foreskin prematurely, you are ripping apart these delicate tissues that nature has "glued" together.

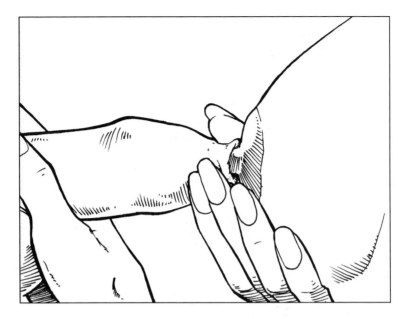

A young boy will often push his foreskin away from his body. As he gets older, he will begin to pull it toward his body. A number of males don't fully retract their foreskins until they are teenagers. This is normal and will usually happen without any coaxing or encouragement from mom and dad.

Parents do need to tell their teenage sons about cleanliness. They should explain that once a boy is able to retract his foreskin he should clean it every day in the shower. As for whether that daily cleaning should include soap, one of our urology-consultant physicians is himself uncircumcised. He is concerned that soaping the retracted foreskin daily might destroy the protective bacterial mantle and actually result in foreskin odor. He suggests only soaping it a couple of times a week, while retracting it and washing it with water the other days of the week. Other healthcare providers recommend retracting the foreskin and washing it with soap every day.

Reader Comments

"I'd never even seen an uncircumcised penis until my current lover, but I've decided now that it's the best thing since sliced bread. The foreskin makes hand jobs 100 times better and easier because it slides over the penis so you don't need lube. I was kind of nervous about it at first but then I realized how stretchy the foreskin is even though it looks kinda fragile. For blow jobs, I pull the foreskin down to the base and massage it there and go to town." *female age 18*

"I love the way his cock slides in and out of his foreskin when he's inside me—it not only stimulates me physically, but the thought of it also really turns me on while we are having sex." *female age 30*

"The only Jewish guy I ever slept with was also the only uncircumcised guy I ever slept with. He seemed to have more stamina than any of the others, but that might just be a coincidence." *female age 21*

"For a blow job, pull the foreskin up over the head and stick your tongue down inside of the opening and swirl it around."
female age 38

"Just ask the guy how he likes it. Some guys like you to pull the foreskin tight; others say this hurts." *female age 20*

"I use my foreskin to massage her clitoris. This might only be possible with a partner who has a larger-than-normal clitoris. You need to be able to get hold of it." *male age 65*

"Once my wife and I are ready for penetration, I roll my foreskin all the way shut. I press it gently against her labia while spreading them slightly, and push the glans in just a little. Then, I withdraw the glans back inside the foreskin, never exposing it to open air. What this does is spread her lubricant all over the first half of my penis. After several strokes like this, I am able to slip inside easily. Sometimes we find this so pleasurable that we continue a good long while before penetrating farther." *male age 38*

"A partner should know that the inside of a foreskin is where there is the most feeling, so gentle movement of it over a cockhead and down the shaft feels great. The best part of getting a blow job is what a tongue and mouth can do with that inside lining of a foreskin."
male age 59

"One thing I find particularly stimulating is to lubricate a finger or thumb, slip it between the foreskin and the head, and massage the glans. It feels really, really great." *male age 19*

"When did I first retract it? I was around ten. I would slowly pull it back every day in the shower. After about two weeks I was able to pull it all the way down." *male age 22*

"Letting the foreskin balloon is quite nice both when peeing and when enjoying the pool jets." *male age 37*

"I like to do the trick of clamping the end shut while peeing and making it swell up. Also, a similar and a more satisfying experience is to leave just a bit of the end open and put it under a strong flow of water so that the water flows in but has a place to get out." *male age 20*

"My fiancee does all the foreskin movement for me. It's such a turn-on when she pulls it back and then returns it to normal. She does this with her mouth constantly while she gives me a blow job." *male 19*

"There is nothing worse than cracking an erection in your pants and not being able to make it go away because your foreskin is retracted and the head of your cock keeps on rubbing on your pants." *male 18*

"The very tip of the foreskin (like the rim of a volcano) can be very, very sensitive when you're soft. A light, caressing finger running around the edge can feel electric... If she's giving you a handjob and her ring isn't tight around her finger, the flesh of the foreskin can get caught in between and pinch like hell. On the flip side, there's something pretty erotic about handjobs while she's wearing your engagement ring." *male age 23*

Resources:

National Organization of Circumcision Information Resource Centers (Includes a list of foreskin-friendly physicians)
www.nocirc.org/

Circumcision Information and Resource Pages
www.cirp.org

No Harm
www.noharmm.org

Circumcision Resource Center
www.circumcision.org

Doctors Opposing Circumcision (D.O.C.)
www.doctorsopposingcircumcision.org

Very Special Thanks to Marily Minos of NOCIRC and Doctors Opposing Circumcision.

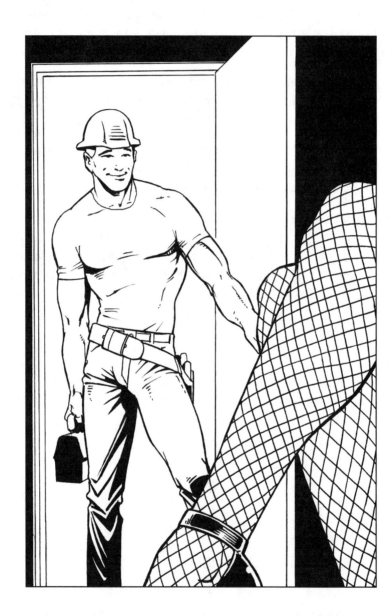

27
Sex Fantasies

Given how sex fantasies are nearly universal, it's surprising we tend to be embarrassed about them. On the other hand, why bother fantasizing about things that everyone else approves of?

Some people know they're horny because of the sexual fantasies they've been having. Some have a single reliable sex fantasy that they go back to time and again. Others have a virtual toolbox of scenes and images that help get them off. The vast majority of people have fantasies during intercourse, and a lot people find it difficult to masturbate to orgasm without an arousing sexual fantasy.

The content of sex fantasies varies; some are sweet, kind and silly; others are weird, kinky and bizarre. Some are action-packed and exciting; others are really boring. Some sex fantasies are populated with past lovers, rock 'n' roll singers, people in uniforms, movie stars, teachers, priests, family members, total strangers and even furry friends from another species.

One of the most popular sex fantasies involves doing stuff with your current partner, but that's when couples are having sex together. When people masturbate, guilt is not so much in your face, and all bets are off as to who or what you are fantasizing about.

Given that our fantasies get their fuel from the deepest recesses of our being, there is virtually no limit to the scripts we create for our sexual selves. Those scripts can be very incongruent from the person we usually are or who our friends and partners know us to be. Within those scripts we can be active or passive, devil or angel. There's nothing that says an obsessively neat surgeon can't be masturbated by a pair of smelly feet, or a faithful and loving wife can't be banged so hard by her husband's brother that she imagines blood dripping from her vagina—all in the theater of the sexual mind.

Fantasies of Rape

It is not unusual to have fantasies in which sex is forced, nor is it unusual to fantasize about sex with people in uniform. Consider the following passage from Betty Dodson's fine book, *Sex for One*, Harmony Books:

> "A friend who considered herself a radical feminist got concerned that her sexual imagery wasn't politically correct because it wasn't 'feminist oriented.' I assured her that all fantasies were okay. Lots of people imagine scenes they never want to experience. I also pointed out that we can become addicted to a fantasy like anything else, and suggested she experiment with new ones. One of her new assertive fantasies is about moving her clitoris in and out of her lover's soft wet mouth while he's tied down. Whenever she gets stuck or is in a hurry, she brings out her old fantasy of being raped by five Irish cops and always reaches orgasm quickly."

Sometimes being raped in fantasy is a way to enjoy pleasure that would otherwise cause guilt. Sex that is out of your control keeps you from having to feel responsible for wanting it. It is also a way to feel sexually desired and valued, since the perpetrator would do anything to have you.

Why the Rape in "Rape Fantasy" Isn't Really Rape

If you ask most women who have rape fantasies to describe the man who is "raping" them, you'll find he's not exactly what we picture when we think of a violent felon, unless the guy has been spending six hours a day in the prison weight room or reads Shakespeare to Bubba his cellmate.

The perpetrators in most "rape fantasies" are actors, musicians or bodice-ripping hunks—someone who the woman might want to have sex with anyway. Missing is the terror, violence, confusion, rage and disgust that makes rape RAPE. The woman with the fantasy is in control by virtue of who she has "raping" her or because she's the one scripting the scenario, while control is the last thing that a woman who is being raped has any of.

Even if the woman's rape fantasy involves her being degraded, humiliated, or left bruised and bloodied by an anonymous aggressor or gang of men intent to do her harm, her fantasy doesn't make her fear men in real life like an actual rape often does. It doesn't make her afraid to go out of doors. Even if her fantasy is a way of processing something overwhelming or abusive from her past, we would never suggest she walk alone at night in dangerous places to get an even better handle on the psychology of it.

No doubt, there are cultural, religious and perhaps biological reasons for why so many women have sexual fantasies where they are "taken" by a man instead of being the taker. But there are significant differences between that and the realities of an actual rape. Women needn't feel guilty or ashamed of their "rape" fantasies, because they aren't really fantasies of rape. The term pseudo- or pretend-rape fantasy is more accurate.

Men's vs. Women's Sex Fantasies

Young girls in our society are raised on fashion magazines that highlight gorgeous female models—gorgeous if you don't take into account how many meals these women barf up to stay slim and how much silicone they have surgically packed into their chests. As girls look through these magazines, they often think about other women's bodies, particularly the ideal woman whom they hope to someday become. Boys, on the other hand, often grow up fantasizing about doing things; for instance, being firemen, sports heroes, musicians, stuntmen and eventually stud lovers. It seems our society wants its girls to be admired for how they look, and its boys for how they perform.

Psychologist Karen Shanor believes that when women see an erect penis in their fantasies, they often relish it as a sign that the man finds them irresistible, as opposed to being in awe of the penis itself. Shanor speculates that many young women learn to include men in their fantasies as an after-thought, with the fantasized male being little more than a woman retrofit-ted with a penis. Perhaps this is one reason why teenage girls so often fawn over totally androgynous male rock'n'roll singers, not that older women don't as well. (Teenage boys tend to look androgynous before puberty, so maybe the teen-girls' fantasies are right where they need to be in an age-appropriate sense.)

When a woman walks into a formal affair like a prom, the first thing she often notices is how the other women look and how she feels in comparison. The first thing a man notices is often the same thing: how the other women look. Men usually aren't concerned with how the other men look, unless they are actors or gay.

As focused as women sometimes are on other women, Shanor's theory does have its limitations. It doesn't explain why some women clearly prefer the sexual touch and feel of a man's body over that of a woman. It doesn't explain why a lot of women enjoy the way a penis feels when it's inside of their bodies, or why they might find a male's butt or shoulders to be sexy.

Your Lover's Sex Fantasies

Every once in a while, one partner will tell the other about his or her private sex fantasy. Stranger things have happened. But don't expect to see the fantasy plastered on a billboard surrounded by neon lights. Most of us are a little embarrassed by our sexual fantasies, sometimes with good reason. As a result, we don't reveal our fantasies in a way that's particularly direct, nor should we.

You Only Get One Chance

Let's say you are a guy and your sweetheart casually or jokingly makes an off-the-cuff statement that she likes seeing guys in jock straps. Boom, ball's in your court. Now, if you have half a brain, and not many of us do, you won't laugh and tell her how much better you feel in boxers than wearing some old athletic supporter. Instead, you will consider buying about a dozen or so new jocks, maybe in colors, maybe one with a cup, what the heck. So there you are later that night, your sweetheart's warm familiar fingers are slowly popping the buttons on your blue jeans and bingo—she discovers that you are wearing a jock underneath! Before you know it, she's in sexual orbit and you are the happiest jock on your block! Or she might discover that her fantasy was best when it was only imagined and that it feels silly or degrading, or loses its erotic edge when acted out in reality.

Odds & Ends

While it's great that you and your partner might be open to hearing each other's fantasies, this doesn't mean that you need to act them out. When one partner has a jones to do something that the other finds loathsome, you might try working out a compromise. It's likely that there are plenty of videos depicting whichever fantasies are currently oozing from the darkest recesses of your sexual mind. Why not rent one and test drive it as a masturbation aid? At other times acting out your sex fantasies can be great fun.

People occasionally have sexual fantasies about someone other than their partner. Sometimes it is prudent not to share these fantasies, e.g., "The reason I got so hot is because I pretended you were Mike." Other times your partner might find these fantasies very arousing.

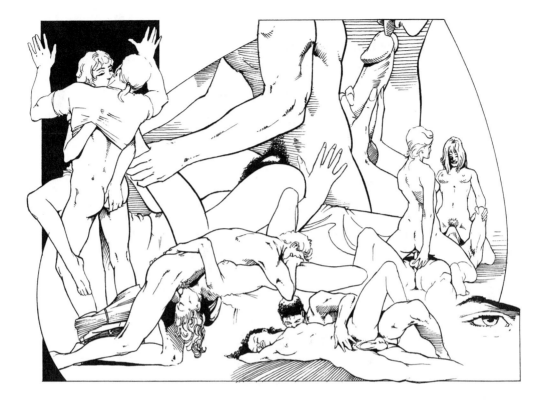

If you are going to make your own adult videos at home, keep in mind the fate of the poor sheriff from the Midwest who accidentally returned a custom-made X-rated video of him and his wife to the local video store. Think "Password Protection" the next time you burn your own DVD or send your lover images of an intimate kind.

By taking a few extra steps, you are safe even if your 6-year-old accidentally grabs your homemade fantasy orgasmo-shoot instead of the latest fare from Pixar or Dreamworks. You won't have to worry about the kids in the neighborhood going home and saying, "Mommy, Mommy, you'll never guess what we saw Emily's mom and dad doing on DVD!"

Responsibility

Knowledge of your partner's fantasies is a trust that remains with you for life. This trust holds true even if you break up and otherwise find yourselves hating each other. No one forced you to be in a relationship with the person, so don't go blabbing personal stuff just to be hurtful. In the long run, it reflects badly upon you.

To put it another way, people who gossip about a current or former partner's sexuality are both shallow and deceitful. The laws of karma will someday haunt them, assuming there are laws of karma.

Readers' Comments

"At work I daydream a lot about sex and what it would be like with certain people that I am especially attracted to. Since I am about to get married, I sometimes feel bad thinking of others, but as long as you don't act on it, you're pretty much okay." *female age 30*

"My sexual fantasies always involve my current real life lover. We're making romantic love somewhere that is new to us, a beach, forest, remote island, in front of a fire in a cabin." *female age 34*

"I probably have similar fantasies to anyone who watches the Sci Fi channel too much." *male age 30*

"My fantasies don't play a huge part in my life, except that I get confused why I have fantasies about other girls when I love penises and my boyfriend very much." *female age 23*

"I had always fantasized about my girlfriend being totally naked with her legs spread apart when I came into the room. One day she actually did this! It was awesome!" *male age 21*

"I don't have any clearly defined fantasy. They are more fleeting feelings and don't affect my life much." *female age 38*

"As a working mother, I get sex and orgasms, but I rarely get romance, so that is what I fantasize about." *female age 36*

"My husband and I have been married for 10 years and still love to act out our fantasies. Last month he was a customs agent and I was trying to sneak something across the border. After he completely searched me, I had to bribe him with sexual favors until he let me go. Later, I was a physician and he the reluctant patient. Acting out your fantasies can be great fun, and it keeps your sex life young!" *female age 33*

"I'd love to see my girlfriend get it on with another woman and I know it would be a turn-on to see her get it on with another guy, but I don't know if I could keep from getting jealous." *male age 39*

Have you ever had homosexual fantasies?

"I used to fantasize about women all of the time. Finally, I decided to give it a try and had sex with one of my best female friends, who is mostly heterosexual. It was fun and every now and then we play with one another. I have never developed an emotional attachment to her or any other woman, and I no longer fantasize about women."
female age 26

"I fantasize about being with another woman often, but I also fanta-size about my boyfriend and Brad Pitt!" *female age 25*

"I am aroused by images of women with women; also by stories of multiple partners. On occasion, I use these fantasies to help me reach orgasm." *female age 32*

"I've had no fantasies or gay experiences, although I wonder some-times if I could get turned on by another guy." *male age 30*

"Gay fantasies? I've never even considered being gay. I'm not gay. I swear it." *male age 22*

Recommended Resources

The Ultimate Guide To Sexual Fantasy–How To Turn Your Fantasies into Reality by Violet Blue, Cleis Press (2004).

Who's Been Sleeping in Your Head—The Secret World of Sexual Fantasies by Brett Kahr, Basic Books. (2007/2008).

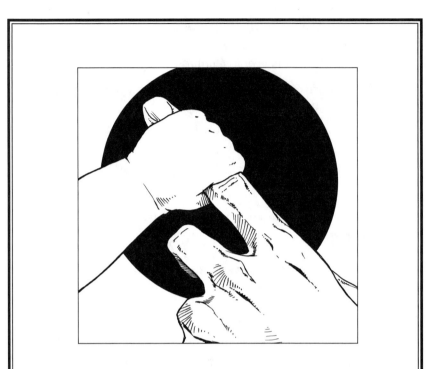

Whether it's your first time, or number 5,000...

Before having intercourse, please discuss with your partner what you will do if you become pregnant. (While condoms are incredibly helpful, 12% of couples using them will become pregnant after a year of having intercourse. The odds go up to 85% if you don't use birth control at all.)

With the advances in DNA testing, most bio-dads will be paying monthly child support until junior turns eighteen years of age.

And as unfair as this is, it's usually the girl who ends up having to raise an unwanted child. Are you prepared to be sitting at home with a crying baby while your friends are out having fun? Raising a child with two mature parents is difficult enough, will you be able to wing it alone?

28
Goodbye V-Card
Your First Intercourse

There is far more information in this chapter than you probably need if it's your first time. The trouble in leaving parts out is that while they might not apply to you, they might be important for someone else. Also, please keep in mind that couples can become very, very pregnant from their first time, even if you are doing it when a woman is having her period. And a brief legal reminder: *Know the laws about sex; if you are under 18, you may be breaking them if you have sex.*

Now, for the fun part.

Preparing Ahead for a Most-Excellent Journey

"It was very hard to do, but I waited until I was 18 to have intercourse. It was with a guy who cared deeply about me, which made my first experience very fun and comfortable." *female age 36*

Most people's first time is awkward and unplanned. It doesn't need to be that way. Hopefully it's a time you will remember with fondness—the beginning of a most excellent journey.

In Addition to This Chapter

There are many wonderful things about sex in addition to getting a penis inside a vagina—just reading this Guide's chapters on handjobs and finger fucking will put you years ahead of the game.

If you'd like more information about intercourse, check out Chapter 22: "Intercourse—Horizontal Jogging." However, that's for once you get up to speed with intercourse. For your first time, there are different priorities and different challenges.

Who to Do It With Your First Time

It makes perfectly good sense to do it your first time with the love of your life. But no matter how much in love we might have been, not a whole lot of us are still with the person who we lost our virginity to.

"I would have waited until I was in college. I would have saved myself years of painful, uncomfortable, inexperienced, or hurried sex. And while it just felt good to be close to the guy, I realize that I haven't thought of him in years. Girls, you ain't missing nothing!"

female age 32

Think about the difference between a crush and a friend. A friend usually has to earn your trust and respect, while a crush automatically gets it because of the way they look or act. The chances are good that you will still have your friends in a year's time, but you will probably have blown through your current crush and pretty much gag at the mere thought of the person.

This isn't to say you should ruin a good friendship by having sex with a friend instead of with a romantic interest. But at least try to make sure that your first lovemaking partner is someone who has the qualities of a friend.

Doing It Sober

Please, don't do it your first time drunk or stoned. While this is often how it happens, every survey on first-time intercourse is chuck full of horror stories from virgins who did it drunk. Seems that the couples who do it sober have a much better and more satisfying time.

Advice for Girls

This part of the chapter is written mostly for women. Hopefully, guys will read it as well. One of the keys to having good sex is knowing your body well enough to be able to say "That feels good" or "Let's try something else" in a way that a lover can understand. This can take years. Even women who have been around the block countless times still keep discovering new things about their bodies. So consider yourself at the start of a long journey.

Now, to learn more about yourself. Girls who masturbate might have a bit of an advantage, but if you haven't masturbated before, not to worry. Wash your hands and get some water-based lube or use your own spit. Saliva is water-based and works great.

When you've got at least a half-hour to yourself (good luck!), or when you are tucked under the covers for bed, start exploring up and down your body with your fingertips. Spend some extra time on your neck and chest, and on the area from your navel to your knees, except for your vulva and vagina. If it makes it more fun, pretend it's a guy's fingers instead of your own.

Once your fingers have explored up and down your body for at least ten or fifteen minutes, you might start to focus on the area between your legs.

Let your fingertips glide up and down and around your vulva, which is the outside part of what's between your legs. For illustrations, see Chapter 7: "What's Inside a Girl."

While one hand is exploring between your legs, there's nothing written in stone that says your other hand has to be tied to your side. At the very least, see what it's like letting it rest on a breast.

It's now time to venture inside. Get a finger good and wet. Slowly inch it inside your vagina, which is an opening that's buried toward the back of your vulva. It's where tampons and penises go. The emphasis should be on "slowly." You want to feel what your finger is feeling, as well as what your vagina is feeling.

At this point, some girls will want to put their finger in farther; others might be feeling a little overwhelmed, especially if they've been raised in a household that was not safe or supportive of their sexual growth. If you are in the "go for it!" group, let your finger keep going. And remember to keep asking yourself what your vagina is feeling. If you are so inclined, you might try adding a second finger. Given how a penis is most likely wider than your finger, two fingers is a nice goal, and three would be fine.

If you are in the group of girls who might be starting to feel like enough is enough, then this is a good place to stop. Just letting yourself go this far might be a really important step. If you can, try to go just a tiny bit farther next time, but don't be discouraged if you hit a personal wall. Maybe it would be easier to have your partner read this and ask him to explore you with his fingers, although only if he has good enough judgment to know the difference between a finger and a penis!

If and when you feel ready, you might practice guiding a tampon or small, tube-like vibrator into your vagina when you are lying on your back. Also practice doing this when you are squatting, as if you were in a girl-on-top position. Don't assume for a moment that your partner is going to have a clue where the opening of your vagina is. Be ready to help him guide his penis in, unless you don't mind if it ends up in your belly button or bum.

If all of this seems too overwhelming, maybe it's not the right time in your life to be having intercourse. There are lots of other ways that you and a partner can enjoy yourselves sexually without a penis going in your vagina.

Hymens Don't Pop

The majority of women who have taken our survey did not experience bleeding during their first intercourse. Nor did their hymens (or cherry) pop. That's because it's a myth. To understand more about your hymen, please read Chapter 8: "The Hymen."

During their first intercourse, some women don't feel a thing hymen-wise, others feel a stretching or a sting, and some feel a level of pain that you might when you get your ears pierced, or worse. But if you do the exercises with your fingers ahead of time, the chances are good you won't feel discomfort. And if you do feel pain, ask your partner to stop.

Now, for advice for members of both sexes...

Pillows and Lube

Two accessories that might really help are lube and pillows.

You have no idea how much a carefully placed pillow under a woman's rear can help with the angle of penetration and her ability to spread her legs. It allows her to better relax her legs and her vaginal muscles.

As for lube, a few drops on the penis and a few drops on the vulva and you are good to go. If you don't have lube, spit can work really well.

Go Slow and Ask!!!

After you've made out for about an hour and are ready for intercourse, do not just ram the penis in! Start with the head gently pushing against the rear or bottom of the woman's labia. (It can be very helpful if she guides the penis to her vaginal opening.) If she is OK with the head pushing slightly into the opening of her vagina, ease it in just a bit more, and ask again.

Once the penis is all the way inside of the vagina, just keep it there—don't start thrusting. This is the first time the woman has ever had a penis in her vagina. She should spend as much time as she needs to adjust to it being inside before there's any thrusting. This can be the most important moment of your first intercourse. It will be the only "first stroke" that either of you will have in your entire lives. Stop and savor it.

Also keep in mind that a nice sensation can result if the guy pushes his pelvic bone against the woman's while his penis is all the way in and does a slow circular motion with his hips. This may help stimulate her clitoris. She can hopefully guide him with her hands on the sides of his butt.

Orgasms, Anyone?

"Be choosy. Take your time. Touch and explore everything."

female age 36

The chances are good that guys will probably have an orgasm their first time, and girls might not—or not from intercourse alone. To understand more about orgasms, see Chapter 9: "Orgasms, Sunsets & Hand Grenades."

If you are a guy, your orgasm might not feel as intense as when you are jerking off. After all, how many times has your penis been in your hand, and how many times has it been in a vagina? When you masturbate, the sole point of contact is your hand gripping your penis; with partner-sex, your whole body is feeling her whole body. Or how often have you had an orgasm while supporting your body's weight on your arms or elbows? And if you wank to porn, there can be a big difference between staring into a partner's eyes and staring up the crotches of actors. It often takes time and experience to put lovemaking together in a way that beats beating off.

If He Comes Really Fast

Some of us guys can come pretty quickly the first couple of times we have intercourse. Some of us don't even get a penis inside before blowing a wad. Anxiety can do that, and there's nothing wrong with being anxious.

Coming soon might not be such a bad thing. Part of the reason why sooner might be better is because it might be the first time a woman has had a penis in her vagina. There might be a little rearranging or familiarizing that needs to go on inside of her pelvis. As a result, it could be that nature actually intended for first-time boys to launch early.

Still, if you are worried about coming too soon, get some really thick condoms made out of recycled boots or something.

Afterward

The time you spend together after you have your first intercourse can be as important as the time during and before. So don't try to do the deed minutes before your team bus is leaving for the state finals. Spend time together afterward and be aware of each other's emotions. Maybe you'll want to hold each other, or maybe you'll want to run downstairs and raid the refrigerator.

You can't predict how you will feel afterward. Perhaps you will be relieved, maybe happy, disappointed or sad. Perhaps you'll feel extra close to your partner, or maybe you'll feel alone and isolated. That probably depends more on the quality of your relationship more than anything else. Allow for a full range of possibilities and the time to experience them in the hours and days that follow.

What if It Wasn't Mind-Blowing?

"Relax and don't expect it to be like the romance novels." *female age 32*

Who knows what makes for mind-blowing sex, but don't be disappointed if it doesn't happen. And if you are thinking that your first time will change your life or transform your relationship, it probably won't, unless you get knocked up or get an STI.

Where to Do It

"Our favorite place was on the floor in the room over my parent's garage when they were out somewhere. When the garage-door motor clicked on and started vibrating the floor we had just enough time to finish, clean up, button up, and act natural before my parents walked in." *male age 26*

For your first time, a quiet, familiar and comfortable setting might be best. But finding a private, unhassled location can be a challenge any time you have sex! Ideally, find a time and place when roommates, friends or parents won't be barging in. And please don't do it your first time in a spare room at a party. You might not care much about yourself now, but maybe you will in a few years. Thinking back over that could be a big regret.

Once you have lots of experience under your belt, forests, volcanos, deserted islands, sandy beaches and glaciers are fine places to have sex. But for now, safe and familiar is best. If you try it in a bathtub or hot tub, chances are good the water will wash away your natural lubricant. If you do it on a beach, the sand will find its way inside the woman's vagina, which is how sandpaper came to be invented.

No Time for Sex Toys

If you are so inclined, there's plenty of time in the future to bring out your stock of dildos, cuffs, and strap-ons. When it's your first time, why not stick to the lovemaking basics?

The one exception might be a vibrator, assuming the woman already uses one and enjoys it. It might not be a bad thing for her to get herself off right before you try intercourse. This can help her relax and it might help her first intercourse feel really nice. Her partner can always hold her while she masturbates or uses the vibrator.

If You've Waited until Marriage

The average reader of *The Guide* is not necessarily the kind who waits until the first night of marriage for sex, so it's not like we have a huge database of advice to pass on. But if you think about how stressful a wedding and reception can be, the night of your wedding might not be the best time to make it your first time. Then again, all that adrenaline might be just the ticket! Talk it over ahead of time, and if you decide to wait until the next day, more power to you.

Advice for Guys

Look over the following advice that our female readers have for women who are doing it for the first time:

> "Make him go slowly and be sure that you are aroused sufficiently before you let him enter you because it will probably be a little uncomfortable the first time. If he rushes, it will hurt and you won't enjoy it at all." *female age 35*

> "Make sure you really want it and it's not about being pressured. Masturbate together first. Be comfortable together. My first time was painful and humiliating; there's got to be a better way."
> *female age 38*

> "Make him read the *Guide To Getting It On* first!" *female age 30*

Men who are virgins tend to be at a disadvantage their first time because they usually don't have the courage to admit that they haven't done it before. So instead of being honest and trying to explore together, the guy tries to fake it. Hopefully, readers of this book won't be so silly.

Your first time can be special and sweet, but not if you need to pretend that you know what you are doing when you really don't. Here are a few tips for guys who are about to make their maiden voyage:

Positions Your first time is no time to get fancy. Go with the old-fashion missionary position where she is on her back and you are on top. There's plenty of time later for her to be on top. Missionary is better for the first time.

During Intercourse If you are on top, she'll want to feel some of your weight on top of her, but not the full nine yards. So use your arms, elbows and

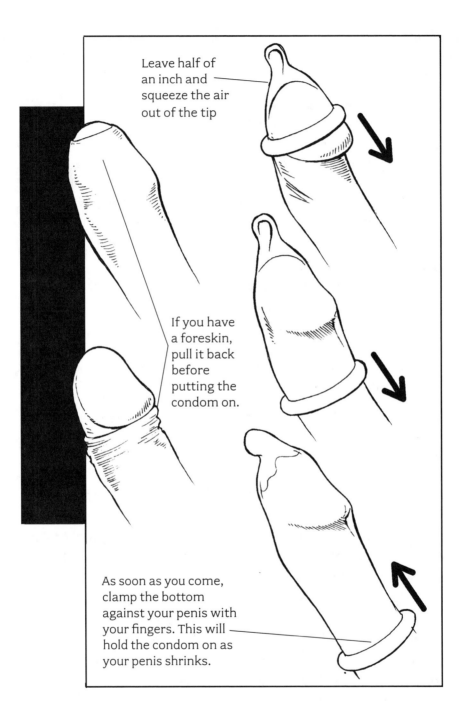

Leave half of an inch and squeeze the air out of the tip

If you have a foreskin, pull it back before putting the condom on.

As soon as you come, clamp the bottom against your penis with your fingers. This will hold the condom on as your penis shrinks.

For the Ride of Your Life!

knees to support yourself and thrust with your hips. Not to worry, you'll get the hang of it. Heck, even your dad did.

Thrusting Speed Contrary to what you might have seen in the movies, thrust slowly. Go really, really slow, and enjoy each and every slip and slide. If she wants you to speed up, she will tell you.

Your Lips You will be hard-pressed to find a single woman on the planet who wouldn't enjoy it if her lover planted some tender, gentle kisses on her neck or lips as his penis is getting to know her vagina.

Porn What makes sex work in a relationship and what makes it work on a TV or a monitor are two very different things. In porn, the camera abhors a tender and loving touch. It comes across as boring. In real life, tender rules.

Oral Anyone? In some situations, it makes perfect sense for you to go down on her before intercourse. In other situations, this would be way too overwhelming. The two of you need to decide together.

Condom Practice Find a condom to practice putting on. Once it's on, jerk off by thrusting your penis into your lubed hand. This is important. See why in the section on rubbers that follows this one.

Erections #1 Neither you nor she should give much heed to an erection that leaves before the big event. Consider it simply as another opportunity for you to kiss and feel each other up, which, if you do what's described in Chapter 15 on finger fucking, will help make it even better when it happens.

Erections #2 One of the bigger motivators for first-time lovers to rush is because the guy might be worried he will lose his hard-on. If he does, he does. It's far more important that you take your time, with lots of kissing, touching, and more kissing. The goal of sex is to share pleasure, fun and intimacy. You don't need an erection or intercourse to do that.

Condoms, Condoms, Condoms

Unless you've really got it together and visited Planned Parenthood, the chances are that condoms will be your default method of birth control. If used correctly, they can be very effective.

If you are a guy, try to get stash of condoms and water-based lube ahead of time. You'll want to study the package, and learn how to open it in the dark. As you are opening it, try to figure out how to manipulate the condom by feel alone. Experiment with rolling it on your dick, leaving a half inch at the top with the air squeezed out. Then put some lube in your hand and try jerking off with the condom on. See what it's like to thrust with your hips into your lubed hand. Thrusting into a well-lubed hand with the condom on will give you a better sense of the condom's road-handling abilities.

Then, after you've blown a wad, look at what happens to your penis. If you are like most of us, it will start to shrink. This is why guys need to crimp the bottom of the condom around the base of their penis as soon as they come, especially if their penis does a rapid deflate. Otherwise, the condom will slip off, and if you keep thrusting, you will push it inside your partner's vagina.

If you are a girl, get extra condoms and try putting one on a banana or something penis-shaped. Learn how to open the package in the dark, and how to roll it on, leaving a half-inch at the end with no air in it.

If it is at all possible, get the morning-after pill (Plan B) in advance. That way, if a condom breaks, comes off before it's supposed to, or you forget it, you'll have a really good chance of preventing an unwanted pregnancy.

This book's chapter on birth control is thorough and easy to read.

16 vs 26

Plenty of people don't lose their virginity until they are in their twenties. The nice thing about waiting is that you tend to be more sensible about it and you have a better experience—for many of the late-bloomers we have heard from, a much better experience. This is from a reader who didn't lose her virginity until she was well into her twenties:

> "I was surprised at how tricky losing my virginity proved to be. The first couple of times my boyfriend and I tried, my vaginal muscles were very tight and penetration was painful. So we slowed down a bit and tried other ways of loosening the muscles (fingers, a vibrator, etc.), I visited the ob-gyn to make sure nothing was wrong (there wasn't), and we waited for a night when I was nice and relaxed. The first couple of times we successfully had intercourse were amazing—I felt a bit of pain with initial penetration, but once my body got accustomed to him the physical sensation was wonderful, and we had a lot of fun trying different positions and experimenting with what felt good!"

A Very Special Thanks to Angela Hoffman for advice and help. Thanks also to Chris, a contented average dude from Canada, and Figleaf.

29
The First Time
Not What You'd Think

Researchers Newlyn Moore and J. Kenneth Davidson questioned hundreds of young women about their sexual experiences and feelings of guilt. Shock of all shocks. Girls with the most negative attitudes about their sexuality are doing it younger, with more partners and in less committed relationships than girls who feel the most positive about their bodies and their sexuality.

Also, the guilt girls are the most likely to have their first intercourse with an "occasional dating partner" or with a "person just met," a pattern they continue to repeat as they get older. They tend to have their first intercourse when drinking or stoned.

The girls who feel the best about their bodies tend to masturbate more. And the girls who masturbate the most and feel the best about sex actually wait the longest before having their first intercourse and they have it with more committed partners. Most importantly, when they do have sex, it's part of a conscious decision. Not so with the girls who feel bad about sex and their bodies. More often than not, they just let sex happen to them, without thinking it through first.

So who are these high-guilt, more-promiscuous girls? High-guilt girls tend to grow up in families where the mother and father are less affectionate toward each other. They tend to regard their dads as being overly strict and they are from homes that are more religious, rather than less religious, than girls who don't sleep around as much.

Perhaps the girls who have the least sexual acceptance at home go searching for it elsewhere. The trouble is, they go about it in such a destructive way that they end up reinforcing the bad feelings about themselves that they grew up with, and they end up with partners who are just as constricted as their dads.

Who knew that the daughters of the self-righteous would be more likely to sleep around and do it drunk than daughters of parents who have a more open, honest approach to sex and sexual feelings. It's certainly not what the self-described moral majority would have us believe. Perhaps there's more to waiting longer than the abstinence-only proponents want us to think.

Girls vs. Boys — Feelings about Sex

For a boy, puberty usually brings freedom. It also leaves a young man feeling more positive about his body, more independent and more masculine. Not so for girls. Menstruation itself often leaves a girl with a feeling that her body is out of control.

According to Karin Martin, who studied teens and puberty: "The girls whom I interviewed gave only negative descriptions of their menstruating bodies. Their bodies made them feel 'yuck' or 'sick,' or as if they had 'shit their pants'.… While plenty of girls look forward to having their first period, a lot become ambivalent after the first couple of periods have come and gone."

Teenage boys may struggle with wet dreams and unwanted erections, but not many would equate these with shitting in their pants. On the contrary, a boy's growing body often makes him feel more grown-up and effective in the world, while a girl's growing body brings parental warnings about the evil intentions of men and restrictions on everything from climbing trees to learning to sit like a lady. These warnings can make the world seem scary.

For a girl, her growing body represents loss as much as it represents gain. For instance, the mere fact that she suddenly has breasts causes changes in her relationship with her dad and every other man she meets. No longer will her dad be as physically affectionate, and no longer will she be as unconscious about her body. Ever hear that upbeat song from the early 1960s, *Sweet Sixteen?* It talks about a girl who was just a normal kid next door until suddenly she grows boobs and hips, and her former big-brother figure up the street has a hard-on and a hit song. Maybe the girl was happier before puberty when the universe didn't revolve around what her body looked like.

Dr. Martin tells about asking teenage girls to describe themselves:

"When I asked girls, especially working-class girls, to describe themselves or asked, 'Tell me about yourself,' they described their bodies and had a difficult time describing any other aspects of who they were. 'Can you describe an important goal you achieved?' 'I love my hair. My hair's my accomplishment…'

'What kind of things make you feel good about yourself?' 'When someone like pays me a compliment on something, you know. Like says that I look nice or have on nice clothes or something.'"

It was totally different for most of the boys. The boys felt good about themselves because of things they had done or things they felt they could do in the world. Of course, if most of these boys were more in touch with the reality of their "effectiveness" rather than their fantasies of it, they might not feel so confident. But still, when boys want to have sex, it is often with confidence and good feelings about their bodies, while girls often feel the opposite. In terms of sexual economics, we're talking the U.S. versus Peru.

So how does this reflect itself in the feelings that boys and girls have about sex?

"Boys thought sex would be pleasurable, and many said they looked forward to it or were curious about it.... No girl said that she looked forward to sex or that she expected it to be pleasurable."

The majority of teenage girls whom Dr. Martin interviewed expected sex to hurt or to be painful or scary. If this is true, why did the girls have sex?

"No matter how you look at a girl's reasons for having sex, the vast majority break down to the same simple reason: they are afraid the boy will leave, they are afraid they will lose him, or afraid he won't like them anymore."

More than half of the working-class girls and a quarter of the middle-class girls in Dr. Martin's study seemed to have an ideal or exaggerated love for the boys they were dating or wanted to date. Feelings like these will make a girl do anything to keep her man. The boys, on the other hand, did not report looking for romance or ideal love. They seemed to want a combination of friendship and sex in their relationships, although it is possible that the boys kept their romantic feelings to themselves. (For a teenage boy to tell an interviewer about feelings of romantic love might be admitting to less-than-manly aspirations. Or as the fraternity boys at Dartmouth might say, "Whadda you, a faggot or something?")

When it comes to teenagers and sex, boys and girls often have different wants and expectations. Far more boys think that the sex will feel good, while far more girls believe it will hurt. More girls idealize their boyfriends and feel they can't live without them, or they need the boyfriend as an affirmation that they are attractive and worthwhile. For this, they are willing to have sex.

As for masturbation, many teenage girls feel it is something that boys do, and do not associate it with femininity. Nor do they seem very interested in exploring their own bodies. As Dr. Martin comments, "Their boyfriends were allowed more access to their bodies than they allowed themselves." And this study was done in the 1990s, not the 1950s.

Perhaps one of the most frightening findings of Dr. Martin's research is that almost all of the teenage girls felt better about shaving their legs than they did about the sex they were having with their boyfriends. It seems that being able to shave their legs provided a happy identification with their mothers or older sisters. It made the girls feel grown-up in a good way.

Few and far between are the teenage girls who feel in control of their bodies and who have sex because they expect it to feel good. But those girls who did tended to have good relationships with their mothers which included lots of conversations about sex. They had good relationships with their dads, and they were also more involved in extracurricular activities like sports or 4-H. They seemed to place more value on the size of their IQs than on the size of their waists. They knew their own bodies better and felt more in control of their sexuality.

Counterpoint A female reader replies: "Sex for me was definitely not because I was afraid of losing the guy. I don't even know if it was really about my feelings for the guy. Mostly it was my curiosity about how sex felt. Few of my friends were dating and none were having sex, so it wasn't about fitting in."

Recommended: *Dilemmas of Desire: Teenage Girls Talk about Sexuality* by Deborah Tolman, Harvard Universities Press (2006).

See also Chapter 28: "Goodbye V-Card—Your First Intercourse"

30
Better Mating
Through Internet Dating?

Internet dating can make good sense for some people, especially if you are over 30. It provides access to others who are hopefully like-minded without requiring you to ever visit a singles' bar or attend a singles' dance or social. It can also give you a much needed assist if you are painfully shy or having trouble walking up to someone and starting a conversation.

On the other hand, is this a better way to meet people than at work or through friends? While the Internet-dating services swear that it is, we're not so sure. Internet-dating services play their "find your soul mate" card in suspiciously high proportions. As for their marriage-success statistics, hopefully they are right, but we at Goofy Foot Press can make stuff up, too.

What they don't want you to know is that the first rounds of Internet-dating service divorces are starting to be filed. They don't want you to know that Internet-dating relationships are just as fragile and the divorces are just as messy as they are for couples who didn't meet online.

Contrary to their ads on TV, there is absolutely no magic to Internet-dating services. Researchers have tried and tried to come up with ways of matching singles. Their results have been dismal failures. Internet dating services cannot match you any better than you can match yourself. They simply allow you to sort through a large pool of single people—some of whom are telling the truth about themselves. Those with better writing skills will appear to be a better match, but couples in relationships need to be able to talk to each other, unless they are texting maniacs.

Virtual Logistics

Before you join an Internet-dating service, take a hint from your old friends at Goofy Foot Press—consider reading two books that have a different emphasis from each other, but are complementary:

I Can't Believe I'm Buying This Book—A Commonsense Guide To Successful Internet Dating by Evan Marc Katz, Ten Speed Press (2004).

Virtual Foreplay—Making Your Online Relationship a Real-Life Success
by Eve Hogan, Hunter House (2001).

Don't let the ancient copyright dates fool you. The Katz book is funny
and well-written. It will tell you what you need to know, from choosing services to creating an effective personal profile. *Virtual Foreplay* takes a more
psychological look at the emotions involved. Eve Hogan is a therapist who has
made Internet dating her area of expertise. She speaks about the need to have
compassion and respect, and many of the tips she offers are excellent. However, people around here nearly gagged at statements such as, "The attention
is placed on aligning your virtual presence with your real essence and using
the experience as a process for growth." Does anybody have any idea what
that means? And if anyone at Goofy Foot Press ever uses the word "soulmate"
in a serious way, nuke us. In fact, be safe and nuke the entire Northwest.

What You Want and Where You Want It

You will be amazed at how many different types of Internet-dating services there are. You will probably want to join a couple. But before you decide
which ones to join, you'll need to decide what it is you are looking for. Are you
looking for a buddy to have fun with on the occasional weekend date, or are
you looking for someone to settle down with? Are you in a "screw the ring, I
just want sex" mode? Find out what people use in your area. By the way, if
you are looking through ads and see "NSA," we would not be talking about
the governmental agency in Washington. In the world of online hook-ups,
NSA means "no strings attached."

After you decide what type of relationship you want, check out a number
of Internet-dating services that fit the bill. There are services that match people based on religion; others try to match people who are into similar kinds
of kink. See if there are plenty of members in your age group and in your geographic area. Just because a service says it has more members than the population of China doesn't mean there are any members this side of Beijing.

You will also want to compare and contrast the features that the different services offer. It's not uncommon for someone who successfully hitches
up to forget to remove his or her profile. So a feature you might want is one
that lists the last time the person visited the site. That way you won't waste
your time responding to a cutie who has moved across the country or a death-
row inmate whose final appeal was denied months ago.

Your Profile

Most services will ask you to fill out a profile that shoppers—uh, members—get to read. It's how you present who you are. A lot of people don't take profile-writing seriously enough. This is where Evan Katz's *Internet Dating* excels. It helps you decide what's important to put in your profile and how to go about it. If the males who have taken our online sex survey are typical of how the average straight guy writes, then some of you boys might consider having a more literate friend help you write your profile.

For How Long and How Much?

Some services say they are for free. You usually get what you pay for. Many of the better services charge between $20 and $30 a month, but they offer discounted three-month and six-month plans. Consider going for a longer plan. Give yourself time for the process to work. If you find the partner of your dreams in the first week, consider the extra money a tip for a service that was well provided.

Time For a Reality Check

Internet dating isn't going to make the competition disappear. Internet dating isn't going to keep you from feeling bad when someone says no. It's not going to make you seem any more appealing if you are short on social graces or high on the kind of behaviors that result in a psychiatric diagnosis.

What will be different is that the process is going to be more private and it may help you to have a more focused approach. It might give you more choices. If you don't do well with romantic cold calling, being able to e-mail back and forth and then talk on the phone might be a great help. But just because you find someone whose profile looks good doesn't mean they will answer back, and it doesn't mean you would want to go out with them if they did.

Assume that you will need several months of solid effort to make the process work for you. Things might start clicking right away, but that would make you the exception rather than the rule.

From Email to Phone Calls to Pressing Flesh

Let's say you find someone with an interesting profile and he or she thinks the same about yours. Where to go from there? While it might be more desirable to e-mail each other several times and then spend a few weeks trying each other out on the phone, someone might come along who is more aggressive and next thing you know, the person you've been having the conversations with is already hitched. When it comes to timing, making the move from online to in-person is a totally subjective call, with risks each way. Learn how to protect yourself. Eve Hogan's book lists several precautions that are a good idea to consider throughout the Internet-dating process.

The Possibility of Being Overwhelmed

It doesn't matter if you are 20 or 50, occasionally someone will write a great profile and he or she will be overwhelmed with responses.

This is a good thing, and don't feel like you have to respond in detail to everyone. As you start to see the type of people who are responding to you, you might want to establish a set of criteria that helps you in making a quick first cut. This way you can form a short list of who you'll want to spend more time responding to. Even then, you might not have the time to do so as well as you would like. Don't be afraid to tell people when you've been overwhelmed. Say that you won't be getting back to them for awhile.

Don't Be the Litter on the Side of the Information Superhighway

It's only the Internet. What's so wrong with stretching the truth a little, like when you say you've got a D-cup or nine inches when it's a B or six? What's wrong with saying you are well-read and sensitive when the only thing you've read this year is the handout at your anger-management class?

Why should honesty be any less important in cyberspace than face to face? Why be an online offbeat? Think seriously about telling the truth, even if it's the Internet. Integrity is an important part of your character.

Next to telling lies about yourself, another form of dishonesty in Internet dating is to say you'll do this but then you do that. If you aren't interested in going further with someone, have the decency to say so. Don't just disappear, and don't keep something going because you feel too guilty to say "no more." Have the courtesy to say "so long" or "it's been swell."

And Then What?

Whether we want to admit it or not, dating is a significant part of a single person's life. When a date truly clicks it can make you feel on top of the world, and when a date misfires it can make you feel deflated. Even if you swear off dating totally, it remains a significant part of your life because you have to work so hard to ignore the importance that our culture puts on it.

Internet dating is like arranging your own blind date. It is an attempt to meld technology with Cupid's bow. It changes the dating process, but it doesn't change the feelings that are involved in that process.

Thanks to Evan Marc Katz.

31
Sex in Cyberspace

The world wide web is part of a vast digital expanse known as the Internet. In January of 1994, there were fewer than 1,000 websites on the world wide web; in April of 2006, there were more than 80 million; in September of 2008, there were 181,277,835 sites, although many of these were bogus link farms set up to trick search engines. Still, it is not unreasonable to assume that the world wide web has seen a bit of growth.

Technology and Sex

There's nothing new about using technology to get sex.

When the author of this book was a boy, the best porn magazine collection in town was in the lobby of the two-story hotel that was named after the founding father. There was one problem. The old man who ran the hotel sat behind a large desk that was next to the wooden racks that held the glossy goods. The old man took seriously his job of protecting the dirty 'zines from the admiring gaze of the town's young. If you were under the age of twenty-one, the town's only porn stash might as well have been on the moon.

Fortunately, right across from the old man's desk sat the only elevator in town. It was an amazing, ornate contraption that was as old as time itself. Using it required the old codger to leave his wooden perch, enter the ancient time machine, pull the shiny brass gates shut, and perform a ritual of knob-turning and lever-pulling that would nudge the lift to the floor above.

Whenever the boys in town needed reassurance about the intimate parts of a woman's anatomy, they would head over to the hotel and hide behind the oversized Morris chairs that populated the west end of the lobby. They would wait patiently until the old geezer had his back turned. Then one of the boys would do a crawl-sprint up the stairs to the second floor and ring the call button for the elevator. By the time the old man minced his way into the elevator and made its big piston ascend, the boys would have two-and-a-half minutes to look through the glossy magazines. That's how long it took for the old man to return with his empty cargo.

Nowadays, if the author of this book wants to see porn, he slaps his keyboard and there it is—an outrageous supply of nakedness and extreme sex. Whether it's the Internet today or the clunky old elevator from years ago, sex and technology have never been strangers.

As for the old hotel with the antique elevator, there were other things of a sexual nature that went on upstairs that were beyond what the mind of a young boy could comprehend. They were curious things that helped some of the town's people keep their sanity, and others to nearly lose theirs.

Flower of the Military-Industrial Complex

If things have parents, then the sperm for the Internet was donated by the Cold War. If they have godfathers, the Internet's might as well have been Sputnik, a transmitter in a tin can that the Soviet Union snuck into space in 1957. The launch of Sputnik put the fear of God into the U.S. government and it triggered a massive race in technology. The foundations of the Internet arose from this national fury which was the technological equivalent of going to the gym, getting buff, and winning the babe back.

The Internet was based on a new idea called "packet switching," which was the communications version of coming in spurts. It's how we upload and download everything from PTA schedules to X-rated streaming videos.

One of the false myths about the Internet is that it was designed as a communications cobweb that would keep working after places like Washington, New York, and Chicago were buried by nuclear bombs with hammers and sickles on their sides. While no one at the Department of Defense would have minded such a stout creation, the Internet seems to have evolved as a way for computer programmers from the major universities and defense labs to share information. This was the womb that would eventually give birth to the world wide web.

Even if it wasn't created to be nuke-proof, thank goodness they designed the Internet to withstand a great deal of abuse. During any given week, millions of people in this country are abusing themselves while they are logged on to the Internet.

Sex on the Internet: Two Different Forks

The flow of sex online takes at least two different forks, one being interactive and one not. In the first fork, you are an observer, a consumer and a downloader, but you don't contribute to the content. In the second fork, you both consume the product and help to create it through what you post, which might be anything from a chatroom exchange, to images, to the creation of your own website or blog.

The First Fork, Sex That's Not Interactive

There are several ways to use the Internet for sexual purposes. Here are some of the ways that Emily does it.

Emily uses the web to get sex information (and misinformation!). Let's say Emily's new boyfriend ejaculates too soon or she catches him wearing her bra and panties. Since she lent her copy of the *Guide To Getting It On!* to a friend, she goes to Google and puts in "premature ejaculation" or "transvestite." Hundreds of resources pop up. Or maybe she wants to know what other women think about swallowing. So she finds online forums that talk about it. Or maybe she wants to learn more about different methods of birth control, or whether women should use pills to stop their periods, or how the drug ecstasy affects people's sexual experience.

Using the Internet is both good and bad. For instance, anything you read about sex in this book has been checked and double-checked by some of the world's experts in their respective areas. But on the Internet, anyone can publish anything and call it fact. Misinformation often masquerades as science; so you get it quickly, but not necessarily right.

Emily also uses the web for reading arousing stories. She goes to the *Erotic Writers and Readers Association* website to read stories about steamy sexual encounters. She gets to read people's personal posts about everything from orgasms to what kind of threesomes they prefer. For Emily, a fast mouse makes for wet panties.

Like a lot of her friends, Emily gets off on good porn, whether it's visual or text-based. There are some sites that she and her boyfriend go to where they rate pictures that couples post of themselves having sex. She can also use the web for buying sex toys that she might be embarrassed to hand to a flesh'n'blood person at a retail store.

The Second Fork of Sex on the Internet — Cybersex

Here are the accounts of cybersex by three readers who tell about two different kinds of experiences: the first being personal between two lovers, the others being more public, in chat rooms and the like:

> "We're in a long-distance relationship, so masturbation in conjunction with cybersex is a great thing. Basically what we do is a 'This is what I'd do to you if I were there and horny.' Most of the time it's describing the various sex acts either one of us would like to perform on the other one, and the 'receiver' making the appropriate typed noises of pleasure. We both use AIM, but through a multi-IM protocol called Trillian. There have been swaps of risque digital pictures too, but that doesn't always coincide with cybersex." *female age 18*

> "In answer to your question, I've tried many sex chatrooms, but they've been disappointing: lots of males chasing a very few females, or just as likely, chasing males who are pretending to be female. A bit pathetic, really. Chat rooms with a webcam facility are as bad: a lot of males getting very excited over a very little exposed female flesh. I've not yet found an intelligent user in any of the sex chat rooms, despite spending what must be many hours looking through user profiles. I'm sorry if that sounds harsh, but it's my experience. The rooms are also infested with advertising bots. Apart from chat rooms, I've found that newsgroups are better for porn than websites."
> *male age 51*

> "From what I've seen in the IRC world, the male-to-female ratio tends to be about 20:1. And I have experimented entering a chat room as a woman just to see what would happen, and yes, you get pounced on." *male age 22*

When people are having cybersex, they are using the Internet to get each other off in real time. The way they do this ranges from typing text on the keyboard to masturbating in front of video cams.

When you compare cybersex to real-life sex, one of the most striking features is how much is left out. In preparing for cybersex, you don't need to comb your hair or brush your teeth. You don't need to shave or shower. You don't need to figure out how you're going to get across town (or across the world) to his place or hers. You don't need condoms or birth control.

You don't need to worry if an online partner snores, has gas, or is seriously out of shape. You don't need to worry if your partner is single or married, rich or poor, male or female, or recently payrolled. Everything is just too perfect for words, as long as you are able to trick yourself into thinking that the hand in your pants is your cybersex lover's and not your own.

In cybersex, people exist as words, sentences, avatars (avs) and lines of text, unless you park a video cam between your legs and let the interface fly. And if you find yourself in a fantasy situation that starts to feel uncomfortable, relief is just a delete button away.

No Scratch'N'Sniff in Cyberspace

In real life, you are able to smell the person you are having sex with. Given that there is no scratch'n'sniff in cybersex, your sexual partner's smell is whatever you want it to be.

In real life, you touch your partner and your partner touches you back. In cybersex, it's you who is touching your body in the exact way you want to be touched. The touch you are giving yourself is fueled by a level of fantasy that is untouched by the problems of everyday life or of living together.

Imagine a woman who finds an eloquent guy online and they go into a private chat room. She is highly aroused by the cybersex fantasy that they are weaving together and she is masturbating. Do you think there's a guy or girl on earth who could touch her genitals in the exact same way that she knows to touch her own at that moment? It makes sense when some people say they have more intense orgasms in cybersex than with real-life partners.

Liberation from the Real Body? Not Really

Some people say that the Internet is a medium where gender and looks are no longer factors. Yes and no.

To paraphrase sociologist Dennis Waskul, when you look at the cybersex profiles that people create for themselves, you start to wonder if the only people who use computers are women with large breasts and guys with 9" dicks. Good luck going through a cybersex chat room and finding someone who is 5'2" and 250 lbs. Good luck finding the phrase, "Oh baby, let me suck your pathetically small dick!" Not only does the body count a great deal in cybersex, we're talking a whole new religion devoted to the perfect person and the perfect lover. In cybersex, nobody comes too soon, can't get it up, or doesn't get wet.

In cybersex, everybody gets an extreme makeover. In cyberspace, looks count a great deal.

Cybersex proves that if given the opportunity, people will recreate themselves in the image that society says is the perfect 10. In cybersex, everybody looks as good as—gulp—the characters in the illustrations of the *Guide To Getting It On!*

Virtual Pubs—A Sense of Community as Well as Role Playing

There are countless numbers of forums, habitats and chat areas on the Internet where people form a very real sense of community. For example, there's a group of woodworkers who have a power-tool forum where they give each other advice on the different kinds of equipment they use, from drills and planers to table saws and dust collectors. There are members whose names you learn to recognize and whose opinions you trust. In each new thread there is kidding and criticism, but always a sense of cohesion. When one member is struggling with a difficult project, other members offer an impressive stream of support and encouragement.

This same kind of community can be found in cyber groups that researcher Lori Kendall refers to as "Virtual Pubs." These are Internet portals where members interact in ways similar to a neighborhood bar. They rely on each other being there month in and month out, and they offer the same kind of intimate support and candor that would happen at any neighborhood bar.

An interesting thing about these non-sexual forums and chat rooms is that members tend to be honest about who they are. The expectation is that you are who you say you are. It's not much different from life offline. However, when the focus moves to sex, that's when the fiction starts to fly.

Gender in Cyberspace

A woman's husband went into a chatroom one night while using her computer. He was logged on with her username. A political discussion occurred, and he presented his views on a subject rather strongly. This was no different than what he does on his own computer using his male persona. But this night he was surprised to discover a strong negative reaction among the other members of the group. They assumed he was a woman because he was using his wife's username, and they didn't like that a woman would have such strong and forceful opinions.

There is very little gender switching in non-sexual forums, although if a woman wanted to be taken seriously in the woodworkers' power-tool forum, she might consider saying she was a guy. But when you are dealing with sex on the Internet, all bets are off. While there might be a hope that the woman on the other end really is 25 years old and wants nothing more than to have oral sex with you, it's just as likely that she's a 60-year-old man with a wife and ten grandkids, or a 16-year-old high-school student who's doing this instead of his physics homework. And you don't want to assume that people with usernames like "8inchElmer" or "StopStaringAtMyCock" are necessarily men, although it's a pretty good bet that they are.

Virtual Deception or a Real Reflection?

It's easy to be critical about the deception in cybersex, but aren't there plenty of precedents in real life?

For instance, in real life, Amy is an engineer who works for an aerospace firm. Amy used to have a bra-cup size that was an A. After $11,000 of cosmetic surgery, Amy's breasts are size D and the bump and bulge in her nose are history. She is wearing make-up, her hair has been bleached and permed, and she's got on $200 of underwear from Victoria's Secret. What's so real about any of that?

Or what about Fred? He works out at the gym three hours a day, leases a $90,000 car, and spends $3,500 at the Laser Hair Removal center each year to keep the hair on his chest and back at bay. He's in debt up to his plucked eyebrows and he drinks more than he should.

Fred and Amy have never tried chat rooms or cybersex, but are they totally real—or do they have plenty of virtual parts themselves?

Beyond Text: Cybersex with a Webcam

If there are two things that will get the hackles up on a card-carrying feminist, one is when a person is reduced to a sexual object and the other is when that "gaze" thing is in high gear—when a guy looks at a woman's boobs instead of straight into her eyes. Yet it is these very things that are the hallmark of webcam cybersex. In cybersex with a webcam, people are reduced to close-ups of their bodies, often just their breasts or genitals.

In cybersex, you've got people crossing a forbidden threshold which can be exciting. The risk isn't anywhere near what a flasher in a park has to face, unless a jealous former lover downloads pictures of you playing with yourself on the web and gives it to your colleagues or e-mails it to everyone who you invited to your wedding.

As for actual identities, it used to be that you seldom saw a cybersex participant's face. The camera was often focused on body parts being grabbed and rubbed. So you had the thrill of watching and of being watched, while feeling safe. But today, both women and men are posting pictures of themselves that include their faces as well as their legs splayed wide open. Likewise, we are putting private content on public blogs–intimate details of our private lives that used to be considered highly personal.

While it is unlikely that the Internet is responsible for our changing ideas about privacy, it's most certainly been the vehicle for that change to occur so quickly and in such a global way.

From Porn to Social Media

Sex in cyberspace has been studied extensively by sociologist Dennis Waskul. For instance, in cybersex, you often see the genitals of the other person first and their face last, assuming you get to see his or her face. Yet in real-life romance, you see the other person's face first and genitals last, or at least that's the way we do it around here.

One of the things Waskul is keenly aware of is how the Internet has made pornography accessible in parts of our society where it has never been. Before the Internet, porn was mostly a guy-thing, often relegated to magazines that could be hidden under the bed. But with the Internet, porn can now be seen at work, in your car, in sidewalk cafes, and even on the bus or train as you commute. Nor is it any longer just a "guy thing."

Two years ago, Waskul was fascinated by the proliferation of websites where people submit naked pictures of themselves that others rate, such as "rate my dick," "rate my pussy" or "rate my boobs." He was surprised at the numbers of women from all walks of life who post pornographic images of themselves on the Internet.

Today, Waskul seems more interested in social media, as do more young adults. While the heyday of porn is far from over, the great majority of Internet porn consumers are males from the ages of 35 to 50. While porn used to be an interesting and innovative player in the world wide web, in a short time it's become a bit boring and staid, perhaps reflecting the mindset of its main consumers.

For more interesting ways of using the Internet for sexual exploration and enjoyment—besides the usual surfing for porn—see Regina Lynn's *Sexier Sex* book that's listed at the end of this chapter.

Privacy in Cyberspace?

> "You already have zero privacy. Get over it."
> —Scott McNeally, CEO, Sun Microsystems

> "Today's satellite-image technology means that even in today's desert, complete privacy does not exist."
> —Google response in the law suit of
> "BORING et al v. GOOGLE INC." July, 2008

If you honestly believe there is a single private thing about anything you put on the Internet, you are one big silly goose! It doesn't matter if you are in a private habitat or in a MOO on Mars. It doesn't matter if it's a blog in Bangkok or a MUDD in Madagascar, if it's on the Internet, it is as public as if you wrote it in spray paint on the side of the freeway. The same is true if you and your cybersex partner are masturbating for each other via a webcam, so pay close attention to the accepted cybersex convention of showing no face when you are spanking your monkey.

Media Reports about Sex in Cyberspace

One of the truly fascinating things about sex and cyberspace are the statistics that people invent about it. Consider this article that was in a college newspaper: "While an estimated two-million Americans engage in cybersex, 200,000 of those people are addicted, which means it disrupts their professional or personal lives." Really? This begs a question or three:

1. Watching porn on the Internet disrupts people's professional and personal lives, but sitting in front of the TV for hours on end doesn't? Hmmmm.

2. There is no way of accurately knowing how many Americans engage in cybersex, so any figures you read, be they 2 or 2 million, are pure fiction.

3. How do you define "cybersex addiction?" Is there a definition that is accepted by Internet-savvy sociologists and psychologists? Or is this the usual prattle of the addiction fanatics?

The hysteria about "OSA" or Online Sexual Addiction is so fascinating that we now include a separate chapter on it that follows this one.

Adultery Online?

Is having sex in Second Life or anywhere else in cyberspace cheating on your real-life partner? And how do you have sex in cyberspace, anyway?

Hurt and angry partners sometimes blame the Internet for problems in their relationships. But if people are looking for a technology to blame, it seems like the telephone and the automobile should be on their lists. How often does adultery happen without a phone or a car being involved?

As for whether cybersex is or isn't adultery—some people say it is, others say that what they are doing is helping to keep in check their inclination to stray in real life. Either way, it takes more effort to keep the sex in a real-life relationship exciting than it does to have exciting sex in cyberspace.

Is having cybersex behind a real-life partner's back any different than flirting with someone in real life? Fire is fire, even if it's anonymous. It is probably best not to do it unless your real-life partner says it's okay.

Sex in Video Gaming, MMORPGs and MMOs

For many years, the annual Consumer's Electronics Show (CES) has been where new technology is showcased. A number of the big companies used to hire Playboy and Penthouse centerfolds to promote their microchip-based products at the CES. This made sense given how both the chips and the centerfolds seem to have so much in common. However, the "silicon" used in microchips is a very different beast from the "silicone" used in breast implants.

To this day, sex is an important part of technology and it is a part of the wonderful world of gaming that technology has helped to spawn. Whether it's avatars flirting in WOW, emerging sexual economies in Second Life, or GTA's Hot Coffee Mod, sex at the crossroads of gaming and cyberspace is a fascinating subject. Brenda Brathwaite's *Sex in Video Games* (Thompson, 2007) does a great job of exploring it. **NOTE:** While a number of our readers are avid and passionate first-person shooters, their sex surveys report that if they had to choose between gaming and real-life sex, they would take the sex.

HIGHLY RECOMMENDED: Whether you want tips for looking your best on a webcam to breaking up with an online lover, THE source is *Sexier Sex: Lessons from the Brave New Sexual Frontier,* by Regina Lynn, Seal Press (2008)

A Broad-Band of Thanks to Dennis Waskul, Ph.D., Minnesota State University, Mankato – one of the world's finest minds on sex on the Internet. And to Mr. Rich "Bare Bones" Siegel for thoughtful and helpful guidance, as always.

32

Online Sexual Addiction Really?

Joe's wife spends four hours a night watching television, and one hour during the day watching her favorite soap opera. Joe spends two hours a night looking at porn on the Internet.

Joe's wife is normal, while Joe is addicted to porn on the Internet. Or that's what Joe's wife's therapist tells her about any man who spends two hours a day looking at porn on the world wide web. And heaven help the poor pervert who spends three hours on Sunday afternoon looking at porn on the Internet as opposed to his upstanding co-worker who comes home from church and spends the rest of the afternoon screaming in front of the television while the Browns get clobbered by the Bears. If the football-watching maniac masturbates later that night, he's normal. But if the porn-watching web guy jerks off to what's online, he's got OSA—Online Sexual Addiction.

Interestingly, when researchers have tried to validate some of the claims that mental health experts have made about how the Internet "is a powerful medium for OSA," the claims have proven to be invalid. Yet scientific refutations of OSA don't make for good media play. After all, we've got an excellent hysteria going here, and we all know there was no porn before the Internet. Porn was a sleepy fringe business: *Hustler, Penthouse, Playboy, Deep Throat.*

Fears about new technologies aren't new. In the 1800s, when printing technologies improved, there was concern that people would stay at home reading newspapers and books instead of gathering in town for their news and gossip. In 1922, the *New York American* reported that "the pathological, nerve-irritating, sex-exciting music of jazz orchestras led to the fall of 1,000 girls in the last two years."

In the 1930s, there was concern that teenagers were imitating the sex they were seeing in the movies. Girls were adopting the flirtatious personas of actresses, and after seeing certain movies, women felt compelled to find men for sex. Boys were learning how to kiss and make love from the movies, and men claimed that the movies of the 1930s had driven them to commit rape.

In the 1950s, it was reported that the new medium of television was lead-ing young offenders to commit sex crimes. Blame *Lassie, The Three Stooges,* and *I Love Lucy.*

So we shouldn't be surprised when today's psychologists warn about the "isolation," "alienation" and "depersonalization" that results from Internet addiction. Of course, none of that happens if you are sitting in front of your television watching crime-show reruns and *American Idol.*

New technology has always had a way of bringing fear. So has sex. But neither sex nor technology have made us any more alienated, isolated, sad, happy, loving or lonely. These are the things we bring to technology, not things that technology creates within us. The Internet does not give people psychological problems, nor is the ability to sit quietly and anonymously in front of it a lightening rod for instability. People bring their problems with them whether they are on the Internet or on the phone. And in the same way that the phone made it possible for people who have never met in person to engage with each other in rich and productive ways, so has the Internet.

The anonymous nature of the Internet allows us to look at sexual con-tent that we wouldn't if other people were looking over our shoulders. But is this content any more damaging than the early silent films which experts claimed were causing the ruin of young women and men, or any more ruin-ous than the early television shows that we now call classics?

Granted, we never saw Lassie humping June Lockhart, and Ricky and Lucy never had group sex with Fred and Ethel, but would our country be any worse off today if our grandparents had seen those things? Mind you, there would be no protest from here if you did something better with your time than jerking off in front of a computer, but we'd say the same to all of the people who sit like rotting potatoes in front of the television each night.

Thanks to Steven Stern and Alysia Handel for their excellent paper "Sexuality and Mass Media: the Historical Context of Psychology's Reaction to Sexuality on the Inter-net," *Journal of Sex Research*, 38, 283-291 (2001).

33

MRIs of Sexual Arousal
Is the Brain Half Empty or Half Full?

While researchers were looking for the parts of the brain that light up during sexual arousal, they actually discovered parts of the brain that were shutting down. You would think it would be the opposite, with sexual arousal causing sparks of activity arcing from ear to ear. However, it appears that in order to get into the sexual moment we need to shut down parts of our brains as well as fire up others. This would validate what women often say who take our sex survey at www.GuideToGettingItOn.com. When asked to describe what intercourse feels like when it's really good, they often say that the rest of the world disappears, for example:

> "When it's really good, I feel like the world just stops and my mind just goes blank and all I want to do is feel every single move, and enjoy each breath. But when its bad, I can't stop thinking about everything other than what is really going on. My mind will be racing."
>
> *female age 22*

It's clear that MRI or neuroimaging studies of the brain and crotch are the future of sex research. However, it's equally fascinating to consider the limitations of brain-imaging technology when it comes to exploring sex on the brain. This chapter will give you an idea of the challenges that researchers have to deal with as they are exploring this virgin territory. Understanding the limitations of current technology is particularly important given the media's tendency to make way too much out of findings that are tentative and have yet to be replicated and validated in other labs.

Problems with the Old (and Still Currently Used) Technology

Before sex researchers started using MRI technology to study our brains and crotches, research about sexual arousal and sexual feelings has often included tying strings around men's penises that were attached to gauges, and sticking plastic tampons containing infrared sensors up women's vaginas. We would then try to make educated guesses about what it meant when the strings got stretched and the sensors sensed. This was particularly fraught with peril when you consider that a third or more of the research subjects would routinely be disqualified because their strings didn't stretch convincingly. There were also questions about how representative a person might be who volunteers to watch porn movies in a lab with a probe stuck up her vagina—while totally sober!

Worse yet, when it came to women's arousal, we've mostly been limited to measuring the changes in the blood flow in her vagina. As some of you may have noticed, women have a clitoris that's involved in their sexual arousal. But we haven't had a very good way of measuring what was going on inside of it other than slapping a glob of KY on the end of an ultrasound probe and pushing it up against a woman's clitoris. So researchers have left the clitoris out of the equation when measuring female sexual arousal.

With the newer imaging technology, researchers suddenly have the capacity to not only measure what's going on inside the entire pelvis when it's sexually aroused, but inside the brain as well. All of this while allowing the subject to remain in relative privacy—if you assume having your genitals stimulated while attempting to lie totally still in a large metal cylinder at a university lab is private.

The Current Limitations of Neuroimaging

As exciting as the new wave will be, for now we need to be mindful that brain imaging in sexual research is still in its infancy.

As for some of the current kinks, a research subject's head needs to be kept perfectly still for several minutes while the images are taken. The slightest movement results in signal changes that threaten to muck everything up. Worse yet, the part of the brain where some of our sexual arousal and orgasms are processed is located in an area of the skull that is next to a sinus cavity that the brain uses for air conditioning. By virtue of being located next to the brain's air-conditioning shaft, even the slightest of head movements is magnified and creates even more unwanted artifacts than if it were located closer to our foreheads.

Fortunately, researchers can use higher-resolution scans with smaller voxels or volume pixels to get reliable data. Still, try to imagine a research subject having an orgasm while needing to keep his or her head perfectly still for minutes on end. Head movements during MRI studies of orgasm are one of the reasons why these studies must be reproduced in another lab before they should be considered valid, yet few studies have been replicated elsewhere.

Also, the subjects are often shown porn clips to make them feel sexually aroused while the MRIs are being done. But how do the researchers know if the subject's brain is processing sexual arousal, or the way the porn actors' bodies are moving (kinesthetics), or the changing frames in the video porn clips or some random thought that popped into the subject's mind?

There's also the question of what happens to the information when it gets inside the brain—is the information being compared to similar information that was stored in the subject's mind years ago, or is it being treated as novel information? Is the subject's brain processing the porn clip based on how the subject feels when he has had sex in the past, or is the turn-on strictly in the here and now, with no prior referencing?

Today's neuroimaging technology is still pretty crude compared to what it will be in another twenty to thirty years. Right now, the equipment doesn't focus on the actual neurons that are firing, but on the blood that drains from that part of the brain. So let's say researchers are focusing on what's happening inside a small part of the brain called the insula. Small as it might be, the insula contains an ocean of neurons. Using the current generation of MRI equipment to nail down the exact neurons that are involved would be like trying to go to the moon using a Nintendo DS Light.

There's also debate about how long to measure what it is you hope you are measuring, and whether you are actually measuring what you think you are measuring. This depends on a researcher's hypothesis about what areas of the brain are going to be activated. Because researchers use different measurements, it makes it a challenge to compare studies with each other.

The next time the media runs a big story saying that men's brains process sexual arousal differently than women's brains, you might wonder if the study actually measured how our brains process sexual arousal, or how they process the porn clips that the researchers were showing the subjects to get them aroused.

Think about the anticipation and erotic edge you feel when you are looking forward to having sex as a partner first arrives, as well as the sounds, smells and actual feel of your partner's skin against yours. Does your brain respond differently to that kind of sexual arousal versus the kind when you are watching porn on a TV screen?[1]

While the current MRI findings are exciting, thought provoking and will be unlocking many of the mind's sexual secrets—all things in good time. For now, researchers are just beginning to break a sweat.

---

[1]While reviewing this chapter, a researcher on the forefront of neuroimaging commented: "For many researchers, it's not clear that they have specific research questions when they enter the scanner. Some of the discussion sections seem like exercises in reading tea-leaves."

A Very Special Thanks to Mr. MRI Adam Safron of Northwestern University, to Serge Stoleru of the Université Pierre et Marie Curie, and to Claire Yang and Kenneth Maravilla of the University of Washington for their very helpful article "Magnetic Resonance Imaging and the Female Sexual Response: Overview of Techniques, Results, and Future Directions" in the April 2008 *Journal of Sexual Medicine*.

CHAPTER
34
Orientation in Flux

Labels for sexual orientation like "homosexual" and "heterosexual" can be useful at times, for instance, in helping you decide what part of town to visit if you are hoping to get laid. Labels are also helpful for people who don't have the same sexual turn-ons as their peers. They let them know where to go for sexual guidance, comfort and fun.

From this Guide's perspective, the biggest utility for these labels is in the discussion that researchers are having about them as new technologies provide new ways to pry under the lid of human consciousness. One of the more interesting things these researchers are finding is that orientation might be a beast of a different color for women than for men.

From the Cutting Edge

Research in sexual orientation is in a state of flux. Actually, it's been a bit topsy-turvy for the past 100 years, and before then, it didn't much exist.

The latest state of flux is being fueled by new ways of looking inside the brain while people are being presented with things that turn them on. This is in addition to the more traditional research, which involves slapping sensors between the legs of college students and seeing what happens when you hand them dirty pictures or show them films of people who are fucking.

It used to be that people thought of "straight male" and "straight female" as being opposite sides of the same coin. No more. Fortunately, some of the top researchers in sexual orientation were kind enough to offer readers of *The Guide* their current thinking about sexual orientation. Consider what researcher Richard Lippa has to say:

"People come in different sexual orientations. It's part of human diversity—like variations in skin color, hair texture, mental abilities, and handedness. An analogy is: although right-handedness is clearly more common than left-handedness, it's equally OK to be right-handed, left-handed, or ambidextrous.

Scientists are interested in figuring the causes of sexual orientation, just as they are interested in figuring out the causes of variations in handedness, personality, and intelligence. When scientists study the causes of human traits, it's not necessarily because the traits are good or bad; rather, it's because it's interesting to understand the causes of human behavior. We're still not sure of the causes of sexual orientation. However, in recent years the pendulum has swung more in favor of biological theories.

Recent research suggests that the nature of sexual orientation may be quite different for men and women. (I've conducted some of this research.) Women's sexual orientation seems to be more fluid and flexible than men's, whereas men's sexual orientation seems to be more fixed, 'black-and-white,' and perhaps biologically wired in. For example, recent studies of people's physiological arousal to sexy male and sexy female stimuli show that heterosexual men are turned on by sexy women but not by men, and gay men are turned on by sexy men but not by women (as you would probably expect). However, women—both heterosexual and lesbian—get turned on by both sexy men and women (which is perhaps not so expected).

Western society has become more open about variations in sexual orientation and has become more tolerant of non-heterosexual orientations and relationships. So it will be really interesting to see how the expression of various sexual orientations develops in coming years."

Here's what researcher Michael Bailey has to say:

"Increasingly, people are understanding that men and women do sexual orientation differently. Men are straightforward. A man's sexual orientation results from what causes him the greatest sexual arousal, what kind of person (or animal or thing) gives him the most intense sexual excitement and the most dependable erections.

Women are different. Increasingly, it appears that women's sexual orientation is not closely linked to their sexual arousal patterns the way it is in men. I even question whether women have something called a sexual orientation, although they clearly have sexual preferences. Women's sexuality seems more fluid than men's, in that it can vacillate between different types of people, and women are known to fall in love with each other and then to revert to a heterosexual identity and life."

Of course, given how the author of this book is a psychoanalyst, he fears these distinguished scholars may have been smoking too much of the Ganja. If men and women do orientation differently, it's surely because of upbringing and environment. And when the author's daughter prefers to play with Barbie dolls instead of Legos—it's all the sitter's fault...

What Do They Mean By "Women's Orientation is More Fluid?"

When sex researchers ask women to put tampon-like probes in their vaginas that measure their genital blood flow, they find that just about any kind of sexual stimulus results in arousal between their legs. Heck, a picture of two hippos humping would probably do it for some women. But before you take a girl to the zoo hoping you'll get lucky, what flows between a woman's legs and what she feels in her heart or thinks in her head can be very, very different. As our Ph.D. female friends so eloquently say: there can be a huge disconnect between cunt and cranium. This means it is a very unwise person who assumes that a woman is interested in sex just because her genitals are showing signs of arousal.

There is also the assumption floating around these days that women are turned on by women. But if you ask them what they actually feel, most women say they would rather have sex with guys as opposed to with other women. And if you look at who women actually have sex with, you will find that only a small minority have had sex with other women.

So just because researchers are saying that female sexuality is fluid doesn't mean that waves of women are going down on each other. Perhaps a better way to put it is to say that when it comes to sex, the theater of a woman's mind tends to have more potential for variety than a boy's brain. How much of this translates into actual behavior is another story, and how much of it has to do with biology versus upbringing and culture is a never-ending source of interesting conversations.

"Mostly Straight" vs "Totally Straight"

If women's orientations are more fluid than men's, it might explain the results of our own sex survey. Over the past years, we have received approximately 6,000 surveys from visitors to our website who have taken its totally unscientific sex surveys. One of the first questions on the survey has been, "Please state your orientation as *totally straight, mostly straight, depends on the day, mostly gay or totally gay.*" Here are the approximate results:

	"totally straight"	"mostly straight"
males	80%	15%
females	20%	70%

Over the years, we've tried to design a safe, nonthreatening question about same-sex interest. We have had to keep making the question safer and safer, as even the possibility of same-sex interest can make male survey takers pissy. In its various states, the question was stated mostly as follows:

"If our society did not care or notice, and if your girlfriend and best friends thought it was perfectly normal and OK and did it themselves, do you think you might ever consider experimenting sexually with another guy to see what it was like?"

[For the women's version of this question, we changed "girlfriend" to "boyfriend" and "guy" to "girl".]

The vast majority of the women replied, "Sure!" or "I've already thought about it and am wondering how to make it happen," or "It's nothing I would seek out, but if it happened, I might go with it."

It was a very different story for the male survey takers. Many of them flamed in all caps, "NO FUCKING WAY" or "I'M NOT GAY!" Around 30% said "Maybe" or "You never know." Most said, "It's nothing that interests me." Of course, we weren't able to see the men's answers after they'd had a six-pack of beer, which some people hold as the dividing line between a guy who is straight and one who is bisexual.

One factor that might be pushing the boys to be uppity about the slightest hint of same-sex attraction is memories of relentless grade-school taunts about being "Queer!" or "a fag." Even the straightest of straight boys in our culture has to face such taunts if he is caught not towing a manly line. (While girls have their own special ways of being cruel and mean, taunts about sexual orientation are not usually at the top of their nastiness agenda.)

Of course, guys who are openly gay faced the same cultural influences, and it didn't stop them from wanting the one-eyed winky. So perhaps culture doesn't hold a candle to biology when it comes to sexual orientation.

On the other hand, consider the possibility that most males come out of the womb with an orientation that says "Seriously Straight" or "Seriously Gay." For these guys, it's the sensation in their dicks rather than anything culture has to say that charts their sexual course in life. But what about boys who come out of the womb sitting on the sexual fence? Perhaps culture has a significant influence on their sexual choices.

As for a man being able to choose his sexual orientation, research seems to indicate that he can teach himself to suppress an erection if his brain says, "Bad choice, you'll have hell to pay." But it doesn't work the other way around. Conservative Christian counseling claims to the contrary, a man who doesn't get hard over women can't will a tent in his pants. He can force himself to wear mental blinders when it comes to checking out dicks in the locker room, but he can't will himself to become a muff man. He has to be born with that potential. It doesn't appear that it can be programmed in later.

Wet Panties Have Their Advantages

If a woman becomes aroused at the sight, smell, or touch of another woman, she doesn't have to worry about being found out. If she's undressing with another woman and finds the situation arousing, she can smile inwardly and enjoy her feelings and not have to worry about a boner sticking up between her legs to give her away. In fact, she doesn't even need to think of her feelings as sexual at all, or as homosexual.

But if a guy gets an erection in the locker room, there's going to be nastiness to deal with. If he even gets caught looking in the wrong direction, there might be repercussions. Even when he is at home alone, his penis still tells him when something is sexually arousing. It's not like he can choose to ignore it, or not as easily as a woman can ignore the stirrings inside of her pelvis.

Having a penis, which is one of nature's more obvious feedback devices, makes sexual thinking more black and white for males than for females. Perhaps this would be true even if guys were born like Ken or GI Joe, with nothing but an ambiguous little lump that hardly hints of maleness. Figuring it out provides an interesting challenge for sex researchers.

Social Factors Influence Girls, Boners Influence Guys?

A psychologist like Roy Baumeister will tell you that women are more sexually flexible than men, and not just in terms of intercourse positions. The reason is because women's sexuality is more influenced than men's by social factors such as religion, education and parental pressures. Perhaps this helps explain why women with college educations are more likely to masturbate than women without. At the same time, women are usually the first to call women who are more sexually adventurous "sluts" or "whores." Perhaps this is because social factors and social prohibitions shape women's sexual beliefs more than men's. Since men's beliefs are shaped more by what creates an erection, they might have more admiration than scorn for a woman who is sexually adventurous. Of course, this varies greatly among individuals.

She Knows It When She Smells It?

Please, don't make too much of the following findings. They are only mentioned to give you an idea of some of the different ways that researchers are studying sexual orientation.

Shortly before this book went to press, researchers in Europe discovered that when straight women smell certain molecules from the sweat of men, parts of their brains light up that don't light up in lesbians or in straight men who smell the same thing.

While this could result from social learning, it is appearing more and more that responses like these are inborn. It suggests that events in the womb influence what turns us on. But we also know that the environment we are raised in can play a wicked game of pong against the brains we are born with, so complexity reigns.

While it is fascinating to think that dude-sweat can light up a straight girl's brain, this doesn't explain why a straight girl may have been thinking about her female friend when she was masturbating last night, instead of the sweaty guys who she was working out with at the gym.

A New View of What Turns Women On

Since the 1960s, sex researchers have assumed that the things that get women off sexually are the same thing that get men off. That's why they thought they had hit the pharmacological pot of gold when they discovered that Viagra worked for men—they assumed it would work just as well for women who had a low desire for sex. Viagra for girls didn't work. Nor has testosterone for girls.

What researchers haven't wanted to accept is that the state of her relationship, and the impact of her past sexual relationships, has a lot to do with whether a woman is turned-on to sex. Her genitals can be pumped up, but it doesn't mean she is pumped up. Just as her way of "doing" sexual orientation is different from the way men "do" sexual orientation, so is the way she becomes sexually aroused.

Jerking Off Together at 12 vs. Jerking Off Together at 21

If a therapist hears about two 12-year-old boys masturbating together, or masturbating each other, or blowing each other, it shouldn't raise flags of concern if the kids are well-adjusted and happy. Whatever orientation they are, they are. You can't talk a child out of one orientation and into another.

If the therapist is trying to ease the minds of the super-straight parents who are paying $160 an hour for the assessment, he or she might say, "Not to worry. It was *parallel sex-play*; your boys were really thinking about girls when they were blowing each other."

If the same boys were doing the same thing at age 21, people will automatically say, "Gay!" But if it were two girls at age 21 instead of boys, we would probably say, "Could just be a passing thing" or "lesbians until graduation."

It is unfortunate how sex that both partners want and enjoy needs to have a label at all, but that's the culture we live in. And when it comes to same-sex attraction, we are much more judgemental about boys.

What Happened to Bisexuality?

The new, more fluid definition of heterosexuality for women makes the concept of bisexuality a bit redundant for females. However, the reality is, if a woman in a church group is romantically kissing another woman during the congregation's annual anti-pornography pot luck, it won't matter how fine her three-bean salad is, she'll have hell to pay.

And good luck if a woman who is a lesbian takes a man to a lesbian-sponsored consciousness-raising seminar and looks at him longingly. Women may be more fluid, but they often see themselves as guardians of the family and champions of the status quo, whatever it might be.

As for bisexual boys, it used to be that 30% or more men were thought to have bisexual tendencies or reactions. Now researchers are arguing between 1% and 5%, which still means millions of men. Some researchers believe that the desire for other men has a stronger pull than the desire for girls, and that bisexual males are on the slippery slope to the gay side of town. Others disagree, especially bisexual males who have been liking both sexes with equal fervor for most of their lives.

One of the problems in doing research on bisexual males is that men who enjoy sex with both women and men know that our society is very polarized, being either pro-straight or pro-gay. Our society is totally distrustful of males who might enjoy sex with both women and men. In most straight circles, it's better to say you are a serial killer than a bi-boy, and in most gay circles, you'll be accused of betraying the gay lifestyle. So we don't yet know if researchers on male bisexuality are sampling a true cross-section. Their ads for research subjects might be netting bisexual males who are more gay-identified and closer to coming out as gay. It would also be interesting to know if guys who sleep with women but who have same-sex fantasies even think of themselves as being bisexual. The men who have sex with the he-she prostitutes who are discussed at the end of Chapter 36: "Gender Benders" think of themselves as being straight.

An interesting finding of researchers is that women with higher sex drives tended to be attracted to both men and women, while men with higher sex drives were not inclined to be bisexual.

Sperm-Drinking Males and Homophobia

While homophobia among males is not a sexual orientation, it is most definitely a strong response to a sexual orientation. So we will close our look at sexual orientations with two different looks on homophobia—one abroad and one in Georgia.

A number of years ago, an anthropologist discovered people on a remote island who believed that in order to become real men, male adolescents needed to drink the sperm of the adult males in the tribe. Given how the adult males didn't exactly have sperm spigots on their penises, the way the young boys harvested the sperm was by blowing the old boys.

Unfortunately, some of the people in the modern world who read these studies assumed that the sperm-drinking adolescents regarded their rite of manhood with homosexual glee. But the reality is, they probably did it as an anticipated experience like a teenager today welcomes the opportunity to take a driving test. It means you achieve a certain level in independence, not that you want to keep taking the test again and again.

A few decades after the initial research, an anthropologist returned to the island to see what was up with the off-spring of the sperm-drinking tribe.

Time had done a number on the people of the island. Many of its members had moved to a more urban part of the island, and Christian missionaries weren't too excited about the magical properties of swallowing sperm. The teenage grandsons of the sperm-drinking granddads were wearing wraparound shades and listening to iPods or MP3 players in front of the island's equivalent of the 7-11 store. Satellite dishes meant that this was the first generation of this people who had grown up under the influence of prime time TV.

When the researcher inquired about rites of manhood and what the boys needed to do to be regarded as manly, they looked at him strangely and wondered if he wasn't talking about some kind of extreme skateboard tricks.

He eventually broached the subject of the sperm-drinking to some of the boys, who became very grossed out and said, "My granddad did what?"

While some of these boys are probably homophobic, it is very unlikely that their sperm-drinking grand dads were. So when it comes to homophobia, it is not a leap to wonder how much it is culturally inspired.

Homophobia in the Homeland

Let's take a look at a study on homophobia that was done at the University of Georgia. The University of Georgia is one of the finer institutions of higher learning, and not simply because they have used the *Guide to Getting It On!* in their sex-education classes, although it does speak well of them.

Psychologists gave a questionnaire about homosexuality to a group of sixty-four men. Based upon their responses, the men were divided into two subgroups: those who were homophobic and those who were not. The testers then showed the subjects hardcore X-rated videos of men having sex with women, and men having sex with men. They did this after placing sensors on the guys' penises to see if they were having a penis response while watching the different videos.

When watching the tapes of gay guys, 80% of the homophobic men had penile arousal, while only 34% percent of the nonhomophobic men did. Naturally, almost all of the homophobic men denied feeling aroused while watching gay guys having sex.

Unfortunately, the penis does not always tell the truth, and studies using genital sensors tend to raise as many questions as they answer. It is also interesting to ask why some men can be homophobic about male-to-male sex, but get sexually excited about female-to-female sex.

Also, keep in mind that men who are homophobic don't care if homophobia is a biological or a cultural construct. They are viscerally enraged and hateful, and one needs to assume that they are dangerous. It could be that they believe their very existence is being threatened by the mere presence of a gay guy, or what they think is the presence of a gay guy.

One might think that they protest too much.

Happy Trails

The next chapter is on same-sex attraction. Before it begins, this might be a good time to return to something that researcher Richard Lippa wanted you to know:

> If you're a young person, remember: There is no good or bad when it comes to sexual orientation. You are who you are. Sexual identity and sexual orientation may not be fully fixed in young people, and this may be particularly true for women. Whatever your sexual orientation is and whatever gender (or genders) you're attracted to, learn to accept yourself and enjoy your sexual feelings. Sex is always a process, but not necessarily a fixed process. So learn to go with the flow—in particular, learn to go with your flow—but do so in a safe, sane, and sensible way."

And what better way to finish this chapter than by leaving you with our most favorite reader response on sexual orientation that we've ever received:

> "I would probably be gay if I didn't find guys so damn ugly."

male age 23

Recommended Reading For a view from the cutting edge, the place to start: *Sexual Fluidity—Understanding Women's Love and Desire* by Lisa M. Diamond, Harvard University Press, 2008.

A Special Thanks to Richard Lippa of California State University at Fullerton, to J. Michael Bailey from Northwestern University, and to Ralph Bolton from Claremont College.

35

Same-Sex
Fun & Luvin'

Most books on sex written for a predominately straight audience have an obligatory Gay, Lesbian, Bisexual & Transgendered chapter. Authors include them like they do gender-neutral pronouns. But the truth is, there is no way this material can or should be covered in only one chapter, or in only ten.

So Paul did surgery on the obligatory GLBTQ chapter from prior editions and included only what made him smile, especially *The Guide's* hard & wet steamy fiction reading list for young adults who are thinking about exploring same-sex relationships. How many respectable, mainstream books on sex include anything this useful?

This chapter now has the goal of getting you to think about just one thing—any one thing—differently about sex than you did before you read it. If it is able to do that, then it has done more than most GLBTQ chapters in most books on sex.

Alice in Sexual Orientation Land

People tend to take their sexual orientations very seriously. Boundaries are staked out and rigidly enforced. So, what would happen if....

...If the head of the Lesbian Women's Caucus found herself being turned on while standing behind the cute guy at the hardware store who was on a ladder grabbing a box of screws? Is she suddenly less of a lez—as she would be the first to accuse any other lesbian who admitted to lusting over a testosterone-drenched male pelvis? And what if she had a fantasy of the hardware boy easing her down on the newly-displayed lawnchair recliners in Aisle C, as she eagerly spread her legs, clutching a Tiki Torch in each hand while he slid his big bolt of a boy boner into her "women's only" area?

...If a gay male cheerleader finds himself looking up a cheerleader's skirt and suddenly wonders about something other than whether she waxed her bikini line correctly? Or what if he feels compelled to sneak a pair of her panties from her workout bag to see what it's like to jerk off into them? Is he in danger of having to surrender his subscription to Honcho and his $2^{(x)}$ist coutour pouch briefs?

...If a totally straight guy gets tossed into the slammer for twenty years and has a non-exploitive, loving and tender sexual relationship with his cellmate, Bubba? And if after the parole board lets him skedaddle and his choices are no longer limited by the situation, he still misses Bubba?

Would any of these people be less of who they think they are if these egregious violations of their assumed sexual identities were to occur?

Jerking Off to the Wrong Underwear Ads!

This book doesn't much care what your sexual orientation is, but in case you do and you are wondering how people with same-sex attraction learn about theirs, here's a very funny description from author Ellen Orleans:

"At What Age Do You Know You're Homosexual? As you might imagine, this varies greatly. Guys seem to be aware of their sexuality early on. A single erection while watching Batman free Robin from the clutches of the Riddler provided many young men with their first clue. One gay friend told me that his childhood role models were Bert and Ernie. For others, it was Skipper and Gilligan.

"Women seem to discover their sexual orientation more from personal experiences. Although I didn't realize it at the time, my first clue was when I zipped up Bobby Wolinsky's fly for him in the second grade. My teacher said this was not proper—that that was a boy's private area. At the time, I didn't see what the big deal was. Guess I still don't."—From *Who Cares If It's a Choice? Snappy Answers to 101 Nosy, Intrusive and Highly Personal Questions about Lesbians and Gay Men*, by Ellen Orleans, Laugh Lines Press

Of the various sexual orientations, which is best? We have no clue. There are times when life and relationships totally suck no matter what your orientation; being straight is no guarantee of happiness, nor is being gay. Straight is what most people think they are, and it's usually easier to be part of the majority no matter what. Easier, but not necessarily more satisfying.

Different Takes on Male Cruising

In case you grew up under a shrub and never heard about cruising, there is an interesting phenomena where guys who enjoy having sex with other guys hook up on the spur of the moment to have totally anonymous sex. Words or names are seldom exchanged. You give or get a quick glance of approval, and one guy's dick is out and the other is on his knees or is grabbing his ankles faster than either man can say, "Thank you, Craigslist!" (Hooking up by computer has become an important part of cruising. The Internet has become the new trailhead, with meeting locations decided online at sites such as adam4adam.com and bigcocksociety.com.)

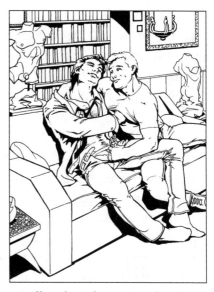

Of course, a lot of straight people shake their heads and say, "Gay thing." But what percent of straight males would suddenly cruise for sex if straight women started dropping their panties for all comers? (Can you say "Hooking-up sex"?) It would be just as high as the percent of gay guys who do it now. In fact, during the 1800s when the brothel was an extension of the American bedroom, the only thing that kept most single men from having sex with different women each night was how much money they could afford to spend.

"Ah," you say, "that's just proof that all males are pigs, straight or gay."

Well hold your horses, little lady.

In our totally unscientific sex survey for the website of this book, we have been asking women a big "what if" question—what if they never had to worry about being pregnant, catching an STI, or being called a slut? Would they be doing sex differently than they are today?

Of the women under age 24 who are in exciting new relationships, the answer is pretty much, "No—well, maybe a little, but I'm pretty satisfied." That's to be expected at the start of anything new that is sexual. But a solid half of women who have taken the survey say they would be having more sex with more men if they didn't need to worry about the things that women need to worry about.

So if you take away the danger of pregnancy, STIs and needing to parent kids, and we stop calling women whores for having the same amount of sex that men have, are you sure we would continue to see such a big difference between the sexual habits of gay men who cruise and straight men and women? Would marriage keep its allure if straight men and women could easily have sex on demand?

With the coming of birth control for men and vaccines against STIs in the next two decades, all bets are off.

There are plenty of people who hold the heterosexual model of marriage as an ideal, and the gay model of cruising as an aberration. However, with a divorce rate approaching 50%, and with a large percentage of married couples staying together just for the kids, some people wonder whether the straight model of monogamy is all it's cracked up to be. And some experts, such as college professor Ralph Bolton, say that while plenty of gay men are monogamous, others find it rewarding and fulfilling to cruise and have multiple partners. He believes that cruising can have as much intimacy and closeness for some gay men as sex in monogamous relationships does for straights.

Straight Male Friends Can Be Important

Contrary to what some heterosexuals fear, the last thing most gay men want is to have sex with a straight guy. While there are exceptions, most gay men would be bored by the concept. And if you are a straight guy who gets hit up by other men for sex, it's quite easy to say, "Sorry, but I'm one of those boring breeder types." If the person is really thick and persists, you might say, "Again, no thanks, but let me describe for you how much I love licking a woman's pussy, and what it looks and feels like." If that doesn't gag the guy on the spot, be careful. He's probably an undercover cop.

Also keep in mind that there are lots of reasons why some gay men value their friendships with straight men. With straight men they are only friends and not potential sex partners, and they can have conversations about things like baseball scores and new car tires without the added postscript of who got the plague or who went home with whom after working out at the gym. Their straight male friends aren't invested in the sometimes vicious politics of the local gay scene. And the stereotype that all gay guys are fems is destructive. There are plenty of gay men who are every bit as masculine as straight men and who desire their company.

As for any particular orientation of men being a danger, the vast majority of serious crimes in this country—from violent attacks, rape and child molestation to bank fraud and illegal drug importation—are committed by heterosexual males. People who are homophobic ought to think about that one.

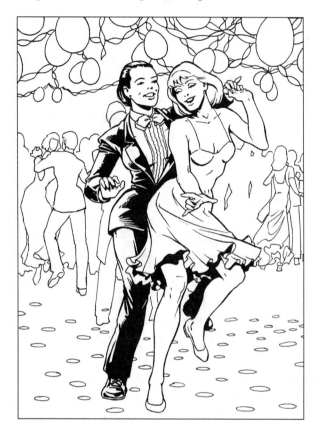

Life As a Lesbian, As If We Had a Clue...

Gay men and women are often grouped together because they are both homosexual. This is like assuming Germans and French are a lot alike because they share a common border. The real question that should be asked about gay men and lesbians is if there are any two groups on the planet who are more dissimilar—aside from the homophobia they receive from straights?

Even their statistics are dissimilar: while the majority of gay males in this country will have sex with at least 100 different partners in a lifetime, the average gay woman has sex with a lifetime total of two to seven partners. And while less than 20% of gay males have had sex with a woman, more than 80% of gay women have slept with a man.

Setting a stereotype for gay women is not possible, says sex researcher Ira Reiss. While common personality traits and pathways to homosexuality have been found among gay males, Reiss has found few among gay women.

Lipstick Lesbians & Diamond Dykes

People sometimes think that all lesbians are bull dykes or ride on Harleys. This Guide is willing to bet its left foot that there were as many lesbians entered in last year's Miss America Pageant as were on the women's professional-golf tour. Lesbians are just as feminine (or unfeminine) as women who sleep with men. A number of very hot-looking actresses and models are lesbians.

Equally off-base is the notion that gay women make love in a delicate or particularly poetic way. Women who love women get it on with as much passion (or lack of it) as women who have sex with men.

Beyond Brown & Yale

In the past, women who preferred women still dated and married men. And women who had lousy experiences with their fathers often replaced them with equally difficult boyfriends or husbands. It was usually expected that women remain in heterosexual relationships even if they preferred being with women. There are at least five reasons why this is not necessarily the case anymore:

1. Mothers used to teach their daughters that it was hugely important to marry a man and have his children. This is not as true as it used to be. 2. Appealing lesbian role models used to be few and far between. There now exists a group of very appealing, successful, high-profile lesbian role models in sports, business, rock 'n' roll, and entertainment. 3. It is now acceptable for lesbian couples to have children by artificial insemination, spawning a whole new market for turkey basters and adoption in most states. 4. It is now the height of academic chic for angst-filled co-eds to have lesbian affairs at schools other than just Brown and Yale. 5. Straight women get no respect at the WPGA golf tournaments.

Mistaken Identity?

Women in our society can hug, hold hands or dance together, and it is not considered a sign of same-sex attraction. As a result, they can have sexual feelings for women without acknowledging them as that. The following statements from two different women help describe how this lack of labeling can impact the ways that women think about their same-sex attraction:

"I never thought of homosexual as relating to women, only to men...."

"Our sexual relationship we kept to ourselves, and I was more ex-cited about it than anything else. I thought it was just a delicious secret. And at the same time I had a mad crush on a guy."

—From *Women's Sexual Development*, edited by Martha Kirkpatrick, (New York: International Universities Press)

Superb Resource

No one in America who is thinking about exploring romantic attraction between women should be without Lillian Faderman's *Odd Girls and Twilight Lovers : A History of Lesbian Life in Twentieth-Century America*, Penguin (1992). This little gem provides an essential historical background that people today have little sense of. Anyone, gay, straight or lesbian, will learn from this book.

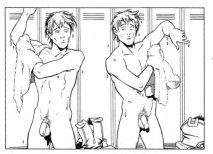

Dear Paul,

I am 17 and am on my high-school football team. I'm also gay. Nobody knows about it. It feels like I'm living a lie. I know that my dad would explode if I came out, and when someone isn't giving 100% on the football field, Coach calls him a fag. What do I do?

Mark in Atlanta

Dear Mark,

One of the books that is most often stolen from libraries is Dan Woog's *Jocks. Jocks* is real stories from young athletes who struggled with exactly the same questions you are. Plenty of guys your age want to read it, but are afraid of being found out if they officially check it out.

Let's break your question down into two parts—the dad part, and the coach part. A lot of the street kids who I used to work with had been kicked out of their homes for being gay. Trust me, you don't want to ever live on the streets. So the first thing I encourage you to do is to stop worrying about "living a lie." There's plenty of time to come out later. For now, consider where you would live if your dad kicked you out. If you don't have a safe place to go, forget any coming-out announcements for the time being.

Then there are your coach and teammates. Yes, there are stories of gay high school athletes who are supported by their team. But here's my guess—

they are few and far between, and they aren't in football unless they are all-league quarterbacks and their team's only chance of making it to the finals. When it comes to protecting star athletes, coaches and teammates have an amazing way of convincing themselves that rapists are decent guys and that gay athletes are just confused and will probably get over it—the operative words being "star athletes."

On the other hand, I recently heard from a university sex-ed teacher that one of the assignments he gave his class of mostly straight students was to write a coming-out letter to their family and friends. This was just an exercise that they were supposed to hand in to him. A few months later, one of the students who was an athlete called him to tell him that his computer had a virus, and that random files had been sent to people in his address book. The "coming out" letter he had written for the class was one of the files that had been sent out.

He found out when he started receiving phone calls from his family members and friends telling him that they loved him and that they were there to support him. What surprised him the most was how supportive and loving they all were!

So it could be that if you don't come out, you will be cheating your family, coaches and fellow players from the chance of rising above it all. You will also be cheating them of the opportunity to defend you as opposing players try to "spear the queer." So if you absolutely must come out while still in high school, why not wait until track season?

I hope that this is changing, but I doubt it. Many guys, especially those your age, define their masculinity by how un-queer they think they are.

According to some people, your chances of being accepted by your teammates would be better if you were in a sport where there are individual performances, like gymnastics or track. Your chances would also be better if you played women's sports, but you didn't mention having gender issues.

If you do come out, you will probably need to deal with your teammates' concerns about what will happen in the showers and locker room. You can laugh and point out that nothing happened before you told them you were gay. Or you might try kidding them by telling them not to worry and that your standards are higher than those of their girlfriends.

[Another book you might try is *Inside Out: Straight Talk from a Gay Jock* by former Olympic swimmer Mark Tewksbury, Wiley (2006).]

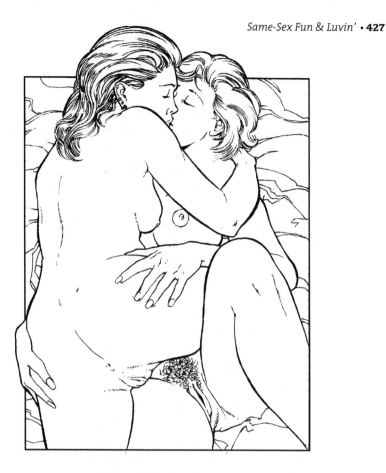

The Guide's Hard & Wet
Steamy Fiction Reading List

Let's say you are a young adult and you would like to explore more about same-sex feelings. If you check with your local Gay and Lesbian organizations, they will probably recommend one of the usual coming out books with pictures on the cover of a white kid, a black kid, a Hispanic kid, and an Asian kid, all smiling and happy. Sorry, but it didn't make our list of suggested titles.

We have devised the following reading list to help you have a fun time exploring same-sex feelings, while forestalling any lemming-like march into gayness or straightness. In constructing this list, one of the goals was to have books that would cause a stirring in your crotch—titles with a hard-on or wet factor that might necessitate one-handed page turning. Many of these titles do, but a few don't. Another important factor was that the books be well-written or intelligent and fun to read.

Of course, there will be problems. For instance, what if you have homophobic friends and parents? How would you explain these books to them?

You'll need to be clever and sneaky—having to keep hidden an important part of yourself. (What else is new?) If you drive or use public transportation, maybe you can take a day trip to a library in another city. Instead of having to check the book out, you can spend the day reading it there. Or maybe you have an aunt or uncle you can trust, or there's a minister or teacher who will keep your secret. Perhaps they can get the book for you and you can read it at their place. Just be sure it's not someone who is going to insist that you "come out" or that you "get help," unless you really do need to speak with a therapist.

Another problem is that there are probably a dozen other books that deserve to be on this list, but aren't. No one would be surprised if we missed some exceptional titles. Also, some of the books will be out of print. You'll need to hunt them down.

Young & Wet

Skim — Mariko Tamaki
Keeping You a Secret — Julie Anne Peters
grl2grl: Short fictions — Julie Anne Peters
Far from Xanadu — Julie Anne Peters
Annie on My Mind — Nancy Garden
Ruby Fruit Jungle — Rita Mae Brown
Fried Green Tomatoes — Fannie Flagg
Valencia — Michelle Tea
The Passion — Jeanette Winterson
Tipping The Velvet — Sarah Waters
Dive — Stacey Donovan
Strangers in Paradise — Terry Moore
Flaming Iguanas — Erika Lopez
The Wrestling Party — Bett Williams
Girl Walking Backward — Bett Williams
Dare, Truth or Promise — Paul Boock
Deliver Us from Evie — M.E. Kerr
Crush — Jane Futcher
Memory Mambo — Achy Obejas
Parrotfish — Ellen Wittlinger

Note The body of lesbian literature for young adults is a bit thin if you include the criteria of "fun" and "sexy." Tragic and angst-filled, no problem; boring and academic—you could fill a library. Fortunately, there's plenty of really excellent panty-drenching lesbian erotica, but that might be a little intense for someone who is just starting to explore.

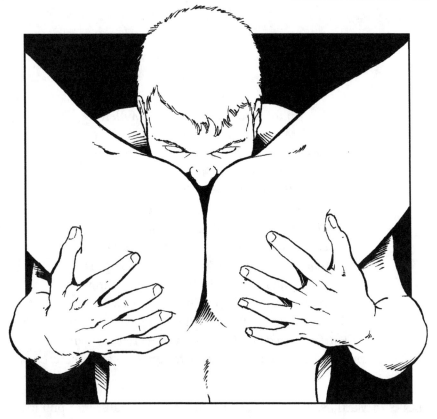

Young & Hard

Dan Woog — *Jocks*

Keith Hale — *Cody*

Perry Moore — *Hero*

Wiliam Taylor — *Jerome*

Will Fellows — *Farm Boys*

Paul Russell — *Boys of Life*

Kief Hillsberry — *War Boys*

Russell — *The Coming Storm*

James St. James — *Freak Show*

Alex Sanchez — *Rainbow Boys*

Mark A. Roeder — *A Better Place*

William Taylor — *The Blue Lawn*

David Levithan — *Boy Meets Boy*

William Corlett — *Now and Then*

Brent Hartinger — *Geography Club*

Brian Malloy — *Twelve Long Months*

PINS — Jim Provenzano

Lawnboy — Paul Lisicky

Diary of a Hustler — Joey

My First Time — Jack Hart

Foolish Fire — Guy Willard

Dream Boy — Jim Grimsley

Boys Like Us — Patrick Merla

Easy Money — Bob Condron

Glove Puppet — Neal Drinnan

My Worst Date — David Leddick

The Persian Boy — Mary Renault

The Boys on the Rock — John Fox

Changing Pitches — Steve Kluger

Smooth and Sassy — John Patrick

Enchanted Boy — Richie McMullen

For a Lost Soldier — Rudi van Dantzig

Harlan's Race — Patricia Nell Warren
Blind Items — Matthew Rettenmund
Boy Culture — Matthew Rettenmund
Absolute Brightness — James Lecesne
Enchanted Youth — Richie McMullen
Call Me by Your Name — Andre Aciman
World of Normal Boys — K.M. Soehnlein
Execution Texas: 1987 — D. Travers Scott
The Milkman's on His Way — David Rees
The Front Runner — Patricia Nell Warren
The Arena of Masculinity — Brian Pronger
Sex Toy of the Gods — Christian McLaughlin
Angel, The Complete Quintet — John Patrick
Telling Tales Out of School — Kevin Jennings
Gay Olympian — Tom Waddell & Dick Schaap
Out on Fraternity Row — Windmeyer & Freeman
Entries From a Hot Pink Notebook — Todd Brown
Someday This Pain Will Be Useful to You — Peter Cameron

THANKS to Matthew Torrey, who consults on gay literature for public libraries, Kayla Strassfeld, former book buyer for Good Vibrations, and Dan Culliane from Alyson Press, and Judith Rosen from PW. If the list has half the heart, intelligence and humor as these three people, it will serve you well!

Thanks also to Eric Garrison, clinical sexologist at The New School and former high school soccer coach. Eric reports, "One time, a student came out to me MID-GAME as I was being yelled at by a referee about a hole in my net. I guess when you have to come out, you have to come out."

A Very Special Thanks to Ralph Bolton, Professor of Anthropology, Claremont College. Professor Bolton is first person in the country who the author of this Guide turns to for help with mind-boggling questions of an anthropological nature, including those about *Magnum PI* reruns.

Highly Recommended *On Our Backs Guide to Lesbian Sex* edited by Diana Cage, Alyson Press (2004), then you might be Here are a few chapters: "Flirting Tips for Fat Chicks," "Pack Like You Mean It," "Rim Like A Gay Boy," "How To Suck Dyke Cock," "Fag Sex That Will Make Your Dyke Dick Hard," and "No Ass, No Tail: Uniform Fetish Aside, Real Military Dykes Aren't Getting Laid."

CHAPTER

36
Gender Benders

The author of this book recently sent the following e-mail to a university professor who is renowned for his incredible sex education course saying, "I'm really struggling with how to present transgenderism. Do you have any suggestions?"

The professor, who has always been generous with advice, replied apologetically that he struggled with trying to understand transgenderism. He said, "Be sure to let me know what you come up with."

Transgenderism has many layers and variations. Its expression can range from when a sexy-looking girl wears her boyfriend's clothes out clubbing, to when a person endures thousands of dollars of surgery and cosmetic hell to become a member of the other sex.

Transgenderism has its own vocabulary and nuances, including words such as "packing," "tranny bois," "tranny fags," "transitioning," "drag queens," "drag kings" and "genderqueer." Even the terms transgender and transsexual are nuanced, with a transsexual being someone who wants to completely change gender by having top and bottom surgery, while transgender is more of an umbrella term whose range extends from the girl who packs a fake set of male genitals in her jeans to the role-bending straight couple where she pegs he in the rear with a dildo.

Rather than trying to provide an overview of the transgender scene, which is still evolving and defining itself, it would be quite an accomplishment if you left this chapter with an appreciation of some of the different possible combinations, and how complex it can be for those readers who live it as well as the for the family and friends who love them. To that end, this chapter will focus on the transsexual part of transgenderism, which is where a person want to change their sex.

Trading in Your Balls and Bat

Around here, when you need help explaining something fundamental about sex, you turn to baseball. After all, what sport in creation has donated as many fundamental sex terms such as *Getting to first base* or *Hitting a home run?* And while the following quote from Yogi Berra wasn't about transgenderism, it was certainly in the ballpark: "90% of this game is mental, and the other half is physical."

So meet Clive Deacon, who spent the better part of eight seasons in the Carolina League. Given that this was the minor leagues, Clive had lots of time to think. Especially during the year when he started with the Lynchburg Hillcats and ended in Winston Salem, with stops at Durham and Myrtle Beach.

Clive Deacon was a pitcher. He was good enough to stay on a roster, but didn't have the stuff to go any further. One of the things that occupied Clive's mind were his feelings in the locker room, particularly during shower time.

While the other guys would be thinking about which of the local girls were going to show up after the game, Clive would be thinking about sex, too. But the sex he was imagining was being done to him instead of by him. And it was being done by one of the better-looking players, and not up the butt. Clive kept imagining that he was a woman who was being sexually ravaged by one of the boys of summer. Clive thought a lot about being one of the local girls who showed up after the game.

Clive knew about gay cruising and baths and gay bars. It's not like any fans would recognize him if he did it. He'd even had opportunities with players, but Clive wasn't homosexual. He had no interest in guys who were gay. That's because he wasn't gay.

As the seasons progressed, so did Clive's awareness that he felt like a woman and needed to become one. More and more, as he soaped his hairy chest and pulled his dick out to pee, it felt like he was touching the body of someone else. These were parts that belonged to a man and they symbolized being a man. Clive had less and less use for them. By the time he reached Lynchburg, it felt like aliens had stuck on the penis and had given him the hairy chest.

What's the Score?—Transgender Possibility #1.

Clive wants to be a woman, and he wants to be fucked like one—in a vagina and not up the ass. And he wants to give that heartthrob second baseman for the Nationals the best blowjob the boy has ever had, but this would be no gay play. The second baseman for the Nationals would be getting it from a woman with a woman's scent and a woman's love and a woman's body. And that second baseman would be putting his penis inside a woman's vagina, Clive's vagina when he could finally get one.

Are you starting to get the difference between gender and orientation? Being a man or a woman is about gender. Being straight or gay is about orientation. If Clive was happy being a guy and wanted to give the Nationals' second baseman a blowjob, it would be about Clive being gay, and that is about sexual orientation. But this is about gender, as in "male" or "female."

Unlike Clive, the Nationals' second baseman is 100% male in body and mind—his psychology agrees with his anatomy. He is the what the woman in Clive's mind longs for: a straight guy with a really good batting average.

Transgender rule #1 Gender trumps orientation. The first question is always "What sex does the person want to be?" as opposed to "Who is the person sexually attracted to." But that will change in the next inning.

Clive's Change-up

Okay, we know Clive wants to be a woman. He feels like he's a woman. More and more, when he uses a restroom, he has to stop and consciously remind himself to go into the door with the figure of the little man on it instead of the one with the girl in a dress.

But this is a new inning in our game of TG-Ball. Since Clive is a character of our own creation, we are going to change what turns him on sexually after he becomes a woman. You might say, "So why not bring in a whole new pitcher?" Sorry, but the only other transgendered pitcher in the minor leagues was called up to the majors. We'll have to make do with Clive. And quite frankly, if this weren't just a little bit confusing, it wouldn't be transgenderism.

Instead of wanting to be a woman and have sex with the Nationals' second baseman, the new Clive still wants to be a woman, but one who has a crush on the Pelicans' scorekeeper, Penny.

"So big whoop," you say. "Clive's a good-looking guy, nice personality, he doesn't chew—why doesn't he just ask her out, get her a little drunk like the other guys do, and fuck her? Penny is a known resource throughout the entire Carolina league."

But Clive doesn't want to fuck her, not with his penis. Clive doesn't even feel like his penis is his. Some mornings he doesn't know how it got there. Clive wants to make love to Penny woman-2-woman style, like two lesbians in love. Well, maybe Penny is not gay, but there's a really good chance she's bi. And Clive feels like he is a woman, once you get past the penis and chest hair.

What's the Score?—Transgender Possibility #2

Never, ever assume that because a person wants to change sex, you can predict what orientation they'll want to be once they get there. In the first example, Clive wanted to become a heterosexual woman who wants to fuck straight men—second-base straight men, to be exact. She has no interest in sleeping with women. After all, she's not gay.

But in this new example, Clive wants to become a woman who is gay. He wants to change gender (become a woman), and the woman he wants to become is a lesbian, which is a change in sexual orientation, as well. Clive wants to have sex with Penny girl-to-girl, rubbing his girl breasts against hers, pushing his womanly lips against hers.

Clive to the Showers, It's Barbie the Batgirl's Turn

We just traded Clive. Now our transgendered attention is on Barbie the Batgirl.

Barbie is a woman of few words; maybe it's the chew; maybe it's the swagger. Some lazy evening, after the Blue Rocks have been swept in three, you can buy their manager a beer and maybe he'll tell you about the night when the Blue Rocks' top reliever tried to get fresh with Barbie. They had to air lift him to a hospital in Philadelphia.

Make no mistake about it, Barbie wants to have a penis, but not in her. Barbie wants a dick hanging from her. She just can't figure why it isn't there each time she tries to whip it out to pee. And she can't figure why she doesn't have big hairy balls to scratch like the other guys. She knows they're there, she just can't find them.

Believe it or not, Barbie has a thing for Penny the Pelicans' scorekeeper. But not as a woman to a woman. Barbie the Batgirl is not looking for some lesbian extravaganza. Barbie wants to fuck Penny like a man does a woman, or like they do in the minor leagues, anyway. Barbie wants to get her a little drunk, and then fuck her till the Avalanche comes to town.

To the very depths of her soul, Barbie the Batgirl is a boy. She and everyone else pretty much knows it. There's just that awkward problem that nature stuck the penis that Barbie wanted for herself on Clive. And Clive wishes he had been given Barbie's clit. That way, he could get off the way that feels right, by rubbing his clit instead of by stroking his penis.

Barbie wants to stroke her own penis to orgasm, while Clive wants to rub his own clitoris to orgasm. Being able to stroke instead of having to rub (or visa versa) can be a very real issue for someone who is transgendered. It's something those of us who aren't transgendered take for granted.

What's the score—Transgender Possibility #3.

"I've got it this time!" you say. "Barbie has the gender thing going on, and gender trumps orientation. So Barbie's best bet is to load up on as much juice as Bobby Bonds, get that manly muscle thing going, and become a man—a heterosexual man who wants to have sex with women." Barbie wants to fuck women as a man.

It's Your Turn to Bat—You Decide Transgender Possibility #4

So, you think you've got it. Before you look at the next page, take a guess at what happens if Barbie wants to change both gender and orientation.

In this case, Barbie the Batgirl becomes a man (changes gender), but becomes a gay man who wants to have sex with other gay men instead of with women. When an F2M woman becomes a homosexual male such as this, she becomes a he who is known as a *tranny-fag*.

Neither before nor after changing genders does Barbie have any desire to have sex with straight men. Sure, she could have had sex with men when she was still a woman, but look what happened to the ace reliever for the Blue Rocks. If Barbie wants to have intercourse with a guy, she wants to have it as a guy who's doing another guy.

Orientation vs. Gender Recap

Keep in mind that 99.9% of most human males, whether they are gay or straight, are just fine with their gender. They love being guys and they love having a penis and testicles. If they wanted any changes between their legs, it would be to have more and not less. Even the queeniest of bottoms who can't be fucked enough each day loves being a man and has no desire to be a woman. So gender has nothing to do with orientation, and orientation has nothing to do with gender. One is meat, and one is fish.

This doesn't mean that a guy might not occasionally wonder what it's like to be a woman during sex. If some men could, they would become a woman for a few days just to see what it was like to have sex. And some women would become men, e.g. a dick for a day, just to see what it's like.

And what about straight couples where the woman pegs the guy in the rear with a dildo or the toy of her choosing? Is this transgenderism? Yes, but it is a reminder that there are degrees. We're not talking about the kind of curiosity where they want to take special hormones, or have their penises snipped off; or their vulvas sewn up.

Gender Benders Who Want To Remain Factory-Equipped

While sex-reassignment surgery used to be at the top of many transgendered persons' Christmas lists, more and more people with genitals that don't match their sense of gender are leaving their genitals as nature formed them. Instead, they are changing the rest of their bodies to look like the gender they feel they are. Think of it as more of a change in packaging and format than hardware.

Some transgendered men want to look like women, act like women, and be women in every way except that they enjoy their penis and testicles. This person might be known as a she-male, or a pre-op who stopped after having top surgery, and not because she ran out of money. And some opt out of surgery because they understand just how little sensation surgically-constructed genitals have. You can look at pictures of them in sex books, especially the surgically created vulvas, and think, "Looks like the real thing." But they sure don't feel like the real thing. As for a surgically-created or "after-market" penis, some people in the transgendered world call it a "Frankendick" due to its lack of sensation. There are incredibly expensive surgeries where a nerve is moved from the arm to the newly created penis. The arm ends up looking pretty mangled, but some sensation can be felt in the penis.

One of the bigger problems with leaving your genitals intact is the law. In most cities, your gender and your crotch are one and the same, no matter how many hormones and cosmetic tortures you have endured. If you've still got a dick, you're a dude according to the law. If you still have a vulva, you are a girl. This can be a real problem when it comes to marriage, real estate, and medical and life insurance.

Odds'n'Ends on TS Theory

Based on records kept in the Netherlands in the early 1990s, one-in-12,000 biologically born males and one-in 30,500 biologically born females were taking hormones to alter or change their sex. Even if it were now three times as high, we're not talking about every third person in your high-school graduating class, although you might have had your doubts.

In the world of male-to-female transgenderism, there is a controversial but prominent theory that MtFs tend to fall into one of two groups—those who become women with a desire to have sex with straight men, and those who want to become women because they are in love with women's genitals and with the thought of being women.

The first group tend to have been effeminate males. As children, they probably played with dolls instead of trucks, and most were a source of angst for parents and teachers who felt that boys should be boys. Most identified as females from day one, and it would be unlikely that any would have been baseball players like Clive, even in the Carolina league. After they change from males to females, one of their greatest self-validations is when a totally straight guy is sexually attracted to them. It makes them feel like women. They usually don't seek out sex with gay males, as it would mean they weren't passing as women.

The second group identified as males from day one and tended to be more like regular guys when they were growing up. A lot dated and married women. The main clue that there was trouble in genderland is that lot of them were seriously into crossdressing. These men had a profound love for female genitals, so much so that the desire to have female genitals eventually became overwhelming. So when they became women, it wasn't because they wanted to be women who wanted to have sex with men. They became women because they love being women and being with women.

This, of course, can stir up a world of hurt among biologically-correct lesbians. Even if the former bio-boy's penis is at the bottom of a land fill, it can be a challenge for lesbians to stop viewing an MtF as anything other than a wolf in women's panties.

While this theory about the two camps of MtFs is widely accepted by some, others think it generalizes too much and doesn't capture their personal experience. Either way, transgenderism is complex. Very complex. Especially for the people whose sense of gender doesn't match the genitals they were born with.

Transsexuals Sometimes Can't Win for Losing.

Strange events bore strange alliances. For instance, there are a number of liberal academics who are upset by the way that transgendered persons sometimes behave like caricatures of ultra-feminine and ultra-masculine stereotypes. The academic-types have long argued that most of the divisions between males and females are socially constructed, yet they feel that transgendered persons are working overtime to reconstruct these divisions.

At the same time, there's nothing that will get the hackles up on a conservative fundamentalist more than a transgendered person. For them, transgenderism is an egregious assault on God's great plan that we all become breeders. They empathize even less with gender benders than they do with homosexuals, perhaps because of the extreme measures that many transgendered persons take to alter their God-given gender. There is at least hope that the demon will be exorcised from between the homosexual's legs and he or she will see the heterosexual light—not so after the surgeon has clipped your balls off or sewn up your vulva.

A She-Male & Her He-Male Client

Here is a she-male having sex with a married male client. The client identifies as being totally straight. The she-male is very attractive and might pass as a model. She has had breast implants and takes female hormones, but still has her bio-born penis and testicles. According to the she-male sex workers interviewed by researchers Joan & Dwight Dixon, all of their male clients are married. None appeared to be homosexual, nor did they see themselves that way.

These men are not interested in sex with a man. They aren't turned on by the fantasy of a homosexual experience. Nor did they show up to have sex with a woman. They are turned on by having sex with a she-male, in these cases, with an attractive-appearing woman who has a working cock. The sex these men have with the she-males ranges from wanting to suck the she-male's penis and being fucked by her, to a more traditional encounter where she gives him oral sex or he has anal intercourse with her.

Some clients tell themselves that because they are having sex with a woman, they are not gay. Other clients tell themselves because they are

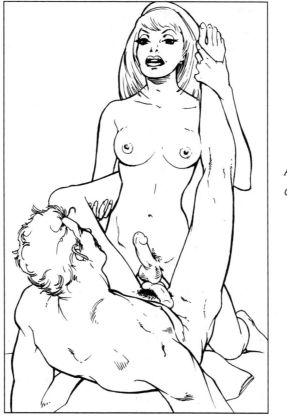

*A she-male
and her client*

having sex with a man, they are not being unfaithful to their wives. However, most clients are fully aware that they are having sex with a she-male because they are highly aroused by a woman who has a penis. They know that they are not with a traditional woman or a traditional man, but with a member of a third sex who they are physically and psychologically attracted to.

History shows that in other cultures at other times, she-males were highly prized, and men were not embarrassed to have sex with them. Today, even the transgendered community rejects them.

There are prostitutes who pretend to have an internal she-male persona, but who are faking it for the money. The Dixons, who have done the research, believe that a true she-male is a member of a third-sex, both inside and out.

One of the challenges for a she-male can be in getting her female hormone dose high enough to make her look and feel like a girl, but low enough so that her penis can still become erect.

Intersex is Different from Transgendered

Our society does "male" and "female" poorly enough, but imagine if you had to negotiate it when your genitals don't shout *PANTIES* or *BRIEFS?*

Intersex is a general term for a variety of conditions in which a person is born with a reproductive or sexual anatomy that doesn't seem to fit the typical definitions of female or male.

People who are intersex aren't to be confused with people who are transgendered. The transgendered are usually born with biologically-correct genitals—their issue is that the emotional self doesn't fit the physical self.

We have a separate chapter on intersex that is next.

Recommended books on Transgenderism:

Normal–Transsexual CEOs, Crossdressing Cops and Hermaphrodites with Attitude, by Amy Bloom, Vintage Books, New York (2002)

How Sex Changed–A History of Transsexualism in the United States, by Joanne Meyerowitz, Harvard University Press, (2002)

The Man Who Would Be Queen–The Science of Gender-Bending and Transsexualism, by J. Michael Bailey, National Academies Press (2003)

A Very Special Thanks to Alice Dreger, medical humanist and, conjointly, a very fine person, to Dr. Ray Blanchard, and to Joan and Dwight Dixon.

CHAPTER
37
Intersex

When we talk about your sex, we're talking about whether you are male or female. It's usually based on what's between your legs and what is in your chromosomes. The interesting thing about a person's sex is that we think of it as an either-or thing—pull down their pants, and either a penis or a vulva will be staring back at you. But that's a distinction people make, not nature.

Nature doesn't feel constricted by pink or blue, "It's a Boy!" or "It's a Girl!". Nature made the sexes on a continuum, with the vast majority of our bodies falling toward one end or the other. However, there are a number of people born with an intersex condition, where their genitals don't shout a simple "Puss!" or "Penis!"

Sometimes a person has an intersex condition where they look typically male or female on the outside, but inside there may be some blending of the parts we call male and female. What about the girl who is a high-school cheerleader and who feels 100% female? Every straight guy within 100 yards gets a stirring in his pants when she walks by. But she has what's called androgen insensitivity syndrome. She has XY chromosomes like most men do but a woman's brain and a woman's body. While her vulva looks like that of most other girls', her vagina isn't quite as deep as that of a woman who is XX and she doesn't have ovaries. Chances are, she won't learn about her AIS until she finally goes to see a gynecologist to find out why all her friends have started their periods but she hasn't. To say that she's in for a bit of a surprise is to put it mildly, but this doesn't change the fact that she's every bit as much a girl as any other female at her school.

Rolling Out Gender

Gender is what it means to be a man or a woman, and it usually lines up with what's in your pants. You know, masculinity and femininity.

Fortunately, some of the more confining gender role notions have been falling by the wayside: we no longer assume that a doctor is going to be male, or that a nurse is going to be female. We no longer assume that "the wife" does the cooking at home while a master chef in a restaurant is a man. We do, however, still assume that only male soldiers can be on the front lines during combat, which is based on our gender-role idea that only men's bodies should be shot at and blown up on the battlefield.

Born With It vs. Taught

Until not too long ago, psychologists assumed that we learned our gender roles as we were growing up, as opposed to biology having a strong influence. And since they believed our male and female gender roles were strictly learned, they were sure you could take a baby boy, remove his testicles, make his genitals look female, and raise him as a perfectly happy little girl who would never know the difference.

And that's what they did to a lot of children who were born with ambiguous genitals. You knew a kid had ambiguous genitals when there was a painfully long silence in the delivery room while the doctor said, "It's a..... uh.... hmmm.... Can I get back to you on that?" Then it would only be a matter of time before the doctors would strongly suggest to the parents that they raise the baby to be a Katie instead of a Kyle. That's because it was easier to cut the gonads out and remove anything else that looked like a penis, and then shoot the kid full of estrogen at puberty.

While that might have worked just fine for doctors and parents, they didn't bother to check in with Mother Nature. It turns out that our gender roles aren't as socially constructed as we thought they were. Sure, the part about girls being more helpless than guys and wanting sex less than men do—that's a big load of hooey. But whether you are sexually attracted to men or women, and whether you feel yourself to be a man or a woman—that's mostly determined by the time you are born. It's shaped by whether there was a big wave of androgens in the womb at a certain time during the pregnancy, and the impact that this wave of androgens had on your fetal brain.

So what we ended up with was a number of biological boys with ambiguous genitals who had been raised as girls, who never felt like girls. And once they started going through puberty, they particularly did not feel like girls. Ditto for bio girls who were raised as boys.

Today we know to leave well enough alone. While there will be social hurdles, kids with ambiguous genitals will probably do better if their genitals are left for them to decide what to do with. Their parents can raise them as boys or girls based on best guess, the way we were all raised. And if those kids decide to reshape their genitals later, that will be their choice. As we have discovered, only a very small percentage of intersex people who are raised this way go on to change gender or feel bi-gendered.

This is particularly important to know, now that there are so many chemicals called estrogen disruptors in the environment. These estrogen disruptors seem to do a number on the sexual development of the human fetus. We should probably brace ourselves for a lot more intersex babies in the future.

Teens and Young Adults with Intersex

The following thoughts for readers of *The Guide* are from William Reiner, MD, a professor of urology and psychiatry who works with children and teens who have intersex conditions:

"Often, teens with intersex conditions have been afraid of their sex organs, embarrassed by them, and they have had them examined by doctors far too many times. They tend to think that their sex organs make them freaks or weird. In fact, their sex organs are designed for pleasure just like anybody else's, even if theirs look a little different (typical penises and vaginas actually look a little bizarre anyway)."

"For teenagers in particular, how they feel about themselves and how they feel about their bodies can be very important to their happiness and sometimes even to their successes in relationships. Most typical teenagers have fears about being rejected by the person they are sexually attracted to. Teenagers with intersex conditions often have these same fears, but they may be far more than in other kids."

"Teenage boys and girls fall in love with a person (so do adults). They do not fall in love with penises or clitorises or vaginas. I try to help teenagers with intersex conditions learn how to talk about their sex organs to their lover, before they touch each other's genitals or try to have sexual intercourse. And I let them know that they must ask what makes their lover feel good. How else would you know? Sexual relations among teenagers, as among adults, is all about relating to the one you are in love with."

Intersex vs Transsexual

When your feelings of being a man or a woman don't line up with what's in your pants, you fall into the area that's called genderqueer or transsexual. The official medical term is Gender Dysphoric or GID (Gender Identity Disorder).

GID is usually very different from being intersex, given that people with gender dysphoria usually have typical genitals and the "right" chromosomes. There's nothing ambiguous about what's between their legs, and their factory equipment is just fine.

The gender issue for people with GID often seems due to how their brain was either feminized or masculinized while they were still in the womb. As a result, the big head above the shoulders may feel like that of a woman, but the head down below shouts "I'm a guy." Or, the head up above says "I'm a dude," while the vagina down below says, "Uh, we've got a bit of a disconnect going on here." Chapter 36: "Gender Benders" is entirely about that.

Highly Recommended: These are excellent and highly regarded resources:

"Intersex in the Age of Ethics" edited by Alice Dreger, University Publishing Group, 1999.

"Hermaphrodites and the Medical Invention of Sex" by Alice Dreger, Harvard University Press, 2000.

"Intersex and Identity: The Contested Self" by Sharon Preves, Rutgers University Press, 2003.

Sugar and Spice and All Things Nice to Alice Dreger, Ph.D., from Northwestern University, who was very helpful with this chapter, and a few puppy dog tails, too, for Bill Reiner M.D., Director, Psychosexual Development Clinic (Child and Adolescent), University of Oklahoma Health Sciences Center.

38

Sex & Breast, Brain & Ball Cancer

After seeing the title of this chapter, you are probably thinking, "Just the upper I've been wanting to read!" Actually, you might be surprised.

When we have sent questions about sex to cancer experts, their responses have been along the lines of, "People with cancer are more concerned about living than orgasms!" You would think we had walked into an AA meeting with a twelve-pack of *Anchor Steam*. So if you are wondering about the subject of sex and cancer, the following account of a 37-year-old reader with breast cancer might be helpful. The reader accounts that anchor this chapter tend to be long, but they contain tips and suggestions that are far better than what's in much of the professional literature.

> I hate cancer, hate having lost a breast. I went through a horrid jealous phase, envying other women their whole breasts, their health, their fertility (treatments put me into early menopause). But that's a draining response, so I don't dwell on it. Now, I just try to appreciate beauty when I see it.
>
> Treatments for cancer can cause discomfort, fatigue and intense pain. Still, it's possible to be sexual throughout treatment, just differently than before. Self-pleasure through masturbation is easiest because you set the pace. Try masturbating even if you have a partner because then you can guide them as to what feels best. I started with self-pleasure for sleep and pain relief a few days after surgery. Later, masturbating in front of my partner also helped be a turn-on at times when I didn't feel up to active sex.
>
> Relaxing with a bath set the stage, lighting a few candles in the bathroom for mood, then a warm tub filled with epsom salts to relieve aches and detox skin. I used lots of lube for self pleasure. I started this bath ritual about a week after surgery, keeping water away from the scar area and drainage tubes until healed.

I talked with my best friend about sex and body image. She said, "You know, no man has ever pursued us for our fabulous cleavage. We both have small breasts, so we are beautiful and desirable for other reasons," and then she gave this wonderful dirty chuckle.

Imagination helps create sexuality beyond what your body is actually capable of expressing at the moment. Erotic talk and guided fantasies help me meet my partner's sexual needs. Often, I put my head on his chest and cup his balls and tell erotic tales when I don't have energy to do more. He touches himself and is happy because we are close.

Tenderness is now more important to me than carnality. My former enjoyment of raw fucking just faded away. I think my partner misses the erotic she-beast who morphed into a cuddle-kitten.

During treatment, I started using light taps and code words to signal when I needed to move, stop or pull away due to pain or discomfort. My favorite position became the couvade, or twisting my pelvis to rest on one hip for side entry, legs sandwiched around his, and supported by lots of folded towels and an extra sheet. The extra towels served another purpose. Nausea and incontinence are common responses to chemo and radiation. Having the towels there to wrap around made me feel more confident about bed play.

Lube is hugely important. Drink extra water a few hours before sex. All mucous membranes (especially the mouth) get sore with chemo and radiation, so during treatment, I added plastic condoms, even for oral sex, to help prevent any infections while my immune system was down and out. Semen made my skin burn and get rashy, so I cleaned up fast. I learned that I liked not having a bush of pubic hair so I continue to trim it even after it started growing back. Being bare makes me more responsive.

Alcohol upset my stomach, but pot soothed my nausea and made me feel relaxed enough to be sexual. I think medical marijuana should be legal for cancer patients to help sexual healing and getting a groove on as well as combatting nausea.

Lace is itchy against the scars on my chest and under my arms where lymph nodes were removed. I won't wear underwire bras anymore because they are too constricting. But I do put on cute camisoles that are soft and stretchy enough to take off without tugging.

Sexual confidence comes and goes more readily. Sometimes, I don't like being exposed, and will drape a sheet over me during sex to cover my scars. My partner has to be patient with that. If I have a hot flash during sex, I'll ask for oral sex instead, so there is a lot of back-and-forth during sex. Continuing joint pain makes me move positions a lot, so I use small pillows and bolsters for support. Yoga helps with pain management, too.

Interestingly enough, I now get aroused through massage of my inner foot arches. It's nice to have discovered a new erogenous zone to take the place of lost nipple sensation. A foot massage is a sweet way to get started relaxing and wiggling around in my partner's lap; it's fun.

My lover is an amazing partner who helped me do all the hard stuff: shaving my head when my hair began to fall out, going with me to meet the doctors when I felt afraid, or offering a helping hand to steady me as I stepped into the tub or shower. I am lucky to have such love and care.

The following is from another reader who was diagnosed with breast cancer at a very young age:

I was diagnosed with breast cancer at the age of 31. My boyfriend asked me to marry him ten days after that. Knowing that he still loved me and wanted to marry me after hearing such devastating news was so incredible to me.

I elected to have a double mastectomy which was a scary thing to do because the thing that defines you the most about being a woman is your breasts. It was strange thinking that the thing that I had criticized the most about my body was now feeling like the most precious part of it. I immediately had reconstructive surgery after my double mastectomy so I never experienced life without breasts, but the ones I woke up with were made of silicone and had no nipples. My skin was ultra sensitive, and at first I didn't want to wear a shirt let alone be touched. After a few days I had no sensation in my breast area at all.

Before my surgery I had LOVED having my nipples played with and I used nipple clamps frequently. It was so devastating to lose such an important part of my sexuality to cancer. It was hard to imagine enjoying sex as much without my nipples and the sensations they had produced in my whole body – a tingle that goes from your head all the way to your toes. I felt so ugly and disfigured. I really couldn't fathom that my fiancé would even want to have sex with me. Proving to me yet again what a wonderful man he is, we ended up having sex just a few days after I was discharged from the hospital. It was one of the most therapeutic parts of my sexual healing. Just seeing the devilish sparkle in his eyes as he looked at me with so much love and longing warmed me from the inside out!

It's been almost two years since my surgery and I feel sexy despite my cancer and reconstructed breasts. My husband has continued to be turned on by me and we've found other areas of my body that are as sensitive (if not more sensitive) than my nipples used to be. It really goes to show that being sexy is more a mental attitude than a physical trait and that facing your fears about sex after such trauma can be a very positive experience."

Dating Someone Who Has Cancer

One of the things that's different about dating someone who has had cancer is that you are with someone who has had to fight hard to be alive. Outside of combat veterans, not a lot of us know what having to fight to stay alive is like, and how it changes your perspective on a lot of things that we ordinarily take for granted.

If you are dating someone who has had cancer, they will most likely want you to know as soon as possible. This is not for some perverse kind of bragging rights, but because they don't want to have to deal with starting a relationship only to find you suddenly bailing once you find out about the cancer. This is especially important to people who can no longer have kids because of the cancer treatment or who have surgical scars or other cancer-related challenges to cope with. We live in a society where even models and athletes can be wickedly self-conscious—imagine someone who's got scars or something missing.

Outside of the effects of chemotherapy and the invasiveness of treatment, there's nothing about cancer itself that makes a person want sex any less than anyone else does. In fact, the latest study on this subject expected to find that certain cancers or certain kinds of treatments would be correlated with having less sex a few years down the line, but the biggest factor turned out to be the quality of the person's relationship. No doubt, chemo was a bitch and took a toll, and missing certain key hormones can be a challenge, but at the end of the day it was the relationship that counted most when it came to having and enjoying sex.

Advice from Anne

Sex educator and cancer expert Anne Katz recently phoned with some thoughtful reminders for readers of *The Guide:*

 Medical students get about two hours of sex education, with most of it focusing on penis problems. It's easier for many oncologists to talk about dying than sex. You, the patient, will need to be the one to ask about sex.

 Lack of desire and lack of libido can be huge in cancer patients, but it's not only from having your body nuked or poisoned. Imagine what it is like for a patient with cancer in her pelvis to lay there with her legs wide apart and a bright beam of light shining on her anus or vulva while several strangers crowd around to administer treatment? In order to cope, she learns to go somewhere far, far away in her mind. It is not always easy to come back when it's time to have sex with a partner.

 Body image issues are immense—how do you tell a perspective mate you are missing a certain body part, or you have this large scar? When do you tell a date "I can't have children"?

 With childhood cancer survivors, their whole lives have been medicalized. Some can more easily tell you their white cell count than how they feel. Many often have to face lifelong screenings for secondary cancers.

Making Adjustments

One of the things that makes sex enjoyable is that it's fun. But when you hear the word cancer, "fun" is one of the last things you think about. So the job for a cancer patient and his or her partner after the diagnosis is how to make sex fun again. This you will both need to work on!

So let's get the bad news out of the way first. A healthcare provider named Peggy McKeal, Ph.D. LMHC, who has lots of experience with sex and cancer sums it up for us. While she talks about women with cancer, what she says applies just as much to men with cancer:

"Remember, women are often the family caretakers. Nothing is supposed to happen to them. And then they need time to deal with the treatments. Imagine surgery that yanks out organs that produce the hormones that help make you want sex. And then imagine having what you are told all your life is a huge part of your sexuality disfigured. Now let's go one step farther; imagine erogenous zones that aren't erogenous anymore. Nipples that are gone and a scar left; desensitized skin, or skin that feels uncomfortably odd.

"Abdomens that have a running scar and your tummy no longer sends rushes of desire when caressed, but feels numb right down into the mons pubis. Desensitized erogenous zones all over the body due to hormone loss. (That nibble on the neck no longer makes goose bumps.) Think about body image from weight gain that will absolutely not go away due to hormone loss and cancer treatments. Think about wanting to want to have sex, be sexual, but not being interested, unable to fantasize due to hormone loss. (Yeah, that actually happens.) And then imagine trying to, but not getting turned on, and when/if you orgasm it is an incredibly quiet whisper instead of a shout. Imagine damage done to your body by radiation that makes touch or penetration painful and provokes anxiety. There are solutions that help improve things. Silicone dilators, lubricants, vibrators, time, time, time, and compassionate understanding from a partner. There are hormones that can be replaced IF your cancer is not fed by estrogen. Women who have been diagnosed with cancer and undergone treatment may be experiencing all of these things, or only some. And they feel sad, guilty and angry. They want to want. A lover who is blissfully calm, understanding, nurturing and incredibly patient is a wonderful human being."

Okay, so you see what you are up against? You'll need to both explore and find new places where touch feels good. Reread the accounts of the women at the start of this chapter. That's exactly what they did. Look at how important love and sex has been to them. The question is how the two of you approach it, your patience, and your ability to make sex fun again.

Next, if you are boyfriend or husband, get yourself a copy of *Breast Cancer Husband*. In fact, the following suggestions are from Marc Silver's rock-solid and highly-recommended book *Breast Cancer Husband, How to Help Your Wife (and Yourself) Through Diagnosis, Treatment and Beyond*:

A husband is often concerned about flirting with his wife who has cancer, for fear she will think he is pressuring her for sex. But not flirting with her can easily become a signal that she isn't sexy anymore. His hesitancy to touch and play with her remaining breast if she had a mastectomy can also become a signal to her that she is no longer attractive to him. Or he might fear hurting her if she's got drainage bulbs hanging out of an incision following surgery.

She has breast cancer, not dementia. She knows her partner's sexual desire didn't suddenly melt away with the discovery of her cancer, and the chances are, hers didn't either. At some point, hopefully sooner than later, the two of you need to talk about sex. Get your signals straight that it's okay for him to pursue sex with her, and for her to pursue sex with him, and that it's okay for either of you to say "yes" or "no" without feeling uncomfortable about it.

Adjustments will need to be made in the way you have sex, but maybe that will be one of the hidden pluses in all of this. Maybe you'll start exploring new ways to enjoy sex with each other, in addition to the old. (You'll see that in the next section, where a guy with brain cancer and his partner use sex to feel closer in times of fear and distress.)

Radiation can do a number on the skin of a woman's chest. If it feels okay, it might be a nice way for the couple to keep physically connected for her partner to rub lotion on her chest a couple of times a day. (The same can be true with radiation in her pelvis. Rubbing her vulva and vagina with lube or an oil that her healthcare provider approves of can help with tissue that's lost its elasticity.)

For some women, chemo can make intercourse extremely painful. No matter how wet she might have gotten before, have a couple of different kinds of lube handy for when you start having intercourse (each has a different feel, which is why you should try a couple of different brands). Be sure to coat both the head of the penis as well as the insides of her vagina. Otherwise, if she has painful intercourse, it might start a nasty chain reaction where her vagina automatically tenses up whenever it senses an erect penis in the neighborhood. (Semen is actually somewhat corrosive on a good day. So don't hesitate to start using a condom if that helps.)

If you have access to a swimming pool, swimming-pool sex can be really nice. (As is mentioned elsewhere in *The Guide,* sex in water can actually end up being dry sex because the water can wash out a woman's natural lube. An excellent work-around is store-bought silicon-based sex lube or a vegetable oil. Coat your respective genitals with it before getting wet, so to speak.)

Sexy, short lingerie like a silk camisole or peignoir can help her feel less conscious about any missing chest real estate.

If she's receiving chemo and she feels like having sex (which might not be too likely) the man should probably wear a condom for the first day or two. That way, he won't risk getting a rash on his penis from any of the chemo that is in her vaginal lubrication. For the same reason, he should avoid giving her oral sex for the first couple of days after she receives chemo, unless he's got a tumor himself and you're doing couples' chemo.

Think about her physical state now compared to a few weeks before her diagnosis. If she's undergoing chemo and has had surgery, chances are she's bald and missing a big part of what Hugh Heffner tried to convince the world is the most sexy part of a woman's body. She may have scars that she didn't have and she isn't exactly feeling like she did when she was twenty and the tease of the town. While it would seem weird to her if you didn't acknowledge the new realities, this is also no time to hide your sexual desire for her. And if she's way too tired from chemo to even think about sex, ask if she'd like a foot rub or if she'd like you to massage her fingers.

If you end up going for months when she doesn't want sex and you've been masturbating a lot, still try to keep a physical and sensual connection. This will make it easier to reconnect sexually when the effects of the chemo and/or radiation are starting to fade.

One of the biggest casualties to breast cancer can be romance. It's hard to be romantic when so many new and mostly unwelcome things are suddenly intruding on your lives. Keep in mind that if you put romance on hold during the worst of your cancer saga, you'll need to rekindle it as soon as you and she are able.

 Life can have its unfortunate contradictions. One woman who loves her pubic hair might lose it all during cancer treatments, while another who goes through the hassle of shaving herself bare every day won't lose any of it!

When there is sexual desire but little energy, think about ways to make adjustments. For instance, what if you find a comfortable position where he can have his penis inside of her vagina without thrusting while she uses a vibrator? He might then need to masturbate after she's had an orgasm, but you still get the sexual and physical intimacy without her needing to expend much energy.

If a woman is feeling bad about the way she looks and particularly unsexy, she should try not to assume that this is how her partner feels about her. And he should know that even if he still finds her to be sexually desirable, she might be so turned-off by her current condition that she assumes he is as well. This is one more example of just how important it is to talk to each other about sex.

If her vagina is too tender to handle but a minute or so of intercourse, she can get him close to coming with oral sex or by hand, or he can jerk himself off until he's just about to come, and then they start intercourse. Also, a finger on or in his anus during intercourse might help him to come sooner.

You might need to change your thrusting depth and rhythm during intercourse. Experiment and give each other a lot of feedback.

Birth control is a must for any woman who is not past menopause. Check with your physician(s), as they probably won't want you using hormonal methods.

Squeezing your breasts, sexual touching, and sexual activity will not spread cancer or impact your recovery in a negative way! Having orgasms does not alter or negatively impact your estrogen balance. Being wet sexually and having orgasms are just as good for you during and after cancer treatment as before.

From a Young Couple

We recently received an email from a young woman whose boyfriend has brain cancer. He's 20, and she's not yet. He's had multiple brain surgeries, radiation, and now chemo.

Because of his nausea and problems with stamina, she's on top during intercourse more than before. And some of the things he used to love her to do before his cancer can make him feel nauseated now. But she says as long as they give each other lots of feedback, they still enjoy sex, which shows that you can cut into a person's brain, nuke it and poison it—it won't necessarily stop them from wanting sex. In this case, his orgasms help him to feel better after chemo, assuming he's able.

She says, "Sometimes we have sex just to feel closer in a hard time like after we heard he was going to need a second surgery. It's comforting to be that close to the person you love and know that nothing is going to happen to them right then, even if outside of those moments you are living in constant fear. Sex has shifted to being almost totally focused on what feels best for him and I wouldn't have it any other way."

She didn't mention anything about her own emotional journey, but it's worth noting that modern medicine is, by necessity, so focused on the person with the cancer that we sometimes forget that his or her lover can be suffering just as much. The lover may feel way too guilty to even allow themselves to be conscious of how much emotional pain they are in. (This is a reminder to healthcare professionals, who are sometimes pretty overwhelmed themselves.) As for the details of how this couple approach sex and cancer, here it is in her own words:

"We ended up trying me on top more because he didn't have to move as much and it can be less physically trying for him. He has less stamina so it's nice for him to be able to have sex without ending up completely exhausted. I was tentatively afraid that I would cripple him if I were on top, but it turned out to be a very successful position. He actually likes it best out of all the positions we've tried.

"Communication has turned out to be key because he has sudden nausea or pain sometimes, but if sex is done correctly (with proper communication and being cautious not to over-do it) it can actually make him feel better. Sometimes we start but he needs to rest and then we keep going in a few minutes. He lets me know if something I'm doing is good or if it's making him feel worse because some of the things we did before aren't good anymore (for instance I used to kiss him on the stomach and back and he used to love it but now it can make him nauseated.) Sometimes things like that feel good and sometimes they don't.

"He has good days where he we can try different positions and places and bad days where we stick to me on top and we have intercourse in kind of a soft, relaxed setting. We discuss what he would like to do that day before we even start any foreplay and then he tells me if he's changed his mind anytime after that based on how he's feeling. That way we almost always avoid nausea, and intercourse can be great even with restrictions.

"During his chemotherapy, sometimes he has close to no sex drive and then we don't do much at all sexually, but he'll still do things like finger me just pretty much to be nice, since he's not so much up to anything sexual.

"I'd say if anything has increased it would be the number of blowjobs I give him because that's another thing that gives him pleasure but lets him remain pretty much still and comfortable. We don't have as much intercourse because he's just not up to it all the time."

Cancer of the Testicles

Please see the chapter "Balls, Balls, Balls" for a discussion on the nuts and bolts of cancer of the testicles.

The people who worry most about their sexual appeal after cancer of the testicles tend to be younger straight guys, as well as gay males. Hopefully, the gay males won't put up with a partner for whom only one ball would be a deal breakers. As for the straight guys, we hate to burst your bubble, but based on how women have described the scrotum when we asked them about it on our sex survey, it's hard to think that they are going to dump any guy because he's one nut short of a full load. Seriously, there aren't too many women who sit around fantasizing about men's balls or scrotums. So if you are the girlfriend or wife of a guy who's just been diagnosed, please let him know that it's unlikely you'd even notice 99.9% of the time.

Unlike other male cancers, it's a rare day when a man with cancer of the testicles won't be able to get an erection after surgery. His equipment will work just fine and he'll have the same wad he had before. Believe it or not, a lot of guys who have lost a ball to cancer don't have it replaced with a fake one, and are quite happy with their decision.

As for the psychological aspects of any and all things regarding cancer of the testicles, we defer to a man who knows a bit about it from firsthand experience, Mr. Doug Bank of the amazing Testicular Cancer Resource Center: http://tcrc.acor.org:

"I would like to stress that testicular cancer is not contagious and it cannot be transmitted via sexual intercourse. There are a lot of reasons to be afraid of cancer, but this is not one of them."

"Regarding sex drive, testicular-cancer survivors we have spoken with have told me everything from having sex the day after their surgery (ouch!) all the way through having to go on hormonal therapies to re-establish their desire—which would only be the 2% to 3% of guys who lose both testicles. In those cases, supplemental testosterone takes care of everything. The desire is still there and the ejaculation is still there.

"Just as each one of us is different going in, we're going to be just as different coming out, too. If you feel different, or just out of whack, let your doctor know. They cannot read your mind, and they definitely cannot diagnose anything if you do not tell them that something is wrong!"

Other Cancers

This chapter mostly focused on three of the B cancers—breast, brain and balls. Hopefully you won't feel left out if you have one of the other cancers. We tried to make this chapter helpful regardless.

Highly Recommended: *Breast Cancer Husband, How to Help Your Wife (and Yourself) Through Diagnosis, Treatment and Beyond* by Marc Silver, Rodale Books (2004). If your partner has breast cancer, GET THIS BOOK!

Ann Katz has written a book on sex and cancer for healthcare providers. The title is *Breaking the Silence on Cancer and Sexuality* from the Oncology Nursing Society (2007).

For a very helpful explanation of how to help your vagina after chemo or radiation, see *Vaginal Recuperation after Cancer or Surgery*, on the website of A Woman's Touch: www.a-womans-touch.com

CHAPTER

39
Bashful Bladder

Finding the right home for this unusual subject was such a struggle that we decided to provide it with its own separate chapter! It didn't fit in with the chapter on sex fluids, or with sex at all. But if you struggle with being pee shy, you will be relieved by the discussion that follows.

Being Unable to Pee in Public

You wouldn't believe the number of people who have trouble using public rest rooms, and not because they don't like the smell or hygiene issues. Being unable to relieve yourself in a public rest room is a very real problem that can be extremely limiting.

Being pee-shy can get in the way taking a urinalysis at work or for a job interview. It's a problem any time you need to pee on demand, like at the doctor's office for a physical exam. People with this problem can even find it a challenge to urinate in a private bathroom while at a friend's home or when at a party.

We recently heard from a college student who was worried because he had enlisted in the Marine Corps and was soon going to ship out for basic training. He would sometimes walk up three flights of stairs in his college dorm to find an empty bathroom where he could pee. He had no idea how he was going to manage in basic training, where there would be next to no privacy at all.

This problem is called paruresis or bashful bladder syndrome. For readers who don't have a bashful bladder, imagine what it's like never being able to pee while you are at a concert, baseball game, or when dining at a restaurant. Imagine what it's like when you seriously need to relieve yourself and your bladder freezes up whenever someone walks into the rest room.

For millions of Americans, this happens each and every time they try to urinate when they are not in their own home. The only safe place they can go for vacation is to the beach. Or maybe someone else's swimming pool.

Paruresis comes in different degrees: some people who have it can pee in a public rest room as long as they are in a closed stall. Others are unable to go in a rest room if anyone else is there, and some can't urinate at all if they are anywhere but home. They won't even try to enter a crowded rest room after a movie, between classes, or during an intermission at a large event.

You might have the idea that this is a wimp's disorder, e.g. "A real man could just whip it out and pee." But plenty of guys who have this problem are tough enough to take on any and all comers. They have no shortcomings with women or sex, and are in high demand on both scores. Not only is it impossible for them to go in a public bathroom, but some need to sit when they urinate at home for fear the stream will make noise and someone will know they are peeing. This is in stark contrast to the independent and able men who they are in other parts of their lives.

The problem often starts before adolescence. Some people with shy-bladder problems can remember back to a specific event that triggered the anxiety. For instance, a kid having to use a group urinal in a football stadium with a bunch of grown men who are standing around him peeing out two quarters' worth of beer. For others, the causes can be more unconscious.

Far more men have shy-bladder syndrome than women, but few women are asked to urinate next to each other without being in an enclosed stall. Guys are expected to go where other guys can watch, casually discussing the weather with each other while whipping it out and doing their business.

The problem can be severe enough that some people need to carry a catheter in order to relieve themselves. But the best way to deal with the problem is with desensitization techniques. For most people, these exercises can provide a decrease in the severity of their bashful-bladder problem. These exercises are described in an excellent book which is recommended below.

HIGHLY RECOMMENDED: "Shy Bladder Syndrome—Your Step-By-Step Guide to Overcoming Paruresis" by Soifer, Zgourides, Himle and Pickering, New Harbinger (2001). Also try visiting their excellent website at: www.paruresis.org This website provides a bladder-stretching list of articles and help.

40
Sex & Diabetes

You're not going to believe this, but nowhere on the website of the American Diabetic Association do they discuss whether swallowing when giving a guy oral sex impacts your blood sugar level, or if diabetic girls taste sweeter. At least they were kind enough to intimate that nobody's diabetic penis is going to get gangrene, although you might hold off on wearing a cock ring. Decreased circulation and numbness can be a problem with diabetes, and why risk making it worse?

As for aerobic activity, just about anyone who has ever done a finger stick knows about the importance of exercise. Exercise increases the number of insulin receptors in your cells. This can help your insulin work better and make your diabetes easier to manage. Fortunately, there's no rule that says exercise can't be done while you are naked at home with your sweetheart rather than at a gym. Like with any exercise, check your BG and have a snack if needed.

Unfortunately, exercise that's sexercise needs a diabetic caveat or two. For instance, one reader had a nasty experience while performing oral sex on her boyfriend. It was her first time, so she assumed the funny feeling she was having was from being nervous. She was kneeling over the boy when she fainted from low blood sugar, almost choking on his penis. At least she thinks the culprit was low blood sugar.

Checking your blood sugar before, during and after sex is the last thing anyone feels like doing. But until you understand your body's reactions while making love, especially with a new partner, taking frequent readings is the only way you will learn. Also keep in mind that the emotional part of being with a new partner can add to the blood-sugar lowering potential.

You will want to learn about your body's reactions in the minutes and hours after sex. The muscles in a horny pelvis eat up extra glucose, especially when it's been rocking back and forth. And hormones like adrenaline, noradrenaline and prolactin are released during orgasm. They can change your blood sugar, sometimes dramatically.

A healthcare provider or diabetes educator can help you with lovemaking-management strategies. Should you adjust your insulin downward? Is it a good idea to inject yourself in the abdomen instead of your thigh before a love-making marathon, or does the bunny-like thrusting of hips cancel any slow-down in the insulin-absorption rate that you might hope to gain? Should you eat something other than your partner before, during or after having sex?

Since high blood sugar and ketones are best managed by drinking lots of water and exercise, highly-aerobic sex might be just what the doctor ordered. And peak insulin times simply require a food snack before your sex snack.

It is also essential to educate your partner about diabetes, and how he or she can recognize your hypoglycemic episodes and other possible problems. They need to know how to be in charge when you aren't, and what to do. It will be much harder to explain after the fact. Since most diabetics feel good as new in a few minutes to a few hours, it won't be long after treating a low when you and your partner will be back in the saddle.

Here are a few of many other sex-matters to consider:

💡Safe sex for diabetics includes keeping a pack of Lifesavers or glucose tablets next to the condoms and lube.

💡Women should watch out for blood-sugar weirdness a few days before and after their periods. If you can find any menstrual-related patterns, make adjustments in your diet, exercise, insulin, and sexual robustness.

💡High glucose in the blood means that more glucose is available in the urine. This can trigger an infection. Plenty of women discovered they were diabetic as a result of recurrent urinary-tract infections. If you get yeast infections, avoid lubes with glycerin.

💡Sugar binges from marijuana munchies can be a problem, although some people claim that marijuana helps even out their blood sugar. There aren't any studies on this, so please discuss it with your endocrinologist. Ecstasy can make you think you have boundless energy when your body is on its way to a blood-sugar low, and people on Ecstasy tend to drink lots of water, which lowers BGL. Problems from alcohol are the most dangerous of all. Alcohol raises BGL and can also result in dehydration. Alcohol-related lows usually come from being too polluted to eat or to remember to eat. When you have been partying, others around you will assume that any unusual behavior is from being drunk or stoned. You might not get the help you need. Be sure that friends you party with know what to do, although their responses might not be 100%, either.

💡Decreased vaginal lubrication and erection problems are common side effects of diabetes, especially in sex-crazed seniors. These problems can be due to an interruption in nervous-system feedback, problems in circulation, or a combination of both. Store-bought lube without glycerin is a great equalizer for women, and Viagra-like medications are helpful for many males. Even if they aren't, this Guide is full of suggestions for pleasing your partner without needing to have an erection. If you do take erection medicine, don't get it over the Internet. Be sure to consult with your healthcare professional, and get a prescription from him or her.

💡Peeing before and after sex can help reduce urinary-tract infections. If you are a female diabetic who gets frequent urinary-tract infections, consider shacking up with a partner who is into golden showers. Going on your guy will be killing two birds with one stone, or stream, although women who are kinky and infection prone should only be the doers and not the receivers of the golden stream.

💡Be sure to wear a medical ID bracelet or tag, and if you're a man who cruises the parks or trails, you might put an extra tag on the waistband in the front of your briefs where it's more likely to be seen.

💡If you can't live without getting your love parts pierced, the chances of getting an infection are higher when your blood glucose levels (BGLs) are elevated. Infections will increase the scarring around piercing sites and they will make your BGLs shoot even higher. Get thee to a health-care provider at the slightest indication of an infection. Also, tongue piercings will make your tongue swollen and sore, which will inspire you to skip meals, which can lead to a hypoglycemic episode.

💡We hate to mention the following little nastiness, and hope it applies to no readers of *The Guide*. But rumor has it that some girls will skip their insulin in order to keep their BGLs high. This results in decreased appetite. This kind of "weight-loss program" is dangerous and dumb.

As for inspiration, one of the founders of sex therapy had diabetes for most of his life. Management had been so difficult that he has to inject himself twice a day. His name was Albert Ellis and he recently died at the age of 93. He said that while staying on top of his diabetes had always been a pain, the bigger pain was if he didn't. Ellis had been quite the sex radical during his 93 years, and he was even a fan of *The Guide*. Out of the blue, he sent a very kind e-mail saying it was one of the best sex books he had ever read. Imagine that, still reading and writing sex books when you are in your 90s!

Diabetes doesn't mean you can't be as good or bad as anyone else in bed. As with everything else in life, it just means that you've got to plan ahead and jump through a few more hoops.

A Special Thanks to Ricky Siegel, a sex educator, therapist, and member of Planned Parenthood, and to Barry McCarthy, an author and leader in sex education who also has diabetes. Also, to Bill Taverner, for putting the word out!

41

Sex When You Are
Horny & Disabled

A story appeared on the Internet about a 22-year-old man with cerebral palsy who has virtually no control over his body's movements. He started using his wheelchair antisocially, as a ramming device. He was running over anything he could. Eventually, this young man wrote on his word-board that he was so horny he couldn't stand it anymore. Although his body has the same sexual urges and desires as an able-bodied 22-year-old, he has no ability to walk, talk or masturbate like the average 22-year-old. He can't even download porn or surf adult websites.

As quickly as they began, this young man's wheelchair tantrums stopped. The reason? A nurse's aide mercifully began giving him handjobs. But then she was caught and fired instantly. The board-and-care home threatened to file a complaint against her for sexual abuse.

Sexy & Disabled?

If you think you are fair-minded about sexual matters, consider a quadriplegic who wheels by in an electric wheelchair. The person drools a little and steers the chair with a joy stick that's strapped to his forehead. Do you think of this person as being sexual? Do you think he has the same sexual needs and desires as you? Chances are you'd wonder how good his jump shot is before you'd think of him as being just as horny as you are.

Many people not only disapprove of sex for the severely disabled, but find the concept offensive. They might even feel that we need to protect people who are disabled from sex.

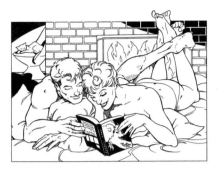

Dear Paul,

I'm a paraplegic. From where I sit, I have women's rears and crotches in my face all day long. You have no idea how much restraint it takes to keep my hands to myself. Last week I copped a feel but apologized and blamed it on my "bad driving" and "spastic hand."

Dude from Dubuque

Dude,

There's not an able-bodied guy on the planet who could come face-to-tail with as much anatomy as you do and not want to reach out and touch some. You must consider a crowded elevator to be a gift from God, as well as one of life's great torments. **Counterpoint** I recently received a letter regarding my response to Dude because I didn't chastise him for his inappropriate actions. "I am really disappointed that you suggest in your response that a man couldn't be expected to withhold his sexual desire and that it's fine to occasionally use a woman's body for your own purpose."

One reason why so many of us blanch at the idea of a disabled person having sex is because the advertising industry spends billions of dollars each year trying to narrow our concept of what sexual attractiveness is. Never do advertisers tell us that sexual appeal might have something to do with integrity and character, given how those can't be paid for with a credit card. Forget even existing sexually if you are missing a few fingers or an entire leg, slur your words when you talk or are paralyzed from the chest down.

A huge hurdle for many disabled people is being able to accept themselves as being sexual. If you don't accept yourself as being a sexual person, it is unlikely that others will.

Roll Models

"Prior to my becoming blind, the only person who was blind that I had seen was a beggar. I was horrified to think that this was the only option available to me as a person who was blind." From an article on women who are blind by Ellen Rubin in *Sexuality and Disability*, 15(1), 1997.

One of the more discouraging aspects of having a disability is that positive role models are few and far between. If you ask people to name a famous

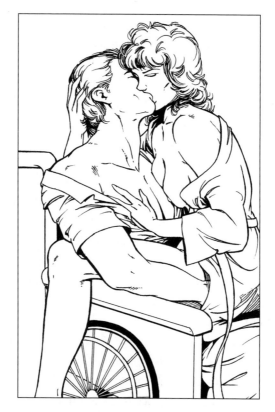

disabled person, just as many will say the Hunchback of Notre Dame as Frank-lin Delano Roosevelt. Of the two, FDR was a real-life American president who provided people with a real sense of sanctuary, although he was unable to walk unaided. There were reasons why FDR tried to hide his disability. When he was a young man, disabled people were considered a success if they could get a job in the circus.

Different Ways That Disabilities Happen

When people are disabled from crashes and accidents, it is often because the spinal cord was damaged. About 85% of spinal-cord injuries happen to men, many in their teens and twenties. That's because men have a penchant for doing things that involve speed or collisions. For instance, if a boy says he needs "pads," you might assume he's talking about something to put under his football jersey. If a girl says she needs "pads," it's likely that she's referring to sanitary napkins or something to stuff into her bra. In addition to sports and car crashes, disabilities might come from gun wounds, stabbings, fist-fights or a serious bonk on the head.

Diseases that cause disabilities include arthritis, which can make intercourse painful or cripple your fingers so much that you can't masturbate. Polio can make it nearly impossible to walk or breathe and can result in problems later in life (post-polio syndrome). Diabetes can hamper an erection or vaginal engorgement, but usually not orgasm. Multiple sclerosis can be mild and manageable or severe and debilitating. Cancer and the treatments for it can impact a person's ability and desire to have sex.

There are many genetic or congenital disorders that can cause disabilities. Certain chromosome disorders can damage a person's physical growth and/or mental development. Congenital disorders might result in dwarfism or being top-shelf challenged. (There's a recent TV series that follows a family with dwarfism who seem just as "normal" as their tall neighbors.) Medications taken during pregnancy can result in the birth of infants with severe disabilities. Parental exposure to pollutants and chemicals can cause birth defects. Disabilities can also result from strokes and heart attacks or cerebral palsy and muscular dystrophy.

Spinal-Cord Injury (SCI) Shorthand When people with spinal-cord injuries are talking to other people with spinal-cord injuries, they sometimes use a shorthand such as "I'm a C-4 quad" or "I'm a T-3." This code refers to the location on the spine where the injury occurred. For instance, a C-4 injury occurs higher up on the spinal cord (in the neck) than a T-3, so it is likely that a person with a C-4 is paralyzed from the shoulders down (quadriplegic), whereas a T-3 has the use of his or her arms (paraplegic), and an L-4 most likely has more use than a C-4 or T-3 because the injury happened at a point on the spinal cord between the ribs and pelvis. Another factor is whether the injury was complete or incomplete, with the latter supposedly being less severe.

Quad Note Thanks to Tom Street for this info. Tom is a C-4 quad from an auto accident in 1988. Tom manufactures a computer mouse for quadriplegics called the QuadJoy. This special mouse, combined with extra software that Tom has written, allows the user to run the entire computer, including keyboard, by mouth. The full range of clicking and dragging happens by virtue of puffing and sucking on the end of the joystick. This can be particularly helpful for a quad who would like to interact with others in chat rooms or who would like to see Internet porn in PRIVATE and without the help of an attendant. Tom can be reached on the internet at www.quadjoy.com.

Chronic vs. Acute

There are disabilities that happen all at once. They don't keep getting worse. This is true of most spinal-cord injuries. There are other disabilities, usually caused by diseases, which have symptoms that worsen over time.

For some people, it is easier to have a disability that starts off worse but stays the same. For instance, once people with spinal-cord injuries are able to learn how to deal with their disability, they can be pretty sure that their condition won't worsen and they won't have to learn a whole new set of skills just to stay even. People with chronic illnesses have a more uncertain future and may have to constantly readapt as their illness progresses. The uncertainty of a chronic illness makes it more difficult to get on with your life, as you never know when your disease is going to pull the rug out from under you. Of course, you can say that none of us has any guarantees for the future, but the uncertainty of everyday life is much easier to cope with than the uncertainty of a disease that is getting worse.

Even the recovery process is different for someone with an acute injury as opposed to a chronic illness. Consider a person who had his leg amputated after being run over in the parking lot at the 7-Eleven as opposed to having a leg amputated due to complications from diabetes. Outside of not getting to finish his Slurpee, the person who lost his leg at the 7-Eleven had no pre-existing condition and must face only the problems associated with the amputation. The person with progressive diabetes has to cope with numerous problems caused by the diabetes in addition to those that are specific to the amputation. Mind you, neither situation is enviable.

Also, the treatments for disabilities or illnesses can cause sexual problems. For instance, tricyclic antidepressants are often prescribed to help with the neurogenic pain that can occur after spinal-cord injury. These drugs can decrease the desire to have sex as well as the ability to have an erection and to ejaculate. The same is true for certain cancer treatments that adversely affect the sexuality of both men and women. (See the chapter on sex & cancer.)

Double Your Trouble

As if it weren't bad enough to have your spinal cord injured, accidents that cause the damage are often severe enough to also cause traumatic head injury. Not only does the person have to cope with possible paralysis from the spinal injury, but he or she may also experience low sexual drive, poor impulse control or unpredictable behavior from the brain injury.

Can Men in Wheelchairs Get Hard-Ons?

People sometimes wonder if guys in wheelchairs can get hard-ons, but they don't wonder if women in wheelchairs can get wet! Why's that? Contrary to what you might think, a lot of males who are in wheelchairs are able to get erections. The stimulation for the erection will often need to come from direct physical contact with the genitals rather than from feeling horny, as the link between the horny center in the brain and the genitals is often damaged. Guys with disabilities can often get good erections with the help of vacuum pumps or injections. Men with higher-level spinal-cord injuries (usually quads, not paraplegics) tend to get reflex erections. These happen when the penis is being touched and have little connection to feeling horny. They usually go down as soon as the touching stops, but some couples learn how to keep the stimulation going so they can have intercourse.

Able-bodied men often become aware of their own sexual arousal by feeling their penis grow. Men who are paralyzed have to rely on other signals to know when they are aroused, e.g. nipples getting hard, goosebumps, heavier breathing and a heart that beats faster. These aren't any different from what able-bodied men experience, but how many guys notice subtle physical clues when their dicks are screaming, "Look at Me!"

Women with spinal-cord injuries may find that the sexual wetness in their vagina is decreased or absent. Using a lubricant during intercourse can be helpful. Many women with spinal-cord injuries are able to have orgasms. Bregman and Hadley (1976) interviewed a number of women with spinal-cord injuries and found that their descriptions of orgasm were similar to those of women with no spinal-cord injury. Also, some people with spinal-cord injury have orgasms that are referred to as "para-orgasms," which are different from genital orgasms but are quite compelling. Para-orgasms can be so strong that women who are injured above the T-6 level need to be aware of rapid changes in their blood pressure.

Both women and men who no longer have traditional orgasms can learn to experience a type of orgasm that is called an emotional orgasm. This kind of orgasm results in a rush of relaxation and calm in the rest of the body that's like the afterglow of an orgasm.

Whether a person can or can't have an orgasm, the good feelings that most able-bodied people get from being touched and loved are still massively satisfying for someone who is disabled. One person with a spinal-cord injury reported, "Before my accident I couldn't get enough stimulation from the waist down; now I can't get enough from the waist up!" When a person is paralyzed, areas such as the back of the neck and arms can become extremely sensitive in a sexual way. Also, plenty of disabled people report that watching a partner doing something sexual to them can be very satisfying even if they can't feel the actual sensations. The brain is able to fill in the missing pieces.

Vibrator Note Vibrators can be a helpful sexual aid for men and women with disabilities. They can supply the necessary stimulation when a hand is unable. If you tend to be incontinent, consider getting a vibrator that's rechargeable or has batteries. Urine is a far better conductor of electricity than water, making plug-in models a wee bit risky. If your hands are too crippled to use a regular vibrator, it's possible to embed one in a Nerf ball.

"Will I Be Able to Have Children?"

This seems like a simple, straightforward question. But it is often an indirect way of asking, "Will I be able to have sex?" "Will anyone want to have sex with me?" "How in the blazes do I have sex now that I'm like this?" The answer to all of these questions is usually yes, unless the person stays in a full-time funk and never transitions out of asking "Why me?" Try as they might, nobody but God or nature has an answer to the "Why me?" question, assuming there is an answer.

Most women with disabilities are able to become pregnant. This is why most disabled women need to use birth control, even if they are paralyzed from the shoulders down. Many men who are paralyzed have problems ejaculating. Physicians are having some success helping these men to ejaculate by sticking electrodes up their rears and shocking the crap out of nerves in the prostate region. Some guys with spinal-cord injuries above T-12 are able to ejaculate with the help of a vibrator on the penis.

Born with It vs. Got It Along the Way

Unless they are in a rock'n'roll band, most people who make it to adulthood have achieved a certain level of maturity. But if a person was disabled at a young age, it's possible that this has gotten in the way of achieving the maturity to behave as a responsible and caring adult. For instance, how does a kid who is disabled at age 16 progress through the usual steps toward independence if he or she needs a parent to get them out of bed and dressed each morning? If in a rehab center, how does he or she get the privacy to explore sexually as other kids do? How do they masturbate with crippled hands?

Consider the following questions posed by a therapist who works with the disabled: "How does a young girl in a wheelchair learn how adults are sexual if her parents are afraid to be that way in front of her? How does she explore her parents' drawers when they are out and find books, movies, condoms, sponges, lingerie and so forth—as many youths do—if she cannot get into their bedroom? How can she find her brother's copies of sexually explicit publications if she cannot get under his bed where they are stashed?" [From "Performing a Sexual Evaluation on the Person With Disability or Illness" by Kenneth A. Lefebre in *Sexual Function in People with Disability and Chronic Illness*, Marca Sipski and Craig Alexander, Aspen Publishers, (1997).]

People who are disabled at a young age will become adults with the same sexual drives and desires as anyone who is not disabled. However, they may be missing a sense of appropriate ways to satisfy their sexual urges. To help fill in the missing pieces, parents and educators of disabled kids need to be more open rather than less about sexual issues.

Sex & People Who Are Developmentally Disabled

It is not likely that people who are developmentally disabled will be reading this book, although we know of one such woman by the name of Linda who loves looking at the pictures! People with developmental disabilities have the same sexual urges and desires as people without disabilities. They simply go through the stages of sexual development at a slower pace.

The developmentally disabled pose special problems when it comes to sexual training, because they may need a good deal of repetitive explanation about things that many adults feel uncomfortable saying even once. Also, in their drive toward sexual pleasure, developmentally disabled kids may be even less apt to use birth control than their nondisabled partners in crime.

If you are the parent of a disabled child, or you work with people who are disabled, you might be at a loss for finding good references to help you in dealing with your child's sexual growth. One book that might be helpful is *Doubly Silenced: Sexuality, Sexual Abuse and People with Developmental Disabilities* by Patricia Patterson. Also, *Sexuality: Your Sons and Daughters With Intellectual*

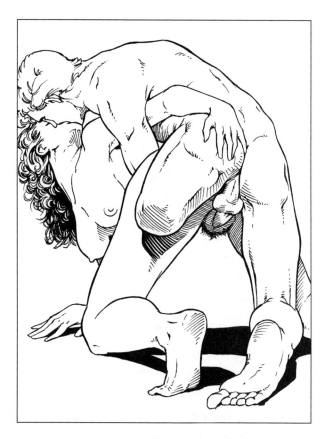

Disabilities by Schwier, Melberg and Hingsburger, Paul H. Brookes Publishing Company, (2000). The Paul H. Brookes catalogue has a number of excellent books on disability.

Body Image

If a person has been disabled for a long time, particularly from a young age, his body image might also include a wheelchair or braces, scars from surgeries, hands that are twisted and not particularly dexterous, a voice that slurs words, a head that doesn't sit straight on its shoulders or other features that aren't always like those of his or her peers. It may be very difficult for a person who is disabled to feel attractive and effective if they can't see themselves as separate from the devices that help them to survive. As a result, they might need plenty of feedback that you value them as a person in the same way that you do someone who doesn't have a wheelchair, braces or disfigurements.

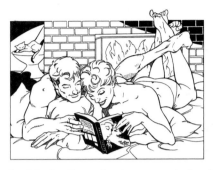

Dear Paul,

We both have spinal-cord injuries and are disabled. Yet we like watching porn that shows able-bodied people having sex. Is this weird?

Rhonda from Rolling Hills

Dear Rhonda,

None of us here have nine-inch penises, last forty-five minutes, come in buckets or have partners who like taking it ten different ways, but we like watching pornography, too. If most of it weren't so boring, we'd watch it more often! Keep in mind that pornography is a fantasy. It helps us go places in our minds where many of us wouldn't go in reality even if we could. Now here's a question for you: I'll bet you aren't worried about watching able-bodied actors in TV or movies, so why when it comes to porn do you suddenly worry about being crippledly correct?

Explaining Yourself & Educating Others

"People do have all these kinds of curiosity, and you have to find ways of making them feel more comfortable around you at first."

Steve, on the videotape *Sexuality Reborn*

Just like people who are able-bodied, people who are disabled need to learn their own sexual strengths and weaknesses and then teach a partner about themselves. For someone who has had a stroke, it might be important to lie on their affected side so they can use their active arm for caressing a partner. Likewise, they might have a "visual field cut" which causes them to ignore one side of their partner's body. The partner needs to let them know about this. (This example by way of social worker Sharon Bacharach.)

When it comes to enjoying sex, different disabilities pose different challenges. For instance, if you can't use your hands in a way that allows you to masturbate, then figuring out how to do that will be one of your first challenges. If you need help breathing but want to give a partner oral sex, you might need to alternate sucking on your partner's genitals with sucking breaths of air from your respirator hose. If you can't have intercourse, then you'll need to work out ways of pleasing both yourself and your partner without it. (This book has plenty of chapters that describe ways of doing that.) Perhaps your disability has left you with little nerve sensation in your genitals, but the opening of your anus is still sensitive; stimulating it might bring you to orgasm. Perhaps your neck, lips, cheeks or nipples are highly sensitized to touch. Maybe it helps if you take a warm bath or shower or to have a beer or glass of wine before having sex. This is just as true for able-bodied people.

Goodbye to Spontaneity

Some able-bodied couples don't like to use a condom because the thirty seconds it takes to put it on destroys the mood for them. Think of how resilient "the mood" has to be when it takes all sorts of preparations and maneuvers to be ready to have sex! Think of how resilient the mood has to be if one partner cries out in pain and adjustments need to be made in order to continue.

One of the things that people who are disabled might lose is the sexual spontaneity that able-bodied couples take for granted unless they are parents with kids who are still at home. Consider the following advice that was recently posted on the Internet:

> "Patience is truly a virtue in disability-related sex. Disability often destroys something in sex, spontaneity for one thing. Drugs, fatigue, depression, neurological impairment can also be a destructive force. Utilizing the turn-on can partially make up for what has been taken away. Sometimes erotic books, photos or videos can enhance the performance. The type and degree of disability often demands traveling that extra mile or two. "   Peter Love

Getting into Relationships

"Why would any man want this body?" "No woman's going to want this!" Some people who have disabilities feel that nobody will find them sexually attractive. As a result, they might push away people who do. Or, at the other end of the spectrum, they might offer themselves to the first person who shows interest, even if it is not someone they like or trust. A disabled person without a solid sense of self might be starved for affection or desperately need to prove that he or she is desirable. Of course, one doesn't need to be disabled to have hang-ups, but it can be extra-difficult when your physical ducks aren't in the same row as everyone else's.

Regarding the subject of dating and people with disabilities, a woman with cerebral palsy recently commented, "I think women are more accepting of differences than men. I see a lot more disabled men married or in serious relationships. I see a lot more disabled women just giving up." There are plenty of disabled men who say it's equally tough for them. Another disabled woman says one of the reasons she fell in love with her husband "was the idea that here was a person who looked and acted OK, wanting to have a relationship with me."

People with disabilities sometimes shy away from dating other people who are disabled. When you are disabled yourself, there can be a kind of hatred of other people who are disabled—an inner need to say, "I'm not like them." There can also be the added problem of social acceptance. Two people in wheelchairs humming down the sidewalk garner far more stares from able-bodied pedestrians than does one.

The Disabled Couple

Perhaps the most difficult aspect of being in a relationship where one or both members is disabled is that ultimately, the couple has to face the same kinds of fights, squabbles, disagreements and difficulties as couples who have no physical disability! As for how disability affects a couple, some able-bodied couples stay in love with each other only as long as each partner is able to mirror the other's sexual attractiveness. If one member starts to look older than the other, slows down or becomes disabled, the relationship may quickly dissolve. With other couples, there is a deep love and friendship that transcends physical change.

When there is a new disability, it is not uncommon for both partners to experience frustration, anger, fear, disappointment, and helplessness. Roles within the relationship may change. Neither the able-bodied member nor the one who is disabled should be afraid to seek help and advice from social workers and rehab staff.

When it comes to sexual intimacy, a couple with a new disability may need to learn anew. This might actually be a relief to your partner if you weren't as good in bed as you thought you were! The good news is that couples who had a rewarding sex life before the disability usually find a way to have a good sex life after.

If you are a couple whose primary expression of sexuality was through intercourse, you may have a good deal of adjusting ahead. It will be easier if you are a couple whose sexuality included a full range of sensory experiences, like enjoying the beauty of a sunset, holding hands and caressing each other.

Also, if you can afford it, it would be wise to hire an attendant to perform caretaking functions. Otherwise, a parent/child dynamic can evolve between you and your partner which can intrude on feelings of sexual passion.

With a Deaf Ear & Twinkle in His Eye

A woman who is a friend of the Goofy Foot Press works with deaf people and has also had sex with one or two deaf men. She said that she never realized how much she relies on verbal cues from a partner until she was romanced by a deaf man. Whether it's being in another room or looking down when you are having a bowl of soup, the usual conditions for connection are suddenly missing when a partner can't hear. With a deaf partner, there is no hearing without seeing. She said that the lack of verbal give-and-take is particularly noticeable during sex, whether it's oral sex or intercourse.

People who are deaf are obviously more comfortable with verbal silence during romance and lovemaking than are people who can hear. If our friend is sleeping with a man who is deaf, she lets him know that she needs more input than he might be used to giving a partner who is also deaf. She also says that it is important to have some of the lights on when you are making love to a deaf person, so they can either see you sign or read your lips. On the other hand, deaf people sometimes sign on each other's skin, or if they are in a spoons position, the person in the back can reach around a partner's body and sign in front where the partner can see.

Attacking Their Own

While many people who are disabled would welcome an increased awareness that they are just as sexual as anyone else, some clearly don't. A few years ago, when a mainstream glossy magazine for disabled people ran a story on sex and the disabled, some disabled readers were so upset that they canceled their subscriptions. You might think that the story was *Hustler*-like and included photos of the naked disabled doing things that would have pleased Caligula. In reality, the article was so tame that it could have been published in *Parade* magazine or *House & Garden*. Perhaps the subject of sex brings up huge amounts of frustration and sadness for some disabled people, to the point where they simply get angry at sex itself.

So You Won't Have to Read the "Sex during Pregnancy" Chapter Unless You Want To

Women can get pregnant in a wheelchair just as easily as they can get pregnant in any other chair. Don't think that because you are disabled or paralyzed from the shoulders or waist down you somehow can't get pregnant. Be sure to speak to each other and to your physician about birth control.

Note Until recently, it was believed that birth-control pills, shots and implants might be unsafe for some women who are in wheelchairs. It's not the wheelchair that's the problem, but proneness to circulatory problems and blood clots that can be increased by the birth-control pill. If your gynecologist isn't used to working with women who have disabilities, check with the *National Spinal Cord Foundation* for a referral.

Attendants and Caregivers —The Good and Bad of It

Powerful feelings can develop between people who are patients and those who are hired to care for them—both loving and hateful. It is beyond the scope of this book to explore the different possibilities, except to say that it does little good to turn a blind eye to the dynamics that can arise between caretaker and caregiver.

If you are able-bodied, consider for a moment the issue of privacy. The kind of privacy that able-bodied people take for granted might not exist for someone who is disabled. This can range from bathing and completing bowel movements to preparing for masturbation and sex. It may be necessary for a disabled person to share private aspects of themselves with an attendant that some able-bodied people don't feel comfortable sharing even with a partner of many years.

Considering the level of dependency that some disabled people have, opportunities for abuse by attendants are rife. This is a huge issue, and abuse is unfortunately quite common. It is important that disabled people speak up against assistants who are abusive. If this is a concern for you, please contact your local center for independent living.

Helping the Helpers

To have fulfilling sex lives, people with disabilities need the help of several different medical subspecialties. These might include neurology, psychology, urology, oncology, endocrinology, physical and rehabilitative medicine and sex therapy. Unfortunately, getting medical specialists to work together in a collaborative effort requires that professional egos be set aside. The problem multiplies when the issue is sex, since many of the professionals who need to work together might be uncomfortable with the subject at hand.

If you are a disabled person who is struggling to get assistance with your sexual needs, maybe it will help if you give your healthcare provider a copy of this book opened to this chapter. Perhaps it will help them feel more at ease in aiding you with sexual matters. After all, it's quite likely that they, too, enjoy sex and would be more than happy to help you if they were just able to feel more comfortable.

Rehab Note When rehab therapists get around to mentioning sex, it is usually in combination with discussions about bowel and bladder functioning. This is most unfortunate. People who are newly disabled need access to positive information about sexuality early in their rehabilitation. Even if they reject the information, it is something positive that will remain in their consciousness, to be accessed at another time.

Stroke Studies — Interesting for a Number of Reasons

Stroke survivors, as a group, experience a drop in sexual activity. Until recently, this was thought to have physical, rather than emotional, causes. However, a study of stroke survivors by Buzzellie, di Francesco, Giaquinto and Nolte concluded that "psychological issues, rather than medical ones, account for disruption of sexual functioning in stroke survivors."

It is especially significant that the researchers found no differences in the sexual functioning of people with right-brained lesions as opposed to left-brain lesions or contralateral lesions. This contradicts our modern tendency to view behaviors as coming from one side of the brain or the other. This study indicates that sexuality is neither "right-brained" nor "left-brained."

Recommended Videotapes

Sexuality Reborn is an excellent video in which four likeable and articulate couples tell about their personal experience with sex and disability. At least one person in each couple is wheelchair-assisted. It is very helpful for both disabled and able-bodied viewers. College instructors who use the *Guide to Getting It On!* in their classes are highly encouraged to show this tape to their students. A great deal of humanness is conveyed without a moment of pity or self-absorption. There is something about the honesty and genuineness of the couples who speak in this video that gives able-bodied people a more realistic and grounded perception of people who are disabled. There are parts of the tape where the couples are naked and having sex, but it isn't in a way that's going to ruffle the feathers of your dean or regents. The only criticism that reviewers had was that the occasional comments by the talking-head medical specialists seemed unnecessary and detracted from, rather than added, to the tape's effectiveness. To order, call (800) 435-8866.

Untold Desires shows interviews about sex with people who have all kinds of disabilities. This award-winning documentary contains no nudity and makes an excellent companion tape for *Sexually Reborn*. We seriously hope that anyone going through a rehab program would get to see both tapes. Included is a wonderful interview with a woman who has severe cerebral palsy. She is astute, funny, and energetic. The tape provides subtitles when she speaks because her speech is so CP-involved. The interviews with other disabled people are equally valuable. As an additional bonus, there is spectacular footage of one chair-assisted man skiing down a steep mountain and a disabled dude racing down stairs and streets. Redefines the term "No Fear." Highly recommended for people with disabilities as well as those without.

HIGHLY RECOMMENDED: *The Ultimate Guide to Sex and Disability,* by Miriam Kaufman, Cory Silverberg and Fran Odette, Cleis Press (2003 & 2007). This is the sex bible for people living with disabilities, chronic pain and illness. It is full of helpful suggestions and ideas, and should be on the shelf of any individual or couple who is experiencing disabilities or chronic pain.

Citations—Both quotes in the section "Getting into Relationships" are from "Dating Issues for Women with Physical Disabilities," *Sexuality and Disability,* 15, no. 4 (1997) by Rintals, Howland, Nosek et al.

CHAPTER

42
Snoring & Passing Gas

The best love-making techniques in the world will take you only so far if your sleeping self passes enough gas to blow the sheets off the bed, or if you snore so loudly that your partner has to check into a hotel, without you. Do both, and your relationship is in double jeopardy.

Flatulence

People with the healthiest diets tend to pass more gas rather than less, but then again, so do people who drink a lot of beer. Whether your gas is from granola or *Three Floyds Dark Lord Russian Imperial Stout,* there are things that you can do to keep your co-workers from calling you the human crop-duster.

The average bum releases from one to three pints of wind each day. But the real killer is that not all air biscuits are created equal. Some are little worse than musty turnips; others can fell men in uniform.

No matter how burly or dainty your lover is, he or she has between fourteen and twenty events a day. Pound-for-pound, girls pass as much gas as guys. It is foods full of complex carbohydrates that make the foul winds blow: everything from fresh fruit to beans and broccoli–virtually anything that's good for you. The thing that creates the ghastly odor is foods that contain sulphur.

Since the array of bacteria in our large intestines varies from person to person, a food that hardly causes a ruffle in Bob's boxers might blow Betty's dress up to the ceiling. And Brooke might be a poster child for the Milk Advisory Board with nary a bark from her bum, while anything more than a cup of milk or a single egg can cause Brianne to clear out an entire gymnasium.

If friends issue a foul-wind advisory whenever you spend the night, try to find what you might be eating that is generating so much gas. You also need to determine if your gas is a normal by product of digestion, or if it is a symptom of a medical condition that can include constipation, ulcers, gastric reflux, irritable bowel syndrome and several other things including cancer.

Only a healthcare professional can help you chase down the medical causes. There are also a number of medications that can cause an increase in gas, as well as sugar substitutes such as sorbitol and xylitol.

If you think the culprit is food, be mindful that it is often combinations of foods rather than just one food that makes a rectum rumble. Start eliminating foods on a trial-and-error basis, although we suggest you keep the chips and tequila until the very end. Also, below a certain threshold, things like onions and mushrooms might be fine, but serve yourself a second helping, and you're a poop-chute flute.

As for things like Beano, simethicone, and holistic approaches such as peppermint and ginger, don't hold your breath. What might work for one person won't stop a single toot in the next.

One of the best articles available on the subject of gas or flatulence is by Margaret C. McDonald, *The Facts About Flatulence*. It can currently be found online at www.spectrox.com/flatulence.html.

Also, there is a highly-effective carbon-embedded seat cushion that not only filters out the bad smell, but muffles the sound. It's the same material that is used in Haz-Mat operations, but packaged so well that no one at your office or sorority will know. You can fart to your heart's content while sitting on the thing, and offend no one. Their website is www.gasbgon.com, and their phone number is 877-GASBGON. Talk about a Christmas present that will blow your loved ones over! We test drove two of them here at Goofy Foot Press. We threw everything we had at 'em. Here's the official Goofy-Foot review: "Tired of your loved ones searching under your chair to make sure the cat didn't die? The GasBGon seat cushion works well enough that you don't sound like such a fool when you blame the kids or the dog. And you can take one to bed with you, much to your partner's relief."

One thing that we learned in researching this pressing problem is that there are people with serious physical problems who are unable to control when, where and how much they fart. This now explains the author's entire sixth-grade year in Sister Justina Isabel's class. Some people with serious gas problems are so mortified that they never go out in public, but that never stopped her. The GasBGone company makes carbon-embedded underwear and seat cushions that can help free people with these disorders from their gastric confinements. And if you're a guy who has trouble thrusting without kicking out some serious smells, cut a hole in front of the Haz-Mat Depends to pull your penis through. Too bad GasBGone doesn't make them with a built-in cock ring to help prevent blow-by.

By way of summary, don't let gas put a cloud of uncertainty over the future of your relationship. In the order of things in life, the fart is mightier than the desire to have sex, at least in people who you might have sex with. Fortunately, there are things most of us can do to get it under control.

Snoring

At least with gas, you get a measure of your own medicine. Not so with snoring. Snoring is on the short-list of problems that cause sexual partners to sleep in separate bedrooms. Unless the snorer has sleep apnea, he or she is unlikely to be impacted by the snoring, except for wondering why his or her partner is so cranky about it.

Snoring is an acoustical nastiness that happens when your breath collides against tissue that's inside your nose or throat. It mostly happens during sleep, because muscle tone in the throat decreases after the sandman pays a visit. The air rushing past the sagging tissue causes vibrations that can make your sleeping self sound like a drowning donkey.

Another culprit might be a blockage in your nasal pathway. This could be from a broken nose, a chronic allergy, infection, or structural defect. It can either be the sole source of your snoring (called nasal-based snoring), or it can cause you to breathe through your mouth, which gives you the snoring capacity of a level-5 hurricane.

Your tongue can also be contributing to the problem, but you don't have to be asleep for your tongue to get you in trouble.

Being overweight, drinking, smoking, and taking drugs are at the top of a long list of snoring stimulators. Hopefully, you are starting to get the idea that snoring can have an array of different causes. Until you determine the specific cause or combination of causes, you will have better luck milking a moose than finding a cure.

You might also have sleep apnea—which is at the Mayday end of the snoring continuum. This is when your breathing stops for more than ten seconds at a time. When that happens, the sensors in your brain suddenly say, "Oops, looks like we're dying!" and they generate a snort that sounds like feeding time at the pig farm. This can happen hundreds of times each night, with periods of dead silence followed by wickedly-loud snorts.

Sleep apnea is always a sign of danger and needs evaluation by a sleep specialist. It can be a forewarning of heart problems, high blood pressure, and diabetes. It can also cause extreme fatigue and depression because it interferes with REM or dream sleep. Treatment might include a special type of mouth piece or a device that blows air into the sleeping lungs, as well as dire warnings to lose weight, start exercising, and stop smoking and drinking.

There are all sorts of people who are happy to take your money for snoring cures. There are also physicians who will hack up the back of your throat in the name of curing the problem, even though there are few studies on the safety or long-term effectiveness of these procedures.

Why not get a voice-activated tape recorder and a mic to put on the headboard or wall above your head? Also, get a clock that speaks the hour. This will activate the recorder so you can learn what part of the night your snoring occurs. Conventional snorers will often start sawing logs as soon as they fall asleep, while snorers with sleep apnea tend to build steam later in the night. Sleep experts can get important clues about the cause of your snoring based upon its pitch, frequency and timing. The tape recording will help them and you to understand more about the problems.

Once a sleep specialist is able to pinpoint the cause of your snoring, research the heck out of it. UNDER NO CIRCUMSTANCES should you agree to any surgeries or throat injections without getting a second opinion by a specialist who doesn't work with the first one. Spend lots of time on snoring forums reading the posts of people who have had the various procedures.

Recommended: One snoring aid that looked promising was exercises for strengthening the muscle tone in the throat. These were designed by Alise Ojay, a singing instructor in England. They seem to be quite helpful when the problem is caused by lax throat muscles. Why not give this a try before letting a doctor cut up the back of your throat or inject funky substances into it? Read the articles on this woman's website: www.singingforsnorers.com.

Take Heed!

If loved ones at are their wits end do to your snoring, please don't ignore them because you can't hear yourself. Hook up the tape recorder as we suggest, so you can get an idea of what has them in such a state. And then, for the sake of your relationship if not for yourself, set out to learn all you can about the problem. Put together a plan of action, and see if you can't improve the situation.

43
Sex & Hysterectomy

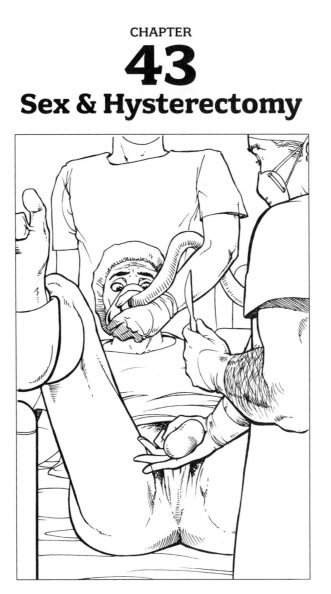

Does the Thought of This Make You Uncomfortable?

If a woman in our society has her reproductive organs removed, no one takes much notice. It's an everyday surgical event. But if a man has his testicles removed, we gasp in shared pain. Are a man's organs more important?

Until the 1990s, when managed health care started taking a closer look at surgeries, approximately 665,000 hysterectomies were performed each year on women at an average age of 42.5 years. A university professor who was a second-opinion expert for Blue Cross reported, "The patients who had the recommendations for the hysterectomies either had no pathology whatsoever or had pathology that was so minimal it was inexplicable to me how anybody could have recommended surgery."

There are times when hysterectomy is necessary to save a woman's life, as in cases where cervical or ovarian cancer is found. Hopefully, if your physician recommends a hysterectomy, you will seek a second opinion. It is your body and your right.

Hysterectomy & Sex

There is nowhere near the kind of solid research on hysterectomy and sex that you would think, given the large number of hysterectomies that are done each year. To help with any decisions you might need to make, Annie Bradford, a researcher from the University of Texas at Austin, has been kind enough to off the following perspective to readers of *The Guide:*

"If I were a woman who is preparing to have a hysterectomy, there are a few things I would want to be asked. First, I would like my physician to discuss the possibility of less aggressive/less invasive treatment alternatives—hysterectomy isn't the only option for an increasing number of diseases. I would want my MD to check in with me about my general well-being in life at that moment, because the literature shows that depression and anxiety going in tend to predict poorer outcomes. I'd also want to know that my MD cared that I had the support of friends, family, and/or significant others; this is another thing that seems to influence outcomes. If my MD suggested that I should have my ovaries removed, I would want a very good reason for it. The idea that I should remove organs that I supposedly 'won't need anymore' on that basis alone is preposterous!

"After hearing from many women about their hysterectomies, the main thing I have learned is that most of them just want information. Even if the MD can't guarantee a particular outcome, they really want to know the pros and cons of all of the treatment options. Contrary to what some paternalistic doctors might tell you, they really can handle that information! Several studies have demonstrated that patients tend to want more information, sometimes a lot more, than their doctors think they want or need. The bottom line is that women want to CONSENT to every aspect of their treatment, and that means they understand why they're taking one approach over the other, etc. Informed consent is not just 'this is what you need, now sign the dotted line.' It's an agreement to a collaborative treatment decision (thus the word 'informed').

"The jury is still out on to what extent hysterectomy affects basic sexual physiology. I would guess that any given outcome is a combination of the surgical technique and the individual woman's composition. I've heard some women say that they have lost some sensation after hysterectomy, or their orgasms aren't as intense as they used to be, but there is no 'typical' hysterectomy experience as far as I can tell. Whether any woman would do it all over again given the chance depends on a lot of different factors. Women whose sex lives are disrupted because of huge, basically inoperable fibroids are likely to still be mostly satisfied when penetration no longer causes sharp pain, and I suspect that for many this would be true even if the cost were a slight change in sexual sensation or the intensity of orgasm. The thing is, though, we can't KNOW what that potential trade-off would mean to any individual woman unless we actually ask her! So, if I were a doctor, I would say, "Look, these are side effects that some women have reported," and summarize the latest research to give her an idea of how common the side effects actually are. It would be up to her to decide if the risk, however small, was worth the potential gains associated with hysterectomy, which themselves are not 100% guaranteed either, of course! It's a cost-benefit analysis, and even though there are a lot of women who want their physicians to make the final decision, I've never heard anyone claim that they got too much information about what might happen to them.

"I *have* heard from a few women who said that they put off their hysterectomies needlessly because of scare tactics, and this is the other side of the story. There are activist groups putting out some pretty wild claims. According to them, hysterectomy can cause asthma! They don't do women any favors with their misinformation and pseudoscience. Ultimately it's a hard decision to make, and women simply need the facts. I am fairly convinced at this point that, for an otherwise healthy, well-adjusted, well-supported woman who lives in a community or in a relationship that won't see her as losing her femininity, hysterectomy is not necessarily a bad thing for sexual function and in some cases might be exactly what she needs. If less invasive treatment options have been ruled out and the main issue is painful intercourse caused by the disease. Otherwise, the picture can be more complex. One of the most consistent findings from past research, though, is that the worse off you are to begin with, both sexually and emotionally, the less likely it is that your outcome will be a complete success. When women ask me about their treatment decisions, I ask them right out: are you emotionally, mentally, physically, and spiritually ready for this? You'd be surprised how seldom women get asked this question.

"No matter how healthy you are to begin with, losing the ovaries IS a big deal, especially for premenopausal women, as it changes the hormonal profile and forces further decision-making about hormone-replacement therapy and so forth. The choice to remove the ovaries should be carefully justified. The medical opinion on this issue has shifted back and forth over the years, but there are many experts who would tell you that, for healthy women with no significant risk factors for ovarian cancer, the cost of losing ovaries is greater than the potential benefits. Sometimes removal of the ovaries is an easy decision to make because of cancer or other factors, but more often than not it should be deliberated very carefully. This is a time to get second opinions."

A Physician Gets Mad

A friend of *The Guide* from way back when is one of the top sex researchers in the country. She is also a physician. Recently, she became so angry with her own private gynecologist that it appeared she was going to rip him a new—uh—vagina. She was diagnosed with cancer of the cervix, and she felt his handling of it was neither sensitive nor professional.

The reason for reporting this is not to dump on gynecologists. There are many excellent ones. It is simply to remind you that even an MD can become an angry and frustrated patient. So if you are feeling overwhelmed by your dealings with modern medicine, you are not alone. Don't hesitate to get a second opinion. If it appears that you will need to have surgery and you don't feel comfortable with your physician, find a university health center to get another opinion. That is what our physician friend recommends after her personal experience with hysterectomy.

A SPECIAL THANKS: To Annie Bradford of the University of Texas at Austin for providing readers of *The Guide* with some of the best advice available for women who are considering a hysterectomy.

44

Techno Breasts & Weenie Angst

People who feel sexually inadequate sometimes focus their angst on body parts. For women, the focus is often on breast size or body shape; for men it is on the penis and sometimes height. Of course, it is silly to obsess about something that you had no say in getting, yet that is what many of us do.

When generating a physical balance sheet, it might be helpful to remember that even Man-O-War had his weaknesses. It might also help to remind yourself that sexual attractiveness is not like a steel chain, where one weak link makes the whole thing useless. All of us have weak links sexually, as part of our bodies and minds.

This offers little solace to people who are convinced that their body parts are deficient. They will keep telling themselves, "Everything would be better if I just had a bigger this or a smaller that." To address such fears, this chapter offers a lengthy discourse on men's genitals, then ruminates on breast implants and ends with a few suggestions about alternative strategies.

Body Concerns: Guys & How They're Hung

While most books on sex say that penis size doesn't matter, there are two groups of people to whom it does matter. One group includes almost every male alive. The second group includes every woman who derives sexual pleasure from intercourse.

In years past, women weren't supposed to care about the size and shape of a man's penis. That is because they weren't supposed to be interested in sex. But wouldn't you notice the size and shape of something that was about to get stuck into your body? As for how women respond to the actual dimensions of the thing, it clearly varies.

For instance, some women regard the penis as a trophy—the bigger the better; others couldn't care less. Some women prefer the feeling of fullness that a beefier penis has to offer; others prefer giving blowjobs to a partner who isn't particularly well hung, and some even prefer a smaller penis for intercourse. Plenty of women get the bulk of their pleasure from what a man is able to do with his hands, heart, tongue and intellect. They view the penis as just another body part.

For some women, a lover's penis becomes her penis or a part of her body when it's inside of her. Does this mean that she necessarily wants the biggest one in town? Not usually. After all, when women buy dildos, they tend to select medium or smaller units. (Sorry, but they sometimes upsize later.)

Of course, this isn't to say that women don't have their favorites. Ask a woman to tell you which lover's penis was her favorite, and she will probably be able to give a direct and clear-cut answer such as, "It was Alex's" or "There are two or three that stand out, but I'd have to say Todd's takes the prize." However, if you ask about the men behind the penises and which ones she loved the most, Alex or Todd might not be at the top of the list. Maybe the guy she was happiest with didn't have a memorable penis, but was able to put it together in other ways.

So while women might prefer one penis over the other, penis size usually isn't a deal-breaker when it comes to choosing a man. It is sometimes disappointing, but usually not the deciding factor.

Irony: While some guys grow up worrying if they are hung well enough, women sometimes grow up worrying that guys will be hung too well and might cause them pain. Maybe we humans were programmed to worry.

Weenie-Enhancement Techniques: Surgery That Makes Your Penis Fat

There used to be a surgical technique for penis plumping in which fat cells were harvested from the lower-stomach region and injected into the penis. The author of this book called three offices that advertised this procedure and was hit by a wave of sales pitches that he hadn't encountered since joining a health club. The heavy sales pitch, which tried to capitalize on every sexual doubt known to man, made sense when you consider that these clinics were charging $3,000 to $7,000 for a simple outpatient procedure that takes half an hour.

One clinic in Beverly Hills refused to even mail out information about the procedure. They claimed that a brochure had fallen into the hands of a child, resulting in great embarrassment. To prevent such a hideous event from ever occurring again, each caller had to make an office appointment where he could read the brochure and talk to a specialist. "Why an appointment?" "Because we process over forty men a day." As it turned out, the dreaded brochure contained no pictures or drawings and was embarrassing only in how it insulted the consumer's intelligence.

This fancy medical clinic insisted that it needed a social-security number and health-insurance information before discussing the procedure. Each visitor was also required to fill out a separate page about his penis. The wording was designed to make a man feel sexually insecure and blame it all on the size of his weenie. It was the forerunner for today's spam and TV commercials that promise a bigger dick with pills instead of surgery—with probably the same people being involved.

The interview was with a clean-cut salesman masquerading in a physician's coat, perhaps so wouldn't be confused with the salesmen who populate used-car lots. None of the three offices offered any studies on the long-term safety of the procedure, they didn't agree on where the fat actually went, and none was willing to say exactly how a penis feels that is encased in a layer of fat.

The best anyone could conclude about this procedure is that a man paid $5,000 to give his penis cellulite. The biggest benefactors of the procedure have been the attorneys who specialized in lawsuits from men who had their penises surgically enhanced. Since that time, there have been ads stating that there is a "new procedure" that is vastly improved over the one used in the past. If you are considering such a surgery, remember that only a few years ago the ads for the "old" procedure used to boast about how safe and successful it was.

If you are considering such a surgery, spend some time at the library and do a search in the *Journal of Sexual Medicine* and various urology journals on penis-enlarging penis enhancement surgeries. Forewarned is forearmed.

The Vacuum Pump

There is an X-rated video called *How to Enlarge Your Penis* in which porn star Scott Taylor pumps himself up with a vacuum device that is supposed to make a guy bigger. Taylor uses the pump to plump his penis up fatter than a grain silo, which he then maneuvers into the apparently spacious vagina of porn starlet Erica Boyer. At no point does Scott's big salami actually get hard; he has to hold his fingers around the base to keep the pressure in. In spite of this "self-help" video, the vacuum pump is one of the options that urologists offer male patients who are having trouble getting hard. Also, inside-industry sources have informed Goofy Foot Press that the *How to Enlarge* infomercial took several hours to shoot. Even Scott Taylor couldn't stay hard that long.

The penis pump was first patented in 1917. About sixty years later it became popular in the gay community, both for sex play and for organ enhancement. Some pumpers even started clubs, along the lines of Kiwanis or Rotary, where guys get together to pump. Straight men started using the pump in the mid to late 1980s. Pumping provides a sensation that some men find enjoyable. It also causes the penis to plump up bigger than usual. Most urologists think that there is no way a guy can make himself permanently bigger with a vacuum pump and that short-term gains occur because the penis is swollen. However, the people who manufacture the pumps claim that long-term gains are possible. They say that the vacuum pump expands the width of the penis by stretching the walls of the chambers that fill with blood during normal erection. The increase in penis length apparently comes from stretching the ligament that holds a third of the penis inside the body.

To achieve a "permanent" increase in size, pumpers say that a man has to pump at least a half-hour a day for almost a year. As for the safety of the vacuum pump, it has been approved by the FDA for use with erection problems, but not for use as a weenie-enhancement device, not that anyone has applied. Can you imagine the lab studies that the FDA might require, with hundreds of white rats having their penises pumped for hours on end to see if they got bigger?

For safety's sake, check with a physician before pumping for long periods of time. That's because there might be a difference between pumping for a few minutes to get hard and pumping for an hour to get bigger. Also ask yourself why you might be focusing so much insecurity on your penis. You would think that the majority of men who pump for size would be those with smaller penises. Not so. A lot of pumpers are well-endowed to begin with. Go figure.

The Bottom Line...

"I once had a lover with an enormous penis. It was a turn-on to look
at it, and an ego trip that a man that huge was my partner. But the

actual feeling of it inside me didn't give me one one-hundredth of the pleasure that my more modestly-sized present partner's does. While the size of a man's penis does create different sensations, it is the relationship I have with the man who is attached to the penis that determines what those sensations mean to me." *female age 47*

Before rushing out to get either a pump or surgery, consider the following: If your penis is average-sized or more, why do you need to be bigger? What's your problem anyway? And if your penis is closer to a finger than a phone pole, keep in mind that couples frequently have intercourse before the vagina is fully engorged with blood. When that is the case, the penis with the bigger girth will probably fill the space better. However, when a woman's vagina is fully-engorged, this helps even the playing field. So make sure you take the time to fully prime the pussy's pumps.

Learn to give great back and foot rubs and become sublime at the art of loving a woman with your lips and tongue. Do this and it is likely that you will be admired by many women, assuming you are a decent human being to begin with. Also try using intercourse positions that cause the penis to be hugged more snugly, and those that might focus more stimulation on the parts of your lover's vagina that give her the most pleasure. A bantam-weight penis might feel longer if the female bends her knees during intercourse. This results in deeper penetration if that is what she wants. Keeping her legs together will help it feel more snug. A couple of positions that accommodate this are rear-entry intercourse with both of you on your sides (aka spoons) and where the woman is on her back and her ankles are resting on the man's shoulders instead of around his waist. If it helps, the most sensitive areas of a vagina are often located in the first inch or two beyond the vaginal opening.

And finally, try to avoid women who are confirmed size-queens. There's no sense in humiliating yourself needlessly.

As for being embarrassed in front of your locker-room buds, it's not fair to compare nonerect penises. Penises that are smaller when they are soft tend to grow more when they are getting hard. So it isn't a fair comparison, unless all of you have hard-ons, and what kind of gym would that be? But reality checks are of little solace to a guy who is feeling insecure in the showers after football practice. Hopefully he will learn that there are other ways of earning respect besides having a big penis, assuming that big penises earn respect rather than envy.

Perhaps it might be good to remember that many things in life have a purpose. In case you are here on earth to learn something, your less-than-memorable member might be one of the keys that helps you find it, especially if it's a bit of humility.

For the Extra-Well-Endowed

Some men feel angst because they were especially blessed between the legs. Others just smile. For those guys whose girlfriends scream in horror the first time they see the penis erect, relax. Talk about it before you get undressed or hand her a copy of *The Guide* and point to this chapter. Flatly rule out the possibility of intercourse for the first couple of times. This will allow time for your lover to become comfortable touching and playing with your trunk—uh—penis. Ray Stubbs's *Erotic Interludes Part 2* is a tastefully done videotape which shows a woman massaging the penis of a man who doesn't give much ground to a race horse. And no matter what its diameter might be, a partner can get you off quite nicely with the oral-sex technique that doesn't require her to take your whole penis into her mouth. It is shown in the chapter on blowjobs. There's also a question at the end of this chapter about sex with a well-endowed lover. It is crammed full of information on the ways of the big weenie.

The Sound of Leaking Breasts

"I tried out for the cheerleading squad when I was a sophomore in high school. 'This isn't a beauty contest,' the advisor had told us, but we all knew better than that.... But you weren't beautiful, Julie Brown, and you knew it. Face facts. You even made a list one time, outlining your numerous faults: breasts too small, buttocks too big, teeth crooked, hair too thin, arms and legs too skinny, feet too long, four inches too tall, nose too bumpy. If you were wealthy, you could make the necessary corrections. If you had enough money, you could have the breast implants you needed, the braces, the nose job, the hairweaving, and with enough money the right cosmetics could be purchased, the ones you saw in the magazines, the ones that would render you flawless..."[1]

Men aren't the only ones who worry that body parts are too small. Women often believe that the world would be a nicer place if only they had bigger breasts. Some women with petite breasts even feel they would get a better job or promotion if their A-cups swelled into majestic Es. Hopes like these have inspired thousands of women to have their chests packed with funky substances.

Many questions have been raised about the safety of breast implants. Silicone molecules seem to leach through the plastic implant pouches. However, it is possible that this isn't any more dangerous to your health than, say, living in Detroit or Los Angeles. Saline implants appear to be safer than the silicone, but far less so than the original equipment that Mother Nature saw fit to provide.

Note Many women who have implants need additional surgery a few years down the line, and even the saltwater boobs make it difficult to screen for cancer. On the other hand, implants are truly a godsend if you have had cancer and are getting them following a mastectomy.

Silicone Sisters[2] and the Men Who Love Them

Here in America, women with plastic chests attract men with plastic brains. What a perfect combination. What a sad perception of womanhood.

Young women in America are raised on fashion magazines that highlight gorgeous female models, whatever gorgeous might mean. Having grown up under the shadow of surgically enhanced breasts, American girls often confuse a combination of anorexia and a fake profile with what femininity is all about. As a result, breast implants and bizarre diets have become a way of achieving the fantasy of perfect womanhood.

Perfect womanhood is a costly and precarious myth to pursue. Even if you are able to achieve the right look, it tends to be short-lived and often comes crashing down by the time you reach age 35 and can no longer suppress that which in other cultures is considered to be a sign of wisdom. It's too bad America's teenage girls don't get to spend time with America's supermodels. They might get over the supermodel fantasy rather quickly.

The Placebo Effect of Store-Bought Boobs

Until recently, some of the biggest proponents of breast implants were the women who got them. Then they had to start spending all that time and energy convincing themselves that the darned things weren't killing them.

One reason women with plastic chests were so excited about their implants was because life did get better for many of them. But the real reason why life improved was that the women's attitudes got better. It's how they

---

[1]By Julie Brown, published in "Beauty" pages 68–70, *Michigan Quarterly Review,* edited by Laurence Goldstein, Vol. XXX, No. 1:91.

[2]With apologies to Bruce Springsteen.

saw themselves that made the difference, not whether their breasts were As or DDs. Otherwise, women with naturally large boobs would seldom feel depressed or have a rotten day, and women with As would all be suicidal.

Feeling more attractive is what made these women be more attractive, but an increase in confidence without the implants would have brought similar results. Granted, there are plenty of men who like the way that big boobs look, and many TV producers won't hire actresses unless they have bizarre-looking breast implants. But is that the kind of person you want to attract?

Microchip Melons — A New Generation of Breast Implant?

Unless there is a major shift in the consciousness of American men and women, it is likely that the medical world will find new ways to surgically enhance women's breasts. As long as that is the case, this Guide suggests that the next generation of breast implants contain slots for video games and a couple of firewire ports—although with the newer MacBooks, firewire appears to be on its way out. Perhaps breast-implanted gaming displays might help the female chest become a full-fledged entertainment center, which is what some men and women expect it to be.

Labiplasty

Labioplasty is the new cosmetic surgery to help a girl's inner lips look like those of a porn star. Think of it as a nose job for your puss.

Different women have different reasons for wanting labioplasty. Some with prominent inner labia find that certain clothes are uncomfortable, or their labia pull when they are taking part in sports, or that they have pain during intercourse because the inner labia are pulled inside the vagina with thrusts of the penis. Other women have no discomfort, but simply don't like the way their inner labia look, or want their pre-childbirth labia back.

A lot of people are critical of labioplasty, but themselves buy teeth-whitening products, get their hair colored, have moles removed that they consider to be unsightly, and have their sons circumcized. And given how this book has wailed and ranted against breast implants with absolutely no impact, we figured we'd simply give you the info you need, and leave the rest up to you.

Women who want to have labioplasty should be shown by their gynecologist pictures of different labia and how normal it is for labia to come in many different sizes and shapes. If the woman still wants the surgery, she needs to find a surgeon who specializes in this procedure and has performed many prior labioplasties. It is not a simple matter of snipping a bit here and there. The woman should be sure that her surgeon knows the different techniques and can describe for her the difference between oversewing the edges, wedge resection and 90-degree Z-plasty. (As of presstime, the latter appeared to be the preferred technique.) Labiaplasty can be performed under general, regional, or local anesthesia. The surgery takes about six weeks to heal. Plan to not have vaginal intercourse for at least six weeks.

Exercise-Video Alert—Truth in Advertising

Exercise videos have been very popular for the past decades. It only seems fair that any actress/model/whatever who does an exercise video ought to list how many cosmetic surgeries she's had to look the way she does. (Breast implants? Ribs removed? Liposuction? Face lifts? Tummy tucks? Breast lifts? Supplemental hormones?) The videos might then post a warning label such as the following:

> WARNING: With $22,000 worth of plastic surgery, a lucky role of the genetic dice, an eating disorder, and the exercises on this tape, you too can look more like your video host.

Alternatives for Both Men & Women

American advertisers spend millions of dollars to make us think, "If only I had this or that, I'd be sexier and happier." It is easy to see why many of us fall for these devious traps. The thought of instantly having bigger, smaller, hairier or balder body parts can be terribly seductive.

If cosmetic surgery is what you need, please choose carefully. Do be aware that if you haven't worked through feelings of inferiority, realigning body parts may not make you feel any better in the long run. You'll simply find new things to feel insecure about.

For alternatives, think about getting your body in good physical shape or dressing better. Breasts that sit on well-developed chest muscles sometimes look bigger, if that is what you are trying to achieve. At the very least, being in good shape makes most people feel and look sexier. A smaller penis will often look bigger if it isn't being dwarfed by a pot belly, or if the eyes are drawn to nicely developed shoulders and pecs. Also, why not find ways to expand your mind's creativity and intelligence? These are the kinds of measures that will make you a better and sexier person.

As for sexual performance, some of the best and most eager lovers are those without ideal dimensions. Since they have less natural endowment to fall back on, they sometimes learn to be extremely attentive in bed.

Considering any kind of cosmetic surgery? Please read Virginia Blum's book on the subject. This book will let you see a side of cosmetic surgery that is well-hidden from the viewers of the *Extreme Makeover*\TV shows. Blum has had plastic surgery and has interviewed surgeons and patients. What would it hurt to read some of the information that you won't find in the glossy brochures at your plastic surgeon's office before making such a big decision? *Flesh Wounds, The Culture of Cosmetic Surgery* by Virginia L. Blum, University of California at Berkeley Press, (2003).

Breast-Reduction Note Some women have breast-reduction surgery because it can be severely uncomfortable to lug huge breasts around all the time. If this is what you are considering, be sure to consult at least two surgeons who specialize in breast-reduction surgery. This is not a simple operation and can leave permanent scaring or disfigurement.

Dear Paul,

My boyfriend and I are both virgins and have been attempting to have intercourse, but we are having a few difficulties. First of all, I have no problem getting wet, but when it comes to penetration I am completely dry. This makes it very painful, as it aches and burns. I am also quite petite, and he, on the other hand, is quite tall and "fully equipped" (8 inches, and rather large in circumference). It seems that penetration is practically impossible as I am rather tight and do not enjoy being fingered. I was just wondering if you have any suggestions as we are getting a little antsy.　　　　　*Tina from Mesa Grande*

Dear Tina,

None of the women I've slept with have had to come up with strategies for inserting an extra-large penis—not when they were with me, anyway. Nonetheless, I'll do what I can.

To put this size issue in its truest, ugliest light, if the Penis Fairy arrived one night and offered to give all men an extra inch of bulge in the front of their blue jeans, or an extra 10 I.Q. points, a lot of us would go for the below-the-belt enhancement without giving it much thought. In fact, until I'd written a book about sex, I never realized that toting around a huge penis can be a liability. We're talking about guys who need to wear specially made underwear, who are forever getting stares in the locker room and at the doctor's office, and for whom hopping into bed with a woman can be a trauma.

On the other hand, I have interviewed a woman who is as petite as can be. Her husband's penis was in the 98th percentile for size, and she never had any problem with intercourse. So you can't predict.

Size aside, medical factors can make intercourse uncomfortable. So I am assuming you have had a recent gynecological exam and have discussed this very matter. If there is a source of pain that is independent of your partner's penis, it is essential that you treat it and resolve it first.

As long as you are OK physically, I would suggest that the two of you call it quits on any intercourse attempts for the next month or two. There are lots of ways you can please each other sexually besides intercourse. At the same time, you can be working on some or all of the following:

1. It sounds as though each time you've tried to have intercourse there's been a fair amount of pain. I suspect that the muscles around the mouth of your vagina are now automatically tightening up whenever Mr. Jumbo tries to land. This would be your body's way of protecting you from more pain. Unfortunately, it is backfiring.

One thing to try is called "femoral intercourse," but it isn't intercourse at all. It is where your partner lies on his back and you lube up his penis. You then straddle him and ride back and forth along the length of his well-lubed penis as it is lying against his belly. (Your vulva is like a hotdog bun, and his penis is like a Ballpark Frank. You slide the bun up and down the length of the dog, enjoying the sensations without him trying to steal home. Be sure to use birth control even if he holds the mayo. His penis is not going into your vagina, but your genitals will be rubbing together and that's reason enough to call out the contraceptives.)

It might help if you could learn to give yourself some orgasms this way or at least enjoy the sensations. You are in complete control and there's no need to worry about intercourse. These pleasant experiences with his penis will help the muscles around your vagina learn to stop clenching in anticipation of pain. This also helps massage the tissues around your vulva, which leads to the next step.

2. Have your partner squirt lube on his fingertips. He can then gently clasp the outer lips of your vulva between his thumb and forefinger and do

a small circular massage on one area at a time. Tell him exactly what feels good and what doesn't. He should massage as deeply as feels comfortable to you, then move to an adjoining spot. His goal is not to stretch the skin, but to get the blood circulating deep inside of the folds. He should do your entire vulva, including the outer lips, inner lips and the clitoral hood. Then, if it's comfortable, he can gently insert a well-lubricated thumb into the opening of your vagina and rest it there. His forefinger should be on the outside, resting on the skin that's between your vulva and anus. He then clasps the tissue that's between his thumb and forefinger and massages. This stimulates the part of your genitals that stretch wider when you have intercourse. (The ceiling of a vagina doesn't stretch as much, as the pubic bone is right above it.)

3. Consider purchasing two or three penis-shaped objects or dildos that range in size from small to large. Start by lubing up your vagina in addition to the smallest dildo. Once you become comfortable inserting that and moving it around inside your vagina, move up to the next size. This process should be done over several weeks and not all in one night. The women who run *Touch of A Woman* (www.TouchOfAWoman.com) can be very helpful with this process. They have products especially designed to help.

4. Once you are comfortable with these steps, have your partner rest the head of his well-lubed penis at the opening of your vagina, but no farther. A day or two later, have him move in about a quarter-of-an-inch if it is comfortable for you. Try just a little extra each time you are together, as long you feel comfortable with it. As for intercourse positions, you'll want to be really conservative. Stay with the classic missionary position where you are on your back and your legs are slightly spread. Avoid rear-entry positions and stay away from anything where your legs are flexed. Any flexing of the knees tends to compress or shorten the available thrusting space in the vagina. Also, you might find that having an orgasm before intercourse helps.

5. One of the top experts on vulvar pain recommends using fresh olive oil for lube. Almond oil and grape seed oil are also on some physician's lists. If you use storebought lube, I would caution you against anything with glycerin in it. While this is not a problem for many women, it does create the potential for vaginal infections. Why tempt the Fates with another negative association to sex?

45

Basic Brain Weirdness

his chapter is about the mental landscape, and parts of it that can get in the way of having a good sex life, or just having a good life. Some people would call these mental glitches; others say they are a normal part of the human condition.

Shyness

Shyness is a funny thing. Sometimes it sits like a shroud over everything you do. Other times it is highly selective, making only certain parts of your life sheer hell. Shyness can take many forms and can be a great deal more mysterious than people give it credit for. For instance, shyness can make you babble like a fool and say really stupid things or it can make you seem cold and aloof when you're really not.

To illustrate what happens when shyness gets the better of you, consider the following true story of Andrew. Andrew is now really old, but he used to be really young.

It was a beautiful spring day about a month or two before the beginning of a somewhat magical time that later became known as the Summer of Love. Unfortunately, Andrew had never even put his hand up a woman's shirt.

None of this stopped him from having an overpowering crush on a very popular young woman who was older than he. This female heartthrob just happened to be the homecoming queen. She was so special that he was too embarrassed to tell even his best friend about his lick-the-mud-off-her-shoes-if-that's-what-she-wants crush. Instead, he focused his energies on trying to act cool whenever she passed by.

To make matters worse, the young goddess was constantly surrounded by senior guys who had their own cars, lettered in football and baseball, and got drunk and never even threw up. He, on the other hand, saw himself as just another underclassman who had less than a snowball's chance in hell of attracting this woman's interest.

One day about an hour after school, some strange and peculiar force caused this special woman to toss her books and pompoms into the back of her car and aim it for the very address where this young man lived. When the doorbell rang he figured it was probably the paper boy or a Jehovah's Witness selling "The Watchtower." When he walked outside and saw who it was, his knees turned to Jell-o, and it seemed like an hour before he was able to take a breath. All things considered, he did well to maintain bladder control.

He stood staring at this babe like a deer in front of headlights. He felt so paralyzed that he couldn't even mobilize the words to invite her inside. After about twenty awkward minutes of trying to deal with the situation, the young goddess blew the baffled boy a puzzled kiss and drove away, never to return.

Many years have passed since this fellow botched the Summer of Love. For much of his life, he continued to feel clumsy and awkward whenever he met a woman who he was attracted to.

On Being a Sex Object

People usually associate "being a sex object" with being a woman. However, this is about a guy named Steve who women treated as a sex object. Steve was tall, blond, blue-eyed and had a perfect body. In addition to being a fine surfer, he was a male model who was actually straight.

Everyone was thrown into total shock one night at Steve's tearful lament that he wished women would stop wanting him just for sex. It was a problem none of us could relate to. Steve was in a total funk because women were constantly diving for his crotch.

It's difficult to imagine that physical attractiveness can get in the way of leading a happy life, but people who are physical 10s are sometimes rather lonely. Friends of the same sex are often envious and sometimes feel threatened by the attention that the 10s seem to get. Members of the other sex often stare or act bizarrely. People who are extremely attractive sometimes marry simply for protection.

What's Wrong with This Picture?

The opposite problem of being a 10 is when you are less than beautiful and have someone who is drop-dead gorgeous show a romantic interest in you. Instead of responding romantically, you might be saying to yourself, "Naw, can't be true. Big mistake here." While the physical 10 may be begging for romance, the less-than-10 is turning a great opportunity into a self-fulfilling prophecy of doom. Sometimes other people can see beautiful things in you that you have no idea even exist.

People Who Claim "The Opposite Sex Is Worthless"

Some people choose sexual partners who can't supply any of their emotional needs. It's as if they would be horribly overwhelmed to find a partner who could be both a friend and a lover, and therefore not quite so "opposite." Perpetual victims such as these claim that they are more mature and able to love more than their moron partners.

The fact is, people who have a healthy self-regard do not suffer the presence of fools and jerks, let alone sleep with them. The perpetual victim is just as immature and has as many problems with intimacy as does the jerk whom he or she dates or marries. Neither has much to brag about.

Giving Friendship a Chance

The male-female relationships that we usually teach our children to value are those with romantic potential. As a result, men and women approach each other as potential sex partners rather than as potential friends.

Platonic male-female friendships are a wonderful thing, but they sometimes become endangered if one person starts to feel sexual and the other doesn't. A lot of male-female friendships never happen because people are unable to work it out when one of them wants sex or romance and the other just wants friendship. Knowing that a friend wants romance when you don't can be uncomfortable. However, if he or she were given the time and understanding to cool his or her jets, the nonsexual friendship might flourish for years to come. As for the person who feels smitten and then bitten, keep in mind that a platonic friendship often lasts for years, while that is not always the case with romantic affairs. You might be losing out on something special if you aren't able to accept the person as a friend instead of as a lover.

Another factor that often destroys male-female friendships is jealous spouses or partners.

Initiating Sex When Holding Is What You Need

Some people find it hard to acknowledge that they need to be held. Asking might make them feel weak or vulnerable. So they sometimes initiate sex when what they really may have wanted was physical tenderness and comfort. Fortunately, the desires for sex and tenderness often overlap, which allows us to receive both at the same time. But sometimes we need more of one than the other. Hopefully you can evolve a set of signals that will help your partner know what you need, assuming you know yourself.

In Love but out of Sync

It's the saddest thing in the world when people have powerful feelings for each other but can't make their relationship work. For instance, one of you might become more settled and grounded earlier in life than the other. You may feel like putting down roots or becoming established while the other is still an emotional tumbleweed who needs to experience the outside world and soak in whatever it has to teach. The lack of synchrony forces a breakup, or maybe there's a level of sensitivity or maturity that one partner won't have for several more years. While you may not have any desire to get back together, there might always remain a place in your heart for the other person.

Breaking Up

Breaking up is the sort of thing that you should write a whole book about. Otherwise, you risk being trite about a phenomenon that can leave even the strongest of hearts totally shattered.

Contrary to what you might think, breaking up isn't always accompanied by a big fight or a hell storm of hostility. In fact, sometimes you spend your last hours together holding each other tight, with a kind of desperate, profound sadness in your hearts. And even if you are the one who is doing the leaving, the final steps toward the door can sometimes feel horrible. Necessary, but horrible.

Forgiving Yourself

Every once in a while we say or do something so stupid that even friends talk about having us committed. This can be particularly devastating when it results in the loss of friendship or love.

The best thing you can do in these situations is to figure out how and why you messed up. Then do what you can to mourn the loss and get on with your life. While there is much to be gained from introspection, there is little to be gained from beating yourself up. On the other hand, if you suffer from a perpetual case of foot-in-mouth, it is possible that there is a chronic confusion or anger in the depths of your soul that prevent you from using good sense. In that case, the input of a respected friend, teacher, colleague, relative or therapist might be an important thing to seek.

Stupid Mistakes—Young vs. Old

If anyone ever tells you that making stupid mistakes is from being young and will pass as you get older, don't make the really stupid mistake of believing them.

True, you usually don't make as many mistakes as you get older, but that's only because your brain doesn't work nearly as fast. As your brain slows down, you simply don't have the opportunity to make mistakes with the same lightning speed that you once did.

The Fantasy of Love & Commitment

When you feel particularly empty inside, it's easy to have the illusion that things will be better if you can just find someone to love.

Love is a special way of sharing friendship that can bring tremendous joy. It allows you to think and worry about someone other than yourself, which can be a much-needed relief. It also lets you know that there is someone who believes in you when you don't believe in yourself. But in spite of all its pluses, it's unlikely that love will take away your fears and insecurities, organize your chaos, cure your bad habits, help you to lose weight, stop smoking, get in shape, or turn you into a better human being—not in the long run anyway. Our personal demons are things we usually need to conquer on our own.

The Dark Side — Nights of Quiet Despair

Sometimes you get hit by a certain mood, one that's a quiet mix of frustration, hopelessness and despair. It's when something deep inside you isn't working right, something incredibly human, but you can't put a finger on it.

Sometimes it becomes a contest between you, the despair and the beer, pills, sleep, food, sex or whatever it is that helps make you feel better. Presidents' wives tell you to just say no, the disc jockey on the all-night radio station never plays the song you need, and a river of pain cuts your heart in two.

Nights of quiet despair sometimes go away by morning.

———————

Dear Paul,

Ever since I graduated from college my sex life has taken a big nose dive. I have had sexual intercourse ONCE between then and today! I had a healthy sex life in high school complete with true love and several short-term physical relationships. That was when I wasn't even an adult. Now I am almost 30, and for most of my 20s my sex life has been NO life at all. I am not at all physically unattractive, although I am somewhat shy and keep very busy. I think my problem is not meeting women. I dislike bars. I do not feel my sex life is representative of a mature, healthy adult male, and the lack of physical intimacy bothers me considerably. Both of my house mates have the same problem, and I know many other guys do. Paul, what is up with this problem, and besides offering your own suggestions, can you direct me to some resources that might help me locate and meet available women?   *Blue in Boulder*

Dear Blue,

Regarding your question about helping you to locate and meet available women, we have chapters on Internet dating, hooking up, and free chapters at www.GuideToGettingItOn.com on dating single parents and sex with someone at work. As for the other matters you listed, here's my personal take.

High school and college may not fill our lives with happiness and bliss, but they do provide an important social safety net. I can remember my own horror at finally having to leave college. I hadn't gotten into medical school, I didn't feel like doing grad work, and my girlfriend had just given me the boot. I didn't know it was possible to feel so awful. I got a job waiting tables—which is the equivalent of leaving school but not really. I wrote and floundered for a couple of years until I finally went back to graduate school when I was about your age. I didn't get laid much during that time. I also made the huge mistake of doing what you are doing—trying to find ways of meeting women. There is no shortage of books on that subject. But I'm not so sure they will help, and I don't know if they are what you need. In fact, I strongly encourage you to do something else with your time than focusing on how to meet women.

Please take a moment to imagine that you only have a couple of hours to live. I am willing to bet that even if you had been a stud lover and had created wet spots on mattresses all over Boulder, memories of your love life wouldn't bring you tremendous amounts of solace in the face of death. I don't think it's sex that would make you feel like your life had been worthwhile. What's more important are the contributions that you've hopefully made in life.

For instance, if you had volunteered in a program where you helped people learn to read, or helped make your community a better place, you would have something to look back on with pride, not that being good in bed doesn't help a community be a better place. Or what if you helped build a park or coached a soccer team—hmmm, not that an affair with a bored soccer mom wouldn't do you both a world of good. Still, what I'm saying is there are more important things to do with your energies than sex, and if sex isn't in the cards, try to turn your focus elsewhere.

So instead of wasting your time trying to find a bed partner, why not do things that will make you a better person? Please, don't think I am suggesting that you take part in altruistic events as a thinly disguised sham for meeting women. There is nothing more obnoxious than people who volunteer for things with the ulterior motive of trying to find love or sex.

Improve yourself, and maybe love will come. Maybe it won't. But it seems that people who are vitally involved in life tend to have an energy that attracts others. This is not as true for people who spend their evenings in front of a TV set or who think mostly of themselves from morning to night.

Not to overdo the death thing, but the best advice I ever received after the age of thirty had nothing to do with sex. It was just three words: "Grow or die." It's something I remind myself of often, especially when the couch potato in me threatens to take over.

Counterpoint I can't tell you how many dying people I've heard from who have begged to differ—not about the solace that living a meaningful life can offer, but about their thoughts as the end was approaching. For instance, I received an e-mail from a dying man who said the thing he was enjoying most in his waning moments was his memories of sex. And I received this:

> "I'm a 58-year-old widower who was married to a supernova of a wife for 25 years. I was a horrifically shy young man. She was the second woman I'd been with. As she was leaving life with stunning poise and bravery, one of the aspects of her life that she specifically named as being valuable and memorable was our love life, so don't be so sure about how inconsequential this is."

I stand corrected if I implied that a good sex life isn't important or valuable. But in the absence of one, I think it's best to use your energies to improve yourself and your community. Who knows what that will bring you or where it will take you, but it's more constructive than focusing on how to get laid.

Dating a Single Parent

There is an amazing pool of women to date that some guys don't realize exist. However, these women come with strings attached besides the ones on the ends of their IUDs—they are called kids.

While plenty of single moms are only interested in long-term relationships, others will say it's the last thing they want. Having a trustworthy guy to meet for sex and conversation every couple of weeks could more than fill some single mom's bills.

While a man who dates a woman without children should be aware of things like restaurants, movies and condoms, a man who dates a single mom needs to know about babysitters. No babysitter, no date, unless it's a family date or the kids are at their dad's. So learn about baby sitters.

The first words out of your mouth after a single mom agrees to go out with you should be, "Can I help pay for the sitter?" and "This isn't the time for me to be meeting your kids, but I can pick up a pizza for them."

The next thing you need to know when dating a single mom is how kids can suddenly spike temperatures or start throwing up, especially when they don't want their mom to go out. And you won't believe the nasty array of colds, coughs and flus that kids bring home from school. So you will need to have the patience of Job, and a strong hand that you can go home to jerk off with. No matter how important you might be in a woman's life, you are not going to come between her and her kid's viruses. And if you do, then you might wonder about her character and take heed.

Until you've been dating for a while, think twice about getting super-expensive tickets for events. It will just make her feel like crap if she has to cancel at the last minute, and it will bother you more than if the casualty were only dinner and a movie. If she suddenly has to cancel because of Junior's croop, you won't be anybody's chump if you leave a bouquet of flowers at the door with a note saying how much you look forward to seeing her soon. Yes, some women are flakes and will use their children as an excuse, but you'll be onto that soon enough. Plenty of women without kids are flakes as well.

Do not try or expect to meet her kids for a long time. It's not fair to them if they become attached to you and you suddenly end up out of the picture. But you can still help. If time and money are in short supply, ask about the things her kids like to eat. The 12-box carton of Mac'n'Cheese and frozen chicken-pot-pies from Costco might be calling. At the end of a date, ask if she needs to stop by the grocery store on the way home. If that's the last thing she wants to be reminded of when she's out with you, she'll let you know. If you do meet the kids, don't go sticking your tongue down their mom's throat when they are around. Don't try to buy them off with gifts. Your friendship and concern about them is more than enough. Do introduce yourself as one of their mom's friends, but nothing else. From their experience in school, they will understand that some friends stick around, and others move away. And if the two of you start having sex, keep in mind that you'll need to become logistical wizards. It's that way when kids are around. And don't assume she remembered birth control just because she is a mom.

We have an entire chapter on *Sex with a Single Parent* available for free at
www.GuideToGettingitOn.com

46

Rape & Abuse
Good Sex after Bad

Some kinds of sex are wicked. Some kinds are evil. That's what this chapter is about. This chapter looks at the aftermath of rape and abuse, with an eye on learning to have good sex after bad. The information it provides is a small drop in a large and sometimes difficult bucket. There is no shortage of information for people who have been raped or abused, and hopefully you will seek it out. Some is recommended in the pages that follow.

While sexual assault is not unique, you are. What works for someone else might not work for you. Be diligent in finding information that is helpful, and be cautious when self-described experts tell you what you should do instead of giving you a wide platter to choose from.

The first part of this chapter assumes that the person who experienced the assault or abuse is female and that the perpetrator is male. That's how it usually is, but not always. The last part of the chapter is for straight guys who have been raped by other men, although gay men get raped as well. If your abuser was a woman, or if your situation is not described here, rest assured you can find plenty of material on it with the right search terms.

Rape Versus Abuse

Rape and abuse are often lumped together, as if the experiences are the same because they are both violent sex crimes. Depending on who you are and what happened, this may or may not be true. Let's consider two women whose only similarity in life is that both had sex forced on them.

The first woman grew up in a safe and loving home. Her parents were there for her from day one. The men she chose for lovers were respectful and decent. The chemistry in her relationships wasn't always the best, but the problem was not because the men lacked character or concern. In times of stress and tumult, this woman's family was a resource she could fall back on. When she was raped at age 24, her family and friends circled the wagons and stood by her. When she was trying to rebuild her sex life after the assault, she had the memory of many satisfying nights with loving men to help her recall that sex could be wonderful as well as wicked.

The second woman had a very different family and childhood. The man her mom remarried sexually abused her from the time she was 8. When her grades began to drop and she started to become isolated at school, her mom conveniently chalked it up to "growing pains." Signs that a less-chaotic parent would have picked up on in a minute went ignored. While the house was well-maintained and she was fed, clothed and clean, home was never a safe place. As the little girl grew into a young woman, her choice of sexual partners reflected the chaos she grew up in.

Mind you, there are plenty of women who are raped who had horrible childhoods, and there are plenty of women from wonderful families whose only childhood blight was their sexual abuse. But in telling about these two very different women, it might give you a sense that the challenges that sexual-assault victims face are not the same. For the second woman, the abuse and emotional abandonment is a part of the mortar that binds her entire psyche. She has no memories of sex being wonderful and loving to fall back on. That is very different from the other woman's psychological challenge, which is to deal with the kinds of issues that one might address after a terrorist attack.

There is also no way of predicting which victims of abuse or rape will have sexual and relationship issues. Some of it has to do with a person's temperament and constitution. It might also have to do with whether she had something good that she could hold onto in her mind.

Sexual Confusion in a House of Abuse

For some women who endured childhood abuse, the times they were abused might have been the only times they were treated with tenderness. Talk about confusing! Even more difficult are situations in which the girl's own mother was jealous of her, as if she were competition for the woman's husband or boyfriend.

We live in a culture where sex is used to influence and control others. Imagine if you grew up in a twisted household where you got treated better for being "daddy's favorite" and your mom was jealous? The idea of having sex for intimacy and enjoyment would be as foreign as wearing a burka would be for a girl who grew up in a beach town with a closetful of bikinis.

Non-abused sons who grow up in situations where a girl is being abused can find it just as difficult to process the twistedness that is unfolding around them. Some are isolated and depressed. Others grow up finding it a challenge to respect the sexual rights and emotions of others.

Learning to Have Good Sex After Bad

Women who have been raped or sexually abused sometimes report that their bodies are betraying them. Perhaps it's just that their bodies are trying to protect them, and the nerves and muscles beneath their skin have no way of knowing that the danger has passed.

For instance, think of what happens in your body when the man of your dreams is tenderly kissing the sides of your neck. As you are becoming sexually aroused, your heart beats faster, you breathe more quickly, and your skin starts to perspire. You might not be consciously aware of it, but your hearing and vision also become more acute.

A woman with no experience of abuse might experience these body sensations as a sign of the good things to come. But for a woman who has been sexually assaulted or abused, her body is apt to confuse these signs with danger. Far from trying to betray her, her body is most likely trying to protect her. Like the Japanese soldiers on remote islands during World War II who were never told that the war was over, her nerves and muscles are still preparing for combat rather than for relaxation and pleasure. The retraining process can be slow. So one of the first things a woman might do is to become aware of sexually-charged situations that cause her body tone to go from "Oh boy!" to "Yikes!" or those that make her feel numb or disassociated.

For one woman, the trigger might be a quick, admiring glance from a man in a restaurant. Another woman's body might be totally into having sex until she feels her lover's penis on her outer labia.

As a woman begins to recognize these triggers, she can take any number of actions. One woman might find it helpful to stay with the bad feeling and observe how it unfolds within her. Another might remind herself the situation isn't the dangerous one that her body is confusing it with. If it happens during lovemaking, she and her partner might have a signal so they change positions or automatically stop. A woman might find it important if her lover says something to her, or maybe they switch on a light so she can physically see his face in addition to hearing the sound of his voice. It might also be helpful for her to have environmental cues going on from the start of their lovemaking, such as certain music or a particular light, or having a special object that she can feel or grasp—a good transitional object that helps her feel safe enough to stay in the here and now.

> "Initially, my now-husband had to learn how to stop and comfort me
> when I had flashbacks during sex. Thankfully those no longer occur.
> I really need to have music on, or something to concentrate on that
> adds to the sex. If it is silent, or we have relaxing sex without music
> or awesome satin sheets or something that provides other sensa-
> tions, then I will have a lot of trouble not disassociating."
>
> *female age 27*

Masturbation to the Rescue

For some women who have been sexually abused or assaulted, masturbation can provide an important bridge to healthy sexual enjoyment. When she masturbates, she can retrain her body to associate a good sexual outcome with the increased breathing and faster heart beat.

For a woman who has never had a good sexual experience, masturbation can be the first step in learning how good sex can feel. For a woman who has had good sex in the past, it can be a safe way for her to remember how good it used to feel.

If she has a trusting, loving relationship with a partner, it might be a huge step for a woman to pleasure herself while he holds her. Hopefully, he can understand just how big of a step this can be for her, and not to feel like she's rejecting him because the site of his hard penis throws her into a panic. All things in good time.

Her partner will also need to be comfortable with masturbation himself, as there might be times when she suddenly needs to put the brakes on during lovemaking. While this might be her need, it could be cruel and unusual punishment for him. He needs to have the option of getting himself off by hand. Hopefully, they can talk about this, and she can appreciate and respect his need to get off, and he can appreciate and respect her sudden need for space.

> "Masturbation had lost a lot of its fun. Isn't that terribly sad? I'm
> finding it again now, and it makes me proud of myself.
>
> *female age 27*

"I was a frequent masturbator before the rape, but for a while after I didn't really want any sexual things at all. But masturbating helped me to start enjoying my body again." *female age 19*

[After being raped at age 12] "I was 14 and my older friend was telling me about how she could have orgasms in the shower. I tried it, and the experience was so amazing and so all-my-own that I began to feel a lot better about what sex and sexuality should be."

female age 18

"Fantasy men were always nice to me—patient, kind, concerned about me, etc. Not like in real life. In a weird way, it taught me what and who to look for in real life." *female age 30*

What Some Women Have Found Helpful

There isn't a right way or a wrong way to have sex after you have been raped. There are many different options, and only you can decide what's right for you. Here are some things that other women have found to be helpful:

Setting Limits & Feeling Safe: If the places and situations where you used to date and have sex no longer feel safe, see if it helps to treat yourself like the nervous parents of an attractive and sweet 15-year-old. Set the kinds of limits you would for yourself that they would for her. Should you be home by 10 or midnight? What about only double-dating with a trusted friend? Don't go to a party without a friend. If you are in a social situation and start to feel unsafe, don't stick around. Go home. If a guy you like asks you to have a beer, there's no reason why you can't say, "No, but brunch on Sunday would be really nice. I know this fun (and really crowded…) restaurant." Decide ahead of time how much physical contact you are going to allow—a handshake, a kiss, a feel above the waist, a feel below?

Note As the women of the Seattle Institute for Sex Therapy so aptly note, if you discover that you are exclusively selecting men to date who you feel safe with, but who you don't feel sexually attracted to, or it's been a long time and you're still not able to get as sexually excited as you used to, it might be a good idea to seek some counseling.

Re-Virginization OK, it was bad enough being a virgin the first time, but now you're just as nervous all over again…. If you are planning on having sex with a guy and think you might need to stop groping each other midway, or will be needing special reassurance, then it's probably best to tell him that you had been sexually assaulted. Otherwise, he might rightfully think you are kind of strange. Most guys will be very understanding and try to help in any way they can, especially once you have given them permission to be something less than he-men. It's perfectly fine to say, "The old me might have been pulling your pants off by now, but with the new me, it could be a couple of months before you even get to feel under my bra. I have no idea how it's going to go, but I need to be able to totally trust that if I say stop, you'll stop at that very moment."

You should also warn him that you might have days when you can't get enough of him sexually and other days when you are certain that aliens have given you the sexual sensibilities of a 90-year-old nun.

On those days when you need to send him off to the bathroom with a stack of porn, let him know that it still might be really important that the two of you do something romantic together, like taking a walk, or going to the bookstore or movies, or flying a kite, or doing any number of things together that couples like to do. And on those days when you need physical contact but need him to keep the snake in his pants, talk to him about cuddling together, holding hands, or exchanging back or foot rubs. If it's not too much for him or you, a warm bath together or dip in a hot tub might feel great.

No matter how passive you might have been before being sexually assaulted, you now need to call the shots, each and every one of them. Perhaps it's something you will keep doing, as one of the few helpful lessons you learned from an education that you paid way too much to get.

If You Have a Partner Your partner isn't the man who raped you, but he can be almost as affected by the rape as you are. First is the little matter that he might try to kill the rapist. That's to be expected when someone intentionally harms a loved one. And then there's the possible "guilt by association" that he might have to deal with from you, by virtue of the fact that he has something similar between his legs as the rapist. Even though you know he wasn't the one who harmed you nor would he ever want to, he is a guy, and guys might not be at the top of your most-favored-sex list right now. He will need to be aware that for some women, it might take months before sex returns to normal. For others, things will return to normal much sooner. You can't predict, and you can't tell. Hopefully, he will read all he can and educate himself as much as possible about the kinds of reactions that victims of sexual assault can have, and learn how to be an ally of the healing process. Patience will have its rewards.

Flashbacks Some women who have been sexually assaulted have flashbacks; others don't. You and your partner need to be aware that flashbacks sometimes happen when you are at the peak of sexual excitement and are orgasming left and right. Your partner needs to understand that flashbacks are not because of anything he is doing that's wrong. Learn about the things that trigger flashbacks and come up with a strategy for dealing with them. Have faith that they will decrease with time.

Recommended Treatment Resources

A book that many therapists and researchers highly recommend is Judith Herman's *Trauma and Recovery* from Basic Books, (1997). For therapists, there's Courtois and Ford's *Treating Complex Traumatic Stress Disorders: An Evidence-Based Guide* from The Guilford Press, (2009).

As for treatment modalities, the two that currently have the highest chances of success are those based on Edna Foa's *exposure techniques* and Patricia Resick's *cognitive-processing therapy.* If you can find a therapist who specializes in one of these treatment modalities, you will be receiving the best methodology that is currently available.

Don't Confuse the Female Body's Protective Mechanism with Being Turned On

Researchers have discovered that there is a difference between what makes a vagina lubricate and what turns a woman on mentally. It is not unusual for a woman's vagina to lubricate in situations where she is frightened or terrified. This will protect her vagina from tearing if intercourse is forced upon her.

This primitive reflex can be very confusing for a woman who has had sex forced on her. For instance, if she had an orgasm while being raped, she might wonder if she has a secret thing for violence and somehow invited the rape. She should understand that other women who have been raped have had orgasms, and those orgasms are the product of a body in terror that's spewing out a flood of adrenalin while physical pressure is being put on her genitals. This kind of reaction is not limited to women. Erections are no stranger to the gallows. It's been known for many centuries that men who are executed by hanging often die with erections, and some even ejaculate. While this may have something to do with the body's response to asphyxiation, terror also plays a role in it. These men were no more sexually turned-on by being in the gallows than is a woman in a violent situation in which sex is being forced on her.

Ways to Help Prevent Rape

Before you read about ways to prevent rape, keep in mind that women who have been raped sometimes go overboard in trying to avoid situations that cause them anxiety. The problem with this is that avoidance merely reinforces anxiety and stress disorders.

So it is important for those who have been raped to conquer the temptation to avoid too much. The key is in using your good sense.

Common-sense ways to prevent rape include not jogging or walking alone, especially at night. Never hitchhike or pick up a hitchhiker. Lock your doors and windows, even if you are going away for a brief time, and do not open your door unless you are certain you know who is knocking or ringing the doorbell. Don't lend your keys to anyone, and do not put your name or address on your keys. Avoid being alone in underground garages, apartment laundry rooms, or offices after hours. Park in areas that are well-lit, and lock your car doors even if it's a quick stop. Lock your doors when you drive, and try not to drive with less than a quarter of a tank of gas.

At parties, open drinks yourself, avoid the punch bowl, don't accept drinks from anyone else or share them, and don't leave drinks out of your eyesight. Even more importantly, never get drunk or stoned outside of the safety of your own home or that of your sexual partner's.

Predator Strategy

According to interviews with incarcerated rapists, they do not pick a victim based on how she looks or how she is dressed. The first criteria is that a predator does not want to get caught. So what he is looking for is a highly vulnerable victim. Can he easily isolate her from others? Can he commit his crime without her noises drawing the attention of others?

Sexual predators—those who often target children—are good con artists. They usually have a well-honed sociopathic personality that gets victims to suspend their sense of suspicion. They seem to know just what to say that makes you feel good. They can often smell loneliness and the need for attention and approval. They excel at flattery.

The sex offender's goal is to find ways to control a victim. He is good at getting women to engage in light forms of romance or sex play, not so much at their invitation, but in a way that she doesn't think to scream "STOP IT!" He manages to take her off-guard, doing things that feel good enough so she gets confused. Then, after it's too late, he's got her. He has managed to physically isolate her and emotionally confuse her. She is suddenly wondering, "Did I invite this?" If she didn't put a stop to it immediately, she is pretty much a goner. He will have invaded her personal space and personal boundaries, and then there's no stopping him.

After committing his crime, his next goal is to not get caught. If you are a friend or acquaintance, he might try to catch you up in the confusion of whether you invited the assault, until you start thinking, "I shouldn't have let him start fooling around with me." Depending on the situation, he might also be able to control you with bribery or threats. And if you are child, he might act convincingly that nothing really happened. You end up distorting your own awareness of what went on.

Date or Acquaintance Rape

An agreement to kiss is not an agreement to have intercourse. It never has been. Fucking requires a separate level of consent than making-out. Likewise, feeling each other up and finding a vagina to be wet is not consent to put a penis in it.

Until the last twenty years, people thought of rape as something that was committed by a stranger who lurked in the shadows or pried a woman's bedroom window open. No one used to think of it as something your date did after you agreed to go upstairs to his bedroom and didn't push him away when he started making out with you. But as researchers interviewed more and more women, they started hearing accounts of when men would not stop in spite of the woman's protests.

Unfortunately, in the hands of some researchers with their bizarrely worded surveys, frightening "statistics" were generated that made every male who ever had an erection in a woman's presence look like a perpetrator of date rape. This over-zealousness on the part of researchers cast a shadow where no shadow should have been cast.

There are men who are adept at engaging women in kissing or petting, and then raping them in the same manner as "traditional" rapists who lurk in corners. Men like these can come from wealthy families who are on the social A-lists. They can be sports heroes, or divinity students at a Bible college.

The emotional impact of date rape can be every bit as great as if a woman were raped by a stranger. To help prevent date rape, the courts have had to push the limits of what consent is into a somewhat artificial and awkward place. Until we find a better solution, the new definition of consent will be the law of the land.

The onus of stopping sexplay now rests on the male the moment a woman says, "Stop!" or "Maybe I should go" or "This doesn't feel good." She may have agreed to have intercourse, but if she changes her mind after 300 thrusts, the man had better pull out on thrust number 301 as opposed to number 306.

Males who do not take this seriously should read the recent decision for the State of California Supreme Court called *People v. John Z.* In that case, a woman had agreed to have intercourse, but at some point during the intercourse, she indicated that she might want to go. She didn't say "Stop" or "I don't want to keep doing this." The court found that she was raped because the man did not stop the moment she indicated a change of heart, or change of pelvis. Interestingly, it was a female member of the court who dissented.

Making sure that a woman is legally able to consent to sex is now the job of the male, and it is very different from what you might think. For instance, even if a woman bought the first two rounds of drinks or brought the pot and rolled the joints, she is not legally able to consent to sex if she has been drinking or smoking. This can be true even if she's the one who went down on the guy until he got hard and she put his dick in herself.

Also, it doesn't matter if both of you were equally drunk or stoned: this does not excuse the male from the burden of realizing that a woman who has been drinking or smoking cannot legally consent to sex. Just the fact that she has been drinking before intercourse makes it sexual assault in some states. Also, it is not legal in many situations to have sex with a woman if you are her boss, her teacher, her minister, her physician or her coach.

Do not assume a woman is playing a game when she hesitates or says "No." And never, ever try to win her over with pressure or persuasiveness. The courts have made it clear that this will not be tolerated.

In the absence of a woman making it completely clear that she wants sex, a man needs to assume that sex is neither desired nor is it legal.

If You Have Been Raped—the First Hours After

The thing you don't want to do is to disturb any of the evidence, and unfortunately, the evidence is on you and in you. Much as you might want to, do not shower, douche, wash your hands, change your clothes, drink anything or even brush your teeth. Saliva can be used to identify a rapist as well as his semen. Try not to pee. If you think you might have been drugged and you have to urinate, do so in a bottle and take it with you to the hospital. Be sure to tell the doctor about any suspicions of being drugged. The way they find out if you have been drugged is through testing your urine, and some drugs pass through your system quickly. (In some states, the threshold of evidence is lower if it is discovered that the victim was drugged.)

If you are a minor, you don't need to have a parent's permission to have a "rape kit" done at the hospital. So there's no reason to fear going to the hospital if you've been doing something that would make your parents want to kill you.

You should take extra clothing that you can change into after they have collected all the evidence at the hospital.

If you can, ask a friend to go with you or to meet you at the hospital. If you live in a dorm, ask a resident advisor to go with you as well. It's OK if the friend stays with you during the exam and during your entire hospital visit. Your friend will be able to be your ears, eyes, and brain in case your own are feeling fried. And your friend will be able to be a—friend! If you or your friend has it together enough, call RAINN (800-656-HOPE). See if there is a victim advocate who can meet you at the hospital.

As a victim of a sexual assault, you have priority over just about everything other than life-threatening illnesses. So unless you see a bunch of people being wheeled in with panicked-looking doctors hovering around them, you should get in sooner than later. If a long time has gone by, ask your friend to remind the person at the desk that you are a rape victim and haven't been seen. If you prefer a doctor of your same sex, let them know. If they can, they will get you one, but it may take more time.

Going to the hospital doesn't mean you need to speak to the police or press charges. But it's essential to go to the hospital for a couple of reasons. If at some point you do decide to press charges, they will have the necessary evidence. It will be much harder otherwise. The people in the ER can give you the morning-after pill to help prevent pregnancy, and they can tend to any physical trauma. Going to the hospital right away greatly increases your chances to receive victim's services if you should need them, and in a lot of states, the state will pay for your expenses. The people in the ER should be able to explain your options and connect you with counseling and other help. It is a very, very good idea to visit a hospital emergency room right away. There are virtually no downsides. As with a car accident, you have no idea of the kinds of emotional or physical trauma that might present itself in a couple of days or weeks. Having everything on record at the ER will make it easier for you to get free services if you should need them in the future.

How People Act after Being Raped

There is no manual for how to act after a sexual assault. Some people will be hysterical while others will be unusually calm. Some will be agitated, others will be numb. It is unwise to judge a person's emotional experience of a sexual assault based on their behavior following it.

Rape in Marriage

People have the idea that rape in a marriage isn't really rape, and it's less serious than if the sexual assault is caused by a stranger. But given all the baggage and history of a married couple, it makes sense that spousal rape might be even more devastating than stranger rape. After all, the stranger never said, "To have and to hold, to love and to cherish, till death do us part."

Women who are raped by their husbands are likely to be raped a number of times before finally leaving. The rape can be oral, anal and vaginal. Dealing with it can be a particular challenge when the wife lives with the rapist.

Further Humiliation

Some rapists will force their victims to pretend they are enjoying the rape. Rape experts indicate that it's is a good idea to go along with the rapist on this one if he is so inclined. It seems that if the rapist is unable to complete the act, he is more apt to seriously injure his victim, and think of how seriously imbalanced he is mentally if he wants you to pretend you are enjoying it.

Whether to Report—If It's Child Abuse

While it is very important if a child who is being abused can find a trusting teacher, counselor, minister or parent to tell, it's an unfortunate comment on our society to say that reporting doesn't always improve the situation. For some girls, it makes it worse, as dysfunctional families will often try to make her the problem. There is also the reality that while some state protective-services agencies are top-notch, others are as dysfunctional as the families they are supposed to be protecting children from. Between failures of the criminal-justice system and an overwhelmed social-services system, good outcomes are sometimes the exception rather than the rule.

If you are an adult who suspects a child is being abused, you are often legally required to report to your nearest child-protective-services agency.

Unfortunately, you wouldn't believe the number of grandparents and relatives who suspect abuse is occurring, but don't report it, and not because they are concerned about how well the system will or won't work. They will be the first to tell you what a shame it is the child is being abused, but blood is thicker than sperm. They wouldn't want to upset the family.

Equally disturbing are the number of divorces where one angry parent accuses the other parent of abuse out of revenge. If they are so sure the other parent was abusing the child, why didn't they say something about it before the divorce? This shouldn't be confused with situations where the divorce came as a result of learning that a child was being abused.

Whether to Report—If You Are an Adult and It's Rape

It's no secret that few rapes are actually reported, and that the percentage of reports is even lower in the nearly two-thirds of all rapes where the victim knew the offender prior to the sexual assault.

There are reasons why women don't report. A very common one is if the rapist is an important member of your social circle or your mother's favorite cousin. Or if he's your sister's husband or a popular guy at work or school.

Aside from social realities, it's hard to talk about a sexual assault. Other reasons for not reporting include fears that you won't be believed, fears that you will be blamed, and fears that the accused will somehow retaliate.

Some women believe that if they didn't put up a fight, the state won't consider it rape. This is not true. Not fighting may have been the best way to prevent further injury or death. The fact that you are still alive indicates that you did the smartest thing that you could have. While fighting may have stopped the rape, it could have just as easily ended up in your being killed or seriously injured beyond any sexual trauma.

So why should you report? There are three very good reasons:

1. Rapists tend to be bullies who may see your failure to report as an indication that you liked what they did, or that you are an easy mark for a repeat offense. Reporting a rapist tends to protect you from re-assault rather than putting you in harm's way.

2. One of the greatest regrets among women who don't report is knowing that their lack of action may have made it possible for the rapist to sexually assault other women. This fact, even more than the rape itself, is what haunts some women the most.

3. Even if the man is not convicted, your report puts him in law-enforcement radar. It makes it much less likely that he will get away with it the next time. Even if he is not convicted, your reporting is what might save his potential victims.

Reporting—If He's In Your Social Circle

Reporting is socially easier if the rapist isn't part of your social circle. If he is, be prepared for people taking sides, and not necessarily yours. On the other hand, if you don't report, he will know you are an easy target, and you will have to live with letting him get away with it and with victimizing others.

Don't waste time trying to warn him or threaten him. Your actions in not reporting him are all he will hear.

If you have reported someone from your social circle, it's probably best not to discuss it. Don't try to defend yourself or to say anything negative about him. Technically, the only people you should be speaking to about it are the police, the DA and your healthcare provider or counselor if you have one. Keeping these boundaries will probably make it easier for you in the long run.

Reporting—If You Are in a Sorority

Hopefully things in the Greek system have evolved and justice is more important than keeping quiet to maintain the social order. But understand that if you were raped and report a fraternity member to the police, his house brothers will likely feel that you have reported them—all of them. And that sorority sister of yours who had a secret crush on the guy? Get ready to meet your new worst enemy.

You won't read this advice in the "Welcome To Our Wonderful College!" booklets, but if you've been raped by a fraternity bro and decide to report him, get thee to the psych library and read about what happens in dysfunctional families when a child reports that she's been abused. Knowing how strange it can get will help you maintain a sense of irony and perspective that could be necessary if a psychodrama were to unfold around you. People join fraternal organizations with the hope of being a part of something that's bigger and better than they are. In accusing a fraternity man of rape, you are not only threatening the relationship between your sorority and his fraternity, you are taking to task the very system that has been the spawning ground of presidents, senators and supreme-court justices.

Does this mean you shouldn't report? Heck no. But it does mean that you will be standing out as an individual in an organization that is not exactly the Walden Pond of free thinking. The priority of some sorority sisters is to party with boys with pedigrees. They are as likely to see you, rather than a fraternity man who takes uninvited liberties with his dick, as the problem.

If you are in a sorority and you report a fraternity boy for rape, or if you are in any tightly-knit organization and report a fellow member, be prepared to move out and move on. But think about it—in a world where people are tortured and killed for speaking the truth, is it such a huge price to pay for doing the right thing? Is it such a huge price to pay for helping to protect other women this person might victimize throughout his life, because that's who will suffer if there is no price to pay for sex that is forced. In the long run, wouldn't you rather be known as a woman not to mess with, rather than as an easy target for forced sex?

If you are raped by a fraternity member and your sorority sisters stand by you, understand that you have found something that is truly precious.

When Straight Men are Raped by other Men

Most of us believe that rape happens to only women and gay or imprisoned men. We assume that any man who doesn't want to be sexually assaulted is able to defend himself and fend off the attacker. But just because you are a guy, it doesn't mean you should be able to win a barroom fight, thrash a mugger or fend off a rapist.

Rape is first and foremost about violence, power, sadism and hatred. The rapist didn't choose you because he thought you had a cute butt. He chose you because he thought he could.

When you've got a gun to your head or a knife to your throat, you suddenly have other priorities than saying, "Excuse me, Mr. Rapist, you've got it all wrong. I like girls!" Your job is to survive, and even if that means having to go down on the guy, you should do it and not think twice. Think of how many girls have done it for you—and hopefully lived.

In addition to being blind-sided with a lethal weapon, a man can be sexually assaulted by a group of men he doesn't stand a chance against. Sometimes the rape can be the result of blackmail or of being drunk or stoned. The last thing a guy who is drunk is going to be able to protect is his rear end.

Male rape can happen in other ways, as well. Not too long ago, a former National Hockey League Player revealed that he was sexually assaulted by one of his coaches when he was a teen.

Unfortunately, a man who has been raped has fewer options than even a woman who has been raped. Think about it: how many guys are going to find it cathartic to tell their friends they were raped? Sad but true, the chances are good his drinking buds will be doing all they can to keep from giggling.

If you are a guy who has been raped, call a rape-crisis center or, even if you are the epitome of straightness, consider calling a gay-men's health center. They tend to be understanding and helpful about sexual violence against men. The advice they give you will most likely be the best to follow.

One thing that can be really confusing is if you became hard or came when you were raped. The truth is, it is not unusual to have an erection and orgasm when the body is under extreme stress or panic. As mentioned earlier in this chapter, plenty of guys who go to the gallows meet their maker with an erection and ejaculate in their pants, and not because they thought it was sexy to have a noose around their neck.

Some rapists are aware that you might get an erection. They will intentionally stroke you to orgasm just to mess with your mind even more. So what's the big deal if you did get hard and came? The important thing is in understanding that you were violently assaulted. We should all have erections and orgasms in such situations. At least you lived to think about it, which is a very good thing.

Men who are bisexual or gay sometimes worry that being raped or abused is what gave them their same-sex orientation. Or if you know a straight guy who was sexually assaulted by another male, you might wonder if this will impact his sexual orientation. Studies have never shown that sexual abuse or rape influences a person's sexual orientation, yet this is a myth that persists.

While you might want to keep it all inside, it could be that the rape has been causing you to deal with others–especially intimate others–in strange ways. What do you have to lose by speaking to a counselor about it for a session or two?

As for reporting, the big issue is how strongly you feel about the guy being able to do this to other men, because it is likely that he will if he can.

Resources:

National Center for Victims of Crime
(800) 394-2255

Rape, Abuse, and Incest National Network
(800) 656-4673   (800) 656-HOPE

National Domestic Violence Hotline
(800) 799-SAFE

Your state or county may have excellent resources as well.

Judith Herman's *Trauma and Recovery* from Basic Books, 1997.

Therapy treatment based on Edna Foa's *exposure techniques* and Patricia Resick's *cognitive processing therapy*.

A Very Special Thanks to Alessandra Rellini from at the University of Texas at Austin, and now Yale University. And to Cindy Meston for finding her!

Readers Speak

"I was seriously dating one guy for four years (I was 16 when it started). Over time he became more and more thoughtless during sex until the point where it had crossed the line into violence. If sex was painful he would not stop, and there was emotional violence. We started out using porn to enhance our sex lives, but after a while he would position us so he could ignore me during sex and just watch the screen.

"I did two years of being single without sex after that to pull myself together. When I began having sex again I had flashbacks and would panic. I used to be so sexually outgoing and playful. I would enjoy oral sex. Now I don't do any of that anymore. For a long time I could not joyfully give my partners oral sex because of the negative associations with it, and sometimes I still have trouble not choking, even when it is barely in my mouth. Things are slowly improving, but I am worried it will never have that carefree way about it. It is hard to relax and not over protect myself. I've been married for a year now to a wonderful and gentle man that I've been intimate with for five years…. That's how long it's taken." *female age 27*

"I have been raped twice in my life by two separate men. The first was during my 16th birthday. After the party I went to my friend's spare bedroom to sleep. My then-boyfriend came in and lay next to me. We started fooling around but things started going too far. I asked him to stop but he didn't. He kept pressuring me, saying he wouldn't do anything serious. It ended with him just shoving himself in me while I was sobbing. That was how I lost my virginity. The saddest part is that I stayed with him for two more months.

"The second time I was at a friend's house. Drinking and playing Dungeons and Dragons. (Yes, girls are nerds too.) I drank far too much and lay down on a mattress that was sitting in the middle of the living room. All my friends went into the den to watch TV while this guy lay next to me. I should have figured it out then, but I was really drunk. I asked him to leave me because I was too drunk to be near anyone, let alone a guy with 'intentions.' He didn't leave. He started with the foreplay. I alternated between liking it and asking him to go away. It ended with him on top of me while I told him to stop. I suppose this one was partially my fault. Needless to say, the friendship ended there.

"Sex since then? I've never orgasmed. That may be due to the fact that I can't trust men. I'm never comfortable being naked around anyone. And to be completely honest, I don't really like sex. I think I'm just expecting men to mistreat me after having it. To just use me. Recently I have been in a relationship with a man who was a virgin before we had sex. His love and trust have gone a long way toward helping me believe that a guy might like me for more than just sex. It's helping me to enjoy myself more." *female age 20*

"I was continually abused growing up (emotionally, spiritually, verbally, mentally, sexually), so much so I don't remember much of it. I continued the abuse voluntarily by getting involved with men who abused me. For instance, I have two kids as a result of 3-a.m. encounters when I was three-quarters asleep. I'm still pretty badly messed up and have a hard time seeing when someone is trying to be decent. I have never had normal sex. I discovered recently (in the past two years) that what I thought was normal was far from normal. I never knew that you were supposed to have feeling inside. I thought it was normal to be numb inside. My former partner could stick any number of fingers up inside me, and I could never tell him how many there were. He could even put a whole fist inside, and I didn't know. He could scratch and wiggle–nothing, nada, zip, zero, zilch. Still have that problem. Maybe I'll figure it out someday."

female age 31

"When I was in middle school, and my body was just starting to mature, my step-dad was going through a rough time with work. He was pretty stressed. My mom was around, but she had a job as well, so obviously I was left alone with a man who I wasn't exactly fond of. He started getting a little too close and intimate for comfort. I told him I didn't like it. When he didn't stop, I told my mom. She didn't want to believe me. One night while she was out with her friends, I woke up and he was on top of me. I tried to scream. He stifled me. "It'll feel good, I promise," he told me. It didn't feel good. I screamed and flailed my body until I could get away. I ran and tried to hide. He found me and hit me so hard that I don't remember any more of that night. I was 12.

"I was ashamed of my body for a long time after that. But at the same time, I still really wanted the fellas who were my own age to take notice of me. I think I was looking for someone who would try to protect me. Eventually, I found myself in a good relationship that was much more about the emotional connection than a physical one. When we finally did get to that point, I felt so at ease with him that it was completely natural, pure and honest [and way good!]."

female age 18

"I was 9 years old. My karate instructor gave me a lesson in oral sex and other such matters. This was 32 years ago. I was not in a huge hurry to lose my *official virginity*. But then I had a great boyfriend for my *first time*, so it worked out. Get someone to talk to—a professional—and don't stop until you find one that helps you to release the pain or anger. It's not only possible; it's probable for good sex after bad IF you take it slow and find the right person. I think about sex not as something that is being done to me, but as something that I am giving to someone else." *female age 41*

"I was molested by my dad & younger brother. It took years of therapy to overcome self-destructive behavior. The abuse took a seemingly wholesome, enjoyable act, and made it ugly. I became psychotically self-destructive with sex, alternating between frigidity and promiscuity. I was able to find good therapist and a good man who loves me. I can finally breathe and trust, relax, have fun, and enjoy sex. (We're getting married later this year.)" *female age 30*

"It was seven years ago. In my room. My cousin's husband attacked me while I was sleeping. I never had sex before then. I look at sex as something that I don't need. Sometimes it just brings back the night of the bad. My advice? Take control next time. You'd be surprised at how much better it can be the next time that way! If it's happened to you, don't hesitate to tell someone else. I didn't, and I'm still paying for it. It took me four years to come to the reality of it. Don't hide anything. If you've been raped, don't think of sex as bad. Think of it as a way to better yourself." *female age 20*

"Recognize and accept what you can morally live with. If I'd had someone to turn to/talk to when I was a kid, things may have turned out differently. Now'days there are people, places, and/or Websites you can contact to help you adjust. It's not your fault. Masturbation has been the one saving grace which has helped me adjust to my sexuality." *male age 68*

"Report it right away. My biggest regret is that I never did. The man who raped me raped others. Maybe if I had said something, they would never had to experience that. And get counseling. Don't just sit there and blame yourself. Always remember it wasn't your fault, and it doesn't make YOU a bad person." *female age 20*

"When I was about 7 or 8 years old, I was masturbated by an uncle. He gave me a dollar to "not tell." I never did. I began having sex at age 13 and was quite promiscuous. I believe I've had about 50 sexual partners, but only 6 or 7 of those in the past 10 or 12 years. I now realize that my behavior probably has something to do with the experience. I've learned to forgive, and to realize that people are better than their worst moments." *female age 33*

"I can't imagine a single situation in which rushing out and boning the first willing, semi-attractive person with a pulse is a good idea to help you overcome an unfortunate sexual encounter."
female age 18

"Relax and take your time. My fiancee & I weren't exacting rockin' the first few times. I needed to build trust and security, and then I could relax and truly enjoy myself." *female age 30*

"When I was 6- to 8-years-old, my best friend's dad molested me. He would make me give him oral sex, and touch him, and he'd touch me.... I try not to make too big of a deal about it. I have good relationships with women and like to think I am a relatively emotionally stable person. You can't let yourself be a victim. However, I still have frequent dreams about him abusing me, and sometimes I have sex fantasies about him as well. These disturb me because he abused me. I was so young that I think I repressed most of the negative thoughts. All I can remember are the way things felt." *male age 21*

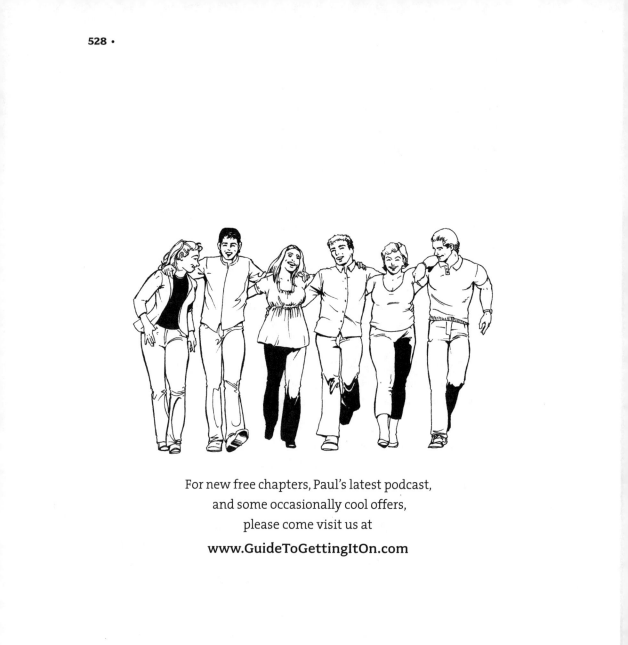

For new free chapters, Paul's latest podcast,
and some occasionally cool offers,
please come visit us at

www.GuideToGettingItOn.com

CHAPTER

47
On Needles and Pins
Piercings, Tattoos & Sex

In the first edition of *The Guide*, piercing and tattoos didn't even get a mention. In the last edition they rated three pages in the section on kink. Now they have a fairly substantial chapter of their own.

Tattoos, which used to be the hallmark of bikers and bandits, have become the body chic and new mainstream cool. Who knew that tattoos called "tramp stamps" would show up on more girls' rear ends than anchors on sailors' arms or cobwebs and tear drops in prison-yard tattoos?

A recent study in the Journal of the *American Academy of Dermatology* found that 24% of people ages 18 to 50 have tattoos and 14% have body piercings. For young adults between 18 and 25, the number of body piercings increases to between 35% and 50%, and this doesn't include pierced ears.

However, according to a large study of students at Texas Tech, Baylor, Notre Dame and Purdue, less than 2% have piercings through their nipples or genitals. So while this chapter may focus on genital piercings, please don't assume that masses of people have them or that getting one is necessarily a good idea. This chapter is in response to questions about nipple and genital piercings, but is not a recommendation to get nipple or genital piercings. We sense that if nature wanted you to have extra holes through your nipples or between your legs, she would have put them there.

Warning & Disclaimer: While this chapter discusses some of the safety and health issues surrounding piercing and tattooing, it does not provide medical information and should not be viewed as a substitute for such. In two large studies, between 17% and 45% of people pierced had resulting medical problems ranging from local tissue trauma, bleeding and bacterial infection to endocarditis and hepatitis B. Before getting a piercing, please consult the website of the Association of Piercing Professionals, and be sure to read and follow all of their safety guidelines (www.safepiercing.org). Before getting a tattoo or piercing, understand that there's not much difference between an unsterile tattoo or piercing needle and the needles that junkies use to shoot up with.

If you have diabetes, take antibiotics when you go to the dentist, or have any other health-related conditions, please consult with your healthcare provider before getting a piercing or a tattoo. Also, placing metal posts through highly innervated parts of your body such as your genitals has the potential to result in permanent nerve damage, serious infection and severe bleeding.

Keep in mind that a piercing site that is healing is an open wound and needs to be treated as such. It can easily become infected, and is a source of infection to others. Follow the instructions that the piercer or tattoo artist gives you regarding your healing site, including when you can resume having sex.

Penis Piercings and Other Male-Genital Adornments

There are no scientific studies about the effectiveness of penis piercings in increasing a man's or his partner's sexual pleasure. Those who do speak up seem to be happy with their piercings. The men often say that the piercing helps to increase their own sexual pleasure as well as that of their partners. Some men particularly like the increased feeling in their urethra when they have a piercing that goes through it, although there may be a price to pay in terms of how your pee and ejaculate comes out. Piercings might also make it even more fun when you masturbate.

Here are a few of the different penis piercings:

Prince Albert or PA: This is probably the most common penis piercing. It is where a ring is threaded through the urethra and out through the frenulum or part of the shaft where the foreskin attaches to the glans (see the illustration on the next page). It is said to heal sooner than most. Given that a man doesn't usually arrive for a penis piercing with an erection, it is important that the ring has a large enough diameter that the urethra doesn't rip when the penis gets hard. The gauge should be large enough to prevent tearing, and the ball should be big enough that it doesn't drop down the urethra if it comes undone.

Reverse Prince Albert: Same as the Prince Albert, but the ring goes through the top part of the penis glans instead of the frenulum side.

Apadravya or AP: This is a vertical piercing through the head or glans of the penis. It can run through the urethra, or avoid it by sitting higher on the head of the penis. Strangely enough, APs that go through the urethra are said to heal sooner. It seems the urine helps to clean the wound, and with the urethra in the middle, there are two smaller tunnels to heal rather than one

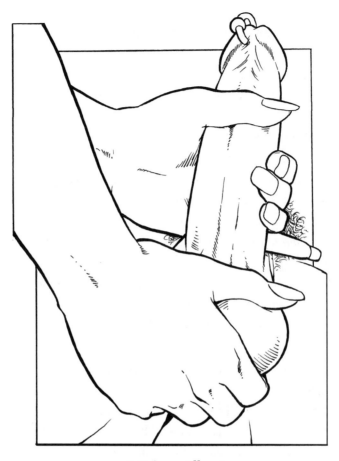

A Prince Albert

long one. If done correctly, the apadravya can be very comfortable because it has so much flesh around it. When there are problems, they usually occur because of how it impacts the corpus cavernosum of the penis.

Pallang: This is a horizontal piercing where a barbell-shaped piece of jewelry runs through the head or glans of the penis. It can go through the center of the urethra, or above it.

Magic Cross: While not nearly as popular in evangelical circles as the name might imply, the magic cross consists of a pallang and apadravya through the penis head which forms a cross. If done with one stacked on top of the other, the two bars can touch or meet inside the urethra.

Dydoe: This is where small rings or barbells are placed around the edge of the head or glans of the penis. It can hurt like hell and is prone to more problems than other kinds of piercings. If the man is not circumcised, he will need a baggy foreskin for this to work.

Infibulation: Where the foreskin is pierced in a way that jewelry connects the two sides of the foreskin to prevent intercourse or the glans from being exposed.

Frenum: When the shaft of the penis is pierced along the raphe, sometimes in a series which is called a frenum ladder.

Scrotal: Any piercing that passes through the skin of the scrotum. These piercings can be difficult to heal, given that ball bags perspire, and clothes, thighs and the penis can rub and irritate the piercing site.

Scrotal ladder: A series of piercings that are aligned to make a ladder up the scrotum.

Guiche: A piercing of the perineum, or area between the balls and bum. Can run in the direction of thigh-to-thigh, or scrotum-to-bum. Perspiration and rubbing from underwear can make this kind of piercing a bear to heal.

Beading

This is where small beads are implanted under the skin on the shaft of the penis. If a sexual partner doesn't like the feeling of studded dildos or studded condoms, it is unlikely she will jump for joy when you pull out a penis with beads under the skin. It never hurts to discuss with your partner any genital alterations that you might be considering well in advance.

Meatotomy, Genital Bisection, Penis Splitting and Subincision

These terms are body-mod speak for slicing a penis in two. Some of the most popular photos on the Body Modification Ezine (www.BME.com) are of this very modification. Perhaps it's due to disbelief rather than admiration ("We are so not in Kansas anymore!")—although you never know.

Penis Piercings and Your Partner's Pleasure

Aadravya (beads at 12:00 & 6:00) vs. the Pallang (beads at 3:00 & 9:00): With the AP, the beads at the ends of the little barbell are at the 12:00 and 6:00 position on the head of the penis. This means that the apadravya has the potential to stimulate a partner's G-spot area, assuming she has a G-spot area and likes being stimulated there with small metal balls. As for the horizontal pallang, it's hard to see how this would add to a partner's pleasure, unless she likes extra stimulation on the walls of her vagina at 3:00 & 9:00.

Ampallang Impact on a Partner's Vagina: It can take quite the cocksman to get a penis with a steel bar through its head to slide inside a vagina in a way that is comfortable for a woman. Expect a learning curve for both of you. Also expect to use a lot of lube, possibly a condom, and you'll want to make sure the bar is no longer than is absolutely necessary.

"Slowpoke" on the BME website has done a great job of reporting on the adjustments he's had to make for intercourse to work with an ampallang:

1. He uses a condom with lots of lube. The barbell does not usually tear the condom, and the condom helps his accessorized package get inside his lover's love tunnel. Experiment with whether a tight-fitting condom works better for you and your partner, or a condom with a baggy head.

2. Experiment with different kinds of jewelry to find a combination that feels best for you and your partner. A titanium barbell helps minimize the heft which can decrease cervical bruising for your partner. Also, try to decrease the length of the bar as much as possible. You don't want your penis looking like a tightrope walker carrying a balance bar.

3. Experiment with different kinds of thrusting. Slowpoke found that his girlfriend liked it best when he used shallow strokes that maximized the way the ball on the top of the barbell rubbed near her G-spot area.

4. Your partner might be nervous, which can cause the opening of her vagina to tighten. Spend as much time as she needs before you try to slide your accessorized penis into her vagina. Slowpoke tries to go in while still a bit soft. He cautions against pulling all the way out while thrusting.

5. Cleanliness afterward is important, as his AP has made him more susceptible to getting yeast infections.

Cervical Abrasion

Due to the way the cervix is innervated, the woman won't necessarily feel the surface of it being abraded by the top ball or bead of the apadravya. (There would be reasons nature made the head of the penis more like a cushion than a metal ball.) Your partner will usually know if you caused cervical abrasion by drops of blood afterward and discomfort the next day.

Showerhead Effects & Ejaculation Effects

Any piercing that intersects with the urethra can cause urine to spray out of the penis instead of come out in a stream, or in the case of a Prince Albert, the pee can cascade down the side of the jewelry. Some men are able to minimize the problem by rotating the penis 90 degrees or more when peeing. Others say a finger pushing against the lower hole can help to minimize the problem. Lord knows, you'll have plenty of opportunity to experiment and find what works best. The bottom line: If you have any kind of piercing that goes through your urethra, there is a good possibility that you'll end up needing to sit when you pee.

Your ejaculations are unlikely to paint the ceiling once a metal bar is running through your urethra. If you used to squirt, you might now ooze.

Ring Tossing

Jewelry on the end of a penis can case a diaphragm, cervical cap, or NuvaRing to dislodge (aka "ring tossing"). Fortunately, a NuvaRing is easy to take out before intercourse and to put in after. Doing so can be a fun part of your sexplay. The NuvaRing can stay out for three hours before you need to worry. If a woman who wears a NuvaRing has a partner with a penis piercing, at the very least she or he should check after intercourse to make sure it is still in place.

Chip & Swallow

Make sure that the balls on your boy's piercing jewelry are firmly attached before sucking on a penis that is accessorized. And while wearing a mouth guard is not necessarily called for, be mindful that teeth have been chipped by jewelry that's on a pierced penis. Back teeth are vulnerable as well as front.

Clitoris and Labia Piercings

Women often report that their genital piercings help them feel a greater sense of pride and ownership in their vulva. If done correctly and in synch with sexual preferences, piercings can also provide welcome sensations, as well as provide a fun frame of reference for vagina dialogues with a lover.

Girl piercings are dependent on each woman's particular anatomy. Decisions about what to put where need to be carefully coordinated with an experienced piercer who understands vulva landscapes. Jewelry with a larger gauge can provide more stimulation and is less likely to pinch or tear delicate tissues. You should also purchase the finest jewelry possible, as harmful bacteria can collect in any pittings that might be on the surface of the jewelry.

Most clitoris piercings are really clitoris-hood piercings. Here are some of the different clitoral and labia possibilities:

Vertical Clitoral Hood Piercing or VCH: This is where the piercing runs in the direction of nipples to knees and stimulates the clitoris directly. While not piercing through the clitoris, the jewelry lays on top of it and touches it directly. A woman who doesn't like her clitoris to be touched should beware, as a VCH is going to provide a lot of clitoral contact. The jewelry that goes in the piercing can be a barbell or a ring. A barbell will probably be more stimulating, as the top sits on the shaft of the clitoris while the bottom ball kisses the tip of the clitoris. **Note:** One way to see if you've got enough hood for a hood piercing is to lubricate the head of a Q-Tip and see how easily it can fit between the hood and your clitoris. The piercer will need to insert a receiving tube under the hood in order to keep the needle from skewering your clitoris. If there's not enough room or if the ring is too tight against your clitoris, consider other kinds of piercings.

Christina: This is a surface piercing that is mostly for decoration. It goes where the mons pubis joins the outer labia. It is easily rejected, does not provide sexual stimulation and can be a nightmare if you are wearing tight jeans. There needs to be some thick tissue here for this one to work, as this part of a woman's crotch often flattens out or moves with her normal range of motion. It carries with it a greater risk of infection.

Nefertiti: This piercing runs vertically under the clitoral hood from the top of the vulva where the large lips meet and exits where the clitoral hood hangs over the tip of the clitoris. Given how long the piercing is, a flexible bar made of tygon or nylon is often used, and it can take a long time to heal.

Isabella and Princess Albertina: These are dangerous piercings. Avoid them at all costs. You do not want a piercing to invade the female urethra, nor do you want to risk severing the dorsal nerve or puncturing the artery of the clitoris. Nuff said?

Horizontal Hood Piercing: A woman's clitoris and hood tend to retract when she stands, and the placement of horizontal piercings needs to take this into account. Otherwise, discomfort can occur. Placement is said to be optimal when the bead rests on the tip of the clitoris. Larger beads tend to be more stimulating. Jewelry with a thicker gauge might be preferable when a woman enjoys more pressure during intercourse. Women with a narrow pubic area or large labia or thighs that rub might not do as well with a horizontal hood piercing.

Triangle Piercing: This is where a ring is passed under the nerve bundle of the clitoris at the base of the hood. It requires an extremely experienced piercer who can locate the nerve bundle and negotiate the jewelry behind it. It can look like a sexy door knocker, assuming your clit is hung well enough to handle it. This is the only piercing that stimulates the clitoral tip from behind, and it can seriously ratchet up the sensations during intercourse. Not that many women have a clitoris that sits out far enough for a ring to be safely passed under it. A narrow crotch or big outer labia can cause the ring to twist. If that's the case, a teardrop-shaped ring might work better than a circular ring. **Note:** Piercing people refer to the clitoris in the usual "what you see is what you get" way that most of us do. However, as you can see in the chapter "What's Inside a Girl," this is only referring to the clitoral tip. The rest of the clitoris wraps around the vagina and occupies much more space.

Inner Labia Piercing: The success of an inner-labia piercing will depend a good deal on the thickness of the labia. Anything less than an 1/8" wide is likely to fail. Also, the piercings need to be placed far enough from the edge of the outer labia so they don't pull against the outer labia as a woman walks, runs and bends over. As with most genital jewelry, a thicker gauge will usually feel better and is less likely to tear these tender tissues. If a labial piercing is placed closer to the vagina, a woman's partner will be more likely to feel the sensation during intercourse. If it is placed closer to her clitoris, she might feel more sensation during intercourse.

Outer Labia Piercing: Given how outer labia have sweat glands, perspiration can be a problem as these piercings try to heal. To keep these piercings from getting irritated, let your outer lips flap free. The jewelry can also rub unpleasantly against tight panties and even your other labia.

Fourchette: This is a piercing on the bum side of the vagina that goes from the bottom wall of the vagina into the perineum. We're not talking much room to work with. This can be uncomfortable for women who enjoy intercourse, as the ring can get pulled into the vagina with incoming thrusts.

Pierced Clit: Some women have a clitoris that's beefy enough for piercing (minimum of 1/4" wide and the hood can't constrict the jewelry). Piercing an actual clit seems worrisome when you consider that the part of the clitoris that would be pierced has small chambers that become engorged with blood during arousal. Putting a post through the clitoris itself seems like it's playing Russian roulette with some pretty important neural pathways.

Female Genital Jewelry and Pregnancy

Most women with genital piercings have no problem getting pregnant. The problem can be with what happens when the kid decides to come out. Talk it over with your obstetrician or midwife. The time to NOT get a new piercing is if you are pregnant or trying to get pregnant. Your body will be changing a great deal, and what was a well placed piercing during your first trimester might not be so during your third.

Beware the Naval Piercing

You would think that of any piercings, the naval would be a piece of cake. But if there is one place where you truly want an experienced piercer, your belly button is it. Wrong angle, wrong jewelry, and you are staring at six to eighteen months of healing. **Hint:** while you might have been dreaming of there being a cool little ring in your navel, consider a curved barbell instead. And keep in mind that not all navels are made for piercing. For instance, an outie navel most likely contains a herniated umbilicus, and there are some asymmetrical parts of innies that do as well. The problem with this is if your site becomes infected, the infection might go straight to your liver via one of these blood vessels. If that happens, we're talking the likelihood of getting your next piercing in the afterlife.

Nipple Piercing

As with genital piercings, nipple jewelry can bring its owner a sense of pride as well as being a great distraction for a partner to play with. But nipple piercings also come with a serious "ouch factor," and unless they are done right, they can migrate faster than a wildebeest across the Savannah.

The jewelry that's best for nipple piercings will depend on the size of your nipples and breasts. Also, men and women alike need to let the piercer know if their nipples are soft or erect at the time of the piercing. Jewelry that is placed in an erect nipple that later goes flat can be uncomfortable. (Jewelry that's more flexible like tygon or nylon might work better with flat nipples.)

In case you haven't noticed, female nipples tend to have a bit more going for them than male nipples when it comes to being pierced. So unless a woman has flat nipples, the piercing should go through the base of the nipple where it meets the areola, but not through the areola. (You don't want to court a case of mastitis.) It's different for boys. Unless a guy lives to be Super Sized, his nipples usually aren't as robust as a woman's. The piercing will often need to go through his areola to avoid being rejected. He also doesn't have a mammary-gland situation to contend with.

Other Nipple Piercing Considerations

Males usually don't need to worry about menstrual soreness, but a woman should weigh that before getting her nipples pierced.

Women who are planning to have their nipples pierced should inquire about the kinds of fabrics they will be able to wear. How will your nipple rings look under a conservative business suit? Lacy bras will probably be out, since the ring will constantly catch in the lacy material. Ditto for the kind of shirts you will be able to wear to work.

Wearing a bra during the healing process can put pressure on the piercing site and prolong healing, and a woman who thinks she might have an infection at her nipple site should seek medical care immediately. As stated earlier, mastitis can be a bitch.

Nursing and nipple piercings is a topic you should research if you are planning on having a baby. The advice is often contradictory—perhaps because different women have had different experiences. So look up several sources and be prepared for a number of different scenarios. (What if your normally stoic nipples become terribly tender during your third trimester? Should you remove your nipple jewelry for the duration while nursing? What if the scar sites on your nipples becomes extra sensitive?)

Tongues, Lips and Labret

A tongue piercing is something you should enjoy the feeling of in your mouth. A lot of people have tongue piercings, so be sure to ask around and get their advice. You'll want to have a sense of how far forward or back you want your piercing. Street wisdom has it that if you enjoy going down on women, you'll want your tongue piercing more forward, and if you like to give blow jobs, get it farther back—but this depends on your technique. Other considerations with placement include how much you want the outside world to know it's there. Some women change their tongue jewelry to match certain outfits. And you can get small silicone caps that fit over the bead of a barbell. These are soft and are used for decoration and for giving oral sex.

Also research the angle you want the piercing to be. The straighter it is, the more the ball will rub against the top of your mouth. Be aware that the post will angle just a bit to the side in order to avoid the web on the bottom of your tongue. The piercer might initially put in a post that's longer than what you'll need. This is to help accommodate the swelling during healing.

Tongue piercings don't usually hurt a whole lot, but expect your tongue to swell up like a weather balloon soon after. Don't expect to be talking right for the first week, and remember that eating can be a challenge with a sore and swollen tongue. The healing period will normally take a week to two weeks. The piercer might want you to avoid certain foods during the healing period, including sugars. The folks at BME caution that tongue piercings are susceptible to genital warts, and a tongue piercing might increase your chances of giving and getting sexually transmitted infections. **Note:** If a woman who gets frequent vaginal infections has a partner with a tongue piercing, bacteria in her partner's piercing might be causing the infections.

A labret is a type of lip piercing, of which there are many variations. The inside of the lip can sometimes grow over the jewelry, and gum recession and chipping of tooth enamel can be problems. Be sure ask if there's a special kind of backing you can use that might help prevent these complications.

Piercings to Avoid

Surface piercings can easily reject and can leave a scar. Hand webs are piercings in the skin between the thumb and forefinger. Not a great idea. And under no circumstances should you ever attempt a uvula (throat) piercing, unless you have no gag reflex or aren't concerned about choking.

Abandoning a Piercing

Always check with an experienced piercer about protocol for pulling out a piercing and letting the skin grow back together. And if the piercing is on your face, seriously consider getting the advice of a plastic surgeon before pulling out the post for good.

Airport Security

With a couple of recent notable exceptions, airport security is unlikely to discover your piercing jewelry. One of the reasons is because it's usually made of high-quality metal that isn't magnetized. As one woman on a web forum remarked, airport security didn't catch her rather stout nipple rings, but they did find a penny in her pocket. Nonetheless, the government recommends that you take out your body jewelry before going through airport security. However, you should probably try to put it back in as soon as you clear security, as holes can start to close almost immediately.

Some people who are screened frequently, such as pilots with Prince Alberts, elect to replace metal jewelry with acrylic jewelry. Other options include jewelry made of glass or medical-grade plastic.

X-Rays and Medical Procedures

You will usually need to remove all metal rings and body jewelry before having an MRI and certain medical procedures. Think metal in your microwave. You can always put in a nylon post to keep the site from closing.

Tattoo, Tattoo!

Studies done at Texas Tech found that both male and female students with tattoos were "substantively and significantly more likely to be sexually active" than nontattooed college students.

Tattoos can be very sexy, so if that's what you want to do, why not put some serious thought and effort into it and get the best you possibly can? Learn about the different styles, the different inks, and healing times and sterilization. Don't just rush out and do it, especially if you have been partying and are still trailing tequila vapor. Save your money for the absolute best tattoo artist you can possibly find. Research, research, research. Spend a few hours reading every line on the tattoo FAQ from the rec.arts.bodyart newsgroup. This incredibly well-organized, helpful, gold mine of information is lovingly maintained by Stan Schwarz. Don't be put off by the wicked URL:

http://faqs.cs.uu.nl/na-dir/bodyart/tattoo-faq/part1.html

Tattoo Logic

The first thing to consider about getting a tattoo is that it is forever. It's highly unlikely it's ever going to go away. If the reason you are getting a tattoo is because your lover's nickname is Cyclops and you think it would be cute to have a cyclops tattooed on your chest with your nipple as his eye, keep in mind that Cyclops might someday get an eye for another babe, and what do you do then? Even if he doesn't, boobs sag. Maybe not today, maybe not tomorrow, but you will blink and gravity will have suddenly gotten its mitts on your perky breasts. It won't let go, and your cyclops tattoo will start looking like things do in those curvy carnival fun house mirrors. (The same is true for the skin on every other part of your body, not just breasts.)

Or what if you are truly and totally bonded to your lily-white bros in your white-supremacist street gang, and you get a racist tattoo across your entire back, and in two years' time you fall head over heels in love with a wonderful girl who is Jewish or black?

Hopefully, your reasons for wanting to get a tattoo are well thought out, and you are going to spend some time and money getting the best and most interesting tattoo you possibly can.

Tramp Stamps and Ass Antlers

A tramp stamp is a lower-back tattoo that rides on the pants line. It peeks out at you when the owner—usually a woman—wears low-rise jeans or a cropped T-shirt that shows her midriff, or she bends over and her pants go low and her shirt goes high. The tattoo is often V-shaped and points down in a way that signifies the anatomy below. Tramp stamps are the kind of tattoo you can hide when you're at work if you need to. Designs range from flowers, butterflies, dolphins and tribal art to unusual symbols, geometric shapes and even sentences, although this is probably not the spot for biblical quotations.

Some women are offended by the term "tramp stamp" because they feel the expression is derogatory and suggests that women who get this kind of tattoo like sex more than most. One can only hope. When you consider other possible terms such as "fart art" or "lower lumbar tattoo," the term "tramp stamp" starts to sound downright endearing.

There was a brief blogging frenzy when a blogger from Northern California discovered that rub-on tramp-stamp tattoos were being sold in the vending machines at Toys'R'Us, next to the Hannah Montana stickers. All things considered, seems like perfect product placement.

Removing a Tattoo

A study of people who have tattoos removed showed that while twice as many women as men wanted their tattoos removed, at least a third of these women wanted to get new tattoos on another part of their body.

Tattoo removal will cost you dearly, and is unlikely to be totally successful. It can be painful, and you may need to opt for a cover-up instead of removal. Do lots of research and ask tattoo experts as well as a dermatologist or two their opinion before deciding on a removal process. A botched removal can leave an unsightly scar. If you go for a cover-up instead of removal, find a cover-up specialist who comes highly recommended. There are some cover-up specialists who do it often and do it well. There are others who will only make the tattoo look worse.

Reader Suggestions

Here is advice for men from female readers on using their body jewelry to sexual advantage:

Kissing: Unless you are careful, you can bang and perhaps chip your partner's teeth. So go easy and be aware that your tongue needs more tooth clearance than one that is less accessorized. Also, women don't seem to enjoy being kissed by guys who slobber. But having a post through your tongue may keep you from sucking the saliva from it as well as you did pre-op. And some women aren't crazy about having foreign objects in the back of their throat. So when you French kiss, don't stick your tongue in very far, and remember to swallow.

Nipple Play: One woman says that dragging a steel ball across her nipples can be "a bit gnarly." Assuming your partner likes to have her nipples licked or sucked, make sure that you've coated her nipples with a heavy layer of saliva. Extra saliva on her nipples may help your ball glide rather than drag. Use the tip of your tongue when playing with her breasts and nipples. This will help keep the steel ball at bay. The best solution is to talk to your lover about this, with her giving you plenty of feedback.

Oral Sex: Here's where the real skill comes in, ball or no ball. It is possible to give wonderful oral sex, but only as long as you know where your ball is and what it's up to. Try flicking your tongue across the palm or back of your hand. This will help you learn to steer your ball better. The last thing you want to do is bang a steel object against a woman's tender nerve endings. You will need to flick your tongue more delicately than a guy who doesn't have a steel ball attached to the end of his. To paraphrase a woman who has dated a couple of different guys with pierced tongues, flicking a pierced tongue across a woman's vulva can feel really cool, but only if the man is extremely gentle and acutely aware of the impact that a pierced tongue has. She also cautions against probing inside a woman's vagina with a tongue that's pierced.

Special Thanks to Dr. Jerry Koch at Texas Tech, to the people who maintain and contribute to BME (Body Modification Ezine) at www.bmezine.com, to Anne Greenblatt, manager of the rec.arts.bodyart Piercing FAQ, to Stan Schwarz, manager of the rec.arts.bodyart Tatto FAQ, and to Dr. Myrna Armstrong & The Body Art Team.

48
Threesomes

***D**ear Paul,*
I was originally writing for advice about having a three-some. But my husband and I have recently met up with a third person for sex, and the experience was great!

Bonnie from Bonneville

Dear Bonnie,

Back when I was doing my psychoanalytic training, threesomes were thought to be a very bad thing.

A few years later, a female patient told me that she and her boyfriend had decided they were going to try out threesomes, an *MMF* and an *FFM*. Having been a Freudian black sheep, I didn't sound any warnings, but I did make sure that we explored the fantasies and unconscious motivations.

As far as I could tell, the *FFM* went off without a hitch. But there was a problem with the *MMF* that threw my patient's poor boyfriend into an unexpected funk. Seems my patient ended up making the exact same noises when she was having sex with the new man as when she and her boyfriend made love. Her boyfriend was horribly depressed, realizing that "his" special magic could easily be supplied by another.

So the first advice that I have for any couple who is thinking about inviting a third for play, besides talking it over for a couple of months and doing lots of research, is how you would handle it if you discovered that the new person gave your partner as much or more pleasure than you usually do? How would you feel if your partner was lavishing more attention on the third person than on you, although for some people, watching their partner doing it with someone else is one of life's little pleasures.

I would consider a threesome only if it's something that both of you are truly interested in, as opposed to when one partner does it just to please the other. Also, it's a bad idea to try a threesome if your purpose is to help repair a relationship that is struggling. Your relationship needs to have a foundation of trust and love for threesomes to work. Of course, plenty of you are thinking, "How could there be love and trust if my sweetie wants us to get naked with someone else?" To that I would say, love and trust are best defined by the beholders.

One of the first couples I ever interviewed about sex were in their early 70s and had been married for more than 35 years. They were church-going pillars of the community. The most important thing in their lives were their kids and grandkids. When I sat down in their tastefully-decorated living room, the woman said, "Why don't you look through the photo album of our last vacation that we took with some good friends?"

Within minutes, my grad-student mouth nearly fell off its hinges. Not a single person in the pictures had a stitch of clothes on. Their vacation had been on board a special cruise for swingers. Then they said that just last weekend six couples had been going at it in this very living room. And then the man looked lovingly at his wife and said to me from the depth of his heart, "Mama here is the best little cocksucker of any woman in the group!" His wife beamed with pride and gratitude.

The second couple I interviewed wasn't into swinging. They were soon to be married. They were madly in love and very pleased with each other sexually. They even invited me to their wedding, which was held in a fine church. They had a traditional relationship and would no more have had a threesome than the Pope would. We stayed in touch for the next two years, when their marriage suddenly split up. I never heard from either again.

A few years later, I was having a conversation with a young woman about computer software. She eventually asked me what I did. After I told her, the volume on her voice suddenly dropped. She told me that she lived with two men and was having sex with both of them. One was her husband, and the other was their roommate. This had been going on for a couple of years, and she said they were all very happy together.

So I gave up long ago on trying to predict what makes a relationship work or fail, and whether having a threesome was a good idea or bad. I figured it is a good idea for some couples, and a bad idea for others. I also gave up on any notions that swinging was for liberals and monogamy was for conservatives. One of the complaints I've heard from people in the swinging lifestyle is how conservative other swingers often are politically. A sizeable number of the couples are in the police and military, as well as grade-school and high-school teachers—all hazardous professions, as far as I'm concerned.

How Many Wives Can Fit on the Head of a What?

Having a threesome is not an unusual fantasy. But what about those adventurous souls who actually want to try it? It's not like you can walk up to the reference desk at your local library and say, "My wife's birthday is coming up and she's always wanted to do a guy with a bigger dick than me—do you have any books on that?" or "The three of us live together and share the same bed; do you have any books that can help our parents understand?"

Threesomes can evolve in many different ways. They can be a once-in-a-lifetime event when your husband's old college roommate visited for the weekend, or it might be something you do a couple of times a month.

Adding a third person in sex isn't like adding another cherry to your banana split. Threesomes are a declaration of war on two-thousand years of marital tradition—namely, that if you want to include another person in your sexual mix, you are supposed to lie to your partner and cheat on the side. So caution is in order. A threesome revolves around the emotions of three people instead of the usual two. The potential for everything goes up—from the level of sexual excitement to the degree of hurt and anguish.

The Definitions

There are many ways that people have sex in numbers. So before visiting the land of three, let's consider the following:

Threesome—This usually means two guys and a girl, or two girls and a guy. One of the *Ms* and one of the *Fs* are frequently in a committed relationship, with the third *M* or *F* being a free agent.

Open Marriage—This is when a primary couple agrees that each other can hook up with outsiders for sex. The past decade has seen an increase in couples who agree on the open-marriage option from the start. However, they usually don't announce this addendum at their wedding ceremony.

Swinging or *Being in the Lifestyle*—This is when an established couple gets together with a larger group to have sex. It has many variations, from when two couples enjoy getting it on in tandem, to sex in large party rooms where almost anything goes. While the swinging couples often form friendships, it is the recreational part of sex that initially draws them together. (The term *swinging*, which replaced *wife swapping*, is now being replaced by *lifestyle*.)

Polyamory—This has been described as a fluid state of friendship, love and sexual intimacy. Poly-people don't just get horny and fuck. They tell us they are able to have simultaneous romantic relationships without the usual encumbrances of jealousy, pettiness and divorce lawyers. Must be sweet.

Wife Swapping—Wife swapping used to be the catch-all term for anything that couples did that they wouldn't tell their priest about in confession. But the term got to be politically incorrect, and it implied something that wasn't true. As the authors of *Considering Swinging* point out, "It's the women who usually run the swinging show."

Let There Be Three

Why do people have threesomes? For starters—alcohol. Plenty of threesomes occur when three friends have been drinking enough to lose their inhibitions, but not enough to lose their erections. Threesomes created on the vapors of ethanol are seldom planned and seldom repeated. Threesomes that endure usually take forethought and planning.

Threesomes are often structured like the food pyramid that the U.S. government publishes. At the base of the pyramid or threesome triangle is a male-female couple involved in an ongoing love relationship. They are the whole-grains and green-leafy-vegetable part of the food pyramid. The third person is the forbidden food at the top—the sugars, desserts, and fats.

The possibilities for what three people can do when they are together could fill a book. Why they decide on an *MMF* or FFM could fill volume two, although there's no reason why a threesome can't include three males or females. If you don't know what you'd like to do and need a menu of possibilities, then maybe it's not the right time to be trying a threesome. While some successful threesomes just fall out of the sky, most take a great deal of planning and thought. Here are a couple of hundreds of things to consider:

In *MMF* threesomes, the chemistry between the men can range from "I'm fine with you doing her, but touch me with your dick and you're dead!" to "Oops, it just kinda slipped into my mouth!" The following chapter on DP discusses how if the two guys are seriously homophobic, things can get a little strange. At the other end of the spectrum, guy-doing-guy play can work out well if the men are willing and the woman is turned on by everybody doing everybody. It won't work so well if she's thinking, "My idea of fun is not sitting here watching my husband with a man's cock in his mouth!"

In *FFM* threesomes, the over-riding dynamic is often the desire of the women to experience more than the usual girl-hug and kiss. This kind of threesome is often about letting the women explore, with the man providing a safe, solid, masculine backstop.

There are many ways that the man can help same-sex exploration feel safer. The women might want him to be lying on his back, with one of them sitting on his penis while the other is sitting on his face. Both women are facing each other and they can kiss and caress while being connected to a man sexually. (This combination might be more comfortable when all three are on their sides.) Or maybe the women will be happier if he just watches and strokes himself, or if he joins one in doing the other.

Unless both women are totally into it, it's usually not a good idea for an *FFM* to focus around pleasing the man. *FFM* threesomes usually work better if the man takes a background role and allows the ladies' to lead. He should never try to script the threesome or try to set the tempo, unless it's a BDSM scene with a master and his two naughty slaves.

In a threesome, the women's orgasms are seldom the end of anything. They're more like the "fasten your safety belt" sign. However, the men's orgasms in a threesome can put a definite dent in the sexual build up. This may be one of the reasons why members in an *FFM* threesome often spend the night together, nestled in each other's arms, while in *MMF* threesomes the third-wheel guy usually goes home after the final wads are fired.

The Plan

Spontaneous sex is a special gift of the gods that is bestowed upon young couples who have undemanding jobs with predictable hours, no children, and friends and relatives who live on other planets. For everyone else, planning and compromise are as important to a good sex life as the twinkle in your eye and bulge in his pants. Triple that for sex with three.

The next part of this chapter is about some of the planning and logistics that are involved in having a threesome. It is divided into four sections:

1. *More Than a Fantasy, But Not Yet a Plan*—things to consider when considering a threesome. 2. *The Pre-Penetration Plan*—from how to find a third wheel to pre-penetration negotiations. 3. *Let the Party Begin*—possible positions and positions on what's possible. 4. *The Morning After*—don't let the dawn get you down.

More Than a Fantasy, But Not Yet a Plan

This chapter assumes that your threesome is made up of an established couple and a third wheel. That isn't how it needs to be. There are debates about whether threesomes are best when they are made up of three individuals versus a primary couple and a third wheel. There are also debates about whether the third wheel should be a friend, an acquaintance, or a stranger. There are no studies on these options, only opinions, and good luck finding any two that fully agree. These next sections are written as if the primary couple is the main audience. A separate section for "the third wheel" follows.

A number of these suggestions are from Suzy Bauer's e-book, *Step By Step Threesomes*, Nina Hartley's *How-To Threesome* series of videotapes, and from Violet Blue's chapter on threesomes in her book, *The Ultimate Guide To Sexual Fantasy—How to Turn Your Fantasies into Reality*.

💡When you are first discussing the possibility of a threesome with your partner, avoid blurting out a list of potential lovers, such as "Your friend Ally would be sensational!" or "I'm sure Jason would add a great deal!" What your partner will hear is that you can't wait to screw someone else. If your partner is receptive to the idea of a threesome, you might ask who he or she thinks would make a good third.

💡Anticipate that the threesome could sour your relationship. And what if one of you fell for the third wheel? Be sure to discuss these possibilities and strategies to deal with them ahead of time.

💡Try to imagine the sight of someone attractive and alluring having sex with your partner. Your partner is laughing, flirting, sighing, and enjoying intense pleasure with this person. How will you deal with it when it happens during your threesome? Are there ways you can signal your partner if jealousy is getting the better of you, so she or he can help reassure you?

💡In a threesome, an erotic connection can sometimes build between two of the participants, with the third person being left out. This is fine as long as the third person enjoys watching, but can result in a major pout if he or she feels excluded. How will you deal with this when it happens?

💡What if your threesome is an *MMF*, and when the third-wheel guy drops his drawers, you and your partner drop your jaws? What if nature blessed the boy with a package of penile perfection? Ditto if you are a woman, and the second female has the kind of body that a woman only gets when she's cut a deal with the devil? Are you prepared for this kind of situation?

Before trying a threesome, why not rent some videos that show the different positions and possibilities?

If you are considering an *MFF* threesome, you can simulate it by going to a upper-end strip bar where you can pay one of the girls to do a lap dance for you. It might give you a sense of the buttons that are pushed. However, think three times before taking a nude dancer or prostitute home for a threesome. She might be so experienced that it gets strange. It's better to stick with someone whose sexual perspective and experience level is closer to your own.

If you are considering an *MMF*, both of you might see what it's like to be in a strip bar where male dancers are the ones who get naked. Since they usually don't allow other males in the audience during male stripper shows for women, you might need to visit the gay part of town for this. Even if your guy isn't into the same-sex aspect of an *MMF*, it will give both of you a sense of what it might be like to have another naked male in your presence. Besides, it could be worth a chuckle to see other guys trying to pick up your husband.

Whether the dancers at a strip club are male or female, keep in mind that these places are seldom equal-opportunity employers. It is unlikely that the third wheel in your threesome will be quite so uninhibited or look like he or she spends hours each day at the gym.

Your Pre-Penetration Plan

To prepare for your first *MMF*, the woman might consider getting a dildo and butt plug for practice. She can simulate different penetration scenarios with her partner and the toys, which can help the actual threesome to be more manageable rather than overwhelming. (Most *MMF*s don't do double penetration. But just having a penis in your mouth at the same time that you've got one in your pelvis will provide a lot more man than most women are used to.)

Having a threesome with a friend can deepen your friendship, or it can seriously mess it up. And while it might be good to have a threesome with someone you know and trust, it's not such a good idea if he or she has a secret crush on you or your partner. Likewise, an ex boy- or girlfriend could make a good third, or a horrible third.

🔆 To find a third wheel who is not a friend or an acquaintance, swingers have clothes-on munches which you might check out. Male strip shows can be excellent trolling-grounds for MFFs. The women in the audience are usually amped and uninhibited. Plus, the male dancers are often gay and more interested in the money than the honey, so they aren't competition. One strategy is for the female to show up at the start, spotting potential women from the audience. Her male partner joins her after the strippers are done and the regular stiffs are allowed in. Other possibilities for meeting a third wheel include the Internet and ads in magazines or papers, although print media should be a last resort. The ads need to be carefully worded and carefully placed. Also, keep your eye out for single moms. After doing threesomes for a number of years, Suzy Bauer and her husband were thinking back over the numerous women who had joined them, and it suddenly hit them that the majority were single moms.

🔆 If the prospective third wheel is an unknown entity, protect your identity. Only provide a cell-phone number or an e-mail address. If they then contact you, set up a face-to-face meeting at a neutral location where you can meet with your clothes on. Discuss things like setting up personal boundaries, safe-sex precautions, and what you hope to get from your threesome. If the pre-penetration meeting doesn't increase your desire, or the chemistry doesn't feel right, consider it a message from the heavens above that you don't have the right combination.

🔆 Before your clothes-on pre-penetration meeting, decide what is and isn't off-limits. For instance, one woman might be fine with a third wheel giving her husband a blowjob, but will morph into a psychotic puddle if the third wheel and her spouse French kiss. So she needs to set love-making limits that encourage the third wheel to kiss her husband anywhere from the Adam's apple down, but nowhere above. Make a list of the things that you'd like to encourage and discourage. Discuss them during your pre-penetration meeting.

🔆 If a man is being invited into a threesome with an established couple, he needs to have a thumbs-up from the primary-couple's male partner, as in "Don't worry, I won't kill you if you fuck my wife." One way to do this is for the male of the primary couple to bring up the subject of a possible *MMF* threesome to third-wheel male candidates. Likewise, if an *FFM* suits your fancy, the alpha female needs to invite the other woman to join. There are exceptions to these rules of the jungle, but respecting them will serve you well.

☞As with any situation where a new partner is involved, you need to protect yourself against sexually transmitted infections. Do not take a stranger's word that he or she is disease-free. Be sure to use condoms, plenty of lube, and any other safe-sex precautions that the situation warrants. Also be sure to protect against unwanted pregnancy. And if you are having an *FFM*, and the M is going to be double-dipping into the FFs' vaginas or rectums, he'll need to change condoms when going from one girl to the next, and from one orifice to the next. So have a bunch of condoms and lube handy.

Let the Party Begin

First and foremost, consider the following advice by Nina Hartley from her *Nina Hartley's Guide to Threesomes* videos:

"Start slow, with lots of teasing and foreplay, kissing, petting, massage. It's likely two of you will be part of an existing couple where you know each other's sexuality better than the newcomer, so don't rush. Take your time bringing the newcomer into the situation. Unlike us [porn stars], you aren't making a movie. You don't have to be so goal-oriented. Let things unfold naturally instead of pushing for the kind of acrobatics you see in porn. It may take more than one get-together to make it all work, so don't be discouraged if the first threesome ends up with a double blowjob or handjob. It may take time for the three of you to get comfortable enough for actual intercourse. It is not necessary for all three partners to be equally engaged at the same times. Kicking back and watching can be exciting, too. Don't assume that dicks in every hole at all times is a measure of a successful threesome. Do the easiest things first, and see what develops. Don't forget to talk about your feelings afterward. You'll want to learn as much as possible from each experience."

☞Be sensitive that you are inviting a perfect stranger into your love-making lair. Don't assume that he or she has a clue of what to do or how to be. This is the moment of truth when what used to be 100 percent fantasy becomes 100 percent reality, which is not always the prettiest of transitions. Be gracious, kind, and offer the level of reassurance that you would want someone to offer you. The third wheel is not a fuck-bot who is there at your convenience, unless you are paying by the hour.

☞Just being naked together, feeling relaxed, and opening up sexually is a major accomplishment. Pay attention to the chemistry of the threesome rather than to your own need to get off. Don't try to script your threesome. It may take a couple of times together before the three of you find your groove.

🔆Your primary concern in any relationship should be that your partner feels loved and valued by you. This may mean paying more attention to your partner than to the third wheel—unless you agree that one of you mostly wants to watch. This doesn't mean you should be anything less than welcoming to the third wheel, but the chances are good that you didn't have children with the third wheel, and you don't share a mortgage and car payments.

🔆Be sober enough to legally drive. If you are too anxious to proceed without getting stoned or plowed, consider it a sign that this isn't something you should be doing.

🔆Don't be afraid to stop half way through the lovemaking to talk about what's going well and what could be going better. With three, you need to huddle often.

🔆There could be a time during an *MMF* when the woman is on all fours and is doing oral on the guy who's in front of her while the other guy is behind her and thrusting, aka "spit roasting." The male who is thrusting into her vagina or rectum needs to check in with her about rhythm and depth, since his thrusting might be causing her to gag on the penis of the guy who's in front. Likewise, the guy in the front needs to establish with her a comfortable pelvis-to-face distance. Both males need to be aware that the woman is between a rock and a hard place. You will probably need to work out a nonverbal signaling system, given what's in her mouth and all. Likewise, during an *FFM*, if the man has his penis inside one of the women who is giving the other woman oral sex, he needs to check in with her about the best speed and depth for thrusting. Otherwise, his thrusting might be making it difficult for her to keep her lips around whatever it is they are around.

🔆Be sure you have amassed a threesome-sized stash of condoms, lube, towels, props (eg. cuffs for tie-ups or harnesses for dildos, if you are so inclined), toys, vibrators, and whatever else floats your sexual boat. Have the entire scene set-up beforehand rather than searching at the last minute.

🔆Make sure your cell phones are turned off and the kids are safely away at their grandparents'. Use a hotel or another location if there's any chance that teenagers might show up, and don't even think about doing this when you are on-call.

The Morning After

No matter how enjoyable your threesome may have been, expect that you will wake up the next morning with worries and bad feelings. After all, you've just violated the expectations of a society that values monogamy. If some people in this day and age still feel shame after they masturbate, imagine what you might feel after having two penises in you at the same time or your first same-sex experience while your spouse was watching. Hopefully these memories will bring a smile, but don't bet on it.

No one should leave the morning after with self-doubt. Take the time to express your thanks and gratitude to one another—to both your primary partner and to the third wheel. If you enjoyed the experience, it's important to send the third wheel flowers if she's a woman, or something manly if he's a guy. Be sure the card has both of your names on it, and maybe even a separate line from each of you if you are an established couple.

While you have each other to talk over any morning-after doubts with, the third wheel has only him- or herself. The flowers or gift will help with that process. Do not slip up on this one. Talking it over with your partner the next day and doing something nice for the third wheel are as important as all the planning that went into making the threesome click, especially if you had a good time.

When You Are the Third Wheel

There is a certain freedom in being the third wheel in a threesome. If things don't go well, you can avoid seeing the others again. They probably live together and won't have the option of avoiding each other. On the other hand, they still have each other and can comfort each other. Or at least that's the fantasy that singles often have about couples, unless it turned out to be one of those "Who's Afraid of Virginia Woolf" evenings.

If you are a woman, it's likely that a big part of an *FFM* threesome is for you to explore sexually with the other woman. If it ends up being all about pleasing the man, consider bailing early, unless he's the chair of your dissertation committee. Be sure to discuss it with the couple ahead of time.

Always meet with the couple ahead of time to get a sense of your chemistry together. Talk about the things the three of you might like to try. Whether you are male or female, it's an important time to discuss the kinds of things you will and won't do. Come up with safe words that will either slow or stop the action if you find yourself feeling overwhelmed. Discuss everything from sexually transmitted infections to birth control. Don't assume that because they are a couple they have their act together.

You will most likely be joining an established couple with lots of history together. As a third wheel, you will need to deal with the reality that you won't be coming first, or not metaphorically, anyway.

💡Keep in mind that you will be having an experience with three separate entities as opposed to two. You will be dealing with each of the others as individuals, as well as with them as a couple. The couple may have its own dynamics that are different from those of the individuals who make it up. This is not a problem in some threesomes, but in others, the mind-fucking can outpace the body-fucking. You didn't sign on to do couples therapy. If you find yourself being placed into that role, BAIL!

💡Things might go spinningly well, or they might get very weird. If the threesome starts to get weird, don't hesitate to suddenly remember an important meeting or a sprinkler in the yard that you are sure you left on. Do not be afraid to call it a day, no matter what stage the threesome is in. Do not for a moment be intimidated because it's them against you. If you suddenly start feeling that this is the wrong time and place, don't hesitate to grab your pants or purse and make yourself history. Be sure to drive to the location separately, or have an escape route that doesn't depend on them.

💡Unless the couple wants you to be a total stud or stud muffin, the three of you will have a much better time if you don't feel the need to prove what a sexual all-star you are. This is a time to blend, rather than stand out, unless they have specifically asked you to have your way with one member of the couple while the other watches.

💡If you are a third-wheel guy in an *MMF*, seek the main man's approval before trying something with his partner, even if she's inviting you to do it. It's not like you need to pull out your cell phone and check with his attorney, a simple moment of eye contact and confirming nod are all that's needed. Likewise, if you are a woman, you're not there to upstage the other woman. Be respectful, and the chances are good you will get pleasure back in spades.

💡Ah, the single-dude dilemma. It is going to be significantly more difficult for a single man to find a willing couple for a threesome than it is for a single woman. It's the same problem with almost every species on the planet, be it a single bull elk, sea lion or homo sapien. Life can be hard on single males who don't have their own herd of cows—almost as hard as it is on the poor male who does have his own herd of cows!

💡This is probably just a bunch of psychobabble nonsense, and even if it isn't, it's no reason not to have a great time. But try to think about any less-than-conscious reasons that might be propelling you, as a single person, to have sex with an established couple. Freud might wonder if it has something to do with unconsciously wanting to outdo one of your parents. Some of Freud's followers might wonder if it has to do with wanting to be loved and taken care of by an idealized mommy and daddy. Again, we all do sexual things with motives that could fill anyone's psych book. That's no reason not to enjoy them. But being more aware of it can sometimes help us from getting stuck in situations that aren't always the best.

Make sure that someone knows where you are going, including the address and phone number. You don't have to tell them the truth about what you are doing, but leaving a trail and an expected return time is never a bad idea. This is just as true for males as for females. The only exception would be if you already know the people. While joining an unknown couple for sex is probably no more dangerous than joining an unknown single for sex, taking precautions is in order.

Just because they are married and say they are disease free, don't believe it. Be sure to bring your own condoms and lube.

The Routine "Slut Disclaimer"

One of the first things you will often see from female writers about threesomes and other forms of sexual swinging is the slut disclaimer. It goes something like this: "Just because we enjoy having frequent threesomes does not mean we are sluts." Au contraire.

When you write a book describing how often you pick up guys at bars and how the vast percentage of women who you have threesomes with are single moms, you are the Sears of sluts. So why not be proud of it? How many men would feel the need to apologize for bringing so much pleasure to so many? Instead of worrying about what others think, why not just smile and wink? You don't need to tell your boss or the other parents at school how many different guys you were doing last night.

When it comes to being judged, men aren't the ones you usually need to worry about. Keep it low-key and wear something conservative to work, and most guys are cool. The ones you need to worry about are other women. One of the reasons why they might judge you so harshly is because they fear you will steal their husbands and sons from their grasp. It's been that way since the beginning of time. Hopefully, you have bigger and better fish to fry!

Resources:

Diana Cage's book is definitely worth getting if you are exploring threesomes: *Threesomes, Fulfill Your Ultimate Fantasy,* Alyson Books, (2006).

Suzy Bauer's *Step By Step Threesome* e-book is very helpful. However, huge blocks of text from Lori Gammon's *Threesome* mysteriously appear in Bauer's e-book. Hmmmm. The focus of *Step By Step Threesome* is mostly on MFF threesomes. Again, while it is very helpful, Bauer's e-book, should have been less than 100 pages instead of 236. Do people really need quotes from Mark Twain and Dr. Seuss when they are trying to learn about threesomes? Many of the book's generalizations should be ignored. Still, it is money well spent if you are thinking threesomes. Be aware that Bauer uses the Internet marketing hard-sell approach, and you might be hammered with ads if you sign up on her Website at www.StepByStepThreesome.com.

While Lori Gammon has plenty of things to say in her book *Threesome,* she has a need to quote studies from *Cosmo* like it was *Scientific American,* and her enchantment with the so-called superiority of women in all matters of sex is a bit much. If women's brains and sexual nature is so darned wonderful when compared to men's, why include men at all in a threesome?

The *Nina Hartley's Guide to Threesomes—Two Girls & a Guy* and *Nina Hartley's Guide To Threesomes—Two Guys & a Girl* videos will show you many of the possible combinations, as long as you realize these are porn and not *National Geographic.*

Violet Blue has a helpful chapter on threesomes in her book, *The Ultimate Guide to Sexual Fantasy—How to Turn Your Fantasies into Reality* from Cleis Press,(2004).

While Luna Grey's *The Kinky Girl's Guide to Dating* from Greenery Press, (2004) isn't about threesomes, it is a fine read for anyone who is thinking about stepping outside of our culture's traditional parameters for sex.

For an introduction to the swinging lifestyle, you can't do better than Dana and Ed Allen's *Considering Swinging* from Momentpoint Media, 2001. Don't let the low price confuse you, this book is recommended by many.

A highly regarded resource that goes beyond threesomes and explores lifestyle issues is Tristan Taormino's *Opening Up–A Guide to Creating and Sustaining Open Relationships,* Cleis Press, 2008.

49

Double Penetration[1]

Some women will tell you one penis is trouble enough. But if you've got two in your crosshairs, or shorthairs, then this might be the chapter for you. Double penetration is for the woman who wants a pelvis full of penises. It requires two guys and a girl. One penis is in her top bunk (vaginal intercourse) while the second is in her bottom bunk (anal intercourse).

Is Double Penetration (DP) Safe?

There have been no studies done on DP and there is little in the medical literature about the safety or danger of it. The tissue between the vagina and rectum isn't exactly made of Kevlar and could possibly tear. It's thin enough that if you put a finger in a vagina when you are having anal sex, you can clearly feel the penis. The same is true with a finger in your bum when a penis is in your vagina. (If you enjoy this kind of exploration, remember to scrupulously clean anything that's been in the bum before it touches a vagina. This includes changing condoms. We're talking two different caverns with two different sets of microbes. Brown should never see pink.)

As for the advisability of whether to try DP, that's between you and your healthcare guru. There's little in the literature about DP being dangerous, but there's little about it being safe.

Oh Nina, Oh Nina!

As sometimes happens when you are looking at life on the sexual fringes, the search for information on double penetration has unearthed some basic truths that apply as much for monogamous couples as for those who like their sex in numbers. Let's review those truths first, before we get to the DP basics.

After watching and rewatching porn star Nina Hartley's *Guide to Double Penetration* video, a couple of universal truths began to appear. These truths

---

[1]It was only with the greatest of restraint that this chapter was not named after the gonzo DP porn series, *One in the Pink, One in the Stink!*

had nothing to do with double penetration, but with how Nina Hartley handles sex on the set. Nina Hartley gives the other actors verbal cues about what feels good and what doesn't. You would think it would be just the opposite. Here's a highly-intelligent, porn pro like Nina Hartley. She has hand-picked her co-stars. You would think she wouldn't have to say a word to them about what feels good. Shouldn't veteran porn stars automatically know? But as you watch Ms. Hartley and the big boys go at it, the opposite is true. Nina Hartley doesn't expect anyone else to know what's going on inside of her body. She makes her suggestions with humor and respect, but she lets the people who she is having sex with know what feels good to her and what doesn't.

This is especially important when you consider that what feels good one day might not feel good the next. How is someone else supposed to magically know? So here is some very helpful and basic sex advice for any couple, whether their sexual tastes are missionary-position pure or devilishly DP:

1. When it comes to sharing sexual pleasure, only beginners think that others should automatically know how to please them.

2. It could be that a woman needs a couple of years of having sex before she's able to tell her partners what works. Being able to instantly convert physical sensation into words takes time, experience, and a partner who can appreciate the challenge. (Perhaps Nina Hartley hand-picks her porn partners not so much for their raw physical skills, but for their ability to listen.)

Hopefully you won't think this book is encouraging you to try double penetration—even Nina Hartley avoided it until she was more than forty, when her backers "encouraged" her to do a *Nina Hartley Guide to DP.* But if it is something you are interested in, the most important thing is for a woman to know her body and to be able to communicate what is going on with it. If she can't do this, there's no way she should be hosting a double penetration.

One That Worked and One That Didn't

Consider the experience of a woman who has tried Double Penetration with two different sets of guys. She hated it with the first set, but liked it so much with the other men that they've repeated it a couple of times.

The first pair of men were homophobic, so it became all about their need to avoid touching each other rather than being three partners in sync. They had a macho "slam-her-hard" thing going on as well. She thinks these boys had watched way too much porn.

One of the things that worked so well with the second set of guys is that they weren't afraid to make physical contact with each other, so they could work as a team instead of as two men who were trying to out-straight each other. This allowed them to focus on what was and wasn't working for her.

If you are a man who would have an identity meltdown if another guy's arms, legs and testicles were touching your own, DP is not for you. If you would be uncomfortable feeling another guy's penis through the thin wall between a woman's vagina and rectum, forget the Robin-Batman thing.

The position this woman liked best was for the man who was doing the anal insertion to be lying on his back. She gave the example of where she faced his feet and sat on top of him while sliding his penis in. She then lay all the way back. That way, she had the full weight of her body pressing down on his, and she didn't have to worry about him getting too aggressive with his butt thrusting. The other man stood at the edge of the bed or knelt in front of them and entered her vagina that way. This is different from the DP position that's often shown in porn movies. But in porn it's all about the camera angle rather than what's comfortable. You don't see any of the preparation and planning that was done ahead of time.

Maybe the position that works best is for the three of you to be on your sides, or maybe with her on all fours, straddling the guy who's in her vagina while the buttman kneels or stands at her rear. You'll need to try different positions and rhythms.

Also, if you have been watching porn movies, keep in mind that most porn pros have rectums that can handle a rig from Roto Rooter. Yours might not be that practiced.

Then there's the matter of thrusting. Maybe the woman will want one man to be thrusting while the other is inside but still. Or maybe she'll want one to thrust slowly and stay shallow while the other thrusts hard and deep. She won't know what works until both boys have their luggage in the station.

A woman might be so overwhelmed by getting twice the bang from her bucks that her command of the English language becomes less than optimal. So before zippers get unzipped, work out a simple signaling system. If she doesn't know her body's cues for when it is getting overwhelmed, she shouldn't be trying double penetration. It's no time for passivity when all of that male energy is coming at her from both sides.

This is also no time to be drinking or getting stoned. It will keep you from being aware of important body signals and sensations.

All three of you need to agree that your goal is your mutual fun and pleasure, and not double penetration. If the chemistry is right but DP feels like a stretch, you can always try to make it work during your second or third time together. If the chemistry isn't right, why force it?

A woman might start preparing a couple of weeks in advance by popping a butt plug into her rear while having vaginal sex with a real live partner. Doing it the other way around sometimes results in the dildo turning into a missile and shooting across the room once her vaginal muscles start contracting. She should also be comfortable receiving anal.

Things to assemble ahead of time include towels, condoms and lube. Be sure to banish your cell phones and arrange plenty of uninterrupted time. Since a double penetration involves three people, you might find the previous chapter on threesomes to be helpful. It has information about everything from hooking up with a third to the dynamics of three people having sex together.

If you have a DP fantasy but aren't into all that extra sperm, consider cuddling up in front of your new plasma display with your sex toys, a bowl of hot popcorn, and the double penetration videos from Michael Ninn. The titles to date are *Double Penetration" #1, #2, and #3*. Despite the lack of creativity that went into the titles, Michael Ninn's productions are as high-end as porn gets. Be prepared for pretty.

Resources:

Nina Hartley's Guide To Double Penetration from Adam & Eve (thanks to Sinclair Intimacy Institute for sending this DVD). More porn than how-to. The face-to-face interview with Nina Hartley is interesting.

Michael Ninn's *Double Penetration* (2004), *Double Penetration 2* (2005), and *Double Penetration 3*, (2006); not yet available at Costco.

50
Kinky Corner

Readers will hopefully appreciate that vanilla is *The Guide's* favorite flavor. So rather than being an introduction to BDSM, this chapter is an attempt to explain a little of this and that. If you want to venture further into the world of sexual power play, some excellent resources are on the *Kinky Corner* part of our website at www.goofyfootpress.com.

This chapter could have easily been turned into two chapters: one on kink where two or more people are involved with each other, and one on fetishes, which are more of an individual turn on. As you will hopefully see in the pages that follow, BDSM is often about an exchange between two or more people. It's the creation of a scene that both participants find to be a turn on. A fetish can be a way of insulating yourself from other people. It's a way of getting off within an erotic world of your own creation.

Men vs. Women

On the surface, it seems that men in our society are more into kink than women. But maybe that's because we define kink differently for men than for women. A woman who wears her boyfriend's boxers or briefs is at the height of fashion, but if he wears her underwear we consider him to be weird. Our society relishes her kink, but gets very uncomfortable with his.

In our society, women touch each other at will. However, if men were to touch each other with half the frequency that women do, they would be called queer. Once again, our culture labels men as being strange for something that women do all the time.

A woman who routinely undresses in front of an open window is thought to be a neighborhood resource. Double that for a woman who plays with herself with the window shades up. But a man who does these things is considered to be a pervert and may even be locked up. There is also the biological fact that women can masturbate without being noticed. Guys can't masturbate with that kind of subtlety. The male who gets himself off in a public place is at much greater risk of being caught and labeled a pervert than the occasional female who does the same thing. A reader comments, "Not only is he labeled a pervert, but if convicted he would be forced to register as a sex offender."

Bondage Lite

The United States was originally settled by religious outcasts, malcontents, criminals and slaves. The fact that we are not all into some form of bondage is a little amazing.

Bondage is the application of pain, humiliation or restraint in a way that some people find erotic and satisfying. It's an endorphin rush like a runner's high. It is an intense shared fantasy that frequently includes one person taking power and the other giving it up. It's about physical or psychological surrender, helplessness and trust. If you are into BDSM, this is a combination that brings far more comfort than pain.

People who are drawn to light bondage enjoy being rendered passive. They have no choice but to enjoy what a partner is doing to them. They don't have to worry about being a "good" partner who provides pleasure in return. Performance anxiety is virtually eliminated. This can especially appeal to someone who has to be in charge and in control the rest of the time.

One form of bondage includes having your arms or feet tied while being kissed, tickled, caressed or otherwise made love to. In parts of Los Angeles, New York and Chicago this type of activity isn't considered bondage, but merely good bedroom technique.

Safety Note If you are into light bondage, be aware that scarves and ties form tight knots that are hard to undo; wrists and ankles can be permanently damaged. Bondage enthusiast William Henkin says that professionally made cuffs may seem expensive to couples who simply like to tickle and spank, but they are much safer than the restraints that people improvise at home. In the event that professionally made cuffs aren't available on your TV's Home Shopping Network, check with places like Good Vibrations, Blowfish, JTs Stockroom or The Pleasure Chest.

Painful Pleasures

Spanking is a form of sexual kink that can be considered either light or heavy bondage, depending upon how it's done. For instance, some participants like their spanking hard and with a hostile edge, while others enjoy a little spank here and there when highly aroused.

Why do some adults enjoy being spanked? One theory states that people sometimes sexualize their childhood shame or humiliation. Turning shame

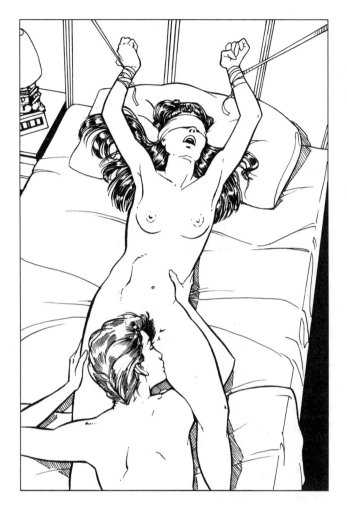

Look at how her wrists are bound. This can cause wrist damage and is NOT the way you want to do it. Splurge and get some fake-sheepskin cuffs.

Or better yet, try the very cool Sports Sheet Bondage Bed Sheet Set. See it at Sportsheets.com

or humiliation into erotic sensation helps it to become more bearable and even fun. Another reason why some people enjoy an occasional swat on the rear is because they find that it feels good, as long as they are sexually aroused and it is their own personal choice to be in the situation. Who can argue with that?

Bondage by Choice—A Feminist Contradiction?

People who are feminists or socially progressive (whatever that means) sometimes feel that they are deserting their own cause if they enjoy being submissive or have masochistic fantasies. For instance, consider a feminist lawyer whose favorite fantasy is being tied up and sexually violated. She occasionally acts out this fantasy with her male lover. Does this contradict her political beliefs? No, since the relevant issue is the freedom to choose rather than what's being chosen.

The lady lawyer believes that each person should be able to choose what to do with his or her own sexuality. In acting out her bondage fantasy with her lover, this woman chooses to give up her position of equality, and she chooses the man whom she wants to give it up to. In the criminal-rape cases that she handles in court, the rape victim had no choice. The act was forced upon her, rather than being part of a shared fantasy between two consenting adults.

Note The term "feminist" is rife with contradiction. For instance, some feminists are opposed to pornography and feel it demeans women, while other feminists believe that women should be proud of their bodies and free to display them sexually if that's what they want to do. Some feminists hate men, others don't; some embrace lesbianism, others are alienated by feminist groups who are more concerned with lesbian issues than with those of straight working moms. Some feminists think that intercourse is a form of oppression that women have been brainwashed into having by the patriarchy (straight white guys). Other feminists view intercourse as a satisfying activity where a vagina is as active and powerful as a penis. Some feminists consider motherhood to be a form of slavery for women, while others welcome motherhood. In fact, most women in this day and age describe themselves as being feminists, regardless of their political views.

Heavy Bondage — A Little Like Life?

"Maddie's path to discovery was a gradual process. She'd been kinky for pretty much as long as she could remember. She remembered the teacher finding her tied up to the swing set at the end of recess. She didn't just play 'doctor' as a young child, she played mad scientist. Her vision was pretty dark, involving elaborate punishment scenes in a neighbor's basement. Not surprisingly, she was usually the one who got punished. She has a half-formed memory of having a bucket of coal poured over her crotch while she moaned and writhed in semi-protest. She can still remember the absolute feeling of erotic surrender, the feeling of loss of control. That memory has a sexual charge for her even today. These dirty little games continued until the inevitable discovery by a parent, at which point they

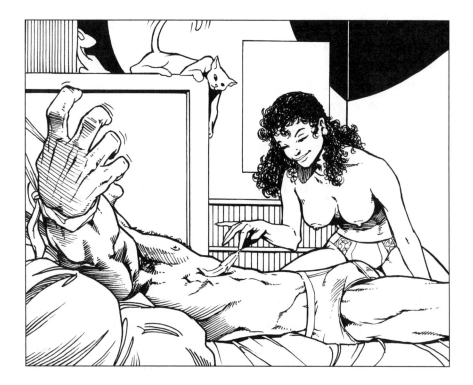

abruptly ceased. She doesn't remember seeing those kids much after that.... During the teenage years, her sexual awakening seemed to always involve some sort of power exchange dynamic. She chose older boys, the dangerous ones, who would use her. And she submitted to this, sometimes with great drama, but some weird little part of her loved it.... The pain of losing her virginity was one of the hottest moments of her life. Unhealthy? Hell, yeah. Self-destructive? Absolutely." —From the funny and fascinating *The Kinky Girl's Guide to Dating* by Luna Grey, Greenery Press, (2004).

Heavy bondage can get fairly brutal. It can be a world of whips and chains and devices that might put a chill up the spine of even the average high-school PE teacher. (Acronyms: B&D = bondage and discipline; S&M = sado masochism; D&S = dominance and submission; BDSM is a blanket term for all of it.)

In heavy bondage, having an orgasm isn't nearly as important as the bondage scene itself, with its undercurrent of domination, submission and sometimes humiliation. People into heavy bondage process pain differently than people who aren't. Bondage lovers find serious doses of sexual pain to be invigorating and intimate. They speak about sexual pain with the same kind of clarity and relish as religious pilgrims who are describing a visit to a shrine or the Dalai Lama.

If you have an irrepressible need to get into heavy bondage, please consider the following advice: don't pick up a stranger who enjoys beating the crap out of people and confuse that with bondage, even if you are a woman who loves too much. In heavy bondage there are established rules and etiquette that keep the participants from getting seriously hurt. Mind you, the definition of seriously hurt is a personal matter. If heavy bondage is what turns you on, learn the rules and make sure that your partner knows and respects them.

In almost every large city in the United States you will be able to find an established bondage club. These clubs often have extensive calendars of events, including talks, demonstrations and social gatherings. Generally speaking, you will be far safer in joining one of these established clubs than by experimenting on your own. You might also be amazed at how many educated, kind and helpful people you will meet at the established clubs.

Even if you aren't into bondage, don't get roped into thinking that mild-mannered people prefer being bottoms (slave role) and that aggressive types prefer being tops (master/dominator/dominatrix). There are plenty of business executives, lawyers, doctors, politicians and policemen who prefer being on the bottom when it comes to sexual kink. In fact, it's a problem in the bondage community that a good top is hard to find. It's also true that a number of people into BDSM enjoy alternating roles between top and bottom.

Lite or Heavy Bondage — Safety Considerations

No matter if you only use bondage once a year or are a full-fledged bondage brute, the S&M book by author Jay Wiseman titled *SM-101*, Greenery Press, makes the following suggestions:

💡Anytime a body part that is tied up feels numb or goes to sleep, untie it immediately. And never tie anything around a partner's neck.

💡In anticipation of catastrophes like fires, earthquakes or an unexpected visit from your mom and dad, be sure that you have a flashlight and a

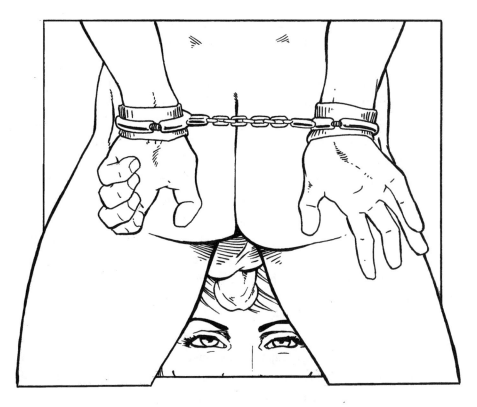

pair of heavy scissors handy. *SM-101* recommends paramedic scissors, which can be found at medical-supply stores. They cut through almost anything except handcuffs. Keep the scissors and flashlights in a place that you can readily find in the dark. Ditto for the handcuff key if that's what you are using. Better yet, tie the key to the handcuffs with a string.

Never leave the person for long, and check them often. If any injuries were to occur, you would be legally and morally responsible.

Always establish a safe word or gesture which means to stop. Some people use "red" for stop and "yellow" for easing up a little. No one who is seriously into dominance and submission uses "stop," "don't," or "no more" for safe words, since any good bottom says them often but doesn't mean them one little bit.

Breath Play or Erotic Asphyxiation—Do Not Do This

A reader recently reported that he puts his hands around his partner's neck and squeezes tightly when they are having sex—at her request. She says it makes the experience feel more intense. He is now concerned because she wants him to use a leather belt from one of her coats to get a better grip.

This kind of sex is called breath play or erotic asphyxiation. It's also referred to as scarfing or terminal sex. The side effects include death and brain damage. There are two groups of people who enjoy their sex this way. One groups is made up of boys and young men who put plastic bags over their heads or tight ropes around their necks while they masturbate. They are known as baggers or gaspers.

Baggers are often white, straight and middle-class. They fit in well socially. They keep their sexual secrets well hidden. Up to a quarter of them wear women's underwear while they masturbate on death's doorstep.

It is thought that several boy baggers die each year in this country. Their deaths are often reported as suicides, but people who are trying to kill themselves don't hang from door knobs and they don't design safety releases into their death devices. Boy baggers fully intend to free themselves after squeezing out their blurry-eyed orgasms.

Horrified parents will often spruce up the death scene before the ambulance arrives. Instead of being reported as masturbation gone awry, the coroner thinks it's a suicide and none of Johnny's friends can understand why a kid who seemed so well-adjusted would want to off himself.

The other group of people who are into breath play are normal-appearing couples. They have no fear of the boy-bagger's fate. They assume that the person who is applying the pressure is like a designated driver who can put the brakes on before it's too late. "Not so!" says Jay Wiseman, the Tiger Woods of BDSM and author of *S/M 101:*

> "As a person with years of medical education and experience, I know of no way whatsoever that either suffocation or strangulation can be done in a way that does not intrinsically put the recipient at risk of cardiac arrest…. If the recipient does arrest, the probability of resuscitating them, even with optimal CPR, is distinctly small."

You could be hooked up to state-of-the-art heart monitors and have a partner who is a board-certified cardiologist, breath play would still be Russian roulette in your birthday suit.

Another thing that has healtcare providers concerned is the risk of brain damage. Those like Charles Moser, a physician who is highly respected in the world of kink, worry about the long-term consequences of breath play. There's also the matter of those pesky murder charges. "Honest, your Honor, she asked me to choke her when we were having sex."

Fetishes: An Overview

Several years ago, a singer named Randy Newman wrote a song whose lyrics entreat his lover to take off all her clothes, except her hat. If Mr. Newman couldn't enjoy sex unless the woman had a hat on, then we might say he had a hat fetish. The Glossary at the end of this book offers the following definition of fetish:

> FETISH—1. Reliance on a prop, body part, scene or scenario in order to get off sexually. 2. The prop can either be fantasized or exist in actuality. 3. One philosopher has described "fetish" as being similar to when a hungry person sits down at a dinner table and feels full from fondling the napkin.

If both people in a relationship enjoy a particular fetish, then acting out the fetish will be a welcome event. But if only one partner is into the fetish, the other person might feel that she or he is not nearly as important as the fetish itself. For instance, if the woman in the above-mentioned song loves wearing her hat while otherwise naked, then she has found the perfect man. Otherwise, she may start to feel like a human hat rack.

Fetish Specifics

Fetishes come in many different forms; some include objects, others include actions that need to be repeated over and over.

For instance, some couples enjoy saying dirty things while having sex. But what if one partner can't perform sexually without hearing the dirty words? This takes it beyond simple sex play and hints of a fetish, especially if the other partner feels stupid screeching things like, "Fuck me harder, fuck me harder, you big stud, Mama wants it all," or degrading things like, "You miserable, worthless little turd." Particularly troublesome are situations where the partner with the fetish needs to say degrading things to you, unless of course, you find something endearing about being called a smelly old cow, fat whore, or pencil-dicked imbecile.

Unbeatable & Untreatable

Men with certain conflicts might deal with them one way while women sometimes give them a different spin. For instance, more men probably have foot fetishes than women, yet women seem to obsess about shoes more often and spend more money on them than men usually do. An obvious, time-honored solution is for men with foot fetishes to work in women's shoe stores.

People with fetishes usually love them immensely and resist giving them up. Therapy is seldom effective in loosening the love for a fetish. As long as the partner is fine with the fetish and it causes no harm to others, there seems to be little reason for abandoning it. On the other hand, if it violates criminal statutes and the wishes of others (e.g., flashing or being a Peeping Tom), or it introduces a level of weirdness that a partner won't tolerate, then the person with the fetish will face sad and serious consequences.

Normal Sexual Turn-on vs. a Fetish

Let's say your boyfriend loves to feel your legs when you have pantyhose on. He's a really sweet guy and you enjoy the extra attention, but your mother says it's a fetish.

As long as it feels like he is more turned-on by you than the pantyhose, they are probably just a fun prop for him. He won't go into sexual mourning if you swear off pantyhose for bobby sox. But what if your boyfriend can't become aroused unless you are wearing pantyhose, or he gets off more and more by your pantyhose and you feel like a mannequin? Rather than being an erotic accessory that helps to spice things up, the pantyhose would be way too important. That's when you're talking a fetish.

Some people have fetishes for objects or materials like leather, rubber, latex, underwear, shoes, socks, boots, smelly feet, hair, breasts and even diapers. There are websites with adults wearing diapers, and not because they need to. Other people with fetishes have scenarios or fantasies that get them off, e.g., the guy who likes his partner to pee or crap on him. Or the fetish might be as hidden and subtle as the kind of haircut his partner has. He suddenly goes bonkers if she changes it. (Ever notice how some guys date or marry only women who are the spitting image of each other? Is it the woman he loves, or a certain look that she has?)

People with fetishes get comfort from the fetish that they can't get from human beings. The fetish becomes the missing piece that completes their sexual circuit. The fetish gets turned into a sexual partner, an unhuman one who isn't demanding or humiliating. (It's far easier to control a pair of pantyhose than to control the woman who is wearing them!) The fetish provides an exciting sense of relief.

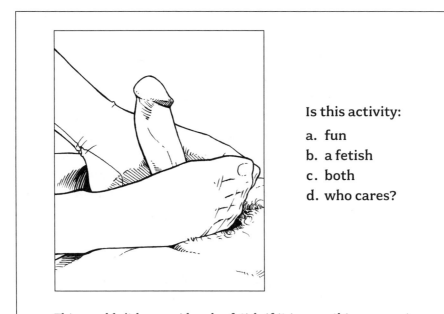

Is this activity:

a. fun

b. a fetish

c. both

d. who cares?

This wouldn't be considered a fetish if it is something you enjoy doing but can also do without. Psychologists would call it a fetish if the man couldn't become aroused without seeing or touching the woman's feet, or if her pantyhose were so important to him that he needed them rather than her to become sexually excited. How do psychologists know? Because they are as kinky as anyone else.

One problem with having a serious fetish is the loneliness that can sometimes be a part of it. No matter how many times you fondle them, a pair of rubber panties or a woman's feet can go only so far in providing the closeness or friendship that many of us value in a sexual partner. In fact, some people refer to the fetish as a compromise between the fear of human closeness and the need for it.

Crossdressing

Some women occasionally dress up like men, to the point of wearing a fake penis. This is a form of accessorizing known as "packing." One woman reports that if she's been packing for an extended amount of time she even stops having her period—without taking a single male hormone. Once she is through packing and the fingernail polish goes back on, her periods become regular again.

However, crossdressing usually refers to a type of obsession or need that some men have to dress like women, aka "transvestism." This might be fine with the guy's wife or girlfriend, but problems could arise if he keeps stealing her favorite bra and panties to wear.

Crossdressing could have been included in the chapter on gender-bending, but gender benders don't consider crossdresses to be part of their tribe. It could have been considered in the same-sex chapter, but most men who crossdress have a straight sexual orientation. It was placed here because none of the other parts of this book wanted it, which is the dilemma that most crossdressers face. Their dilemma is described brilliantly by Amy Bloom in her book, *Normal–Transsexual CEOs, Crossdressing Cops, and Hermaphrodites with Attitude:*

> "Heterosexual crossdressers bother almost everyone. Gay people regard them with disdain or affectionate incomprehension, something warmer than tolerance, but not much. Transsexuals regard them as men "settling" for crossdressing because they don't have the courage to act on their transsexual longing, or else as closeted gay men so homophobic that they prefer wearing a dress to facing their desire for another man. Other straight men tend to find them funny or sad, and some find them enraging....."

There are thousands and thousands of transvestites or male crossdressers in the United States, although they prefer to be described in the millions. Many are straight and appear quite masculine when they aren't wearing a bra and panties. Some appear quite masculine when they are wearing a bra and panties. As men, they are often heterosexual, married and the last guy you'd imagine would dress up like a girl. Most crossdressers value their macho side as much as their feminine side, but struggle with finding ways to enjoy both at the same time.

Contrary to what you might imagine, male crossdressers aren't drawn to professions that welcome a guy's feminine side. The average crossdresser is as likely to be a baseball player, fireman, policeman, auto mechanic or business executive as a hairdresser or florist. They go for manly professions to help hide or counter the feminine side of themselves.

A crossdresser gets sexual excitement by identifying with a woman, but he's still got the straight-guy consciousness going on. Perhaps the bra symbolizes having breasts, and the panties symbolize having female genitals.

So there he stands, in front of the mirror, admiring his "breasts and vulva," while sporting a fully masculine erection. Sexually, he's got his bases covered.

Therapy will not change a crossdresser's need to crossdress. However, if a man is compulsive about crossdressing, therapy can help him with that aspect. Many crossdressers hope that marriage will cure them of their desire to dress like a woman. But the envy and allure of their wife's underwear drawer will soon rear its satin head, and so much for good intentions.

Men who are reading this book while wearing their favorite DKNY dress might be concerned about being found out. This is a fear shared by many crossdressers who are not out of the closet. Please check out some of these: www.tri-ess.org, www.tgfmall.com, www.pmpub.com, www.brendat.com.

As a wife or girlfriend who suddenly discovers that her man has a secret cache of frilly garb, try to give yourself a three-month chilling-off period before doing anything drastic. Talk to your partner about what he does and why. He must love you a great deal if he's worked so hard to hide something that's so darned big. If you can, check out the site of the Society for the Second Self or Tri-Ess at www.tri-ess.org. This national organization is for crossdressers, their wives and their families. Search out anything written by Francis Fairfax, particularly the *Wives' Bill of Rights*.

Given how this is not the sort of thing you can call your mom or sister about, see if there is a support group in your area for wives of crossdressers. The folks at Tri-Ess can help you find them. Talk to these wives about what they will and won't put up with. There are plenty of things you don't need to agree to, like meeting your man for lunch when he's dressed like Britney Spears. And if for some reason he thinks he can dress up in front of the kids or gets so deep into the crossdressing scene that he stops being a good husband or dad, crossdressers' wives will offer all the support you need to confront him. In other words, you don't have to condone what he's doing, but you don't need to divorce him either.

For a lot of women, it would be easier to accept their husband if he said he were gay. But to see him dressed up like Little Bo Peep and hear him say he's totally straight…. Wives tend to fear they will lose the manly part of their crossdressing man. This usually won't happen. He'll be the same man he was in bed before she found out about the heels and A-line dress. Part of their fear may have to do with humiliation that someone else will find out.

After chilling off, a wife or girlfriend might see that there are worse things a man could do than wear women's clothes, fashion crime that it might be. She might also realize that he has the same good characteristics that he had before she found out about his hidden side.

There is no shortage of publications on crossdressing. Some people value the books by Peggy Rudd, a therapist and the wife of a crossdresser. Others aren't so comfortable with her crossdresser-as-visionary point of view. Your public library may have them, but perhaps you'll want to try Amazon.

HIGHLY RECOMMENDED: Amy Bloom's *Normal–Transsexual CEOs, Cross-dressing Cops, and Hermaphrodites with Attitude,* Vantage Books, (2003). Knowledge may not make it hurt any less, but it does give you more options than simply saying goodbye. If you need a gift for a man who enjoys wearing women's clothes, don't forget: www.wayout-publishing.com.

Phone Sex—When 911 Isn't Enough to Put Out Your Fire

Ever wonder what goes on in phone sex, when a man pays several dollars a minute to get a good talking to? A young woman who worked as a phone-sex operator after graduating from an expensive private college was kind enough to offer the following description:

"The fantasies ranged from men who wanted me to physically beat myself on the phone with a hairbrush, to those who wanted me to force them to have oral sex with other men and those who just wanted to hear me have an orgasm. What struck me is that men have more gay fantasies than I would have expected. There seems to be a correlation between men who have powerful jobs and their sexual fantasies. One client, who I later found out was a senior partner in a financial firm always wanted me to 'force' him to do things, mostly to other men and sometimes to me. Others wanted to escape from their life, shed their responsibility and their maleness—they explored their imagination with me and pretended I was their dominatrix, their she-male, their whore. I gave them permission and encouraged them to be who they wanted to be and that's what they needed.

"I always wondered about clients. I was madly, madly curious. I wanted to know who they were, how much money they made, if they were married, if they were straight and if they were the kinds of guys I knew. And often, I'd 'interview' them and I'll admit that I looked up what

I could find on Google. I couldn't help myself. I wanted to know why they were calling me, how it played into their real sex life and what I was to them. In some instances, I was the woman on the phone who was their mistress, but in the most controlled way and they would call on a regular basis. Some got attached to me and I was fired and then rehired and in my absence, I was missed (as I learned later)."

Vaginal Fisting (Handballing)

Vaginal fisting is finger fucking times five, and then some. This Guide first became aware of the concept when reviewing lesbian tapes produced by and for women. It seems that some women enjoy having a partner's fist inside their vagina.

But that kind of fisting is being done by women to women. Most women have significantly smaller fists than men. A fist the size of a man's could take a potentially pleasurable experience and turn it into something akin to childbirth in reverse. On the other hand, a leading sex therapist has informed us that a number of straight couples are getting a fist up.

If vaginal fisting is something you want to try, please plan far enough ahead to read a book or two that covers the subject. Greenery Press publishes *A Hand in the Bush: The Fine Art of Vaginal Fisting* by Deborah Addington. This subject is also discussed in the *Good Vibrations Guide to Sex* by Anne Semans and Cathy Winks, Cleis Press (2002) and in the *On Our Backs Guide to Lesbian Sex,* edited by Diana Cage, Alyson Press, (2004).

Please check with a health-care professional before attempting any kind of fisting, and in no instance should you proceed if you experience anything but the slightest amount of pain. Perhaps you can find the name of a physician or nurse practitioner who is familiar with fisting through a gay and lesbian health center, since your local HMO might not be particularly well versed in the practice. You should never attempt fisting if either of you has been drinking or doing drugs, and you certainly shouldn't try it before reading the advice of women who do it.

Anal Fisting

Some couples, straight as well as gay, are into anal fisting. You shouldn't even think about trying this unless you really, really, really know what you are doing. Technically, this act is possible without causing physical damage, since surgeons occasionally stick an entire hand up a person's rectum. On the other hand, receiving an entire fist up the bum requires the kind of relaxation that is beyond the capacity of the average asshole.

Couples into anal fisting often recommend a book on the subject by Bert Herrman, *Trust—The Hand Book*, Alamo Square Press, (1991). Tristan Taormino's *The Ultimate Guide to Anal Sex for Women, 2nd edition*, Cleis Press (2006) is also an excellent resource. There might also be organized groups of fisters in the nearest large city who give talks and demonstrations. Please check with a health-care professional before attempting any kind of fisting, and in no instance should you proceed if you are not completely sober or experience anything but the slightest amount of pain.

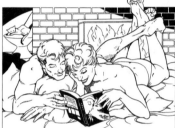

Dear Paul,

Do you have any advice about going to a dominatrix?

Policeman by Day, Schoolboy by Night

Dear Officer,

To help answer your question, I called my friend Lorrett, who runs a house devoted to BDSM and fantasy play. She offers the following advice:

1. BDSM is about creating a fantasy scene, and then acting it out. In creating the scene, you need to talk to the person you are hiring about things like boundaries, safe words, and how you want the scene to play out. You should feel comfortable with the person, and feel that they are comfortable with you in negotiating the scene. If they come off as being abrupt or domineering when setting up the scene, then what follows isn't going to be play. Instead, you are going to be acting out their agenda, and what follows will be anything but consensual.

2. Trust your instincts. It's fine to be nervous or anxious, but if you feel frightened or uncomfortable, go elsewhere.

In domination and fantasy games, the dominatrix doesn't actually get you off. You are free to get yourself off in her presence, but she won't actually give you an orgasm the way a prostitute will. That's why it's not illegal for you to hire a dominatrix.

Special Thanks to Lorrett at Fantasy Makers in Berkeley and Janet at Greenery Press—two of the nicest people around.

51
Vulva Care
Keeping Your Kitty Happy

You wouldn't believe the questions we get at Goofy Foot Press, including those from guys about how some of the women they'd gone down on didn't seem to be paying a lot of attention to general crotch care. When we forwarded an inquiry to our gynecology expert, she went on a rant:

> "It fascinates me how many women come to the gynecologist with a smelly puss. For heaven's sake, give the kitty a little wipe-down before you spread your legs."

Then we thought about what some college healthcare providers have communicated—that they're seeing young women who won't use the Nuva-Ring because they say it's gross to stick their fingers in their own vagina. Ditto for OB tampons.

Let's see, they'll let some guy stick his fingers, face and penis between their legs, but a little self-exploration is gross? Which got us to thinking that if enough women are uptight about their genitals, they might have a tendency to either overly clean themselves in a scrubbing-douching frenzy, or they might just ignore that part of their body altogether and spend the extra time getting a new set of nails. So we figured it was time offer the Guide's Guide to a Happy and Healthy Crotch.

Crotch Care Basics—From Wiping to Giving Your Puss a Bath[1]

Cleanliness May Be Next To Godliness—But Only in Moderation

Out damn butt bacteria! Always wipe front to back *for pee as well as poop* (our gynecology consultant's very words). If we guys had vaginas and had to wipe from front to back, our vaginas would be one big infected running sore. That's why we've got penises: because butt bacteria does not

---

[1]For women who have vulvar pain, infections, concerns about their vaginal health or any medical condition: please seek out the advice of a gynecologist.

make for a happy vagina, and there's no way you could ever train us to wipe from front to rear.

Do not overclean the puss. It only needs soap once a day at the most, and that should be a bland bar of soap like Basis, Pears or Dove Sensitive Skin. (Just because Ivory says it's pure doesn't mean it's not harsh. Besides, why would you want something *pure* between your legs? The women around here prefer that anything going between their legs be bad to the bone!)

Do not use liquid body gels or cheap washes. Our gynecology experts go nuclear at the thought of using body gels and cheap washes, including the bubble bath soaps:

> "I always tell women not to use bubble baths/bath beads. This is basically like douching with those chemicals. These products are so mainstream and often in gift baskets—it's like, 'Here my friend, have this lovely yeast infection and happy birthday to you!'"

Do not confuse pH with penis size: Let's say your kitty is a persnickety little puss who doesn't like soap every day. Unless your gynecologist says something to the contrary, you should still clean her with water. Part of the reason for her not doing well with soap might be the kind you are using. Consider trying a high-quality, low-pH soap like SebaMed between your legs. Your vulva and vagina are a bit acidic, with a pH of around 5.2. However, most bar soaps are alkaline, with a pH of 10 or higher. Some women who have struggled with vaginal infections swear by the lower-pH soaps like SebaMed. These soaps don't have a lot of alkali in them like cheaper soaps, and they are a bit acidic just like your spasm chasm. They also make a SebaMed Feminine Intimate Wash that's just for the vulva. It has an even lower pH and is especially gentle and mild. Unfortunately, the SebaMed Feminine Intimate Wash is hard to find in the States—which is interesting because you can get it in Europe and Canada.

Your Vulva Is Not a Pot: Never scrub between your legs. Using your fingers instead of a wash cloth is best. It's fine if you have a hand held shower head and know just how to hit your sweet spot with it, and that's water on your vajayjay and not soap, and it feels SOOOOOO good.

Smegma? Isn't that Just a Penis Thing? To help prevent clitoral-hood adhesions or smegma—yes, smegma—from forming where a man likes to lick, pull back your clitoral hood and separate your inner and outer lips while rinsing with water. Again, use your fingers, not a washcloth.

Avoid Run-Off from Above: Shampoos tend to be harsh and perfumy. Make sure the shampoo and conditioner don't stream between your legs and through the lips of your vulva when you are rinsing them from your hair. This can be avoided by bending over when you are rinsing out the shampoo.

Pat, Don't Rub! There's a perfectly good time to rub between your legs, but not when drying yourself after a shower or bath. While some experts advise drying your vulva with a hairdryer on cool, others warn against it. They all agree that gentle patting is good, and not just after a bath!

Wipes, Lotions, Feminine Sprays, Douches & Perfume: Do not use baby wipes after peeing or pooping, and never use powders, lotions or perfume. They tend to be irritating. If nature intended your crotch to be perfumed, she would have planted roses between your legs. Also, avoid feminine-hygiene sprays, douches and talcum power. According to our gynecology experts,

> "The vajayjay is a natural cleansing area and douching makes it smell. Douching is acceptable only if it's right after your period and hot sex is coming that night."

Normal Smells

Sorry to be so blunt, but your vulva is an orifice. It has sweat glands and it's covered with hair. As one of our gynecology experts says, "This can lead to all sorts of interesting smells, most of them completely normal." Of course, our guy crotches never smell anything but wonderful. As for the girl groin, it's normal for a vulva and vagina to smell musky, and it's normal for the odor to change throughout your cycle.

Also be aware that female vulvas and male scrotums have apocrine glands embedded in them. These glands respond to stress situations and are the olfactory version of land minds. There's not a thing you can do about it, except maybe move to a tropical island paradise where you can lounge by the beach all day and forget stress altogether.

So there's musky, and there's bad. If your vagina smells bad as opposed to musky, it probably needs a visit to the crotch doc. So check with your healthcare provider. You might also be more prone to an infection early in a relationship, which is pretty common. This might happen "as his stuff gets used to your stuff." So if your vagina smells bad after your partner ejaculates inside of you, consider the possibility that you have a vaginal infection. (Semen is alkaline, which creates an odor-releasing chemical reaction with the secretions in your vagina if you have bacterial vaginosis.) If this continues and you don't have any signs of infection, your partner might have chronic prostatitis, which a urologist can check for.

Thongs & Pads vs. Going Commando

While our gyno expert from the land of sun and sand admits that thongs can look hot, they abrade and tear up the vulva. She sees lots of redness, rubbing and irritation due to thongs. She recommends going commando (wearing no undies) instead.

She also says that wearing pads or pantiliners to "feel fresh" simply traps moisture and is irritating to the vulva. If leakage is a problem, try using a cotton handkerchief to line your panties with, or a 100% cotton pad.

Our other gynecology expert gets her panties in a wad over girls and women sleeping in their panties. She says that vulvas need to breathe, and there's no way that's going to happen if you sleep while wearing your underwear, even the kind with a cotton crotch.

Both of our gyno experts are proponents of going commando as often as possible. That's because your kitty needs air to breathe. As for the occasional Britney Spears moment, if anyone notices, just tell them you are doing your bit to help beautify the homeland.

Peeing, Shaving, and Popping Hair Bumps

Shaving can be really irritating, and so can hair-removal products. If you want your hair short, try a men's mustache trimmer or trim with scissors. It won't be porn-star bare, but who needs that? In fact, our gynecology expert who is a surgeon thinks that a lot of women would have happier crotches if they hacked away at some of the foliage between their legs, because it would allow more air to circulate.

In our culture we wear underwear so much that any extra air that can blow through your lower lips is a good thing. It's the shaving of the vulva with a razor, as opposed to trimming your pubic hair short, that these physicians don't like.

If you do shave and get little bumps around the hair follicles, NO POPPING. There is a high risk for *staph* infections from doing this. Try warm, moist compresses and antibacterial ointment, and see your healthcare provider if you are concerned or irritation continues. If you have labial adhesions or you dribble after peeing, pull your pants all the way down and urinate with your knees apart to prevent urine from pooling into your vagina.

What to Wear Down There If You Can't Go Commando

Wear 100% cotton underwear. Do not wear underwear that is nylon on the outside but has a cotton liner, as the nylon shell will keep the cotton crotch from breathing.

For workout gear, fabrics that wick away moisture are good, but take off your work out gear as soon as your exercise balls are racked.

Thigh highs (nylons) are better than pantyhose for your crotch, and you don't need to take them off if you are having a quickie at work.

How to Wash What You Wear Down There

Optimal crotch care means more than just what you do in the shower or bath. It also means what you put in your washing machine and dryer.

When washing your underwear, use a mild, unscented laundry soap such as Tide Free, All Free and Clear, Dreft, Ivory and Costco's Kirkland Free and Clear. Detergents like these have earned the Goofy Foot Press *Good Crotchkeeping Seal* that says "Good for Your Lips!"

Use less detergent rather than more, and if your washer has a second rinse option, use it. Do not use fabric softening or antistatic sheets in your dryer when you are drying your underwear as these leave residues in the fabric that can easily rub off on your skin. If you've got static in your panties, may we suggest you masturbate or make a booty call.

A Very Special Thanks to Maureen Whelihan, MD, the gyno-goddess of greater Florida, and to Rachel Pauls, MD, FACOG, Urogynecologist and Director, Center for Female Sexual Health at Good Sam in Cincinnati.

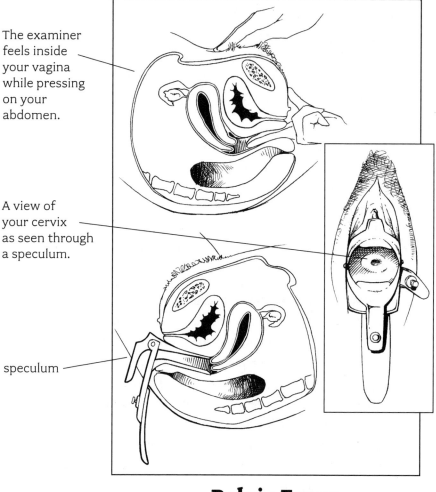

The examiner feels inside your vagina while pressing on your abdomen.

A view of your cervix as seen through a speculum.

speculum

Pelvic Exam

No intercourse the night before!

Dear Paul,

My friends have gone recently to their first gynecologist exam, and the stories they told me really scared me. One girl said it was really uncomfortable, and the other said it was downright painful; she was actually crying. Both mentioned something about the doctor sticking their whole hand inside them; is this true? I am starting to worry because I can't even get a tampon in there: last time I tried it was too painful and I gave up. Do some girls have unusually narrow vaginas?

About to Have My First Pelvic Exam

Dear About to Have,

For the exam itself, you will go into a room and trade your shirt and blue jeans for a paper gown—sometimes purple, sometimes blue, whatever is the latest in disposable gyno fashion. Usually a nurse and doctor will come in for the exam. They will ask you to lay down on an examination table. You will put your heels in metal stirrups and scoot your bum all the way to the end of the table. They will then shine a light on your genitals. The doctor will put a speculum in your vagina to help expand it and insert a little stick-like device to scrape some cells from your cervix. This won't hurt at all, but you still might feel something. The cells will be put on a slide and sent to the lab for testing. Then they remove the speculum, and the doctor will insert one or two fingers inside your vagina to feel your cervix, ovaries and whatever else Mother Nature put up there. She will also feel the outside of your abdomen with her other hand. Most doctors will examine the lips of your vulva and some doctors will do a brief rectal exam. The doctor or nurse will also do a breast exam. Also, it's best to abstain from intercourse the night before, but if you must, use a condom. Here is advice for you from our women readers:

> "I remember how scared I was before my first exam. The best thing to do is to tell the doctor that you are anxious and ask him or her to explain what is going to happen before the exam begins. A good doctor will explain things in as much detail as it takes to help calm your nerves. The worst part for me was the feeling of embarrassment that someone was looking at me. A pelvic exam should not hurt, and if it does for some reason you should tell the doctor immediately so that he or she can stop. As far as tampons are concerned, I have the same problem, and you might want to check out the tampons that are marketed as "slim fit" or even the ones that don't use an applicator. I find that these work best for me. Also try to relax. The more nervous you are the tighter your pelvic muscles will be." *female age 22*

> "It's not that bad, and no MD has EVER put his or her whole hand in me for a regular exam. Your friends are probably being overly dramatic." *female age 18*

> "He doesn't put his whole hand in there, darlin, it just seems like you are very full because of the speculum. It is pressing you open from top and bottom and it is what you mostly feel. Also not all

girls are a straight shot in. I had some discomfort on a regular basis until a male doctor pointed out that my cervix was tilted to the right-hand-side of my body. I now know to tell the doctor about this before going in so I don't get banged in the wrong direction. Unless the doctor is using one of the new disposable speculums, they do come in different sizes as well. I am very petite and know that a smaller size will be more comfortable. Some of this comes from experience, but it is your part to speak out on these issues with your doctor." *female age 33*

"I am a very small woman. My first pap was done with the instruments they use to test small children for molestation, if that tells you anything. I have since had many pelvic exams, all of which have been done with standard equipment. Breathe deeply, and try to think of other things, and let the doctor do her job. And don't let them give you an exam while you're on your period. It's uncomfortable for you, take my word for it." *female age 22*

Last but not least, for a report on getting a pelvic exam from half way around the world (count your lucky stars, girls in America!):

"Each examination room is shared by two doctors. So when I entered, there was another patient splayed out on the table, having a pelvic exam, right next to the door. She appeared to be accompanied by half a dozen people, both males and females; the preceding patient and her entourage were also there, in addition to my coworker and myself, and the two doctors. The door to the lobby was wide open. The first question the doctor asked me was translated as, 'Do you have the sexy life?' (As in, 'Are you sexually active?') Naturally, all eyes turned to me–foreigners are something of a novelty here–and of course, I'd just started dating a guy after six months of celibacy, so I said yes. After several more questions, I was led to a table in the corner of the room and instructed to disrobe. No paper gown, no curtain, no closed door. So, my legs spread for what felt like the world to see, up the speculum went." *female age 24*

52

Surfing the Crimson Wave
From Period Gear to Period Sex

If guys had periods, you could tell when by looking at the color under our fingernails or the stains on the top of our socks. That's because we'd either be checking out our vaginas like they were the Stargate, or because no one's going to stop a game of Halo, Guitar Hero or basketball just because he started bleeding sooner than planned or his flow was a tampon's worst nightmare.

So it's the strangest thing that so many guys act awkward when dealing with their partner's period, or why everyone gets quiet and pretends to ignore it when an ad for tampons or pads is on TV.

Part of the strangeness has to do with privacy because periods are a private thing and that's not a bad thing. But there are ways of respecting a woman's privacy without acting like you've just encountered an alien with a serious slime disease, and there are ways of dealing with tampons and pads without behaving like a dork.

Hopefully you'll find this chapter to be a squirm-free alternative to what you might have been told about periods in a health or biology class—where talk of eggs and Fallopian tubes ruled the day instead of information that might actually be useful in your life and relationships.

In this chapter we'll talk about bleeding, leaking, cramps, period gear, stain removal, menstrual cups, period panties, and more than you'll find anywhere on the planet about having period sex, including why a lot of couples say it feels so good.

Nearly 25% of the Women You Know Are Ragging Right Now

At any given time, nearly 25% of all non-pregnant women between the ages of 15 and 45 are having their periods. That's nearly one-fourth of the women who are skiing, running, swimming and playing baseball, basketball or soccer—women who are students, office workers, doctors, lawyers, accountants, teachers, mothers, dancers, actresses, waitresses.

One of every four girls between the ages of 15 and 45 is oozing blood between her legs at this very moment. When you put it in that perspective, it's hard to understand why people think there's anything unusual or embarrassing about periods.

And more to the point, there is no evidence that a woman's intellectual or job performance is affected by her menstrual cycle. Plenty of women have won Olympic medals and recorded platinum songs while ragging.

The Pad and Tampon Wars

> Two young boys walk into a pharmacy one day, pick out a box of Tampax, and proceed to the checkout counter.
>
> The man at the counter asks the older boy, "Son, how old are you?"
>
> "Eight," the boy replies.
>
> The man continues, "Do you know what these are used for?"
>
> "Not exactly," the boy says. "But they aren't for me. They're for him. He's my brother. He's four. We saw on TV that if you use these you would be able to swim and ride a bike. Right now he can't do either one."

Not too long ago, people believed that women needed to rest during their periods. (Today's females would love the luxury!) The wisdom of the day had it that ladies of the better classes shouldn't exert themselves with strenuous activities or sports during that time of the month. Not so for the maid or cook who was expected to work a full day regardless.

The experts who championed these theories in the late 1800s believed that women were the more delicate sex and that their bodies were more frail than men's. They were sure that women didn't think about sex, and that the female brain was too small for the demands of college and higher education. Then came the first pads (aka "sanitary napkins") and the first tampons, and the "frail woman" nonsense started to get flushed as fast as a used Tampax.

While today's academic feminists are correct to be cramping in disgust at the way women's periods have been portrayed since the start of the pad and tampon wars, they miss a salient concept that a number of these ads championed: that while a woman's period might be annoying and distracting, it isn't debilitating. More importantly, copy from the ads like those below reminded people that the modern woman had social and economic opportunities that her mother didn't:

> "Old-Fashioned ways cannot withstand the merry onslaught of the modern girl..." *Modess, 1929*

> "The Girl of Today demands perfect freedom and comfort. She wants the best and will not tolerate the drudgeries that held her mother in bondage." *Modess 1929*

> "Every Day of the Month Is a Day of Freedom." *Tampax, 1936*

> "Don't Give Up Athletics Any Day of the Month." *Tampax, 1939*

> "You're the Fun in His Furlough... Why let trying days of the month rule your life? You don't need time-out... that is, if you choose Kotex sanitary napkins." *Kotex, 1942*

And what about this over-the-top text from the 1929 Modess pad campaign that championed self-reliance and rejection of old-fashioned ideas:

> "Life is so much more fun when one is not afraid. It is her happy courage—the zest with which she welcomes every new delightful freedom—which is the charm of the modern girl... In a gloomier age, women were resigned to drudgery. Today, young womanhood does not permit drudgery to cloud her joy of living."

These ads refuted ideas from the 1800s that women's bodies and brains were inferior. They took the onus off of the body and put it on the pad—a woman wasn't the slave of her period as long as she bought "the right" tampon or pad. Long before the second-wave feminism of the 1960s and 1970s, these ads were telling women that they could pretty much do anything that men could, with smaller strings attached.

At the end of this chapter, we return to the very first Kotex ad from 1920, and look at how the name "Kotex" came to be. But there's a lot of other things to look at first, from period gear and removing stubborn blood stains to period sex, breast tenderness, period suppression, and a whole lot more.

Menstruation Man's Flow Facts

• Women are told that the normal time for a cycle is 28 days, with the duration of bleeding from 4 to 6 days. That would be fine if one size fit all, but for many women the time from the start of one cycle to the start of the next ranges from 21 to 32 days. The time between periods can be the same from cycle to cycle, or it can be all over the place. The duration of bleeding can vary as well.

• Women are often told that it is normal to bleed between 4 to 6 tablespoons during an average period. Is there a woman on the planet who sits with a tablespoon between her legs during her entire period? Women usually quantify their menstrual bleeding with how many tampons or pads they use. They have no idea how many tablespoons that may or may not be.

• Oh joy! Period cramps are related to labor pains. Both are mediated by prostaglandins. This is why prostaglandin inhibitors like Midol, ibuprofen, ponstel and celebrex can help if you have cramps. The trick is in taking as little as one ibuprofen a day or two **BEFORE** you think your cramps will begin. Birth-control pills can also help because the progesterone in them can quiet the roar in your uterus and might help even you out hormonally.

• For pain relief once your period starts, orgasms can help. Orgasms pump powerful pain relievers into the body and the contractions can help push accumulated fluids out of your uterus. In spite of the benefits, can you imagine a mother telling her daughter, "Honey, if you're having cramps, why not masturbate?"

• The faster period blood drips out, the more red it's going to be. The slower it drips out, the darker it might be. That's because when it flows more slowly, it spends a longer time in the upper part of your vagina and becomes oxidized, which can result in its turning brownish. The reason why period blood often looks brown on pads is because it has mixed with oxygen and has oxidized. If period blood comes out really slowly, it might look like a dark, tar-like paste.

• The clumps in your period flow are from your body's clotting mechanisms. Our gyno consultant said that when there's heavy flow, she likes to see clotting, because it means the body is working to decrease the amount of bleeding. It concerns her when there's a lot of bright red blood that is thin like Koolaid and has no clots in it. She also said that as a woman gets older, "she'll start to shed tissue from the lining that looks like 'strings' of tissue."

• After a woman turns 40 or so, the volume of blood flow might seriously increase, but for only 1 to 3 days rather than the whole time. There might be more clumps, as well.

• If you are concerned about any of this beyond the basic annoyance that it has to happen to you, please ask your physician!

Why Guys Freak Out

There are two things about women's bodies and their periods that have freaked men out (and women, as well) over the ages. First is how a woman's vagina, ovaries and uterus are on the inside. Ergonomically, this isn't nearly as bad as having your balls and penis hanging on the outside, but we still tend to fear what we can't see.

Second issue: blood. We humans are one-tracked when it comes to bleeding. We see it as a sign of injury or disease.

So if you combine monthly bleeding with where the blood drips from—you start seeing cultures throughout the ages that have come up with rituals regarding menstruation to help deal with their fear of the unknown. Some of the rituals were sadly isolating and punitive, while others appear to have been empowering for women.

Women, too, must have wondered about the strange spirits that took over their bodies and made them bleed every month.

From Evil Spirits to Eggs & Fallopian Tubes

Unless she is seriously late or is trying to get pregnant, the last thing a woman thinks about when she's having her period is an egg dropping down her Fallopian tubes. Yet that's pretty much what periods have been reduced to in the way we teach about menstruation in school.

The story of how monthly bleeding relates to reproduction has become the new mythology to help allay our fears about menstruation. Even the Biblical Snake of old makes an appearance in the form of the sperm-spewing penis. It's a scientific narrative that helps reassure us that periods are really OK. But given the silence in the room when a tampon commercial comes on TV, you can't help but wonder about it. Is the silence because the ad is a reminder that a woman has a vagina? That it bleeds? Are people as uncomfortable when an ad comes on for Viagra?

While modern science has better answers about menstruation than philosophers like Aristotle and St. Augustine did in centuries past, keep in mind that we still don't know why women menstruate every month and whether it's a good thing or a bad thing. There is currently a huge debate over the long-term safety of using birth control pills to stop a woman's periods altogether, and we still don't know why some women's breasts get tender at different times in their monthly cycle.

What Girls Really Want to Know, and What Guys Should Know

Are eggs and Fallopian tubes what girls want to know about periods? Of course not. Girls in their teens want to know about how to control the bloody mess, how to control the cramps and low backache, how to get blood stains out of their panties and pajamas, how to better predict when their period will strike and how heavy the flow will be. They want to know how to carry period gear inconspicuously, and how to deal with feelings of embarrassment when boys find out they are having their period and try to tease them.

When girls get older and become sexually active, they also want to know about period sex, and no matter how young or old they are, girls who are having their periods want to know "Why me? Why does this happens to girls and not guys?"

As for guys, once you get into a long-term relationship, menstruation is something that happens to both of you. That's why guys who live with girls will do better in life if they try to understand more about periods. Unfortunately, males tend to relate periods to reproduction or sex, while for women it's about blood, tampons, pads, and for some, cramps, tender breasts and lower back pain. And until a guy becomes a dad who has to pay for tampons and pads, he's usually not aware of how much the things cost every month.

Period Gear

Period gear has come a long way since the days when women wore funky belts to hold thick pads in place–we're talking something just shy of a mattress between your legs. The next couple of sections are about pads, tampons, and period gear. But first here's a story from back when pads had tails:

My mother taught me to read when I was four years old (her first mistake)...

One day, I was in the bathroom and noticed one of the cabinet doors was open. I read the box in the cabinet. I then asked my mother why she was keeping 'napkins' in the bathroom. Didn't they belong in the kitchen? Not wanting to burden me with unnecessary facts, she told me that those were for "special occasions" (her second mistake).

Now, fast forward a few months.... It's Thanksgiving Day, and my folks are leaving to pick up my uncle and his wife for dinner. Mom had assignments for all of us while they were gone. Mine was to set the table.

When they returned, my uncle came in first and immediately burst into laughter. Next, in came my father, who roared with laughter. Then in came Mom, who almost died of embarrassment when she saw each place setting on the table with a "special occasion" napkin at each plate, with the fork carefully arranged on top. I had even tucked the little tail in so they didn't hang off the edge! My mother asked me why I used these and, of course, my response sent the other adults into further fits of laughter. "But, Mom, you said they were for special occasions!!!"

Quick Change Artists & Talking the Talk

While teenage guys need to have certain strategies to deal with unwanted hard-ons, not too many of them have to worry about a friend tapping them on the shoulder and whispering that a BIG blotch of blood leaked through the back of their pants and everyone is looking.

Periods can arrive with little rhyme or reason, especially during the first couple of years, so a girl who has started having her period has to cope with everything from blood leaking out to how she's going to change a pad or tampon during only a five-minute break between classes—all while acting like nothing's up because she's worried guys will make fun of her if they know she's ragging.

On a more positive note, periods give girls an excuse to talk with each other about their own sexual anatomy. Sharing experiences and information about periods can be a source of bonding, not to mention an outlet for sharing personal horror stories, like when the cutest guy on the planet got behind you in the checkout line at the supermarket after you just put a super gigantic sized box of Kotex on the conveyer belt.

Being able to talk with their friends about periods might also help girls share information about their sexual anatomy in a time when parents still refer to female genitals as "your vagina" or "down there," and a lot of teenage girls don't even know what their clit really is.

When a Woman Drops a Tampon

Researchers designed a study where a woman "accidentally" dropped either an unused tampon or a hair clip on the ground. Observers who viewed the woman dropping the objects rated her as being less competent and less likeable when she dropped the tampon than when she dropped the hair clip. (Geez, what do you think the responses would have been if she had dropped a condom?)

Hopefully, readers of *The Guide* will help reverse this little insanity and begin to make fun of women who drop hair clips on the ground as opposed to tampons.

A Sweater or Shirt to Tie Around Your Waist and Period Panties

While some young women wear sweaters or shirts tied around their waists to hide their butts, it never hurts to keep an extra shirt or sweater in your locker or car in case you end up with a blood stain on the back of your pants or skirt. Unfortunately, this is not an option for women who have to wear uniforms. Keeping an extra pair of pants or jeans and undies in your car or locker is also a good idea, as well as some spare tampons or pads.

The cool way to store a stash of tampons used to be to keep them in a Vinnie's Tampon Case, but as of press time, it looks like the Vinnie case is no more. Given that this was such a helpful product, we have started to produce our own tampon/glasses/condoms/cellphone case with the zipper from *The Guide's* cover on them; go to www.GuideToGettingItOn.com.

A lot of women have what they call "period panties," which in some cases were panties they really liked, but have ended up with stains in the crotch that refuse to come out. They only wear them when they are ragging. Others will only wear dark underwear, and some get inexpensive Wal-Mart specials just to wear when they are having their periods.

Period-Related Breast Tenderness

Some women's breasts get really sore when they are having their period. Some women's breasts get sore at a different time during their cycle, like when they are ovulating. And some women's breasts become sensitive in a way that welcomes kisses and caresses during certain times of the month. So if you are in a relationship, breast tenderness is important to talk about.

Period-related breast soreness can be slight, or it can be so extreme that one of our readers said just driving over speed bumps really hurts. Some women say their breasts will feel like they are bruised. Both breasts can become tender, or just one, or hopefully none. This can be helped by taking birth-control pills, or it can be caused by taking birth-control pills. Go figure.

Menstruation Man on Period Sex

Some couples are afraid of having intercourse when Aunt Flo comes to town. Fear not! Period sex causes no harm to either partner. Better yet, it can bring buckets of smiles. Here are some reasons why:

• Period flow is slippery and can make a vagina feel super-lubed. Some couples say the flow feels better than store-bought lube.

• Menstrual swelling can help a woman have a really nice orgasm. Who knows if it makes intercourse feel better, but a woman's cervix drops when she's ragging. As a result, some couples might prefer certain period positions. Explore and see what feels best for you.

• Some women get extra-horny during their periods. This might have to do with a change in hormones, or perhaps they feel more relaxed since it's harder to get pregnant.

Some couples feel all primal and cool being drenched in period sex blood; others act like they've just arrived at a crime scene. You can vary your flow exposure with the following tips:

• Put a towel down to catch the flow, or have sex in the shower.

• Use a male condom or the female condom.

• Wear a diaphragm or use Instead. These are little domes that cradle the cervix and catch most of the flow.

• For period-sex-fantasy fun, turn on a Buffy rerun or have sex while one of the newer vampire shows is on the TV!

• If period sex proper isn't for you, you can always get each other off by hand, with a vibrator or dildo. Orgasms can help ease period pain.

• Anal sex can be an option if both of you enjoy it, but it's hard to think that a woman who enjoys anal sex would have a problem with vaginal sex while she's on her period.

• DO NOT wear a tampon during intercourse! If you do, see pp. 722-3 on fishing out lost condoms. It's similar. Be sure to get any mashed parts out. And you CAN get pregnant from having period sex.

Tips for receiving oral sex while on your period:

• Splash some water into your vagina, then insert a tampon before a partner goes down on you. The tampon will catch most of the flow. If intercourse follows, be sure to take the tampon out first.

• Do it in the shower.

• Wear a diaphragm, Instead or a menstrual cup: Some women get a diaphragm for the sole purpose of having period sex. Some couples start with it in for oral sex, but take it out for intercourse.

• Wrap it! Cover your vulva with a barrier or plastic wrap. A little lube between the vulva and plastic wrap might help.

• Some guys like going down as is, flow and all.

• **Important Health Note:** You can get dangerous STIs like hepatitis or HIV from sucking down period blood, even if the woman shows no symptoms. Best not to do period-oral during hook-up sex.

Getting The Red Out—Removing Period Blood

It's difficult to have periods and not stain things. In fact, if you've been having periods for a while and haven't stained a whole bunch of things, consider getting treatment for an obsessive-compulsive disorder.

It's always best to treat blood stains as soon as possible, but who's got a laundry room handy when most stains occur? However, for triage while on the run, you might try hitting a new stain with a wad of loogie and blotting it up, or if there's some contact-lens saline solution handy, try that. The reason for using saline or spit, which is your own saline with some enzymes and food gunk added, is that saline will help the blood cells float out instead of smearing them on the fabric like cream cheese on a bagel.

So here's *The Guide's* Guide to Getting the Red Out:

 Soak the item in cold water, over night if necessary. If that doesn't take the red out...

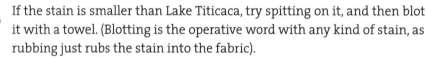

 If the stain is smaller than Lake Titicaca, try spitting on it, and then blot it with a towel. (Blotting is the operative word with any kind of stain, as rubbing just rubs the stain into the fabric).

 If it's too big to spit at, use unpreserved saline solution on it, the kind people use for contact lenses. Or mix one cup of salt in 2 quarts of cold water. Soak for half an hour. Then blot, don't rub.

If Big Red is still there, add a bit of mild bar soap and rub it into the fabric. Rinse with cold water.

If it refuses to surrender, consider this: blood stains can become really nasty when the hemoglobin in the blood mixes with oxygen in the air. This binds the stain to the fabric. Since hemeglobin is made up of iron, what you might be dealing with in a stubborn blood stain is a rust stain. Even the folks at Tide mention using rust remover if the usual removal techniques fail:

 1) Carefully apply Whink Rust Remover or other liquid rust remover following the instructions on the package. Apply over a plastic or glass dishpan, as the rust remover can be a bit gnarly on certain surfaces. 2) Rinse in 1 quart of water to which 3 tablespoons of baking soda have been added. 3) Air dry and repeat the procedure if necessary. Or...

Hydrogen peroxide is often used to get out blood stains. However, while hydrogen peroxide isn't known to harm the color in fabrics, it can make the fabric weaker. That's why hydrogen peroxide is not our product of first choice, as you might end up with crotchless panties sooner than you wanted.

Period Parties & "You Are Becoming a Woman"

This Kotex ad from 1942 shows how period education used to be:

~ Mothers ~

Why get all involved trying to explain the facts of menstruation to your little girls when there's a simple, easy way to do this dreaded task?

Let the new booklet "As One Girl To Another" do this job for you! It will spare you a session that may only end in confusion, and embarrassment.

Fortunately, things are changing. A lot of mothers today are framing a girl's first period as something to celebrate and as an important milestone reached in a girl's life. Some moms take their daughters out to a special lunch or dinner, and some even have parties—which might be a bit much as far as some daughters are concerned. But if parents feel the need to mortify their kid with a cake and party to celebrate their daughter's first period, at least it's a step in the right direction.

How to decorate a cake to celebrate your first period is another matter. We at Goofy Foot Press would most likely edge it with pads and tampons made of marzipan, and a confetti of Midols made from sugar on top. As for the cake's interior, do you stay with a classic white cake with alternating layers of strawberry and raspberry, or do you make a bold statement and go with a red velvet cake mix?

As for saying that a girl has "become a woman" after her first period, that seems to be stretching it a bit when you consider how early girls are having their periods. The concept of womanhood is more social than biological, and to think that a 12- or 13-year-old girl in Western culture has reached womanhood begs a reality check. A girl's first period marks an important biological passage, but it's more reasonable to think of her high-school graduation as a transition into womanhood.

Perhaps the most significant passage a first period marks is it allows a girl to enter into the same "club" that her mom, friends and older sisters are in. This can be empowering and socially important for a girl. Some girls who have their first period later than their friends feel left out of this "club" and can't wait to join it—until they have their first cramps.

Who Put the "Hygiene" in Feminine Hygiene and the "Sanitary" in Sanitary Napkins? And What about Odor?

Toward the end of the 1800s, germs started to become a big deal, not that they hadn't killed billions of people in the years prior. But with Lister's discovery about germs there was no turning back, and the monthly bleed seemed like a perfect target for people who were concerned about contagion.

Some of the greatest perpetrators of menstruation as a hygienic catastrophe were women themselves. Their advice columns for much of the 1900s had the signature of self-loathing and obsessive cleanliness all over it. We have since learned that when it comes to female genitals, cleanliness is next to Godliness only if it is done in moderation. We have also learned that when it comes to germs, your vagina will never be as gross as your mouth or your partner's mouth.

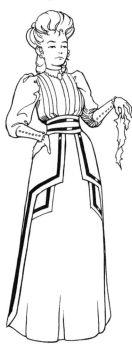

As for the pad people playing the odor card, if there is period-related odor, sanitary napkins themselves may be a source of it. Period flow contains sloughed off or dead tissue. All dead tissue contains organic compounds with names like putrescine. and cadaverine. No one will ever confuse putrescine or cadaverine with Eternity, Shalimar or Issey Miyake. As a result, even tampons can have an odor.

However, a bigger problem occurs when period flow mixes with butt bacteria (e coli). And where's that most likely to happen? In a pad or sanitary napkin that is trapping both blood from your vagina and moisture from your rear end. Disposable sanitary napkins are the perfect delivery system for one to meet the other, although our gynecology consultant doesn't feel that the thong (aka butt floss) is too far behind. If a pad is what you need, consider using a natural cotton pad that breathes. A lot of women use pads like the Luna pad that are washable and can be reused.

For First-Time Tampon Users

"I didn't realize the cardboard was supposed to come out (while the cotton wad stays in). It was a rather uncomfortable first hour, 'til I finally asked a girlfriend, 'What the hell?'" *female age 28*

"I mostly use pads, but they used to get stuck in my pubic hair. OUCH! Tampons are only useful for pools and hot tubs, otherwise it feels really weird walking around feeling like you have a soft dick stuck in you all day." *female age 21 [Editor's note: this could be happening because she isn't pushing the tampon in far enough.]*

"Pads were so horrid, even though I used them for many years. They were just so gross, it felt like wearing a diaper, but I could never get the hang of applicator tampons, so I just used pads. When I got to college we got a free trial pack of OB applicatorless tampons and I fell in love instantly and have never looked back!" *female age 20*

"I hated pads because I felt gooey and gross when I wore them. The blood never absorbs like the commercials say it does. I hurt the first couple of times I put a tampon in, and had to force it, but eventually that stopped and I didn't have a problem anymore." *female age 21*

"I never had a problem using tampons, and I hate it when my pubic hair gets stuck to the bloody pad. YUCK. So I'm a tampon girl—though I have to use the slim kind, as the larger ones hurt." *female age 20*

A number of our female readers have reported strange or painful experiences when they first tried using a tampon, including trying to pull out the tampon while it was still dry. This probably resulted from wearing a higher absorbency tampon than was needed and the tampon ended up sticking to the sides of their vagina. Ouch! Tampons come in a couple of absorbencies. It's best not to use one that is more absorbent than you need.

As for common tampon questions, a tampon can't get pushed in "too far." That's because your vagina ends in a cul-de-sac. Tampons won't ever float away inside your body, so you don't need to worry about doctors having to fish one out from behind your lung. Tampons are not like penises—you shouldn't be able to feel them. If you can, it's probably because you didn't push it far enough inside.

Here are some tips on tampon insertion from our female readers. However, always read and follow the instructions that come with the tampons.

The companies that make these products don't want to get sued, and so the information in their instructions is usually the latest and greatest. Do not leave the tampons in longer than the manufacturer says. If you are concerned about tampon-related sickness, see the section in this chapter on TSS.

Most tampons come with applicators or plungers. Some tampons, like OBs, use the inserting device that Mother Nature provided: your finger.

Putting tampons where they need to go requires three steps: pushing in the applicator, pushing in the plunger, and pulling out the applicator, unless you are using OBs, where there aren't any messy plungers to throw away that eventually wash up on our beaches.

It might help to coat the end of the tampon with a lubricant like KY Jelly. If you can't score the jelly, try dabbing a little saliva on it.

Buy or borrow the skinniest tampon you can find. You might try Tampax Lites or Playtex SlimFit regulars for your first time.

Find your vaginal opening. It's down there somewhere, at the bottom part of your vulva. Spread the lips of your vulva and put your finger in a little way. This is where the tampon will go.

Some women put tampons in while standing with a little squat action or with one leg higher and out to the side. Other women put them in while sitting on the toilet.

Spread your lips with the fingers of one hand, and insert the applicator into your vagina with the other. *Aim it toward your tailbone and not up toward your stomach!*

Insert the applicator so that the wider part of the barrel is almost all of the way in—with just enough sticking out to hold on to. If you don't insert the tampon far enough inside, the ring of muscles in the first part of your vagina can clamp it, making it feel uncomfortable.

Once you've got the applicator in, hold the barrel firmly with your fingers. Push the plunger in. Bingo!

As you pull out the applicator, try not to pull on the string or you'll pull the tampon out and you're back to square one. If this happens, push the tampon back in with your finger.

☀ Make sure the string of the tampon is hanging out of your vagina. If it isn't, don't worry. Squat and push down as if you are trying to take the mother of all dumps. Reach a finger inside your vagina to see if you can feel the critter. You can always use your thumb and finger to pull the string out. If you have no luck, ask your mom, aunt, grandmother older sister, best friend or boyfriend for help, or call your healthcare provider and speak with a nurse. Again, it's not like the end of the world, but you will need to get the tampon out in the next couple of hours. (See pages 722-723 for how to pull out a lost condom. It's not that much different.)

♥ Your vagina might be dry on the last day or two of your period. Don't hesitate to dab some lube on the tampon before putting it in.

☀ Sorry to be repetitive, but do not have intercourse with a tampon inside. While it's not going to end up in the next county, would you want to be that poor tampon getting rammed around your cervix by the head of some guy's dick?

Tampons, Sponges & Toxic-Shock Syndrome

Toxic-Shock Syndrome (TSS) is a rare but sometimes fatal disease caused by the toxins of bacteria that grow in the bodies of both men and women. TSS is now mainly associated with surgery and severe burn cases, but during the early 1980s some women died from TSS following the introduction of a new superabsorbent tampon called Rely.

Contrary to what scientists first believed, the killer tampons were not a breeding site for TSS bacteria. Rely contained two synthetic fibers (carboxy-methyl cellulose and polyester foam) that are thought to have irritated the vaginal lining in ways that triggered the TSS bacteria to produce a danger-ous toxin. Tampons are now made from only cotton and rayon. As a result, the occurrence of TSS among tampon users is rare. Your chances of getting killed in a car wreck are 500 to 1,000 times greater than the risk of death by tampon.

It was originally thought that wearing the same tampon for several hours increased your chances of getting TSS. Not so. But the risk does go up when you use nothing but tampons throughout your entire period, even if you change them every three hours. If you are a tampon user who wants to greatly reduce her chances of getting TSS, don't wear tampons throughout your entire period. For instance, alternate using tampons and pads, or ditch the traditional period gear for a more environmentally sound menstrual cup. Also, some people are naturally more susceptible to TSS. If you have ever had TSS or appear susceptible to it, you are better off not using tampons.

Warning signs of TSS: sudden high fever (usually 102 degrees or more) that includes vomiting and/or diarrhea, fainting or near-fainting when you stand up and dizziness or a sunburn-like rash. Symptoms usually appear very quickly and are often severe. Symptoms can vary, and might include aching of muscles and joints, redness of the eyes, sore throat, and weakness.

If you are on your period, have a sudden high fever and one or more of these TSS symptoms, ditch your tampon at once and make tracks to an emergency room. This would not be a time for modesty—claw your way to the front of the line and let the clerk know there you are ragging and have been wearing a tampon.

There are rumors that tampons contain dioxins that cause TSS. That might be possible if anyone could actually find dioxins in tampons, but the amount of dioxins in tampons is virtually nil. We are exposed to much higher levels of dioxins in the environment than from anything that comes in a box and has a string on the end.

Turning Your Crotch Green

The average woman uses nearly 10,000 or more pads or tampons in her lifetime. If your choice is between pads and tampons, it would seem as though a tampon without an applicator, such as OB, or a pad made of washable cotton, would be the more environmentally friendly choice. Disposable pads contain layers of engineered petroleum products. Tampons are mostly cotton. And it seems that the gynecologists who have consulted on this book aren't exactly big fans of disposable pads (sanitary napkins), especially if a woman is experiencing crotch irritation. A sanitary napkin made of cotton cloth is much preferred for vulva health, but the final decision should be between you and your healthcare provider.

If you do use tampons, please try to use OBs or tampons without applicators. Nature gave you your own applicators—your fingers. If they haven't met your vagina, what are you waiting for?

Also, it wouldn't hurt to investigate using menstrual cups rather than tampons or pads. Women who use them often rave about them for reasons other than having vaginas that are kinder to our landfills. While the learning curve is higher than for using tampons, it is possible you will have a better user experience.

Menstrual Cups—A Cross between a Diaphragm and A Shot Glass

A menstrual cup is a soft, flexible container made of soft silicone rubber or latex that is inserted into the vagina to collect menstrual fluids. It looks a bit like a small, upside-down funnel, although the stem is not hollow and the body of the cup is more rounded than a funnel. There are a number of different brands of menstrual cups, such as the Lunette, Diva, Moon Cup, Lady Cup, Femmecup, Miacup Keeper and and Pink Cup. Most are made of medical grade silicone, with each having a slightly different length, softness, rim, stem and color.

Once it's in place, a menstrual cup forms a seal against the wall of your vagina. This allows it to collect the blood as it flows from your cervix. Unlike a tampon which also absorbs your vagina's natural secretions in addition to your monthly flow, a menstrual cup holds only your period flow until you remove it and wash it out. As a result, it won't dry out your vagina.

Menstrual cups hold enough flow for most women to go for a full day without emptying it, although you might need to empty it a couple of times a day when you are flowing like the Mississippi. Menstrual cups last for around 10 years. They are a little spendy to begin with, but quickly amortize with each new period, as you won't have to buy pads or tampons.

Some women worry that a menstrual cup isn't sterile, as if a tongue, penis, fingers or a tampon are. Depending on the manufacturer's instructions, some women clean them with soap, soak them in hydrogen peroxide, or use other solutions before storing them until their next period. Unlike tampons, they have never been linked to TSS or Toxic Shock Syndrome.

In order to insert a menstrual cup, you need to fold it and then push up your vagina just below your cervix. Different ways of folding them are called the c-fold, origami, "7" fold, and punch-down fold. You can even wear a menstrual cup if you are a virgin or if your vagina is on the smaller side.

A lot of women who are now devoted users say they thought the concept of a menstrual cup was gross or disgusting at first. But they experienced so many advantages in using them that they wouldn't think of going back to pads or tampons.

Some women get the hang of using a menstrual cup the very first time, others require a few efforts. Since menstrual cups don't dry out your vagina, you can experiment with inserting them before you have your period. According to users, here are some of the advantages of using a menstrual cup:

 Tampons can seriously dry out your vagina. Menstrual cups don't. They are soft, flexible and don't absorb your natural moisture.

Once they learn how to make it sit right, a lot of cup users say they don't get the kind of leaking that they did with tampons. With less leaking, the chances are lower that your favorite underwear will be stained and have to become period panties. And some cup users say they experience less cramping than when they used tampons.

No more late-night runs to the store to buy tampons or pads.

You will contribute approximately 10,000 fewer pads, tampons, and their wrappers to the landfills, sewers, and beaches that the average woman uses during her period years.

At the time of publication, there were two excellent websites for women who are thinking about trying menstrual cups:

http://community.livejournal.com/menstrual_cups/tag/faq
www.ecomenses.com

Period Suppression

Period suppression refers to a woman preventing her period from happening by ditching the placebo week of birth-control pills or keeping her NuvaRing in for all four weeks instead of for just three. (You should never attempt this without discussing it first with your gynecologist. It will work with only certain pills, and there might be health concerns that could make it a really bad idea for you to try.)

There is still a lot of debate, which has become quite heated at times, about the safety of period suppression. There are some theories that nature never intended women to have monthly periods and having as many as women do today is not good for you, while other theories claim that the monthly fluctuation in hormones that happens with periods is actually quite good for your body and is one of the reasons why women outlive men by a good five years or so.

One of the problems with menstrual suppression is that we don't have the kind of long-term studies yet to prove that it is or isn't safe.

Women Athletes

It is not uncommon for women athletes to stop menstruating or have irregular periods. One theory is that their body fat is lower than 17%, which might be a necessary level for menstruation to occur. Other theories suggest that menstruation can be delayed due to metabolic reasons. Female athletes and dancers who begin their training before the ages of 9 or 10 often start menstruating a few years later than their nonathletic peers.

It is with restraint that your author tells about the time during his freshman year of college when he lifted weights with the women members of the Soviet National Shot-Put Team. He never thought to ask Olga, Svetlana, and Georgia if they menstruated regularly.

Tipped Uterus Considerations

Some women with a tipped uterus experience period pain more as a back ache than a pain in their abdomen. This could be why these women tend to have more back pain and diarrhea when they are ragging. Some women with a tipped uterus know when their period is coming because they start having loose stools that might be caused by a release of prostaglandins.

PMS

PMS is short for pre-menstrual syndrome. It refers to period-related mood fluctuations. To this day, PMS remains such a loosely defined concept that most men qualify as having it.

During World War II, when the bulk of American males went to war, millions of American women manned the nation's industrial-war machine. Our female-dominated workforce turned out an armada of planes, tanks, ships, and guns that was unprecedented in history. It wasn't until the men returned from war and needed their jobs back that the myth of women's so-called hormonal instability began to rear its head. It fit well with our society's need to get women out of the workplace and back into the home.

An entire PMS industry sprung up during the 1990s that attempted to turn hormonal mood fluctuations into a disease. This helped fuel the notion that women as a group are flakier than men. Just as flaky, absolutely; flakier, no. While period-related mood fluctuations can certainly result in mood swings, this usually doesn't make a woman emotionally unstable unless she's emotionally fragile to begin with. Studies show that men have as many monthly mood swings as women, but there's no psychiatric diagnosis for that.

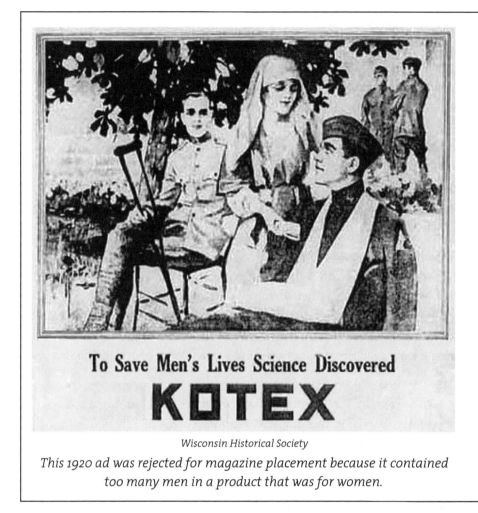

To Save Men's Lives Science Discovered

KOTEX

Wisconsin Historical Society
This 1920 ad was rejected for magazine placement because it contained too many men in a product that was for women.

Something that might help women who have severe period related mood swings that men probably shouldn't try is birth-control pills. Interestingly, while some pills help even out mood swings, others seem to make them worse. Depends on the pill and the woman.

Brief History of the Napkin and Tampon

Kotex, the first widely marketed sanitary napkin, was invented shortly after World War I. Before that, women used rags that they wadded up and pinned to the inside of their underwear.

The modern tampon was born in the late 1920s or early 1930s. It was called an "internal sanitary napkin" because nobody knew what a tampon

⇐ The ad on the left was created in 1920. It is a prototype of the very first Kotex ad ever done.

Kotex had its origins during World War I. Since cotton was in short supply, companies started to make bandages from cellulose. Army nurses found that the cellulose bandaging made an excellent substitute for the menstrual rags that they usually wore. It was cheap, absorbent, and they could throw it away.

As soon as the war was over, Kimberly-Clark, the company that made the bandages, looked opportunity in the crotch and created Kotex, which stood for KOtten-Like-TEXture. They hoped that by using a cryptic name such as "Kotex," women would be able to buy the product without the embarrassment of male clerks knowing what it was. Sure.

Another challenge for the Kotex people was to create an ad for their new product that magazines in the early 1920s would run. We're talking advertising for a product that went between a woman's legs at a time when this kind of item was still new and possibly scandalous.

Look at the headlines that went with this ad. Can you see a similarity with the way we sell products today by claiming that they were "Developed by NASA for our astronauts." Also, whatever the nurse is handing to the wounded officer is about the size of a Kotex, and it is placed in the illustration in front of her crotch. (Thanks to the Museum of Menstruation: www.mum.org, and the Wisconsin Historical Society for permission to use the Kotex ad.)

was. It did not have an applicator or a string. It was wrapped in gauze, which a woman pulled on to remove the tampon.

Another early tampon was called Paz. In 1936, the Tambrands company bought the Paz company and started selling Tampax, which was the first tampon with an applicator. It's interesting that they changed the name of the Paz tampon to Tampax, when Tampaz (TAMbrands + PAZ) would have made more sense. Perhaps it was because the very first tampon was made by another company and it was called FAX. "Tampax" includes Tam+Paz+Fax.

One early problem was that using tampons required women to touch their genitals. There were widespread fears that this would lead to wanton immorality. There were also fears that tampons would devirginize teenage girls. As late as the early 1990s, Tampax ran ads to help dispel this fear. After then, even the people at Tampax gave up the virginity ghost.

As for newer technology, a few years ago we heard about a new menstrual product called the "inSync Miniform." It was about the size of a tampon but fit between your labia. It was supposed to be used on light days, but who reads the instructions? Our research assistant volunteered to try it out. This nearly resulted in a worker's compensation claim against Goofy Foot Press.

NOTE: according to Publisher's Weekly, the classic period book "Are You There God? It's Me, Margaret" by Judy Bloom has sold roughly 7 million copies since it was first published in 1972. It continues to sell more than 100,000 copies each year. This makes it one of the best-selling books of all time.

Highly Recommended—Be sure to check out the amazing *Museum of Menstruation* website: www.mum.org, which rates *Two Tampons Way Up!* or would that be 5 *Panty Liners out of 5?* It includes anything you would ever want or need to know about menstruation. Also, if you are doing research on menstrual products patented in the United States from 1854 to 1921, get a copy of a paper of the same name by Laura K. Kidd and Jane Farrel-Beck, published in *Dress*, 1997 Vol. 24 pp. 27-41.

While the following title is a tad on the academic side, it could be the most interesting and spot-on period book to date. This chapter owes much to it and it should be in the library of any women's studies major:

"Girls in Power: Gender, Body, and Menstruation in Adolescence" by Laura Fingerson, Albany, New York, State University of New York Press, 2006.

Special thanks to Maureen Whelihan, MD, a gynecological goddess, and to Rear Admiral Anne Schuchat, MD, from the Center for Disease Control and Nina Bender at Whitehall Laboratories for their help on TSS. Also, thanks to Harry Finley at the *Museum of Menstruation* for consultation on the history of sanitary napkins and tampons, and to Jane Farrel-Beck for being so generous with photocopies of her articles! The original negative of the 1920 Kotex ad belongs to the Wisconsin Historical Society.

53

Clean Jeans, Tight Jeans & Shaving Down Below

We have managed to put golf carts on Mars. We are engineering cows with genes that nature never intended; but we have yet to find an exceptionally good way to get rid of unwanted body hair. In this chapter, we look at temporary methods for removing unwanted body hair, then at permanent methods. And as long as we're getting up close and personal, we conclude the chapter with a trip up Amber's vagina, where we learn about the fine line between a healthy environment, and one that's ripe for a yeast infection.

NOTE: Both of our gynecology consultants have encouraged our readers to not shave their pubic hair, but to use a mustache trimmer instead. They are not at all opposed to getting rid of pubic hair, but they are concerned about all of the vuvlar irritation they see due to shaving to the skin.

Body Hair Removal

"Shaving is painful and I look about 12 years old, it grosses me out. Trimming works! Borrow a beard trimmer and go for it! One crew cut coming up!" *female age 29*

"My husband really likes to trim my pubic area for me. He gets turned on by this. I think it's highly arousing, too." *female age 45*

"I'm more aware of myself and my sexuality when I'm shaved. It feels sensual, like the first time you wear silk underwear. It's too much trouble to keep up, though. If there was an easy way, I think I'd do it more often." *female age 36*

Women have shaved or plucked their body hair for thousands of years. However, here in the U.S., the current trend of shaving the female frame got its start in the year 1915, when the good people at Wilkinson Sword began an ad campaign to convince women that their arm-pit hair was unfeminine and unclean. This coincided nicely with the introduction of the first sleeveless evening gowns, and razor sales started to soar.

Now, 90 years later, even guys are getting into below-the-neck pruning, with 35% to 50% of the males who took our on-line sex survey saying they trim or shave their pubic hair. It used to be a man who did this was considered limp-of-wrist. Now he's liable to be a member of the football team.

Please don't think *The Guide* is encouraging or discouraging body-hair deforestation. Some people like their lovers furry while others like them bald, and we're not talking about the top of your head.

As for sex differences, a hair follicle is pretty much a hair follicle, there aren't boy ones and girl ones. Some follicles might be more androgen-sensitive and grow a thicker hair, but the underlying mechanism is the same. What is different among the sexes is the timing and predictability of hair growth.

By the time a male is 25, he's got a pretty good idea of how much body hair he is going to have, and where. Not so for women. Mother Nature had reserved the right to play wicked hair tricks on a woman's body at any point during her lifespan. A female reader sums it up quite aptly:

> "I used to have this lovely, neat, wonderfully behaved triangle of pubic hair. And then I turned thirty, and the thing started to spread..."
>
> *female age 32*

Trimming & Shaving the Male Crotch

When we first started asking takers of our totally unscientific sex survey whether men trim or shave between their legs, we expected to see a 10% to 20% "yes" rate. We didn't expect to get blown away with nearly 50%. Nor did we expect to see nearly total agreement between the men's numbers and the women's assessment of their partner's pubic-hair status. (Men and women can't agree on how much sex they've had with each other, but when it comes to the well-coiffed crotch, detente abounds!)

Far more men trimmed than shaved, and when they did shave in their pubic area, it was usually the scrotum. They report that their wives and girlfriends prefer a kinder and gentler crotch for giving oral sex to. And that's exactly what we heard from female survey takers: they went on and on about how annoying it is to get a pubic hair stuck in the back of their throat. Many of them commented on how much nicer it is to lick and suck on a well-trimmed or shaved scrotum, but they thought it a bit weird if a guy shaved off all of his pubic hair, saying it was like sleeping with a Cub Scout. They appreciated maintenance as opposed to scorched earth, and said they rewarded it by giving more oral sex.

"I like it better when they just trim the pubic hair and shave off all the ball hair. It is nicer to suck on then and it shows that the guy takes good care of himself." *female age 24*

Men, likewise, often said they preferred going down on a woman with a manicured mound.

Shaving & The Big Myth

Contrary to what you often hear, there is no truth to the myth that shaving results in a thicker hair follicle or increased hair growth. The reason a hair might look thicker after you shave or trim it is because you are whacking the hair off at the thickest part, at the base. A normal, full length hair is thickest at the base, and tapers toward the tip. So instead of a soft, well-worn tip like that on a fully grown hair, a newly shaven hair stump will look thick and have a nasty, sharp edge. En masse, they create the 5 o'clock shadow.

Shaving is by far the safest method of temporary hair removal, because it does no damage to the follicle. Believe it or not, there are two different kinds of razors to consider, depending on whether you are shaving a large flat area, like your legs, back or chest, or something more rounded, like your face or pubic area.

For chest, back and leg hair, try a woman's razor for leg hair. It doesn't matter if you are male or female, women's razors are often made for large, flat areas. As of press time, a lot of people like the Venus 3, but new technologies are always improving the razor.

If you are shaving your crotch, you'll want a razor with a head that swivels, lke most that are for men's faces. A razor designed to navigate the chin will make small-time of the scrotum, so to speak. These include throw-away razors with one blade, to the vibrating Mach 3, Quatro, or the Gillette Fusion with five blades (rinse it often while shaving). There are also the high-end and highly recommended electric shavers from Braun, as well as wet/dry shavers. You will need to experiment and find what is best for your hair type and skin type. No matter what part of your body you shave, you will need to do it for several weeks before your hair and skin settles into an obliging routine.

If you are shaving between your legs, it is easiest and best to do it in the shower or bath. Or, you can warm the area for several minutes first with a wash cloth. Get it warm and wet to make shaving easier. Use shaving cream that's for sensitive skin, although there is no difference between shaving cream that's marketed to men as opposed to women, except for the fragrance.

For the first month, shave in the direction that the hair grows and not against it. Be satisfied with an OK job instead of a great job. An OK job means just shaving with one stroke or two at most, and never against the grain. After you've been at it for a couple of weeks and want to experiment with going against the grain, give it a try. But not until you get a good sense of the different directions that the hair can grow, and the price your skin might pay.

Doing an obsessively neat job often results in shaving off some of the skin, especially the little bumps in the skin that frequently populate the large labia and scrotum. What you risk receiving is an uncomfortable prickly feeling. It's difficult to pull scrotum and labia skin tight enough to avoid shaving off little bits and pieces. Throw a pair of gonads under the surface, and good luck. So go for an "OK" job instead of a "great" job. Your crotch will thank you and your partner probably won't be able to tell the difference. Newer blades are usually better than those that are old. If it's electric, the people on hair shaving forums don't recommend the shavers with rotary heads.

To help prevent ingrown hairs *(pseudofolliculitis barbae)*, it helps to exfoliate often. Try using a loofah or skin-scrubbing product, or a liquid exfoliant like Tend Skin. Some people say to do it right before you shave, and others say to do it right after. If ingrown hairs remain a problem, try using an electric razor, and shave only every other day if you can get away with it.

In addition to using a loofah on the skin you shave, consider doing your whole body with it, especially your back. It will help take the dead layers of skin off, and it will take off the crusty little whiteheads on your back if you get the type of loofah that's long enough to do your back with.

For the most thorough discussion you will ever find about ingrown hairs, click on the "razor bumps" section at www.hairtell.com.

Here are some other ways to get your hair off :):

Depilatory This is a form of chemical warfare that dissolves the hair at the surface of the skin. You've probably heard of Nair. Depilatories don't do any better job than shaving, but some people like them. Others find they irritate the skin. Be sure to follow the instructions.

Vaniqa This is a prescription cream that started life as an anti-cancer drug. The reason it sometimes works on reducing hair growth is because tumor cells and hair follicles have a lot in common. They have also found that Vaniqa helps cure African Sleeping Sickness. So people coming out of near-death comas might find their unwanted body hair gone as well. Vaniqa only removes body hair on 58% of the women who use it, and only temporarily. The really bizarre discovery is that in clinical tests for Vaniqa, more than a third of the women using a placebo cream also had "improved" or "markedly improved" results with their unwanted body hair. Vaniqa hasn't been tested on men, and its safety and effectiveness hasn't been tested when it is applied to the human snatch. Plus, you need to get a prescription and it is expensive.

Tweezing Contrary to what you might think, tweezing can do some nasty damage to the hair follicle. It can cause hair to grow back thicker, or not at all, which can be a cosmetic bummer if you radically tweeze your eyebrows one time, and find you are stuck with that look for life. The most common body parts that get tweezed are eyebrows and nipples. Warm the area with a wash cloth beforehand to trick the follicles into relaxing their grip. To prevent over-plucking of eyebrows, www.hairfacts.com recommends that you draw the line you would like with a concealer first, then pluck the little turkeys that reside on the other side.

Waxing and Sugaring Owie ouch! You put wax or sticky stuff on the hairy skin and push a special kind of paper or cloth into it. It is then ripped away, with the hair hopefully attached. Infections and broken hairs can result if you are not careful. There is no evidence that waxing decreases hair growth, unless it inadvertently creates scar tissue over the follicles. If you are waxing for the first time, be sure to have it done professionally or by a friend who is highly experienced. If you are a woman, the pubic area seems to be more tender when you are menstruating, so wait until later for waxing.

Rotary Epilators These are electronic torture devices that have rows of tweezers that yank hair out by the root. The Braun model comes highly recommended. You need to pull the skin tight, and the hair has to be long enough for the tweezers to be able to yank them. There are even special ones for the bikini area.

Threading This is plucking with a thread and an ethnic flair. It's a traditional form of removing hair from the faces of Indian and Muslim women.

Bleaching This isn't a way of removing the hair, but trying to make it look less obvious. Contrary to your goal, bleaching can make hair look thicker because the bleach gets absorbed inside the shaft and puffs it up. Plus, it can make the hair stick out more from the skin.

Head Trips? If you are a fan of the naked noggin, you'll find all kinds of head-shaving tips at www.baldrus.com.

Unfortunately, hair-removal methods have something in common with contraceptives—the perfect one has yet to be invented.

Permanent Hair Removal—Electrolysis

There is only one way to permanently zap body hair, and that's with electrolysis. But even electrolysis can fail 10% of the time, and that assumes it is done correctly. With electrolysis, a technician sticks a thin electrified needle into the hair follicle. He or she then zaps it electrically. For a hair follicle, it's the electric chair on the end of a needle.

There are two different kinds of electrolysis, blended and thermolysis or Flash. Thermolysis is faster, but the skin can take longer to heal. You and your electrologist will need to decide which method works best for you. Variables include the intensity and duration of the electrical impulse, and type of needle.

As for pubic-hair removal, an average male might have 25,000 or more hair follicles in the area that runs from his navel to behind his scrotum. If she's lucky, a woman will have fewer hair follicles, and no scrotum. One of the things that makes it difficult to estimate how many hours of electrolysis you will need in order to achieve your goal has to do with density of hair follicles. Jacob might have only 20 active hair follicles in an area that's the size of a quarter, while his girlfriend Bobbi Sue might have 200.

Another problem is that there is a big difference between what your bikini area is showing and what you've actually got growing. Each hair follicle is like a bear. It hibernates. So as soon as you think the skin is bare, a new wave of hairs starts popping up faster than eating disorders in a college sorority. It can take a couple of years of professional zapping to get the job done.

A very knowledgeable electrolysis expert found through the Genital Hair Removal forum at www.hairtell.com offers the following perspective:

> "In the pubic area, there are well over 20,000 hairs packed into that small area, so one would need to remove at least 2,000 hairs just to effect a 10% removal. Proper treatment requires longer and more frequent appointments in the beginning, and tapers off to minutes every 3 to 6 months at the end. If the aggressive schedule is not followed, one could go once a month for an hour for the rest of one's life and only get a minor reduction."

This means that you and an experienced electrolysist need to make a treatment plan and follow it. Don't just go in for an hour or two and think it's going to work. Also keep in mind that removing only 2,000 hairs will take hours of electrolysis.

As for the time involved in doing an entire crotch, figure on at least ten or twelve hours—or several times that—to tame the wild beaver. As for the pain, it can vary from almost none to excruciating, depending on the person who is doing the electrolysis, the person who is having the electrolysis done, and the particular part of your body that's being zapped. For instance, logic might tell you that it's far more painful to have your scrotum done than the hair at the base of your penis, but the opposite is usually true. You will definitely want to talk to the technician about pain-relief options, and don't expect them to be inexpensive or necessarily effective. One cost-effective option might be to have a shot that will numb the area for three or four hours, while two electrologists work on you at the same time.

For a competent electrolysist who will do crotch hair—especially on a guy—visit the forums at www.HairTell.com. You might also search the Internet for suggestions by M2F transsexuals, as they need a lot of electrolysis before they can have bottom surgery.

Between Waxing and Electrolysis—Laser Hair Removal

Laser hair removal works best if you have very light skin with dark hair growing out of it. That's because lasers work by targeting the melanin in the hair follicle. This is the compound that gives the hair its color. The laser emits a very narrow bandwidth of light that can be absorbed by the melanin in the follicle. The heat that gathers in the melanin then radiates to the rest of the follicle and theoretically fries it. If your skin is olive, or the hair is blond or gray, or the laser isn't working correctly or isn't well-matched for your skin type, the destructive energy can be absorbed by your skin instead of the hair follicle and nasty things can happen.

This is why with laser, you should always have a test patch done first and not schedule any appointments for at least a week or more to make sure your skin doesn't become pigmented. You'll then want to make sure that the same attendant does all of your treatments using the same machine.

Also, be aware that no fertility studies have been done to demonstrate the safety of using lasers on a guy's scrotum, and the lack of smooth skin on the scrotum can make for poor follicle frying. And no studies have been done on the impact of laser hair removal on the sensitivity of the clitoris.

Permanent Hair Removal Precaution

Please understand that this chapter has barely scraped the surface of permanent hair removal. If you are considering it, we strongly encourage you to spend hours on the websites www.HairTell.com and www.HairFacts.com. Be sure to read and print out their consultation form. Take it with you if you are visiting a laser hair-removal center. And please read their suggestions on how to select an electrologist and what to ask.

Permanent hair removal can be safe, effective, and satisfying, or it can permanently damage your skin. It can also be painful, and it is almost always time-consuming and very costly. Make the experience work for you by knowing as much as you can before you take off your shirt or drop your drawers and plunk down your hard-earned money and spend your valuable time.

Hormonal Problems that Cause Plentiful Hair Growth

Some hormonal conditions can cause women to have hair so thick on their faces that they need to shave twice a day. Some of these women live in dire fear that they will get into an accident and have to be hospitalized and won't be able to shave their faces. At the same time, there are men who find hairy women to be a sexual turn on, and even porn magazines that feature women with hirsutism, which is defined as *hairy and then some.*

According to Sarah Rosenthal, author of *Women and Unwanted Hair*, the causes of excessive hair growth in women can include too much androgen secretion (polycystic ovarian syndrome), overactive adrenal glands (such as with Cushing's disease), hair follicles that are too sensitive to androgens, certain drugs (including some oral contraceptives, steroids, and dilantin), insulin resistance, hyperthyroidism, endocrine disorders, genetics, obesity and stress.

If you are bothered by the amount of hair you have, or if you suddenly start growing gobs of new hair, try to find an endocrinologist who specializes in hirsutism. Just because the physician is an endocrinologist doesn't mean that he or she is either sympathetic or knowledgeable about hormone imbalances and excessive hair growth.

A Truly Strange Transition—from Shaving to Vaginal Infections

This chapter originally included a few paragraphs on shaving and a few on vaginal infections, along with several other topics on crotch aesthetics. But now, four editions later, the shaving and annoying-infection sections have been greatly expanded, and are all that remain. Keeping them together in the same chapter now makes little sense. So this is the last edition when these two topics will be conjoined, especially now that guys are shaving and trimming their crotches, but haven't started getting yeast infections. For now, the two topics remain bosom buddies, or the crotch-version thereof.

A Trip Inside Amber's Vagina

There are lots of reasons to take a trip inside Amber's vagina. Let's say you want to know what causes yeast infections in a woman's vagina. Or let's say your boyfriend's finger starts to sting when he's had it in your vagina for all of *Desperate Housewives,* and you want to know why. Or maybe you want to know why it is unwise to assume that over-the-counter drugs will automatically make a vaginal infection go away.

Amber's vagina will be our gynecological Ouija Board; the vaginal-version of the Discovery Channel. So let's look at what makes Amber's vagina hum, besides flowers and kisses from her boyfriend.

In order for this to work, we will need to shrink until we are very, very small. So small that we can take a trip up Amber's vagina.

Given how a healthy vagina is fairly acidic, some of you might think of this as an acid trip. If Amber's boyfriend gets his prayers for sex answered before we are done, it will probably feel like an acid trip.

While we could think of Amber's vagina as a warm, wet, heavenly place that lots of guys and some girls would like to visit, it's also instructive to think of it as a massively complex rainforest, an incredible ecosystem with bacterial flora and fauna that keep it all in balance.

One of the most important residents of Amber's vagina is a bacteria called Lactobacilli. There are several different types of Lactobacilli in Amber's vagina, and too much of it can cause as much discomfort as too little. When things are in balance, friendly families of Lactobacilli produce hydrogen peroxide and lactic acid in amounts that are helpful. The hydrogen peroxide helps kill undesirable bacteria when they try to intrude. The lactic acid helps to maintain the acidic environment that's so essential for healthy functioning. It also makes the fingers of Amber's boyfriend sting when they have been basting inside of her vagina. This is a property of all healthy vaginas. Their acidic nature will make most people's fingers sting if they stay in there long enough.

Another positive effect of the Lactobacilli is that they have tiny projections that stick out from their cell bodies. These projections clasp onto the cell walls of the vagina. This prevents other bacteria and germs from attaching at these points. You might think of it as aluminum siding for the inside of Amber's vagina.

If anything happens that causes the Lactobacilli to stop reproducing, the stage is set for infections and uncomfortable conditions. For instance, let's say Amber starts taking antibiotics for a lung infection. This kills off the wicked bacteria in her chest, but it also starts to kill off the friendly bacteria in her vagina. As a result, the lactic acid that's produced by the good bacteria will decrease and the alkalinity in Amber's vagina will increase. The increased alkalinity or rise in pH will cause fewer Lactobacilli to reproduce. A nasty spiral is created where the population of the good bacteria stars falling faster than a dropped ball.

As the population of the good Lactobacilli begins to crash, another of its important by-products (hydrogen peroxide) will suddenly be in short supply. Unfriendly bacteria will have an easier time taking up squatter's rights in Amber's vagina. Also, the Lactobacilli shield that was protecting the walls of Amber's vagina will weaken. Unfriendly anaerobic bacteria with names like Gardnerella and Coccoid will be able to invade the cell walls in Amber's vagina. When this happens, the woman gets what is called bacterial vaginosis or BV. One of the most common symptoms of BV is a discharge with a fishy odor. This can worsen during her period and with the friction of intercourse.

Another kind of vaginal catastrophe can occur from virtually the opposite situation, when the population of Lactobacilli suddenly rises and too much lactic acid and hydrogen peroxide are produced. Natural sugars start being fermented into carbon dioxide, alcohol, formic acid and acetic acid. This causes itching and irritation. The official term is cytolytic vaginosis or CV. When this occurs inside of Amber's vagina, her boyfriend will need more than prayers and flowers to get between her legs.

CV shares the same symptoms as a yeast infection: itching, burning, painful intercourse and a slight discharge. As a result, it is often misdiagnosed as a yeast infection. This is one of the reasons why a woman who is having problems with recurring vaginitis needs both a sharp gynecologist and a good knowledge of how her vagina works. Over-the-counter drugs for yeast infections won't touch CV.

A third problem that can occur in Amber's vagina is when she really does get a yeast infection, commonly referred to as Candida. A fourth type of infection is caused by a protozoa known as Trich or Trichomonas Vaginalis. Yet another kind of vaginitis is known as Noninfectious Vaginitis. Instead of being caused by funky organisms, the source of irritation for Noninfectious Vaginitis can be anything from feminine hygiene spray and regular body soap to perfumed toilet paper, laundry detergent, exercise bikes and tampons.

Coming Down

Well, that does it. This trip up Amber's most wonderful vagina is history. Hope it helps if you are trying to understand the different things that can go on between a woman's legs.

And hopefully, you will now have a sense that an infection isn't just a matter of some foreign germ taking residence inside the vagino-sphere. Like so many things in life, having a happy vagina is a matter of balance, with the sum of the parts being much greater than the whole.

To help prevent vaginal infections, please see Chapter 51: "Vulva Care: Keeping Your Kitty Happy."

Thanks to Andrea James and the formerly hairy forum-fanatics at www.hair-tell.com for an eye-opening education about getting rid of body hair.

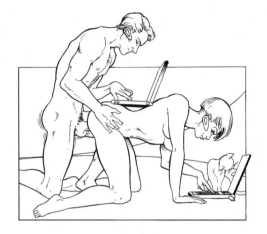

Multi-tasking?

For new free chapters, occasional cool offers,
and the latest on sex in science
and medicine, please visit

www.GuideToGettingItOn.com

CHAPTER

54

Hypospadias

Hypospadias is a condition where the urethra (tube you pee through) doesn't go to the end of the penis. In mild cases, it comes out near the end of the penis, but not quite. In more severe cases, it can come out anywhere from below the head of the penis to the scrotum.

Hypospadias is one of the most common birth anomalies there is, occurring in 1 in 125 to 500 boys. The possible reasons range from genetics and environmental pollutants called endocrine disrupters to diet. (An excellent study released in 2008 cites diet and obesity of the mother during pregnancy as risk factors, with a vegetarian diet or a diet lacking in meat and fish showing a strong positive association with hypospadias risk.)

It makes sense that cases of hypospadias occur on the bottom side of the penis where nature left a long seam. That's because when the penis is forming in the womb, nature zips it up along this seam. The urethra goes inside the chamber of the penis that's just inside the seam. With hypospadias, the urethra got caught in the zipper like your penis will if you are in a super hurry and zip your pants up before your guy is safely out of harm's way.

Hypospadias is usually a minor birth defect that often looms far more massively in the mind of the guy who's got it than in mind of a potential partner. There is nothing about hypospadias that makes a man any less of a man, or any less of a lover, although sometimes it results in a condition where the penis curves more than normal.

The real damage from hypospadias is usually the shame and aloneness that a guy feels when he's growing up. One of the reasons for feeling so different is because he's often got to sit down to pee, given how the pee shoots out the side of his penis instead of the end. The guy knows he's different from other males, and often lives in terror that others will find out and make fun of him. Of course, this never happens, given how kind, understanding and uncruel children are about others who are different...

Aside from feeling like he's got this huge and horrible secret in his pants, most men with hypospadias have a medical history where they had to have their penis repeatedly inspected and examined by this doctor and that. And not being able to leave well enough alone, surgeons are frequently called in to do what often turns out to be multiple surgeries. (While medical intervention is sometimes helpful in certain cases, there are plenty of guys who would have been far better off if their penis had been spared the surgeon's knife.)

As is the case where any kid grows up feeling his body is defective, the most important issues to deal with are often the psychological. Men with hypospadias usually feel great emotional relief when they can meet and talk to other men who have the same condition. Fortunately, the Internet is making this much more possible than in times past.

Men with hypospadias sometimes grow up fascinated by other guys' penises. This makes perfect sense when you consider how often their penis gets handled by parents and doctors, often without a helpful explanation. It also makes sense given how focused a guy with hypospadias can be about the way his penis is different from other penises. However, there is no evidence that hypospadias results in a different sexual orientation unless that's what you were going to do from the start, hypospadias or not.

As for sex and relationships, the main difference between a penis with hypospadias and one without is where the cum shoots out, and that's not going to make a bit of difference to most women. As one female reader said, "I can name you hundreds of other things women are more concerned about in a man than if his pee or cum shoots out straight or from the side—most women wouldn't give a rat's ass. Only guys worry about things like that."

Rest assured there's no reason why you can't become a father, so birth control is just as necessary for a man with hypospadias as for any other guy. The urethral opening for men with hypospadias is sometimes a little bigger, and some guys are prone to urinary tract infections, so drinking extra water and peeing after sex might be a good habit to get into.

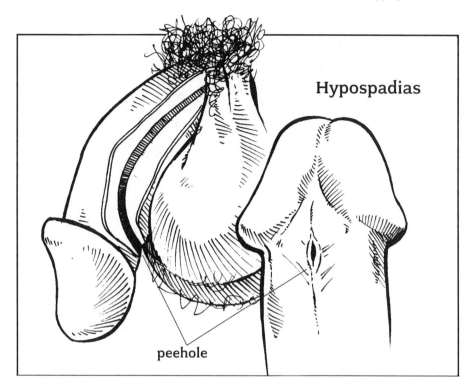

Hypospadias

peehole

Men with hypospadias recommend that you tell a partner about your hypospadias sometime after you've gotten to know each other but before you've got your hands in each other's pants. You can always pull out "The Guide" and point to this page if you need an ice breaker.

And if you are in serious need of a reality check, keep in mind that guys coming back from Iraq and Afghanistan with stumps where they used to have arms and legs would trade for a penis with hypospadias in a heartbeat, and let's not even talk about people born with intersex conditions where a guy's penis isn't much bigger than a clitoris, or where a girls' clitoris isn't much smaller than a penis. This isn't to diminish a man's feelings about his hypospadias, but we tend to make our own little hells in life, and sometimes perspective isn't such a bad thing.

Epispadias

Epispadias is when the urethral opening opens on the top of the penis. The opening can be in one spot, or it can run the entire length of the penis. While it might seem that epispadias is simply a case of hypospadias turned on its ear, it is an entirely different anomaly than hypospadias. It is also very rare. Where approximately 1 in 125 to 500 boys has hypospadias, 1 in 117,000 boys are thought to have epispadias. While they aren't sure what causes it, it is thought to result from a problem in the way the pubic bone develops. Every once in a while, a girl will have epispadias, with it occurring in 1 in 478,000 girls. When it happens in females, the urethra will either exit high than normal, between the clitoris and labia, or as high as the abdomen.

Resources: If you have hypospadias, an excellent resource is the Hypospadias and Epispadias Association: www.heainfo.org

55

Gnarly Sex Germs

Why is it that some men will care for a car or favorite baseball glove with meticulous detail, but refuse to wear a condom when they are at risk for giving or getting a sexually transmitted infection? Why do so many of America's women go nearly insane over a single zit or take hours getting dressed for a party, but throw all caution to the wind about getting herpes or HPV? And why is our nation's rather feeble program to educate its young about sexually transmitted infections little more than a thinly veiled attempt to discourage them from having sex? It is a program that talks about disease, but rarely mentions pleasure. Does it need to be this way? This chapter guides you through the underbelly of sexual infections.

What Crotch Critters Are

VD? STDs? Sexually transmitted infections? They are all refer to the same thing—diseases or infections that are primarily transmitted from person to person by sexual contact.

The Importance of Sex

For many of us, an important part of staying healthy is having sex. On the other hand, there would be a big drop in the number of sexually transmitted infections if people dated for a few weeks or months before getting naked together. By then, you would know more about a potential partner than simply how they fill out their jeans. Perhaps the sex would be better, too.

Defining an Acceptable Level of Risk

Each year more than 40,000 Americans die in car accidents. Thousands more are seriously injured. Yet most of us consider driving to be an acceptable risk. On the other hand, if 40,000 straight people started dying each year from a new sex disease, there would be a great outcry against sex.

Perhaps we believe there is something inherently good about driving and something inherently bad about sex. Or maybe we get more satisfaction from driving. Whatever the case, you can greatly decrease your chances of being killed in a car accident by not drinking or doing drugs when you drive, by wearing a seat belt, and by driving sensibly. The same is true for sex.

Monogamy Only Works for Some People

Monogamy would be fine if people would actually stay monogamous. But for some men and women who have had lots of sexual partners, the chance of remaining monogamous is low.

Don't try to fit yourself into a monogamous space if you belong in a round hole. Whether you are straight or gay, don't stop using condoms in a relationship if there is even the slightest chance that you or your partner might have sex outside of the relationship. If your partner wants the two of you to keep using condoms, do yourself a huge favor and don't resist. "Monogamous" only works for some.

Harm Reduction & Sexual Seduction

Here are some of the more fun things to do in life. The challenge is in finding ways to enjoy them all while reducing your chances of getting a sexually transmitted infection:

Oral Sex (French kissing) Besides being a delightful thing to do, French kissing is a way of contracting anything you might get when someone with a cold or flu sneezes in your face.

Oral Sex (mouth-to-crotch) Yes, it is possible to both give and get a sexually transmitted infection while doing oral sex. Using a condom while blowing a guy makes a lot of sense if you are not in a long-term relationship. Using a dental dam or plastic wrap over a woman's vulva when giving her oral sex also makes sense, but nobody is going to do it. Just be aware that if there is a cold sore on or in your mouth, you stand a good chance of giving herpes to the person you are having oral sex with.

Precum Note Just so you'll know, when it comes to sexually transmitted infections, precum is just as high-octane as a full wad of ejaculate. It carries the same infectious agents.

Oral Sex (rimming or booty lickin') Rimming is when you use your tongue on a partner's anus. If you are in a long-term monogamous relationship, you share many of the same intestinal flora, fauna, and bugs, so there's probably not a big risk associated with rimming. But in more casual relationships, you should be concerned about getting things like hepatitis, E. coli, salmonella, shigella, amoeba, giardia, and cryptosporidiosis. So, if you enjoy rimming but aren't in a long-term or true-blue relationship, get yourself a hepatitis vaccination. It does not matter if you are straight or gay; if you enjoy rimming with casual partners, you are being really dumb not to get vaccinated for hepatitis. As for other bugs and germs, a dental dam would make sense, but tongues that like to rim really like to rim. So a good strategy is to hop in the shower together before the sex games begin. (A post-doc fellow at UCLA did a study on germs and hand-washing. She discovered that if you soap-up a second time after the first rinse there will be a huge decrease in the amount of germs. A nursing student from Portland State University says that the first soaping helps remove the dead layer of skin cells, but it takes the second soaping to get germs that were sitting underneath.)

Handjobs The chances of catching an STI from doing your partner by hand are about the same as breaking your neck from falling out of bed. The exceptions are if you have an open cut or broken skin, and there is research to suggest that HPV can be transmitted from one partner to the next by hand-to-genital contact. What you don't want to do is take a hand with a partner's sex fluids on it and rub it on your genitals, unless neither of you has an STI.

Intercourse (vaginal) Do you really believe that the cute fraternity guy you are about to go to bed with is going to say, "Oh, by the way, I'm totally low-risk except for that little butt-fucking incident last month with the captain of the wrestling team?" Or what about that sweet-looking former high-school cheerleader? Do you honestly believe she will cop to having spiked heroin while going through her rebellious phase last summer? Keep in mind that other people might not be as responsible about what goes on with their bodies as you might be with yours. You simply can't tell what diseases you will or won't get from another person based on promises alone.

Unless you are long term and true blue, you should use condoms all of the time. But especially be sure to use them when sleeping with partners who drink or do drugs, even if it's just brewskis or pot. That's because these substances numb the part of the mind we count on to keep us out of trouble. It's the sober part that says, "I'm not even sure if I like this guy, but he's got one hand under my shirt and the other down my pants; what's wrong with this picture?" But then the polluted part says, "Hell with the condom, ain't nothin' bad gonna happen."

Pulling Out Note Pulling out and squirting off to the side may win you the *Birth Control from the Middle Ages Award*, but it won't keep you from getting a disease. Also, try to put a rubber on as soon as you get wood. A hard penis usually starts dripping before it gets to where it's going.

Intercourse (anal) The only time you might consider having anal sex without a condom is if you are in a long-term, true-blue relationship and you have no concerns about sexually transmitted infections. In that case, barebacking (anal sex without a condom) is probably OK except for three possible concerns. The first is that there might be immune-suppressing factors in male ejaculate that help it in its quest to fertilize an egg. What happens when this sits in the rectum, where it's absorbed into the blood stream? Will it eventually start to impact the receiver's immune system? On the other hand, people have been butt-fucking since the beginning of time. The second concern is that males might be getting urinary-tract or prostate infections due to the high content of bacteria in the rectum. The third concern is that even if you wash the penis, tiny bits of fecal matter still might stay in the peehole and end up shooting into the vagina if you don't pee before having regular intercourse. There isn't a single study we know of that examines these concerns, but you still might be ahead of the game if you bag it before plowing your partner's back forty. Also, you can't use enough lube to help reduce possible tissue trauma.

Late-Breaking Anal-Sex Note Sex educators are now adding the word "trust" in addition to using condoms during anal intercourse. The reason is because if you are not totally relaxed, the anal sphincters can clamp a penis so tightly as to rip a rubber. When done in a trusting, loving relationship, this tends not to happen.

Urine Play If you are into water sports and not in a monogamous relationship, don't shoot urine into any body cavities. Using a partner as a urinal is something that needs to wait for marriage or a long-term relationship.

Drugs Try to eliminate all non-essential drugs from your body, whether prescribed or recreational. This includes anything from meth and cocaine to antibiotics and antifungals. We just don't know what the long-term effects might be on the immune system. Take precautions so you don't have to be prescribed nasty drugs to help clear up something you catch.

Herpes Explained

With each edition of this book, we highlight a specific sexually transmitted infection to look at in depth. For this, the 6th edition of *The Guide,* the garnly sex germ distinction goes to herpes.

Herpes is a virus, not a bacteria. There is no cure for herpes, although antiviral drugs can help with the symptoms. Antibiotics are totally ineffective against herpes. Genital herpes is transmitted through sexual contact including intercourse, oral-genital contact, and rubbing genitals together without being separated by clothing. Condom use reduces the risk of transmitting herpes by half.

The virus can be spread from the mouth to the genitals. So you can get herpes when someone who has a cold sore in their mouth goes down on you.

One of the most difficult things to learn about herpes is that the virus can be transmitted when there are no apparent lesions. 70% of new cases of herpes are transmitted from someone showing no obvious symptoms. Most genital herpes symptoms are mild and easy to miss.

The most common form of herpes is Herpes Simplex Virus 1, which causes cold sores on the lips, nose, chin and other parts of your face. People usually get HSV1 during childhood and most symptoms go unnoticed because they are minor. About 56% of people over age 14 in the US display evidence of a previous HSV1 infection when their blood is tested.

Herpes Simplex Virus 2 is associated with genital herpes infections. About 22% of people in the US over the age of 13 show evidence of HSV2 infection when their blood is tested. Of those infected with HDV 2, only about 10% know it.

Genital Herpes is classified into 3 categories:

Primary: an outbreak in someone who has never had either HSV1 or HSV2. Primary symptoms are sometimes severe and can range from headaches, aching joints, tiredness, fever, pain in the legs, and flu-like symptoms. The lymph nodes in the groin can become enlarged and tender. Lesions and sores may appear in the throat or mouth. Genital symptoms may also include sores, painful urination as well as itching and discharge from the penis or vagina. The sores begin as blisters, then break open to form ulcers in the skin. Women may not notice sores on their labia, and they will normally have lesions on their cervix as well. Men may have lesions inside their urethra. Frequently, a new crop of lesions will appear 5 to 7 days after the 1st batch.

Non-primary: a first-episode infection in someone who has previously been infected with HV1 (cold sores, etc.) and acquires HSV2. Symptoms are less severe and may go unnoticed. As many as 80% to 90% of first-time genital outbreaks go unrecognized.

Recurrent infection: this occurs in people who have had previous HSV infections at the same site or near it. For genital herpes, this includes having outbreaks anywhere in the "boxer shorts" area. A single group of nerves supplies the genitals, thighs, lower abdomen, rectum & buttocks. Since herpes hibernates in the nerves, you don't need to have anal sex for an outbreak to occur around your anus. For some people, outbreaks occur in the same location. For others, the outbreaks move to a new location. The average recurrence lasts 2 to 10 days.

A person could have herpes for thirty years, not know it and then have their first recognized occurrence. When they finally do have an outbreak that they can recognize, it can cause unwarranted suspicions of infidelity. Ouch!

When people have cold sores they should not give oral sex to others. Oral herpes (HSV1) now causes about one-third of the first-time genital herpes outbreaks. At the start, there is no difference between how type 1 and type 2 behave. However, if a person has been infected with HSV 1 in their genitals, they are far less likely to have recurrences. The recurrence rate for genital HSV1 is about one outbreak a year compared to HSV 2 genital infections that recur 4 to 6 times per year.

Prodrome is a set of symptoms that occurs before an actual outbreak is present. Itching, tingling, a crawling under the skin feeling, pain down the leg or in the butt are some of the symptoms. About half of the people with genital herpes experience prodrome. Things that can trigger a herpes outbreak include menstruation, sunlight, pregnancy, birth control pills, diet, friction (prolonged intercourse, oral sex or masturbations), stress, illness, and heat.

Viral cultures are often done to diagnose herpes. The problem with viral cultures is that they give false negative results up to 76% of the time. This means 76% of the time when a viral culture comes back negative the person really does have herpes. All negative cultures should be followed up by a more accurate blood test 3 to 4 months after possible exposure.

Other tests for herpes include a PCR (polymerase chain reaction) which is also a swab test but four times more sensitive than a culture. A Tzanck preparation can also be used for a quick but not terribly reliable diagnosis.

Three antiviral medications are available to help alleviate the symptoms of herpes: acyclovir, Valtrex and Famvir. All three drugs work equally well. Studies with these drugs have found that 80% to 90% of people who take the drugs for suppression have greatly reduced frequency of outbreaks or do not have outbreaks while taking the drug. If a woman should become pregnant while taking an antiviral medication, she should discontinue its use and

The greatest concern sexually has to do with transmitting the virus to another person. Intercourse should be avoided completely during outbreaks for maximum safety when one partner is infected and the other is not.

It is essential to disclose your herpes status to a new sexual partner prior to having sex. Give them the opportunity to make an informed decision about the future of their own health. If you don't tell your partner until after sex, they have good reason to question your integrity and your ability to be trusted.

By far, the best online resource for herpes is the Westover Heights Clinic: www.westoverheights.com/genital_herpes/handbook.html. You can download the *Updated Herpes Handbook* for free, and it really is updated frequently by its authors, Terri and Ricks Warren.

For more information, you can also phone the National Herpes Hotline at (919) 361-8488 or the National STD Hotline at (800)227-8922.

Other STIs—Body Fluids vs. Skin-To-Skin Transmission

Some sex infections are transmitted by body fluids, such as semen, vaginal fluids, anal fluids and blood. Others are transmitted by direct skin-to-skin contact, or contact with an infected sore or area. Depending on how the infection is spread, condoms can provide really good STI protection, (for fluid-based infections) or only moderate protection (for skin-to-skin infections). Regardless of what STI might be present, condoms are the best protection if you are going to be sexually active. Each type of infection is described below.

Chlamydia
Transmission: fluid-based.

With 3 million new cases each year, this is one of the most common STIs today. Four out of five women don't know they have it until they get serious complications such as Pelvic Inflammatory Disease. With males, it's a similar picture, except for the PID. This is why all sexually active people should be tested for chlamydia at least once a year. Men: Few symptoms or liquid discharge and painful peeing. It can cause Nongonococcal Urethritis or NGU. Women: Usually no symptoms, but there can be burning or itching in your vagina with or without a discharge.

Genital Warts See Human Papilloma Virus (HPV).

Gonorrhea

Because it is becoming drug resistant, there is now only one class of antibiotics that can treat Gonorrhea. So it has become a real concern once again. Transmission: fluid-based.

Men: Possible burning discharge from the penis, usually yellow. Women: Often, no symptoms at all, possible green or yellow discharge from the vagina, abnormal vaginal bleeding, or pelvic pain. Pelvic Inflammatory Disease, tubal pregnancy, and sterility are real possibilities if not treated.

Hepatitis A, B, or C

Transmission: fluid-based (B & C) Fecal Contamination (A)

Men & Women: Often no symptoms, possible yellowing of the skin and the whites of your eyes, nausea, fever, and abnormal urine and feces. Liver damage is a common complication. Hepatitis A: Infection usually clears up on its own. Hepatitis B: Can cause serious damage, treatment is not always successful. Hepatitis C: Most who have it are chronic carriers but are not symptomatic. In some, it can cause liver damage and death.

If your sexual boundaries are a bit porous or you enjoy barebacking and rimming, please talk to your physician about getting a hepatitis vaccination.

HIV/AIDS

Transmission: fluid-based

AIDS is a disease or cluster of diseases that involves a shutdown of the immune system. Several factors, including sexual activity, may be involved in its spread. HIV virus is believed to lead to AIDS, however, there is much that we do not know about AIDS. It is one of the most complex and deadly diseases of our time. You are STRONGLY encouraged to learn more about the disease of AIDS. Hopefully you will take the time and effort to do so.

Human Papilloma Virus (HPV) Including **Genital Warts**

Transmission: skin-to-skin

There are more than 100 different strains of HPV that can attack anywhere from your larynx and lungs to your cervix and anus. Some of the strains of HPV can impact your sexuality by giving you genital warts or caus-ing cellular changes. Genital warts are like little cauliflowers. The more seri-ous risk is from strains of HPV that can cause cellular changes on the cervix, penis or anus. Men: Typically no symptoms, or genital warts from HPV can spring up on the head or shaft of your penis, on your scrotum, or around you anus. HPV has also been implicated in cancer of the penis and throat cancer. Women: Typically no symptoms, but warts can be in the vagina, on the vulva, or around your anus. HPV can also cause cervical lesions, which can lead to cancer of the cervix if not treated. These lesions are usually discovered when a pap smear comes back with abnormal or precancerous cells. **The vast major-ity of cervical cancers are related to HPV infection.** HPV can be transmit-ted though any kind of sexual activity, including handjobs and finger fucking. There is a new 3-shot vaccine for HPV (Gardasil) that is currently approved for females between the ages of 9 and 26. A competing vaccine is Cervarix. These vaccines are controversial. The *New England Journal of Medicine* has raised questions about their widescale use. Check with your physician.

Syphilis
Transmission: fluid-based or contact with infected area

Men & Women: First stage is a painless open sore on the mouth or geni-tals. These are called chancres. They disappear in a few weeks. In the second stage, people often develop a rash all over the body, especially the hands and feet. If left untreated, it goes into a hidden or latent stage for 3 to 40 years. Late Stage or Tertiary Syphilis can result in heart, brain, or nerve damage and death. There are often no symptoms, which is why sexually active peo-ple should be tested every year. (See the history of syphilis at the end of this chapter.)

Vaginal Infections
(Trichomoniasis, Bacterial Vaginosis, or Yeast Infections/Candida Albicans)
Transmission: through sexual activity or in nonsexual ways

Trichomoniasis: Possible foul-smelling discharge, painful peeing, or no symptoms at all. You can get it from sexual activity or in other ways, like shar-ing an infected person's towel or bathing suit. Bacterial Vaginosis (BV): Pos-sible creamy discharge and fishy smell after intercourse, sometimes itching and painful peeing. Yeast Infections or Candida Albicans: Possible itchy geni-tals and a heavy, whitish, clumpy discharge that can smell like yeast. Almost always looks like cottage cheese. Yeast infections can happen on their own, when the woman is taking antibiotics, when she's been wearing tight pants, panty hose, leotards, or anything that doesn't allow her crotch to breathe. Men: With some vaginal infections, it is important that the male is treated also. Guys can get vaginal infections in the penis, even if it is a serious contradiction in terms.

Mites & Lice:

Crab Lice, or Pubic Lice

Transmission: skin-to-skin or in nonsexual ways

Pthirus Pubis or Crab Louse (Ever hear the insult, "You louse" or "He's a louse?") Pubic lice are highly contagious mites. They can cause itching beyond belief. Men & Women: Intense itching or irritation in the genital area.

If you think you have pubic lice, see a healthcare provider to get prescription medication. While over-the-counter concoctions can work for crab lice, it is best to see a healthcare professional to make sure it isn't something else that just looks like crab lice.

Scabies

Transmission: skin-to-skin or in nonsexual ways

A creepy, crawly, burrowing parasitic mite that gets under the skin and lays eggs there. It's like getting chiggers in your crotch. Men & Women: Can cause itchy skin with scabby scratches all over the body.

Other Diseases of Mass Destruction

When it comes to new diseases, we don't know what's out there. So rather than focusing on one type of disease, why not try to keep your entire body healthy? First and foremost, this means never, ever do recreational drugs such as poppers (nitrile inhalants) or shoot anything into your veins. Poppers and crystal meth remain extremely popular. In fact, crystal meth is so popular that even young guys are taking Viagra to help reverse the effects of "crystal dick," or meth-related impotence. The reason for avoiding recreational drugs is that there is a strong association between using recreational drugs and getting sick. People who party and do drugs tend not to use condoms or particularly good judgment.

Keeping your entire body healthy means staying fit, eating well and avoiding all non-essential drugs. It also means using condoms if you are having anal sex, whether you are heterosexual or homosexual. And if you aren't true blue and monogamous, it means using condoms during oral and vaginal intercourse as well.

Anyone who has been in more than one sexual relationship during the past year should take his or her genitals to a clinic or healthcare provider for a check-up. Be sure to include a throat culture if you have been doing oral sex and a rectal culture if you've been taking it up the rear. It's a good idea to get routine checkups even if you use condoms and don't have symptoms.

If your STI symptoms suddenly go away, do not assume that the disease has gone away! Keep in mind that the most common symptom of a sexually transmitted infection is no symptom at all. It is very common to have an STI and not be aware of it.

Know yourself, enjoy yourself, and protect yourself.

Gnarly Sex Germs in History

Some people believe that AIDS is the most deadly sex disease that ever was. Sadly enough, the prize goes to syphilis. Even a couple of popes died from syphilis.

Before 1492, when Columbus came to America, there had been no recorded cases of syphilis in Europe. But syphilis did exist in the part of the New World where Columbus and his crew landed. Shortly after Columbus's return, a vicious strain of syphilis began to spread throughout Europe, quickly killing a sizable portion of the population. Smallpox got its name because the lesions it caused were small compared to those of The Great Pox syphilis.

During its first fifty years in Europe, from about 1493 until 1550, syphilis was a savage killer. It seems that the Spanish army sent syphilitic prostitutes to infect the Italian army, which is one of the first recorded instances of biological warfare.

After 1550, syphilis went from being a quick killer to a slow killer, more like the syphilis we know today. Instead of finishing off its victims in short order, syphilis began to linger in the body for years after the initial infection, eventually targeting organs like the heart or brain. Syphilis remained a potent killer for four hundred more years (from 1550 to 1940). Syphilis is less of a problem today because it can now be treated in its early phases by antibiotics, which weren't discovered until the 1940s.

Nobel Prize Note In the 1920s, a medical doctor received the Nobel Prize for infecting syphilis patients with malaria. The high fever caused by the malaria helped burn out the stubborn syphilis infection. Unfortunately, there was no cure for the new cure. Some scientists speculate that more people died from the attempts to cure syphilis than from syphilis itself. Until the discovery of antibiotics, popular syphilis therapies included treatment with arsenic and mercury.

Lonely Shepherds, Scared Sheep

Folklore has it that syphilis was originally caused by lonely shepherds who prodded their sheep with something more personal than carved wooden staffs. The reason for the sheep/shepherd rumor is a simple matter of poetry. In 1530, a great physician, poet, and scholar named Fracastor wrote a poem about the disease of syphilis which hadn't been named syphilis yet. In the poem, a 16-year-old shepherd boy named Syphilis makes the horrible mistake of building an altar on the wrong plot of land and praying to the wrong gods. This was the 1530s equivalent of wearing the wrong colors in a gang-controlled neighborhood. It angers the god Apollo, who strikes the youth's genitals with a chancre-laden thunderbolt. Fracastor's poem tells about the rapid spread of the "new" disease:

> "I sing of that terrible disease, unknown to past centuries, which attacked all Europe in one day and spread itself over part of Africa and Asia..."

Sounds like AIDS! In 500 years, people will think of our modern efforts to fight disease in the same way that we think of Fracastor's account.

NUMBERS:

National STD Hotline: (800) 227-8922

National Herpes Hotline: (919) 361-8488

National AIDS Line: (800) 342-AIDS

A VERY Special Thanks: to Angela Hoffman, birth control and sex education expert, for help far above and beyond the call of duty with this chapter.

56

Dyslexia of the Penis
Improving Your Sexual Hang Time

Welcome to the Goofy Foot Academy of Premature Ejaculation. Early admissions are warmly accepted!

It's easy to understand why most men would be too embarrassed to call a healthcare provider about premature ejaculation. The receptionist always wants to know why you want to see the doctor. *("Uh, 'cause I jizz in about three seconds?")*

Worse yet, most healthcare provider's know more about the rings of Uranus than they do about premature ejaculation. That's why this chapter is kept as up-to-date as possible, and why some of the world's top researchers are consulted just before going to press. (Maybe you and your healthcare provider can learn together.) We try to provide you with the best knowledge and solutions that are available today, knowing that it might be difficult to find them elsewhere.

In reading this chapter, you will see that there are at least two different kinds of premature ejaculation. We will spend most of our time working with only one of these. That's because the other type isn't really premature ejaculation, but a guy's perception that he has premature ejaculation. It's like a totally decent swimmer thinking he needs to take steroids because he can't swim as fast as Michael Phelps.

We at Goofy Foot Press refer to this as *El Prematuro Loco.* That's because while a guy with a very real case of premature ejaculation might only be able to last for 15 seconds to a minute, a man with *El Prematuro Loco* might be able to last for five or ten minutes or more, which could be longer than most other men on the entire planet. In other words, his problem resides in the head that's above his shoulders rather than the one that's below his belt.

While some researchers don't think it's of value to refer to the stopwatch, a reality check is sometimes in order for today's porn-saavy couple who might assume that every guy can thrust hard for 20 minutes after two girls have been sucking on his cock at the same time. So keep in mind that the average male lasts from somewhere between 3 and 8 minutes. That's it, folks! If you are a male who can last for 5.4 minutes, which is a median of sorts and pretty good, then know that two of the guys on your former high-school basketball team were busting their nuts sooner than you, and the other two took longer to set up their shots—unless your team mascots were Wile E. Coyote and the Road Runner.

Unfortunately, the man with *El Prematuro Loco* has either been watching too much porn or his girlfriend can't have an orgasm from thrusting during that 3 to 8 minute window that nature gave most men to come within. So he figures he must have premature ejaculation because he can't stay in the saddle long enough for her to have an orgasm from intercourse alone.

Fortunately, education and reassurance is usually enough to help a man with *El Prematuro Loco* to stop focusing on what he perceives to be his shortcomings, and to work instead on finding ways to give his partner extra pleasure besides just thrusting. That's what most of the other chapters in this book are about.

As for inspiration, what about the man who can last for only one minute, but whose partner is incredibly satisfied with their lovemaking? Even though he would qualify as a premature ejaculator based on the stop watch, the fact that he isn't distressed by his shorter hang time and his partner is pleased means he's not got premature ejaculation.

Perhaps you are starting to see that there are different dimensions to premature ejaculation, both physical and mental, or hardwired and softwired. So it's not possible to define premature ejaculation based on the stop watch alone. However, it's not wise to ditch the stop watch altogether, because if we did, men with *El Prematuro Loco* would assume they have PE, even if they can last longer than most of the men who are reading this book.

NOTE: Terms like premature ejaculation, PE, and rapid ejaculation are used interchangeably, but they all mean the same thing.

You Really Are a Minute Man, and Wish You Weren't

For most men who can't even last a minute, premature ejaculation feels like a joke that their body plays on itself. Their penis suddenly feels like it's

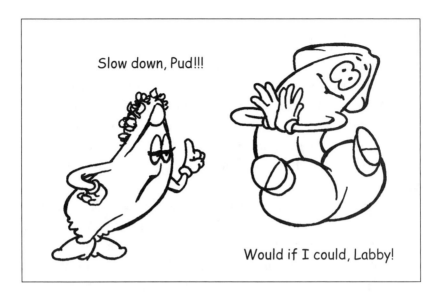

had 10 minutes' worth of hard thrusting before their partner barely has her panties off. As much as they would love to have intercourse, they start to dread it because they feel like such failures.

Unfortunately, some women feel that rapid ejaculation is "his problem," so he's the one who needs to fix it. However, a man with rapid ejaculation can no more will his wad to wait than he can will world peace or stability in financial markets.

While there can be a whole range of reasons why any particular man might come too fast or too slow, there is a basic biological reflex that often plays a key role. Some guys are wired so it doesn't take as much sensation to trigger their ejaculation reflex as it does in others. As you'll see in the chapter that follows, there are men at the other end of the spectrum who require so much sensation to trigger their ejaculation reflex that they and their partners dread intercourse.

While there is no permanent cure for premature ejaculation, there are highly effective ways to deal with it. This means that a man with a 30-second trigger can often last for two minutes or more, and a one-minute man might be able to go for three minutes or longer. How long you will be able to last will depend on the severity of the problem to begin with and your body's response to the solutions that modern medicine and sex therapy have to throw at it.

What The F...?

This chapter has been rewritten from top to bottom since the last edition. Yet the prior chapter was not even three years old. Why the big change?

More and more research is being done on premature ejaculation, especially since the big drug companies realize that they might have a pharmaceutical gold mine on their hands if they could come up with a pill that helps men last longer but doesn't put them to sleep, make their penis feel like a lead pipe, fry some of some of their more vital organs, or cause them to think about suicide.

What this means is that more than 25% of the professional articles on premature ejaculation have been published in only the last two years. But because there has been so little effort to come up with a universally accepted definition of "premature ejaculation," it is difficult to compare studies face to face. For instance, in comparing 14 studies, researchers found that only 2 of the 14 bothered to ask the men about their feelings—it was all about stop watches and seeing how much they could delay each man's ejaculation. None of the studies included input from the men's partners, which should be of paramount concern, and only 1 of the 14 studies had decent enough methodology and validation to be taken seriously. None were designed in a way that's helpful to healthcare providers. So that's what we're working with here.

In this chapter, we combine the newer research findings with some of the older findings, and filter that through what we have learned from our patients in our private practices.

The Hopscotching History of Premature Ejaculation

A good place to begin is to look at what the experts used to believe were the causes of premature ejaculation. Perhaps you still share some of these same assumptions, and maybe it's time put them to rest.

Holy Goat Gonads! Premature ejaculation was first described in medical literature in the late 1800s. Back then, just about everything that could possibly go wrong with a man's mind or penis was blamed on masturbation, or "self-pollution" as they were fond of calling it. Depletion of the body through any kind of sexual release was a concern. To help revitalize and rejuvenate the body, more than a thousand men were given testicular grafts from sheep, monkeys, goats, deer, and other men. Vasectomies also became popular as a way of returning a man's masculine essence back into his own body. Even Freud got one during his declining years.

While it's possible that getting a vasectomy or having a goat's testicle transplanted into your scrotum might cure your rapid ejaculation, modern medicine has come up with less drastic measures to throw at the problem.

Golden Showers: In the 1920s, a psychoanalyst by the name of Karl Abraham suggested that premature ejaculation resulted from a man's unconscious anger at women. Rapid ejaculation was a man's way of symbolically peeing inside of his partner's vagina. How charming. We have since discovered that men with PE are no more or less angry at women than men without PE.

A Headache in Your Penis: In the early 1940s, another German psychiatrist, Bernard Schapiro, speculated that PE was really a psychosomatic illness, like certain anxiety-related headaches and stomach aches. PE was the result of a man's psychological conflict expressing itself bodily. This, too, has been proven false. However, Schapiro was the first to recognize that there were men who'd had premature ejaculation from their first intercourse (lifelong premature ejaculators) and men who had started having it somewhere along the way (acquired premature ejaculation.)

As a result, we now know that if you used to last a lot longer and no earthshaking life changes have occurred that might explain your recently acquired case of premature ejaculation, such as finding your wife and your 16-year-old paper boy in bed together, then it is a very good idea to have a complete physical exam. Your acquired PE could be the result of a prostate infection, an endocrine issue, or a couple of other problems that you should receive treatment for.

PE as a Result of Popping Out Quick Ones: In the late 1970s, renowned sex therapists Masters and Johnson changed the premature ejaculation landscape by claiming that PE was a learned experience. They believed that PE was something guys taught themselves when they rushed their way through masturbation, or had rushed sex in a car, or did it with a prostitute. Fortunately, common sense has resurfaced. We now realize that if popping out a quick one was the cause of premature ejaculation there probably wouldn't be a guy on the planet who could last more than two minutes.

However, it is possible that if a guy was born with a shorter fuse to begin with, then the rushed experiences he had when he was a teenager could have had more of a lasting impact than if he had been born with a body that was wired to go longer to begin with. In that case, the kind of retraining that Masters and Johnson suggested might help a lot.

The retraining treatment that Masters and Johnson helped to make popular is called the squeeze technique which they claimed had nearly perfect success in curing PE. While we have since learned this claim wasn't backed up with a whole lot of science, there is reason to believe it can help some men with PE. You can learn how to do it in the treatment part of this chapter.

From Zero to Sixty Really Fast: In the late 1980s, sex researcher Helen Singer Kaplan proposed the idea that men with premature ejaculation never developed the ability to experience a gradual buildup of sensation in their penis. Kaplan believed that most guys have an early warning system in their penis, and are able to say to themselves, "It's starting to feel like I'm getting close—I'll slow down my thrusting or change positions so I can delay coming." But for the man with the pronto penis, ejaculation is more like a sneak attack. He gets no warning signals until it's too late to do anything to delay. Kaplan also felt that anxiety was what fueled PE.

This theory held sway for many years. But recent research findings argue against it. When men with PE are given medications that allow them to delay their ejaculation, they seem to have the same range of sensory awareness in their penis as guys who don't have premature ejaculation. This would be unlikely if Kaplan's theory were correct. And if anxiety were the fuel for PE, then it is unlikely that some of the new treatments would help. It appears that anxiety is the result of PE rather than the cause.

Research Findings on the Man with the Pronto Penis—Pt. 1

It has been assumed that men with PE either have feedback systems from their crotches to their craniums that are more sensitive or become sexually excited faster than men who last longer. To test this, researchers showed men sexually exciting materials, and expected those with PE to have a more rapid sexual response. Imagine their surprise they weren't able to find any differences?

So they went back to the drawing board and upped the ante so the situation was more like real life. They put pleasure devices on the men's penises, so the men would feel physical stimulation on the penis while they were watching the dirty movies. And that's when they found that nearly 60% of premature ejaculators would blow a wad right there in the lab compared to only 5% of guys who didn't have a problem with coming too soon. This finding helped give credence to the idea that men who are premature ejaculators are wired to come sooner than men who aren't.

There are also anecdotal reports from researchers who have had premature ejaculators and controls masturbate in the lab to get semen samples. The men who were premature ejaculators came out of the rest room holding a cup with their semen sample a lot faster than the men who were controls.

While these kinds of observations hint that there is something about the biology or physiology of a man with PE that causes him to launch sooner than men who can go for longer, they don't show that men who last longer have more control over their ejaculation once they reach the trigger point. Once they get there, they have no more control over their ejaculation than men who are premature ejaculators.

It is also interesting to note that while some premature ejaculators get erect faster, most don't. If anything, guys who come too soon tend to get wood more slowly when they are sexually aroused. It also appears that as many of 50% of men with PE have erection issues. There could be a number of explanations for this, from the man's expectation that sex isn't going to go well for him because it hasn't in the past, to the possibility that PE is a result of whatever might be causing the ED. (There's an especially high association between PE and ED in men who have diabetes.)

This dovetails with the observation of our urology consultant who said there were a number of men in his practice with premature ejaculation who responded well to Viagra—fix the erection problem and they could last longer. While research has shown this to be true for some men with PE, it's not been the case for others. (See the treatment section of this chapter on Viagra.)

Research Findings: Pt. 2—Neurology & Erections

One of the more fascinating research findings has to do with which parts of the nervous system are dominant during sexual activity. After normal ejaculators get erections, their heart rates start to slow down. This is because arousal falls under the influence of part of the nervous system called the parasympathetic. But, when they are about to ejaculate, the other part of the nervous system starts to dominate and their heart rates speed up again.

Not so with premature ejaculators. When a guy who comes too soon gets sexually aroused, his heart beat is likely to speed up from the moment he starts to get hard. For him, sexual arousal tends to be dominated by the "ejaculate now" part of the nervous system. This puts him on the verge of ejaculating from the get-go, and it can make it more difficult for him to even get an erection. However, if a guy with PE is given medication to help him last longer, it seems likely he would show a more normal heartbeat pattern.

Research Findings: Pt. 3—Emotional Reaction

Based on questionnaires, researchers know that men who feel they have control over their ejaculations look forward to sex and are able to focus on actions that can make themselves and their partners enjoy sex even more. However, premature ejaculators mostly focus on their sense of failure. They feel embarrassment, guilt, tension, worry, anger and annoyance about sex. As a result, they aren't able to focus on ways of making sex more fun and rewarding for themselves and their partners.

We used to think these negative feelings were the cause of premature ejaculation—that men with premature ejaculation don't look forward to intercourse and are depressed about sex because they have anxieties about sex to begin with. PE was simply more proof of their unconscious anxiety.

However, we now know that a lot of these negative feelings start to disappear once a man is given medications that can help him feel a sense of control over his ejaculation. Coming so soon takes what should be one of the most intense feelings of intimacy that two people can share, and pretty much negates it. Would you look forward to having intercourse if you were sure you would disappoint your partner? Maybe you'd even feel a little depressed.

Research Findings: Pt. 4—The REALLY Important Part That's Missing

Last year, the results of an FDA trial on a treatment for premature ejaculation that's applied to the penis trumpeted how it added an extra four minutes to the men's thrusting times. However, if you read the actual study like we do here at Goofy Foot Press, you would have noticed that something quite significant was not included in the press release.

In spite of the allegedly great results, the men's female partners didn't report any increase in their own sexual satisfaction. So maybe the problem wasn't as bad as the guys with PE assumed and their partners were just as satisfied either way. Or maybe it was a reflection that the researchers apparently needed to move heaven and hell to just get one part of the trial to reach statistical significance. Of course, we'll never know.

The fact is, sexual problems don't exist in a vacuum. Whenever you read a study about a product or medication that treats one partner, you are missing a big piece of the story if they don't collect information from the other partner. To their credit, at least they asked the men's partner's about their experience in the study above.

When it comes to sexual intimacy between partners, mutual pleasure can't be measured with a stopwatch.

Treatments—Overview

There are at least three different ways to treat premature ejaculation, assuming we're talking the kind of premature ejaculation where a guy doesn't last very long as opposed to the kind we described earlier as *El Prematuro Loco*, where a man just thinks he doesn't last very long.

One of the problems in knowing which treatment to try is that it is very difficult to compare different treatments based on the research. One factor has to do with differences in IELT, which is the time from putting a penis in a vagina to when it ejaculated. Another is how fast the guy thrusts.

Depending on the study, men with PE might have an IELT of 33 seconds, where in another study they might have an IELT of 66 seconds. Are you trying to treat a more difficult situation when a guy launches in less than 33 seconds, as opposed to one who can last for more than a minute? Or is it possible that all the 33-second man needs is a small assist, while the 66-second man needs more? Since PE isn't like a disease with a specific cause, the best treatment will depend on each individual's biology, psychology and relationship, as well as on what's causing him to come so fast. So in exploring different treatment options, you will need to be both flexible and adventurous—two qualities that men are not always known for according to the women who take our sex surveys.

The most logical treatment to try first would be the squeeze technique. It costs nothing and has no side effects, other than needing to ask for and accept your partner's help, and her being willing to offer it. That and the two of you would need to trust each other and talk about your sexual feelings and things like that. OK, we get it. No chance in hell. Best to list the pills first.

Treatments—Pills

New products are currently being researched. By the time you read this, it might not be up-to-date. If anything new comes up, will update it at www.GuideToGettingItOn.com. For now, here are the options we know about.

Keep in mind that none of these options have currently been approved for use as a treatment for premature ejaculation. Using them would strictly be off label and the wisdom of doing so is between you and your healthcare provider. Also, these all have side effects, which might be negligible for some men, but bothersome for others. If the pills alone don't extend your range very far, you might try combining them with the squeeze technique. It could be that the combination will help some men, while just the squeeze technique or a pill alone might be better for others. Unfortunately, there's not much ironclad research to guide us. So it's best to have an agreement with your healthcare provider that this will be a trial-and-error adventure, and adjustments might be needed. It's also helpful to include your partner as part of the discussion.

Tramadol (brand name is Ultram): This might be an interesting choice for PE. It is a centrally acting opiod analgesic, but with few side effects in the doses being used to treat PE. The dose needed to delay ejaculation is only 50 mgs, while the drug is approved for 400 mgs a day. They don't fully understand how or why Tramadol delays ejaculation, other than it does. Research with an on-demand dose of 50 mg had guys who came in 19 seconds lasting four minutes, and a 25-mg dose had men who normally came in a minute going for more than six minutes. It is optimally taken two hours before intercourse. Researchers are currently giving men 150 mg PRN with what they informed us are good results. Time will tell. Tramadol is one of the only opiod drugs that is not a controlled substance, and it is even sold over-the-counter in some countries. People who will abuse a drug will abuse Tramadol, but it has been around since the late 1970s and apparently isn't abused any more than other NSAIDS. The FDA has not approved Tramadol for PE, and you'd need to discuss the advisability of trying it with your healthcare provider.

Clomipramine (brand name is Anafranil): This is a tricyclic antidepressant that has been used for a long time to help people with obsessive compulsive disorders. One of the side effects has been that it delays ejaculation, which is why they started to use it for men with PE. A 25-mg dose taken 4 to

24 hours before intercourse is sometimes recommended. This can be raised to 50 mg, but with that can come increased side effects. A study was done in which a 10-30 mg dose was given on a long-term basis with satisfactory results. As with SSRI antidepressants, there could be an increased risk for suicide among men under 24, although it's not known if that would be the case for young men who are taking it for PE, and who are using it on demand as opposed to daily. As with SSRIs, there might be an impact on your fertility if you take high doses for a long time. Perhaps it's because your sperm are so happy you can last longer they are slam dancing and hurting themselves, but there are apparently other reasons.

SSRI Antidepressants (brand names include Paxil, Prozac and Zoloft): Since a common side effect for SSRI antidepressants is delayed ejaculation, researchers originally assumed that taking a fast-acting SSRI with a short half-life would be a good on-demand solution for premature ejaculation. Then they discovered that it takes several weeks for the medication to have an effect on the part of the brain that results in an ejaculation delay. While one SSRI by the name of Dapoxetine was presented to the FDA as an on-demand treatment for PE, it was not approved because it wasn't particularly effective. This hasn't stopped the manufacturer from trying again. Also, there is an increased risk for suicide in young men under the age of 24 who are taking SSRIs, and there is the possibility of sperm damage in men who take high doses over extended periods of time.

Sildenafil (brand name is Viagra): A number of clinicians who treat men with premature ejaculation have noticed erection-related problems. One of the unanswered questions is whether whatever is causing the erection problems is also causing the premature ejaculation, or if the premature ejaculation causes the men so much distress that they end up having erection problems. Either way, some men with premature ejaculation are able to last a lot longer if they take Viagra. It seems that if you are dealing with PE pharmaceutically, trying Viagra would be an option to consider as long as your healthcare provider is good with it. The side effects tend to be low, and if it helps, it helps. There are also studies which combined Viagra with SSRIs, or with some of the topical creams that we discuss next. But most people wouldn't see a reason for trying that unless they had exhausted the other options.

Treatments—Creams, Sprays and Special Condoms

In addition to using pills, researchers have also been experimenting with sprays, creams and special condoms that desensitize the penis with to help delay ejaculation. The bad news is that these treatments can seriously numb out your penis. Here's a list of what's being used as of press time:

EMLA: This is a prilocaine-lidocaine cream that is available by prescription. Applying it 20 minutes before intercourse is optimal. You need to rub it on the entire shaft, and then use a condom so the residual cream doesn't decrease your partner's sensitivity. Do be careful rubbing a partner's clit with the same finger that you put the cream on your penis with, given how your finger won't exactly be touch sensitive and residual cream will not have the desired effect on her clitoris.

TEMPE: At presstime, the FDA was doing phase III trials on a an a prilocaine-lidocaine aerosal spray called TEMPE (Topical Eutectic Mixture for Premature Ejaculation.) You spray it on the head of your penis approximately five minutes before intercourse. It is not supposed to numb out your partner so you don't need to wear a condom.

SS-CREAM: This is an herbal mixture that contains the extracts of nine natural products. You apply it an hour before intercourse. Korean researchers have been touting it for years. The trouble is, where do you get it?

TROJAN EXTENDED PLEASURE AND **DUREX PERFORMAX CONDOMS:** These condoms have benzocaine gel on the inside and are specially made to desensitize or numb out your penis. It is fascinating to read user comments about these condoms. The reviews tend to either be 5 stars or 1 star, with some guys and their partners loving them, and some hating them. The biggest complaint is that they numb out your penis so much that you lose all sensation, and your erection as well. The biggest praise is that they numb out your penis just enough so you can last a lot longer than you normally do. The beauty is clearly in the eye—or penis—of the beholder. If you don't like one brand, do try the other, as there are reports by men who have tried both brands and prefer one over the other. You might not want to put these condoms on until just before intercourse. Letting your penis baste in the gel for too long might leave it feeling like your gums after getting novacaine at the dentist's office. Also, be very careful not to get the gel from the inside of the condom on a woman's genitals. Plenty of women reported that this did not make them particularly happy. (Be sure to read the instructions.) And as one woman with a numb mouth flamed, do not give a blow job right after a man takes one of these bad boys off.

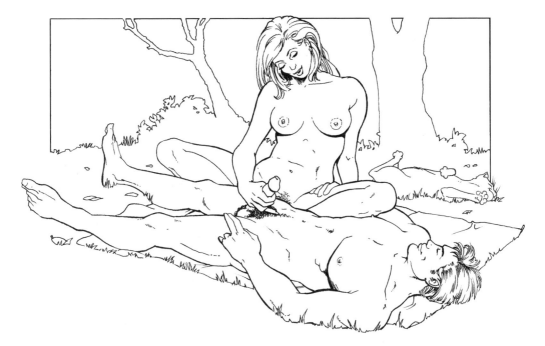

Treatments—Teaching an Old Dog New Tricks: The Squeeze Technique

The squeeze technique for premature ejaculation has been around for a really long time and has had various incarnations. You would think there would be a number of studies investigating its efficacy, but they are few and far between. Part of the problem has to do with funding. Since the squeeze technique is free, drug companies aren't exactly lining up to fund the research. And as you might have noticed, our government rarely chomps at the bit to fund studies on improving sexual pleasure. Abstinence-only and billions of dollars to bail out Wall Street are thought to be better investments.

Two studies that were done on the squeeze technique during the 1980s showed that a number of men had success with it initially, but most of the gains were lost after three years. This is not unusual in the world of sex. Seasoned sex therapists often schedule follow-up appointments for any kind of problem every six months to a year after successful treatment. That's because sexual problems tend to creep back into our lives over time. So don't be surprised if you need to do squeeze-technique refreshers every couple of months. Far from being a burden, this should be fun. Seriously, what's not to like about a partner stroking your penis?

As for squeeze-technique particulars, you both get naked and kiss and fool around. Then you kiss and fool around some more. At some point, which is to be totally decided upon by the two of you, the female partner wags her finger in the male's face and says sternly, "On your back, dude!"

Then she starts stroking his penis handjob style. While it's usually done without lube, there's nothing that says lube can't be used. See what works best for the two of you and happily abuse the little guy with it.

The man's job is to tell his partner what he's feeling in his penis. As soon as he feels like he is reaching the point of no return, he asks her to stop stroking and to start squeezing—right below the head for 10 to 20 seconds. Then, after a minute or so, the man's urge to paint the ceiling should be gone, and she can start stroking him again. Repeat this for three or four times, or even more if you are both enjoying it. When the two of you decide that Mr. Winky has had a good enough workout, she can stroke him until he blows.

A few weeks later, the woman might experiment with switching techniques. Rather than stopping and squeezing when he tells her he's about to come, she might try rubbing only the head of his penis. In other words, she goes from choking his chicken to polishing his helmet.

As for erections, don't worry about them. What you are interested in is trying to tolerate more sensation.

From Squeezing to Intercourse: When the two of you feel you are getting more control over the situation, the woman might try stimulating his penis with her lips instead of her fingers, or by sitting on top of the man and rubbing his penis with her vulva. This is called femoral intercourse. It is where the shaft of the penis glides through the lips of the vulva like a hot dog in a bun. The penis doesn't go into the vagina, but glides through the vulva's lips. The woman can lift her pelvis up when her partner is close to coming.

After another week or two, she might try putting the man's penis inside of her vagina while she is on top. It's good to keep it there for several minutes without thrusting. This helps the man get used to the warmth and other sensations. Keep experimenting from there.

The Point of No Return: When doing the squeeze technique, it is helpful to recognize when a man is approaching the Point of No Return. This is when nothing short of stepping on a land mine will keep him from ejaculating. Signs that ejaculation is eminent include: the veins in his penis start to bulge, his love log gives a sudden throb, the color of the head may darken, his testicles might suck up into his groin, his muscles start to tighten, his hips may thrust, and he might start to groan like a dying bull or invoke the name of God or Allah. Appreciate how well you are doing if you can keep him close to the point of no return for several minutes without letting him go over the edge. With some men this will be possible, with others it might require a pharmaceutical assist.

Also, it helps if the couple can cut themselves plenty of slack. There will be times when a guy reaches the point of no return before his partner can squeeze or pause or pull away. It's no big deal. It's not like this is the first time he's ever ejaculated with a hand around his penis. Doing the squeeze technique should be fun. It's not a reality show competition.

Acquired Premature Ejaculation

Most of the cases where a guy launches in less than a minute are lifelong. However, there are some cases that you acquire. Not to worry, calling it "acquired" is a bit misleading. It's not like you can get it at the store.

As we discussed earlier, if you never or seldom had issues with coming too soon, it's a good idea to consult with a physician if it suddenly starts to happen. While the reason might be physical, it could also be emotional.

For instance, consider the case of Bill, who is a general contractor and who scheduled an appointment with a urologist to deal with his premature ejaculation. Bill rarely had trouble with his ejaculation until recently.

If the urologist who Bill had consulted had been too busy to take a thorough history, he would have missed learning that Bill recently started dating Jenni. Jenni is a corporate CEO. She is high-powered and white-collar, Bill is hard-working and blue-collar. Bill has felt inadequate from the start with Jenni given that she's drop-dead gorgeous and makes about four times as much money as he does. Bill's premature ejaculation started soon after he began dating Jenni. Get the picture?

Bill got his PE along the way as opposed to being born with it. Bill didn't need medication to treat the problem and it's unlikely his prostate or thyroid were the problem. What Bill needed were some sessions with a therapist to help him deal with his conflicted feelings about being in a relationship with Jenni. (Thanks to psychologist and sex therapist Stan Althof for providiing this example.)

What Not To Do

Whatever the cause(s) for coming too soon, men with PE often try to slow it down by thinking about something unsexy, which is about as productive as a race-car driver thinking about golf to help with his anxiety when he's entering a high-speed turn. All of us are occasionally distracted when having sex, but intentionally think about baseball or dead animals along the side of the road is not a good way to last longer. It could lead to erection problems, so you'll then have ED and still come too soon.

The Other 97% of Your Body

It can be helpful for a man with a dyslexic penis to become more aware of the sensations in other parts of his body in addition to the part that he pulls out when he pees. Not enough can be said about allowing a partner to touch you from head to toe while you let your body relax. This kind of non-pressured exploration is often the cornerstone of all sex therapy.

It is equally important for the couple to explore ways that a man's partner can experience high levels of satisfaction besides having intercourse. That way she won't feel resentful, he won't feel guilty, and both partners will get to experience what it is like when she can open up sexually and no longer needs to mute her excitement to help him last longer.

Some couples enjoy using a variety of materials and fabrics to massage each other from head to toe. Good results can be had with feathers or furry mitts, as well as a silk scarf or piece of rayon. Some couples might be into leather, latex or rubber. Others find the feel of a partner's fingertips to be exquisite.

Plenty of men learn to compensate for PE by becoming really good at pleasing a woman with oral sex and different kinds of massage. Perhaps this is why a quick ejaculation does not get in the way of their having and enjoying great sex.

Motivation

It's easy to feel motivated to change at the start of a relationship. But then the desire to change can lose its luster and you fall back into your old rut. In time, the struggle to manage your jobs and family obligations can take all the reserve that you've got. Jerking off in the shower can become easier than confronting problems. Or maybe you are both just as motivated as you were before, but neither of you thinks the other still is.

If you don't find a way to energize and renew your sense of motivation, then the problem will most likely return. None of the treatments in this chapter are a cure. They are simply ways of chasing the symptoms of premature ejaculation. They require motivation and a long-term commitment.

The Most Important Ingredients

In helping a man to last longer, patience, love and a tolerance for frustration are essential for a partner to have. That's because her man is probably fighting a private battle with his own penis that doesn't include much kindness. Chances are, he's more angry and frustrated with himself than she will ever know. And for heaven's sake, don't forget to have a sense of humor. Humor is the sexual lubricant for the soul.

Relationship Fears & Resistances

It is reasonable for a man to be shy about seeking his partner's help with sexual problems. It is also possible that his partner may have resistances or fears about what might happen if her man is able to last longer.

In her book on premature ejaculation, Helen Singer Kaplan said that most of the men who were unable to complete her program for rapid ejaculation had wives or girlfriends who did not necessarily want them to last longer.

The three gentlemen mentioned below were rapid ejaculators as well as contributors to *The Guide*. They were kind enough to share their personal stories for you to read.

Zeus suspected that his wife didn't want him to improve his sexual function and that she would resist helping him do something about it. As it turned out, he was right. His wife didn't enjoy sex, and the faster he came, the better. In addition, she didn't want him having sex with anyone else. She assumed that he would be less likely to have extramarital affairs if his problems remained intact.

Lancelot was afraid that his girlfriend wouldn't want to invest the time and effort in helping him to last longer. He was mortified to even ask. As it turned out, he was wrong. She was happy (and relieved) that he wanted her help in solving the problem. They took on the problem together with historic results.

Heathcliff had a secret and didn't know if Catherine would want to help. While caring greatly for each other, their sex life had never been a central part of their relationship. After several years, he finally asked for her help with his premature ejaculation. He received an unexpected reply. She told him that she often masturbated after he went to sleep, keeping her sexual needs to herself because she didn't think he was interested. They began masturbating together and started feeling sexually intimate for the first time in their lives. They they found many ways to please each other sexually. By this time, Heathcliff had become such a changed man that not even his neighbors could recognize him.

Rather than bulldozing ahead with the treatments that are mentioned in this chapter, why not start by having a couple of long talks about it first? The two of you might do well to talk about your entire sexual relationship and any fears or concerns that you are having.

Get a Grip—Stop Apologizing

Some of the most annoying aspects of premature ejaculation that women report are the constant apologies and self-criticism that men express after coming too soon. They say that this whining and bellyaching puts them off. If you decide to work on these exercises together, the man needs to promise that he will no longer apologize or berate himself for coming too soon!

Stay on Top of the Research

Things are changing rapidly. So if you have premature ejaculation, try to stay on top of the literature. Paul will mention any treatment updates in his podcasts at www.ThePleasureReport.com, as well as at this book's website:

www.GuideToGettingItOn.com

Resources To Consult: *Premature Ejaculation—The New Neuroscientific and Drug Treatment Approach*, by Marcel Waldinger, Routledge, (2009)

A Special Thanks: Donald Strassberg of the University of Utah for his generous contribution of time and experience; David Rowland from Valparaiso University for his generous time, advice and research; Marcel D. Waldinger of University of Utrecht for his responsiveness and excellent research, Joseph Marzucco who has many years in urology under his belt, and Michael Metz who is co-author of "Coping With Premature Ejaculation" and one of the country's most thoughtful experts on rapid ejaculation.

57

Delayed Ejaculation

Some of you might be thinking, "I don't give a rip about delayed whatever-it's-called—it's not relevant to my sex life." But this is one of those less-than-mainstream subjects where you really start to learn about sexuality, such as when an erection doesn't necessarily mean a guy is sexually excited. We'll also be looking at masturbation in different ways than people usually think about it.

For those of you who have delayed ejaculation or are dealing with it in your relationship, be aware that very little research has been done on this subject, and virtually none of it is the double-blind kind that you can hopefully take to the bank. So those of you who are dealing with this problem don't have an abundance of credible resources that are straightforward and easy to understand.

Delayed Defined

Delayed ejaculation is when a guy can usually get a rock-hard erection and can have intercourse for a really long time, but can't ejaculate. What's particularly fascinating is that the majority of men with this problem are able to ejaculate just fine when they masturbate. It's when you put a flesh-and-blood partner between the guy's hand and his penis that he usually has the problem. It can get so bad that his intercourse partner is able to figure out the plot lines to her next three novels before he's even close to coming.

Delayed ejaculation used to be known as retarded ejaculation, until we decided that calling a man a "retarded ejaculator" was a bit harsh. While modern medicine still calls the condition retarded ejaculation, some people refer to it as inhibited ejaculation, and others just call it delayed ejaculation.

How many men have delayed ejaculation? We aren't really sure. The guesses range from 2% to 6%, but even if it were only 1%, that's still a lot of guys whose corks won't pop.

This condition can present itself differently in different men. It can be intermittent or it can happen every time. It can be lifelong or something that crept up along the way. It can be mild, moderate, severe, or super-severe.

If you are stop-watch obsessed and hellbent on quantifying delayed ejaculation, consider that an average guy lasts somewhere between three and eight minutes during intercourse. At least one researcher has cooked the various standard deviations of how long an average intercourse lasts, and suggests if you can't come after 25 to 30 minutes of thrusting, then you probably qualify as having delayed ejaculation. But here's a problem: for some couples, 25 minutes is just getting warmed up, while for others 25 minutes might be a nightmare of sexual excess. So before declaring a dude delayed, you'd want both him and his partner to consider it a problem. And what if a man is able to come after fifteen minutes, but his partner wishes he were done after five? And forget calling it delayed ejaculation if the problem only happens only when you are using a condom. If that's the case, a dab of water-based lube on the head of your penis before sliding the condom down the shaft might help increase your sensation.

As you'll soon see, there can be numerous factors that contribute to how fast or slow a guy launches his load, from the biology that he was born with to how he processes things like excitement and anxiety. Please keep in mind that while one man with delayed ejaculation might respond to X, Y, or Z another man might need A, B and C. So while we'll be taking a shot-gun approach and mentioning a number of possibilities, your job is to decide which if any apply to your particular situation.

Genetically Delayed

Let's start with genetics. If a man has a slow stick for a penis and it's not as sensitive as most other guys, or if his body is wired in such a way that he needs to reach a higher level of excitement than others before it triggers the ejaculation button, then he might be pre-disposed to experiencing delayed ejaculation. He can't do any more to change the way he's wired genetically than you can blink and your Ford turns into a Maserati or your Suburban into a Prius. So what we'll be focusing on are some of the possible work arounds that you might try.

Now, if you are dealing with an ejaculation problem that's at the other end of the speed spectrum and come faster than Hans Solo in a Millennium

Falcon, you might be thinking, What's the big deal—I'll trade my premature ejaculation for his delayed ejaculation in a heartbeat. But unless you've been there and done that, it's hard to understand just how cumbersome and what a burden on a relationship delayed ejaculation can be. It can make sex hard work for both partners.

Even though premature ejaculation and delayed ejaculation are on opposite sides of the cum coin, no matter which ejaculation disorder you've got, the man's ejaculation often ends up taking center stage. Instead of his being able to have fun with his partner and to share sexual pleasure with her, sex becomes more about his equipment and its failure to fire when you want it to.

Delayed Precaution

Here's a caution about delayed ejaculation that you won't read elsewhere. Not many years ago we used to say that a woman who couldn't have an orgasm from intercourse was "frigid" and we gave her a medical diagnosis as if she had a disease. While "frigid" is nicer than "retarded," we now consider ourselves more enlightened. We tell people that a lot of women can't have orgasms from thrusting alone during intercourse, and it's completely fine and normal if they have their orgasms from masturbation and masturbation only. In other words, we've tried to make the female orgasm something a woman is allowed to have by her own hand, rather than it being something she needs to put on parade during intercourse.

We are neither as kind nor as generous with men. If a man can come only from masturbation but not intercourse, we call him a "retarded" or "delayed" ejaculator. He feels horrible about himself, and his partner is sure it's because he doesn't find her sexually appealing or she doesn't feel like she can do anything good for him in a sexual way. So sex can become a source of dread and anxiety for both partners.

If you are a man or a couple with this problem, why not at least try to remind yourselves that there are plenty of ways you can enjoy intercourse and sexual intimacy without needing an ejaculation to signal that you are crossing the lovemaking finish line. What if you agree on a sign the woman can give during intercourse for when she's satisfied and wants to stop? Takes the pressure off him, takes the pressure off of her.

We'd probably be ahead if we just left it that and said end of subject, but let's look at some of the possible causes and treatments of delayed ejaculation with an emphasis on the words "possible" or "perhaps." That's because much of the current information is based on anecdote, which means if it is real science, it's only real science by accident. And please keep in mind that what follows is strictly for information purposes only, and is in no way meant to take the place of a meeting with your healthcare provider.

It's important to be sensitive that this is something that impacts a couple. The couple's chemistry, ability to talk it over and their willingness to deal with the matter is going to be important if you hope to make progress. And if the man's partner prefers to be passive during sex, helping him deal with his delayed ejaculation will require that she step out of her comfort zone.

Patience if Not Prudence

If you're the kind who are looking for a magic pill, it's unlikely the ejaculation gods will be blowing too many sticky kisses your way. If you want it to be like those TV talk shows where guests solve massive problems in the span of two commercials, forget it. And good luck if your goal is to be like porn stars—where the male actors are human thrust-and-come machines who have no emotions, expression, or the need for feedback and communication with their partners. (Actually, one expert who we consulted on ejaculation problems said that he feels a lot of male porn stars suffer from delayed ejaculation; they just managed to make a career out of it!)

Speaking of magic pills, you want to rule out the possibility that the ejaculation problem is a side effect of a drug or medications you might be taking. Various anti-depressants are at the top of a list that includes antipsychotic medications, methadone and other analgesics, tranquilizers, sedatives, medications to lower your blood pressure, various muscle relaxers, poppers, marijuana, alcohol abuse, and possibly cigarette smoking.

Don't assume that drugs that contribute to delayed ejaculation will list this on their warning labels. There are medications that don't list heart attacks as a possible side effect when they probably should, so don't expect them to put "delayed ejaculation" on the side of the carton. If your problem with delayed ejaculation hasn't been lifelong, try to think back if any new medications were introduced around the same time that your ability to come suddenly went. Likewise, delayed ejaculation can be secondary to erection problems, or these conditions might occur in tandem, so if you aren't having good erections, see if your healthcare provider can help you with that.

You also want to be sure that delayed ejaculation isn't due to neurological problems including multiple sclerosis, spinal-cord injury, diabetes, thyroid issues, prostate-related problems, certain surgeries or other pelvic upleasantries. While most cases of delayed ejaculation don't appear to be caused by drugs or disease, it's important to rule out these possibilities.

You also want to rule out diseases that can cause neurological problems, as well as certain psychological states and conditions.

Religion and Abuse?

You might explore whether there were any traumatic psycho-social events that occurred around the time when you started to come slower than a slug in Super Glue. Did you come home unexpectedly to find your wife and best friend going at it on your favorite rug with her screaming, "I've never come like this with that loser husband of mine!"?

Religious prohibitions about sex can be a contributing factor for men with delayed ejaculation. Even without a conservative religious upbringing, guilt and shame can keep a man's semen parked in his pelvis. He might also have concerns about being a dad or his partner were to becoming pregnant.

Is Your Penis a Lying Scoundrel?

One of the first things to appreciate about delayed ejaculation is that the erect penis of a man who has this condition sometimes lies. This can be confusing, because there's often a seriously hard penis between his legs. You'd normally assume the man is highly aroused. But that might not be the case. He might not be allowing himself to experience as much sexual excitement as other guys with hard-ons. To use psychological terms, his erection might be out of sync with his internal state, and the couple may need to work on increasing the level of sexual excitement that he allows himself to feel.

In fact, one of the things that researchers suggest is that the couple focus on increasing the man's awareness of his own sexual pleasure and the sensations that make him feel good. Sometimes men with delayed ejaculation aren't in tune with their body's sensations, and some appear to be so focused on giving their partner pleasure that they won't let themselves be aware of their own sexual excitement, or they don't take in enough pleasure to reach the point of no return when it comes to ejaculation.

Too Much Focus, Too Little Excitement

There are situations in which the man is trying so hard to ejaculate in order to make his partner feel better about the situation that he's focused on his penis at the expense of the rest of his body, and this makes him even more numb to his own sexual excitement.

So consider doing a lot of exploration of the man's body from head to toe—and not just trying to find some magic spot or button that makes him ejaculate. Try to discover some of the subtle things that feel good, and work on talking more easily about them. For some men, this might include long lingering kisses up and down the side of his neck or on his chest, nipples, or back, or maybe a finger up his bum. Again, experiment and explore. Or you can get seriously Cosmo and run silk scarves or soft make-up brushes up and down his body. You might try to stimulate his genitals at the same time that you are kissing his neck. This can help him double up on the excitement and sensation he is feeling.

Again, the goal of this kind of approach is to focus on pleasure rather than on orgasm. You're trying to help him experience sexual pleasure and excitement that he might be blocking out. You're trying to storm the guard that's keeping sensation from putting pressure on the trigger that makes him ejaculate. Of course, you'll need to be sensitive to how much he can handle. While a lot of guys will enjoy whatever you've got to throw at 'em, others will reach a point of overload, after which all you are doing is increasing their resistance.

Note: Some therapists advise that the man not attempt to have intercourse until he can actually feel that he's sexually excited as opposed to simply having an erection.

Harsh, Draconian Masturbation Techniques!

Let's move on to the possible role of masturbation in men with delayed ejaculation. When talking about masturbation, there are at least two factors to consider: one is the physics or mechanics of how you stroke yourself, the other is the fantasy that you call up to help get yourself off.

As for the physics or mechanics, one of the few researchers who has actually studied delayed ejaculation feels that super vigorous or unusual masturbation habits can be a contributor in a number of cases. So he thinks that changing masturbation habits is essential in situations where the guy masturbates face down, or pounds his meat like he's making chicken fried steak. This researcher often tries to get the guy to stop masturbating for several weeks or months, with the hope that he has to rely on his partner to help him come. Also, when the man does masturbate, a goal is to encourage him to make masturbation more like intercourse than a pound'a'thon. He's encouraged to use his other hand, or perhaps to use oil in a way that makes masturbation more like intercourse. You don't want intercourse to have to compete with forceful masturbation techniques. And masturbating face down is thought by some to be a major contributor to delayed ejaculation, although there's not an abundance of good science to back it up.

Masturbation-Gone-Wrong? Or Is This One of Those Chicken-Egg Things?

One trouble with the masturbation-gone-wrong theory is that there are probably plenty of men who pound their meat mercilessly and have no problem ejaculating during intercourse. So if it is a problem, maybe it's only a problem for certain guys who have some of the other contributing factors that we've talked about. Perhaps the guy's penis is less sensitive than most, or his threshold to reach ejaculation is higher, so he learned to masturbate the way he did because it's the only way he could have an orgasm. In that case, his strange way of masturbating isn't the cause of the problem, but the result of it. Still, it's hard to see a downside of a treatment approach that asks him to change hands or ease up on his grip, or turn over the reins to his significant other.

As for the psychological part of masturbation, it is possible that some men with delayed ejaculation have specific fantasies that they need in order to get off, but the realities of intercourse get in the way of being able to call up the fantasy. Let's say a guy has a secret fantasy where his partner is stroking his penis with her feet, or maybe she's dressed in a special corset, or pees on him, or is being gang banged by Dopey, Grumpy, Happy, Bashful, Sneezy, Sleepy and Doc. While these fantasies might work great for him when he's strokin' it alone, how does a guy lose himself in them when he is having intercourse with a real-live partner whose physical presence is a sad reminder that the seven dwarfs are nowhere to be found?

One of the challenges for you and your partner will be in allowing enough of the fantasy to safely emerge to help you get off during intercourse. This means that exploring masturbation fantasies might be fruitful in some cases of delayed ejaculation. This might not be a problem if what turns a guy on is when his partner wears a certain bra or maybe even a pair of pantyhose with the crotch cut out so they can have intercourse while she's got them on. Most women won't be too offended by those kind of requests, and some might even be turned on by them.

But it can be challenging when your fantasies are at the extreme, or when you feel guilty about your fantasies. It can be particularly difficult when you need the same rigid fantasy to get off each and every time, and sex becomes a mechanical ritual.

For That Rare Man Who Doesn't Abuse Himself

There are also situations where a man with delayed ejaculation can't or won't masturbate. If that's the case, you might start to explore the reasons and beliefs that might be behind that decision. This will require some serious introspection, which is not necessarily the hallmark of all males, let alone those with delayed ejaculation. And for some men who are too embarrassed to masturbate, they might try doing it in stages, starting while they are home alone, and working up to where they can do it when their partner is home but in a different room, and maybe eventually when she's in the same room but without any lights on.

The Joys of Pornography

Another thing that some guys rely on to help them ejaculate is pornography. Of course, pulling out your favorite lad mag while you are making love might not sit too well with your partner, although maybe it will help if she understands that this is the ejaculation equivalent of training wheels, and its purpose is to help you learn or relearn to ejaculate during intercourse. So if the woman is feeling a bit used or this doesn't feel all that sensitive to her needs, it might help if she knows that this is for the transition period while you learn how to ejaculate inside of her or beside her.

Threshold Clinging

A consultant to this book who worked in urology for many years had this theory: When most men feel the sensations that tell them they are about to ejaculate, they either cross the threshold and ejaculate, or they slow down or change positions in order to delay coming. But he felt that some of the men he'd worked with who had delayed ejaculation had trained themselves to automatically go the other way once they started to feel an increase in sensation. They would decrease their sensation or excitement even though they were still thrusting away at the same speed. He used to advise these men to stop intercourse if they'd backed away from the point of no return more than three times in one session of lovemaking, because he felt that after that they were just reinforcing this march away from ejaculation and teaching themselves to be even better at delaying ejaculation. Again, this is anecdote, not science, but it might have meaning for readers.

Old Advice vs. New

It used to be that the advice given for dealing with delayed ejaculation was to try having intercourse in novel situations: maybe in the kitchen or in the back seat of the car—in places where there might be additional excitement from the lack of familiarity. However, this doesn't seem to be mentioned in the more recent articles written on the subject.

What this attempts to do is distract the man from his usual M.O. where he's often the master of control. You want to help him relinquish his need for control.

Another strategy that is sometimes recommended is that once the man is able to become more aware of his sexual excitement and more able to allow it to build up inside of him, that his partner brings him close to where he's about to ejaculate either with her hands or mouth, and then he quickly puts his penis in her vagina and begins to have intercourse so he doesn't have much choice but to ejaculate inside of her. This way he's able to see and feel that he can ejaculate inside of his partner without the world coming to an end, or hopefully not coming to an end.

Just Imagine

Something that can be helpful with any kind of sex therapy is for both partners to imagine what would happen if the problem were to suddenly disappear. Is it possible there would be some fears or concerns rather than pure joy? Does the problem keep both partners within a certain comfort zone? Would his partner worry that he'd suddenly want sex more often than she does, or that he'd be tempted to try his newfound skills on other women? Would he be concerned that his partner might make new demands on him, or that he'd lose a sense of control?

As for drugs you might take to help you come sooner, none have been approved, and due to side effects from the few drugs that might be of help, there doesn't appear to be anything on the immediate horizon.

RESOURCES: Some of the best information available as of presstime are Marcel Waldinger's 2007 chapter on delayed ejaculation in the 4th edition of Sandy Leiblums' "Principles and Practice of Sexual Therapy," and Perelman and Rowland's chapter on the subject in Rowland's 2008 "Handbook of Sexuality and Gender Identity Disorders." If you want the latest on the subject from the top researchers, these are your people.

58

When Your System Crashes

While this is a chapter on sexual problems, please keep in mind that it's only a brief overview. You are encouraged to read articles and books on sex that offer a more detailed perspective, and check with a sex therapist or physician as indicated.

This chapter starts with male trouble and ends with female trouble.

Deadwood—The Bummer in Your Pants

It is amusing to look at the impotence ads in the sports section of major newspapers. They are usually located next to the ads for hair removal and hair restoration, above the ads for nude female mud wrestling and sometimes on the same page as the penis-enlargement ads. Most of the men in the impotence ads are older.

Contrary to what the erection ads show, hard-on problems happen to men of all ages, from teenagers on up. For instance, it's not unusual for erection problems to occur at the start of a sexual relationship. Call it performance anxiety, call it fear—it's not unusual for a guy to need a couple of weeks or months to find a comfortable groove. Giving him any less time to get it up is silly and shortsighted, as long as your relationship is solid and there is a strong sense of mutual attraction. The real danger is not with the lack of erection, but with what each of you makes of it. Short-term problems can become long term-problems if the man sees himself as a failure or the woman needs his erection to validate that she's desirable. Consider the following from a young man in his early twenties:

> "Last week we had attempted sex again. Once again I went from an erection down to completely unerect in a short amount of time. It happened when she said do you want to have sex. I had a feeling of uneasiness run through my entire body. It's almost like when you blow past a cop doing 80 and you get that feeling in your chest. It's a penetrating feeling through my body, that I won't be able to get an erection and it becomes self-fulfilling and self-defeating. I don't have control over my body and that is what is so frustrating."

A combination of sex therapy and a Viagra-like drug might be the approach of choice for this young man.

Several kinds of erection failure are discussed in the pages that follow—from those caused by physical impairment to those that are fueled by soft thoughts and limp emotions. Whatever the cause, hopefully a man will be able to utilize these moments of hydraulic failure as an excuse to explore and please his partner with his hands and mouth. At the same time, a partner's lips and fingers can feel incredible on a penis that's soft, and there are plenty of sexual fantasies the two of you can act out that don't require a penis at all.

Rising from the Ashes

There is an interesting sex problem that some men have that is called delayed ejaculation. We talk about it in more in the chapter "Delayed Ejaculation." Fortunately, there are things we can learn about what goes right by investigating what goes wrong.

While the "average man" ejaculates and goes soft in approximately five minutes, these guys can often stay hard for forty minutes or more worth of serious fucking. Some keep going for longer.

So by the way most guys think of it, if five minutes is good, forty would be eight times better. Yet that's not how it is for the men with an Energizer-Bunny penis. They have sex less often than the five-minute men, and they don't enjoy it nearly as much. Even though they have magnificent hard-ons, their low level of sexual excitement makes for one of those, "What's wrong with this picture?" moments.

Likewise, if you look at all of the men who are prescribed Viagra, more than 50% stop taking it, even though it helps them get hard. What we have learned is that it's not always a good idea to give a guy an erection without a few sessions of sex counseling first. When it comes to making love, relationship issues trump penis issues. When you haven't had sexual interaction with a partner in a couple of years, suddenly introducing a hard penis into a bedroom can create as many problems as it solves. The man might be horribly anxious about performing after all these years, and the woman might wonder if he's really turned on by her, or if it's the drug. There can be hundreds of other issues.

So hopefully you will stop thinking that a hard-on can fix all that ails you. Erections are marvelous wonders, but a satisfying relationship they do not make. Unfortunately, when the penis doesn't get hard, or when it comes

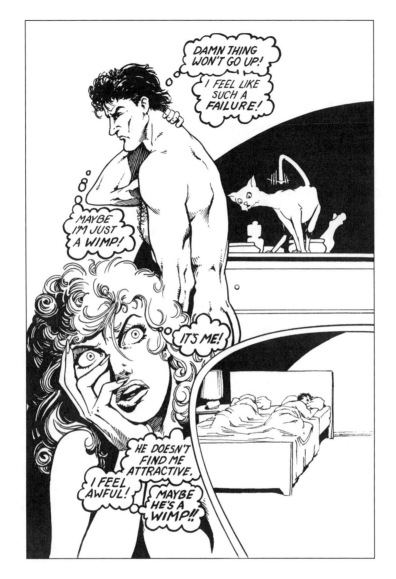

too fast or too slow, it becomes it's own vortex that sucks up all of the energies that a couple could otherwise use in finding ways to please each other sexually. We especially know this in couples where the woman would be perfectly satisfied with her partner if he would allow himself to focus on her instead of on what his penis is not able to do.

Suggestion If a penis stalls out, try not to give it the power to ruin your sexual intimacy. Easier said than done, but what about necking for a long time, finger fucking, oral sex, using a vibrator or dildo, tying each other up, or acting out a fantasy. That way, a potential downer might evolve into something sweet and hot. Success in life is very much about what we are able to make of our shortcomings, even if it's hanging between our legs.

Often, the biggest problems with impotence or coming too soon or not at all isn't the lack of erection. Rather, it's a lack of playfulness and resourcefulness on the part of the man and woman when they are confronted with a penis that's being contrary.

When Your Posse Won't Ride

Books on sex often use terms such as "self-hatred," "self-loathing" and "devastating" to describe how a man feels when he is—gulp—impotent. You know, the horror when he can't get it up. (Just so you won't think you are all alone, guys who come too soon often feel this way as well.)

Perhaps this Guide is way out of step or maybe it's just insensitive, but *devastating* is what happens when your wife or child dies or when you've just been told that you only have six months to live. *Self-hatred* is what you feel if your business flops or if you've just blown your life's savings on something really dumb. *Self-loathing* is what you experience when you've had a major stroke or accident and can't feed or bathe yourself or wipe your own rear.

Call us callous, call us rude, but we can think of about a thousand things worse than if a man's hard-on takes a hiatus, even if it's forever. Sure, it's frustrating and even humiliating at times, but so are a lot of other things in life. The fact is, you still have your fingers and mouth for giving pleasure, and you still have what's in your heart to love your partner with. And if you can't count at least five things in your life to be thankful for, even if your penis never gets hard again or you come in ten seconds, then your priorities are in seriously bad shape.

Contrary to what you'll read elsewhere, penis problems, regardless of the cause, are an opportunity to have better sex rather than worse. Fortunately, there are plenty of ways that modern medicine can help a recalcitrant penis to get hard, but it seems a shame to employ a quick cure without allowing yourself and your relationship to grow in the process. You won't believe how many times Viagra-like pills will result in better erections but not in better sex for either partner.

People who survive heart attacks and cancer learn to approach life differently as a result of the disease. A woman who is overcoming orgasm problems has to welcome a new way of embracing her body and her sexuality.

It's a journey, a process. Impotent men, on the other hand, just want their dicks to get hard—no learning, no journey.

The Sufis have a saying that you have to let yourself die before you are truly born. Sometimes a guy has to give up his penis as a symbol of masculinity before he can get on with his life. Sometimes he has to realize that there's more to being a man than getting an erection or lasting for a prescribed number of thrusts. (Then he sometimes has to convince his partner.)

This is not to say that a man shouldn't inquire about the various remedies that modern medicine has for erection problems. He should also have a full physical to make sure that the erection problem is not a symptom of something else. If there are medical problems, they need to be treated.

Note: No kidding about getting a physical exam. Men who begin to experience a gradual increase in impotency might be seeing the first signs of an impending stroke or heart attack. Impotence may be a greater predictor of cardiovascular disease than the highly regarded stress test. It seems that the arteries in the penis start to gum up before those in the rest of the body. A physical exam may allow physicians to help a man before something really bad happens to his most important organs—the heart and brain. Also, researchers are now finding a high correlation between obesity and impotence. Who knew that the drive-thru at McDonald's could do your dick in?

A Modern Medical Approach to the Great Groin Grinch

If your penis is impotent, it is likely that you are muttering under your breath that we can take our Sufi logic and stuff it where the sun don't shine. You want a traditional Western approach. You want a magic bullet that does not require introspection or lifestyle changes. Good enough. The advice that follows is a spoof on a modern medical approach to fixing erection problems. While it conveys some wisdom, it still focuses on fixing the penis instead of helping the man behind it and the woman in front of it. It is an approach that attempts to turn the clock back to a time when the penis worked just fine. It's a regressive fix rather than a step forward, one that is oblivious to lessons that might be learned or frontiers of trust that are waiting to be crossed.

Dear Dr. Goofy,

My bowling partner recently started having erection problems and is too embarrassed to seek help. Can you offer advice?

Bob from Boston

Dear Bob,

If your bowling partner has stopped throwing strikes for more than a couple of weeks, it's a good idea for him to take his pokey pecker to a physician for a checkup. It's smart to rule out underlying medical conditions.

Modern medicine has decided that more than 99.999% of erection problems are due to physical causes, from diabetes to who-knows-what. We can fix almost anything, unless your friend is a cigarette smoker. If that's the case, he might as well call a mortuary and have himself interred. Cigarette smoking is as bad for your penis as it is for your lungs.

Is your friend able to get erections at all, like in the morning upon waking, or when he jerks off? To explore this further, we might send him home with a device he attaches to his penis when he sleeps. The device won't help to get him off, but it does tell if he has erections in his sleep and for how long. If a man can get a sustained erection in his sleep or while masturbating, the problem may reside in his psyche, although certain types of depression can keep a man from getting an erection, even in his sleep. Yikes. Did I say "psyche?" With the help of our friends in the pharmaceutical industry, we have declared that the psyche no longer exists. There are, however, neurotransmitter issues that we can throw pills at.

Speaking of pills, some physicians will send your friend home with samples of Viagra—or Levitra or Cialis if they have stock in Glaxo or Lilly. If the pills don't work, then they'll do a work-up. Or they might give your friend's penis an injection that's a pecker-picker-upper. Don't worry, no one's going to pull out a syringe with a hollow nail for a needle and say, "Drop your drawers." It's an itty-bitty wisp of a shot that hurts less than getting a pubic hair stuck in your zipper. If the penis gets hard and is able to stay hard, then the plumbing is intact and the problem can probably be fixed with a prescription.

If the shot does not make the penis hard, or it gets hard but doesn't stay hard, then it's likely there is a circulation problem. This can range from hardening of the arteries (strange term for when it happens in the penis!) to leaky valves. More tests would need to be done to peg the exact cause.

It is also possible that there is a neurological problem which is disabling the body's ability to begin the hard-on process. This is similar to when you turn the ignition key on your car and nothing happens.

Another thing we sometimes remember to check is if your friend is taking medications that might be cold-cocking his rooster. Suspicious meds can range from alcohol and heroin to prescriptions and over-the-counter drugs. Some even say that Tagamet can do a dick in. (He isn't one of those meth-abusing party boys, is he? That can be very bad for you.)

Finally, if you insist, we will consider the highly unlikely possibility that your friend's erection problem stems from emotional causes or a combination of something emotional and physical.

To check that mental thing, your friend needs to do some private detective work, or detective work on his privates. For instance, what was going on in his life around the time when his soldier stopped marching? Did his ability to get an erection decline gradually, like the fall of Rome, or did it shut down all at once, like Bear Stearns, Wachovia or Lehman Brothers? Was there a change in his job status? Did his insurance company cancel him without cause? Did his team not go to the Superbowl because of a lousy call in the closing seconds? Was there a change in his relationship with his partner? Did his wife leave him for another man? Did she leave him for another woman? Was he pulled from an important project, or did he lose a promotion he had his heart set on? Did he receive an unkind inquiry from the IRS?

Also, it is helpful to inquire about his relationship with his spouse. If he instantly says, "Naw, it's fine," ask him to describe some of the things that are fine about it. See if he conveys a sense of love and fondness, or if he sounds like he's reading the instructions on a bottle of Kaopectate. If the relationship has fallen on–dare we say–hard times, then he and his wife need to focus on fixing that rather than on fixing his penis, which is merely the messenger.

Don't worry, we're working on Husband-Wife Combo pills for whatever ails them, an SSRI-PDE-5 inhibitor-testosterone cocktail with maybe a little OxyContin thrown in for good measure. In the meantime, in order to treat erection problems that are caused by relationship problems, your friend and his partner might try to forget all that they know about each other and start over again as if they'd just met. This can be difficult, especially if they have had some really lousy times together. They might try taking a month or two doing things like hugging, touching and talking, with no attempt at intercourse. They also might try sharing romantic dinners, movies and the types of things they enjoyed doing when they first met. How about racking their bowling balls and taking a trip around the country in the Winnebago? They might discover that there really is life after bowling. On the other hand, some couples do better when they spend less time with each other. This can be especially true when they are newly retired and suddenly find themselves in each other's face 24 hours a day.

Also keep in mind that the more mature the penis, the more hands-on play and wooing it needs in order to get hard. Lots and lots.

There is also the possibility that your friend had erection problems before he and his wife met. Then he might find it helpful to get some psychological help on his own. And if none of that helps, there's this Sufi saying....

Viagra & Friends

Remember how Barbie had friends like Skipper and Midge? Viagra now has little pill friends, with names like Levitra and Cialis. People often prefer the latter because they last longer. There's something about having to take a pill each time you want to have intercourse that make people prefer Cialis. (As of presstime, there were a condom-full of studies being done on how long higher doses of Viagra last, so the people at Pfizer are clearly aware that consumers want to take only one pill every couple of days.)

One of the finest quotes about Viagra is from the *Boston Globe*'s Ellen Goodman:

"I can't help wondering why we got a pill to help men with performance instead of communication. Moreover, how is it possible that we came up with a male impotence pill before we got a male birth control pill? The Vatican, you will note, has approved Viagra while still condemning condoms."

Now, why is it that such a large percentage of men who get a first prescription for Viagra never get a refill? One reason is because while Viagra can help you get hard, it isn't going to transform your middle-aged or older penis into that of an 18-year old. We're talking an assist, not a miracle.

Also, if you and your partner have been low on sexual intimacy for a few years and suddenly discover that pills or injections can help it get hard enough to get it in, please schedule a couple of sessions with a sex therapist first. You wouldn't believe the number of issues that need to be dealt with before you slide a rusty penis inside a rusty vagina. Questions about intimacy, romance, attraction, excitement, anger and frustration are but a few that might need to be addressed first. On the other hand, if you and your partner have been enjoying orgasms and physical intimacy, but just no intercourse, go for it and see what happens.

Viagra in the Cockpit

Pilots are not allowed to take Viagra for twelve hours before a flight. The FAA does not want the co-pilot to accidentally grab the pilot's erection instead of the landing-gear controls. Viagra inhibits an enzyme in the penis which helps the blood vessels dilate. A similar enzyme in our eyes might possibly be impacted by Viagra. This is why there has been concern that Viagra could result in altered color perception. Pilots who are taking Viagra have apparently seen flying vaginas in the friendly skies. **Note:** the most recent study says that if the pilots are seeing vaginas, it's because a stewardess is dancing around the cockpit naked. Hard as they tried, the researchers weren't able to show that Viagra was impacting enzymes in the eye.

Levitra as a Thrill Pill?

At least the Viagra people have had the decency to market their drug toward guys who might actually need it. No such claim can be made by the makers of the more recently released Levitra, which is clearly going for the younger man who gets it up just fine. In one of their ads, they show a young stud trying to throw a football through a tire. It bounces off to the side. Then, after Levitra is mentioned, the boy gets the ball through the tire several times. He is then joined by his smiling wife or girlfriend, whose tire he has apparently just kicked with satisfying results.

If you honestly think that taking a hard-on pill when you are young and healthy is going to make you a better lover, then you are wasting your time reading this book.

Other Chemicals That Make You Hard

There are some compounds that cause a diehard erection when injected into the penis, assuming the penile plumbing can maintain an erection once the penis gets hard. A compound called Papervine was formerly used for this purpose, but now there are different combinations of ingredients used in the injections. For example, one popular combination includes papervine, phentolamine, and prostaglandin E1.

Also, there is a kind of prostaglandin which a man shoots into his urethra (peehole) before he needs an erection, like one of those fertilizer sticks that you shove in the soil next to your droopy houseplants.

There are other orally-prescribed drugs that can help some men to get hard. One drug that is sometimes prescribed is called yohimbine. Yohimbine is native to Africa. It can often be found in health food stores. Since the cost of yohimbine isn't much more by prescription, why not get it from a urologist? That way you will be monitored for side effects and you can be sure you are getting the yohimbine in consistent doses, which is not true for the yohimbine in health food stores. The doc can also rule out other possible causes of the erection problem. Other drugs for impotence that are being tested include one that is administered in cream form. The problem is getting the cream to penetrate through the part of the penis that surrounds the vascular tissue. Another problem concerns stiffness in the fingers after applying the cream.

"Ejaculate Like a Porn Star," "Add an Inch in Two Weeks," "Natural Male Enhancement," "Recharge Your Libido"— Some Seriously Iffy Ideas

There is probably not a living human being who hasn't seen ads for herbal pills that promise to get you horny, big and hard. Some of these products are cleverly marketed to make them look legitimate.

Aside from some of these companies being shut down for consumer fraud, if the worst of your in-laws wanted to make herbal supplements in their garage where their fourteen cats sleep, they could. And they could sell them on TV. There is no regulation on herbal supplements. They can put strychnine and cow plops in them, the only way the government will test the things is if about a dozen people suddenly die.

If there really was a pill that could put a smile on Bob's face and do all of the things the scammers and spammers say their pills can do, don't you think the multi-billion dollar drug companies would be selling it?

Mechanical Devices for Getting Hard & Surgical Implants

Some men find that the vacuum pump is a useful erection aid. It is a little bulky and cumbersome, but worth a try if you are in search of a lost erection. What do you have to lose, unless there are medical reasons why you shouldn't. There are different suppliers for vacuum pumps. Be sure they include special gaskets which keep your scrotum from getting sucked up into the vacuum tube. (Some of the gay-guy penis pumper companies sell excellent units for less than half of the ones that are medicare approved. Still, expect to pay $100 for a decent rig.)

There are different surgical implants, from semi-rigid shanks to implants with little pumps that give you an erection. Frequent improvements are being made in the technology. Please research this subject carefully before making an incision—uh, decision.

The Warning that Should Be on Prozac, Zoloft & The Other SSRIs

According to the *Journal of Sexual Medicine* (January, 2008), any person who has been given a prescription for an SSRIs should be given a warning such as the following:

> "There is a high probability of sexual side effects while on SSRI medications. There are indications that in an unknown number of cases, the side effects may not resolve with cessation of the medication and could be potentially irreversible."

SSRIs are antidepressants that include Prozac, Zoloft, Paxil, Lexapro, Luvox, Celexa, Effexor, Serzone and Remeron.

More Pharmaceutical Sex Assassins

You wouldn't believe how many over-the-counter or prescription medications can mess with everything from your ability to get wet to your feelings of desire. For instance, just taking a common antihistamine can keep a woman from lubricating. Extending this into a worst-case scenario:

1. The woman takes an antihistamine to help with her runny nose. It dries up her nose, and her vagina.

2. Because of the dry vagina, she starts having painful intercourse.

3. Because of the pain, the muscles in her vagina tense up whenever she sees her husband's penis get hard.

4. The tensing up in her vagina becomes a learned response, and continues for long after she's stopped taking the allergy medicine.

5. Because of the constant pain, she experiences a decrease in sexual desire, which causes her insecure husband to have an affair. She finds out about it and files for divorce. All because she took a couple of Sudafed! Or maybe she's taking an antidepressant which decreases sexual desire. How sad, a divorce due to Prozac.

At the top of the list of sexual suspects should be any medication that says, "May cause drowsiness. Do not drive or operate heavy equipment." Assume when they say "equipment," they are also referring to what's between your legs, or your sex drive.

Whatever your sexual problems or concerns, the absolute first thing to do is to make a list of all the medications you are taking—from simple over-the-counter drugs to prescription medications to herbal teas and vitamin concoctions to heroin, cocaine, pot, poppers, ecstasy, meth, or alcohol. Then check these over with a pharmacist. Medications may not be the cause of the sexual problem, but they're the first and most obvious thing to rule out.

The Tour de France in Your Pants

Urologists have been saying for years that bicycle seats are causing permanent erection problems for hard riders (or formerly hard riders). They've been seeing case after case of young riders with numbness in their crotches and erection problems. It's not so much that riders couldn't get it up, but that it wouldn't stay up. Instead of wanting to study the matter further, the bike magazines went after the urologists. They would have done the cigarette manufacturers proud in trying to discredit these concerned physicians.

But the bicycle industry underestimated the crotch docs who spend hours each day with their faces between mens' legs. The crotch docs wired bicycle seats with more sensors than the Sands Casino when it was demolished. They did studies on bicycle-riding policemen, whose penis heads were connected to oxygen sensors. They found that the typical bicycle saddle robs the penis of 80% of its oxygen and it decreases erections during sleep. Plus, there's a major nerve to your penis that runs between your legs. It takes a terrible thrashing when you are using a normal saddle. You know that tingling sensation? It's not normal. It is from crotch compression, which can damage your *fun nerve*.

When you sit in a chair, your weight is distributed across your entire butt and thighs. Because of the wide distribution of weight, the circulation in your crotch is not compromised. When you are on a bike, the entire weight of your body is bearing down a very small part of your crotch that provides the oxygen and nerves to your genitals. As for the bike seats with the cut-outs? They can actually make the problem worse, as there's even less area to distribute your weight over.

Unfortunately, women are no more immune than guys. Researchers found a measurable decrease in sexual sensation for women who ride seriously. They've also found a condition on competitive riders called "Bicyclist's Vulva" where one of the labia can grow really big due to the thrashing a girl's crotch takes from the seat.

The solution? It's pretty simple, and it isn't bike seats with cutouts. The solution is seats without noses, called no-nose saddles. Inner-city cops who chase criminals on bikes swear by them. For a list of no-nose saddles, go to www.no-nose.com.

Peyronie's Disease

This is a condition that results in a curving or bending deformity of the penis that can range from mild to so severe that intercourse is not possible and there can be pain with erection. Peyronie's Disease or PD results from plaques forming on the tunica albuginea of the penis, but what causes that to happen is not fully understood. The only effective treatment seems to be surgery, with the results being from very good to not great. While there is spontaneous repair in some cases, these would be in the minority. Men who have moderate to severe cases often experience clinical depression, and often describe themselves as "feeling like a freak." The depression can take its toll on a relationship.

A Question of Desire

Some people think that "low desire" is a sickness like the flu that a woman needs to get over. They assume that she's cured of her low desire if she can happily hop on her partner's erect penis. But low desire can mean different things, some of which require a reworking of the relationship outside of the bedroom before there will be any changes between the sheets. The mind-set of trying to recreate what the woman was like in the past is not productive. None of us are the same as we were a few years ago. Our sexuality needs to reflect our current situation, and in some cases of low desire, that is exactly what it is doing.

It is also possible that low desire can result from physical causes or metabolic changes. For some women, taking birth-control pills or certain medications can cause changes in desire that last after they discontinue the pills or medications. We know that anti-depressants can do horrible things to a person's sex drive.

Drug companies are trying very hard to get products containing testosterone approved for women with low sexual desire. This might be helpful if a woman has had her ovaries removed or if she truly has a metabolic disorder, but women should be cautious about these preparations. Their use as an elixor for low desire is controversial at best.

Highly Recommended: Remember the finger that you used to masturbate with? Why not put it to use by turning the pages of Kathryn Hall's helpful book *Reclaiming Your Sexual Self: How You Can Bring Desire Back into Your Life,* John Wiley & Sons, (2004). Dr. Hall treats low desire as a messenger rather than as a disease. Men and women both will be able to find approaches in her book to help them better understand and give meaning to lost desire. She presents a number of ways of approaching desire. Fortunately, she is not beholden to the drug companies and she realizes the short-sightedness of automatically throwing pills or patches at whatever ails you.

When Excitement Is Too Much

Some of us can't tolerate much excitement. Somewhere along the line we got the feeling that sexual excitement is dangerous or disorganizing. As a result, we experience conflicts when becoming sexually excited. People with this problem sometimes numb themselves between the navel and the knees. That way they don't have to face the anticipated dread that sexual excitement holds in their imagination.

Those who want to work through excitement problems need to experience pleasurable feelings slowly and without goals such as having an orgasm. Pressure to feel sexual takes them out of the moment and makes them feel numb. With time and effort, sexual excitement can be tolerated in the here and now, assuming that's what you want.

Some people have trouble managing sexual excitement when they are alone. They can't masturbate or even feel sexual on their own, but do just fine when they are with a partner. Perhaps they need to experience a partner's excitement about them before they can feel their own excitement.

Orgasm Fears & Tears

Although orgasms are usually welcome events, this is not always the case. Young girls or boys who are having their first orgasms can sometimes feel that they have done something wrong or broken something inside.

Adults can have mixed feelings about their own orgasms, especially when sadness, loneliness or guilt are triggered by the orgasm. The sadness can be about a former real-life partner, or maybe the orgasm taps into a deep emotional pain that suddenly gets released. Some people cry after an intense orgasm because it touches a sadness that's deep inside.

There are also people who treat their own orgasms with cold detachment, especially when they feel a need to masturbate. Perhaps the need for sexual relief brings up feelings of weakness or self-loathing. Whatever the case, they are not particularly gentle or tender when handling their own genitals. There are also people who dislike orgasms because they experience them as a form of losing control. It's a fine testament to the power of orgasm that more people in our society don't have problems with them.

Painful Intercourse

Pain during intercourse can happen to both men and women, but more often to women. The pain might not just be limited to the vulva, vagina, or bladder, but can also be a result from problems in the floor of the pelvis.

If you are having pain during intercourse, be sure to check with a physician who specializes in pelvic pain. If the pain is from something that's not related to intercourse, then that needs to be treated first. It is not helpful to treat a pelvic problem as a sexual issue when it needs pain management.

If you are a woman, try to determine whether the pain is at the opening of the vagina or is caused by deep thrusting. Deep-thrusting pain is sometimes caused by constipation or pelvic inflammatory disease. Shallow-thrusting pain has a larger range of possible causes, from adhesions under the clitoral hood or episiotomy scars to yeast infections, herpes sores, or vaginal changes associated with menopause.

Other questions to explore about painful intercourse include whether it happens all the time, how long it has been happening, if it happens with all partners or just one, and if added lubrication helps.

This kind of pain is very real and it can have horrible effects on a sexual relationship. The woman (and couple) who is experiencing it needs the same kind of support as anyone who is experiencing a chronic-pain disorder. Here are some of things that might be going on:

VULVODYNIA: this would be Latin for "a great big pain in my pussy." Symptoms include discomfort or burning pain the vulvar area of unexplained origin, which means that no infections or neurological disorders appear to be present. Often described as a chronic burning or knife-like pain, this disorder is very complex and can be a serious challenge to treat. Most healthcare providers throw their gloved-hands up in despair, which means that the patient will need to do a lot of research and find a specialist who works with vulvodynia. Just to give you an idea of the complexity, vulvodynia can be broken down into pain that is generalized or localized, and these categories are further broken down into pain that is provoked, unprovoked or both provoked and unprovoked. While few physicians who specialize in treating vulvodynia believe it is the result of psychological problems, a lot of patients and their healthcare providers mistakenly do. This isn't to say that stress and anxiety can't make the symptoms worse, but the are unlikely the cause. For an excellent brief summary, see "Vulvodynia" by Goldstein & Burrows, *Journal of Sexual Medicine,* January 2008, pages 5-15, and "The Vulvar Dermatoses" in the February issue.

VULVAR VESTIBULITIS: a form of vulvodynia where the pain or discomfort is localized to the vulvar vestibule, which is the part of the vulva that's between the inner lips. In some cases, the pain has been there since their first tampon or intercourse, in others it started long after. Could be from any of a number of different causes, including the use of oral contraceptives.

VULVITIS: an inflammation of the vulva. There can be as many causes as there are vulvas.

INTERSTITIAL CYSTITIS: pain or discomfort in the pelvis that is related to the bladder. Symptoms often include a persistent urge to pee or the need to pee frequently, as often as a couple times an hour. This is not called "painful bladder syndrome" without good reason, as the urge can feel quite extreme and it can be accompanied by spasms and pressure. People can have pain while urinating, pain while driving, and pain while having sex. In men, there can be painful ejaculation. The cause is not known, although a number of theories are on the table, and it could be there are different things that cause it. There are a number of different treatments, with one of the main goals being in decreasing the pain. People with this disorder are often very depressed as a result, in part due to the pain and discomfort, and in part because it causes such incredible interference in their lives.

PELVIC INFLAMMATORY DISEASE (PID): inflammation of the female reproductive organs, often the Fallopian tubes, which is usually caused by a bacterial infection.

Women's Orgasm Problems

Plenty of women don't have orgasms with thrusting during intercourse. This doesn't mean that they have sexual problems. All it means is that both partners need to explore what gets the woman off and include it as part of their lovemaking, unless it happens to be the man's best friend, though some couples might enjoy that, too.

One of the first things therapists look for in women who don't have orgasms is a history of sexual abuse. Yet plenty of men and women who never had a shred of sexual abuse still have sexual problems. Being raised in seriously religious households can cause sexual problems that appear very similar to those of sexual abuse, including the person's feeling vacant, depersonalized, or numb when having sex. Good luck having an orgasm with all of that going on. Books on this subject that are often recommended include *For Yourself* (by Barbach) and *Becoming Orgasmic* (by Heiman & LoPiccolo).

Vaginismus—Gridlock in Your Groin

Vaginismus is a tightness in the vagina that causes discomfort, burning, pain, penetration problems, or complete inability to have intercourse. The muscles surrounding the vagina can close so tightly that they won't allow anything to go inside. The reaction can be so severe that a woman can't even insert a tampon. Vaginismus can result from many different things from chronic pelvic pain that is unrelated to sex to psychological trauma to a bad experience at the gynecologist's office. The absolute best source of information and help for vaginismus is Lisa and Mark Carter's phenomenal website and online community at www.Vaginismus.com.

Persistent Genital Arousal Disorder

This is an unusual and difficult disorder that has only recently been recognized. It is when a woman's genitals are physically aroused for hours, days, weeks or longer—but she doesn't feel any desire to have sex. Having sex provides no relief, and orgasms don't help her arousal to reside. This would be like if a man had an erection for weeks at time, where he desperately wanted the thing to go down, but the most earth-shaking orgasm and ejaculation would not bring a smile of satisfaction or a dent in the tent in the front of his pants. Some medications can be helpful, but there is no cure.

Excellent Resources:

Principles and Practices of Sex Therapy–4th edition, edited by Sandra Leiblum, The Guilford Press (2007).

Handbook of Sexual and Gender Identity Disorders by David L. Rowland and Luca Incrocci, Wiley (2008)

The Journal of Sexual Medicine, edited by Irwin Goldstein, MD. This is the official Journal of the International Society for Sexual Medicine and the International Society for the Study of Women's Sexual Health

59
Abortion, Adoption

A large percentage of women who get abortions were using contraceptives at the time of intercourse. That's because even the best contraceptives occasionally fail, or sometimes a rubber breaks, or sometimes we forget to take a pill. If you are pregnant, there are a number of different things you can do. This chapter talks about a couple of them.

What If You Just Found Out You Are Pregnant and Didn't Want to Be?

There are plenty of people who will offer advice. Some of it will be helpful. One of your challenges will be in finding someone who will listen and help you think things out instead of needing to tell you what to do. In addition to talking to your partner, you might try to find a level-headed friend, family member, doctor, nurse or teacher who you trust. And call your local Planned Parenthood. They deal with this all of the time and tend to be helpful.

The one thing you want to avoid are "crisis pregnancy centers." These are often run by anti-abortion groups and they have a very specific agenda.

There are many people who have opted for abortion and many who have had unplanned children. Most will tell you that they did the right thing. Whichever way you decide, keep in mind that millions of people have had to face the exact same thing that you are— even though you may feel like the loneliest person on the face of the earth.

In case you are wondering about the emotional aspects of having an abortion, studies show that most women who have abortions don't report an increase in depression (as a group) for any more than a week or two after the abortion, if that. One of these studies was funded by a very biased agency that was hoping to find the opposite result. On the other hand, your own personal beliefs might not allow for abortion, in which case your options will be whether to raise the baby yourself or give it up for adoption. There are plenty of agencies that will help with the latter, but not many that will help the parent of an unplanned child who is trying to raise it on her own.

Please be aware that some of the strongest anti-abortion proponents are highly supportive while you are still pregnant, but are quite stingy and punitive when it comes to helping the unmarried mom of a toddler or older child. To many of these groups, your value is in being the vessel that is incubating the unborn child. Once the baby is born, they won't want to have anything to do with you.

Whether you choose to have an abortion or to have the baby, it's important that you make your mind up as soon as possible. Many people who are faced with unwanted pregnancies are indecisive and don't act as soon as they might. If they opt for an abortion, it is sometimes later in the pregnancy when the procedure might be more complicated. And if they decide to have the baby, they sometimes don't go for prenatal care until later in the pregnancy. This is especially true for teenagers, and it places them at high risk. Delaying prenatal care will endanger both yourself and your baby.

If you decide to keep the baby, make sure you have a support system in place to help after the baby is born.

A Special Note on Giving Your Baby Up for Adoption

There are thousands of loving couples who can't have a baby of their own and desperately want to adopt one. These couples tend to have been married for quite a while. Most have stable homes, good relationships and solid incomes. They will give your child a lifetime of love and care. Unfortunately, many of these couples must wait as long as seven years before they can adopt a baby, since not many single parents are giving their babies up for adoption these days. Part of the problem is that younger moms are often encouraged by their nonpregnant peers to keep the baby (easy for friends to say!). Unwed moms often have the unrealistic fantasy that keeping the baby will make their lives better, or that the baby's father will want to marry them. This seldom happens.

One of the really nice things about adoption in this day and age is that the pregnant mom gets to interview the couples who want to adopt her baby. She gets to decide which couple she wants to raise the baby. That way she will know her baby is being raised and loved by people she likes.

If you have medical questions or want to schedule an appointment with the nearest Planned Parenthood, call toll-free 1-800-230-PLAN.

60
Trying to Get Pregnant

Dear Paul,

My wife and I have been trying to get pregnant, with no luck. They want me to get a sperm count. Do you know anything about this? Hank from Thunder Bay

Dear Hank,

If personal experience is of any use, here's the skinny on getting a sperm count. First, a sperm sample needs to be less than an hour old in order for an accurate test to be done. In fact, the fresher, the better. That's why they may want you to produce the sample on location—where you go for blood tests.

Unfortunately, your sperms don't suddenly appear for roll call and that's that. There's a whole procedure that needs to be followed. Like handing the proper authorization form to a total stranger in a white coat who will automatically yell in a loud voice, "Whadda ya here for?"

That's when you will become acutely aware of just how many people are sitting in the crowded waiting room less than five feet behind you. There will be a mom with a couple of kids, two teenagers, an older gentleman, and maybe even a nun—all waiting to hear your answer just like the people before them waited to hear theirs. You will clear your throat and say as quietly as possible, "I'm here for a sperm count," after which the person in the white coat will immediately say in the loudest voice possible, "SPERM COUNT?" as if for some reason you were really there for a barium enema, but said sperm count just for the heck of it.

The person in the white coat will then yell to another person at the other end of the lab, "Louise, where are the specimen cups for doing a sperm count?" at which point Louise will yell back "WHAT?" to which the person in the white coat will respond even louder, "I NEED A SPECIMEN CUP FOR THIS GUY TO GIVE A SPERM SAMPLE."

Now maybe Louise will yell back, "Top shelf in the cupboard on the right." Or maybe she'll yell "WHAT?" once again, and the person in the white coat will look up at you shaking her head, expecting you to offer a sympathetic nod.

Eventually, they will find the correct cups and hand you one. If you are lucky, they will open the door and direct you to a bathroom down the hall.

Otherwise, they will tell you to have a seat in the waiting room, where twelve sets of eyes will be staring at your face and then at the plastic cup that's in your sweating hand. And then the little five-year-old, who is sitting with his mother, will ask, "Mommy, what's a spurn count?" and the woman will glare at the child with her most intense "Don't-ask-me-that-now—OR EVER!" stare, and the little boy will protest, "But that man has to have a spurn count. Is something wrong with him?"

I am still not sure what the correct response should be when the person in the white coat finally summons you to the bathroom down the hall. Do you smile, make eye contact and say, "Thank God!"? I marvel at the man with gumption enough to look at the specimen cup and ask, "What do I do with this?" or better yet, "It won't be big enough."

Of course, if you are anywhere near to being a normal guy, harvesting your own sperm in a locked bathroom is nothing you need instructions for. On the other hand, when you are producing sperm for an official sample, thoughts may enter your mind that never have before. For instance, "How long should I take?" You don't want to return in two minutes, deed done. On the other hand, you don't want to take half an hour, because you know that Louise and the person in the white coat will be giving knowing glances to each other, as if they aren't already.

To top that, no one has ever given you a grade on what actually came out. This time, not only are they scoring you on the number of sperm you're about to produce, but your wad will be graded on how well your sperm swim and on how full you fill the cup. So suddenly you'll be asking yourself, "Is there some way I should be doing this for optimal results? Should I be squeezing my testicles at the moment of truth? How do I get the most out?" I don't know what to suggest, except if you want to save yourself the embarrassment of scoring in the lower percentile of men who have ejaculated in plastic specimen cups, save up for a couple of days. You'll never believe how large a specimen cup looks when you are trying to fill it with sperm.

Finally, when you are done, you might smile inwardly and walk down the hallway looking for the person in the white coat. That's when you discover she is drawing blood and you'll need to hand the cup to Louise. Oh God. During your entire lifetime there may have been dozens of different ways that you've delivered sperm to a woman, but never in a plastic cup and never has she held it up to the light and swirled it to inspect its contents, and never has she stared so blankly and never have you felt quite so strange.

Anyway, Hank, that's what I know about spurn—uh, sperm counts. Good luck to you and your wife.

P.S. If a couple is trying to get pregnant, it takes an average of eight months before hitting conceptual gold. If a couple is not trying to get pregnant, it only takes one night.

———————————

Dear Paul,

I've heard that couples who are trying to get pregnant are not supposed to use synthetic lubricant, and I've heard that saliva can kill those little guys who are trying to get the job done. I don't lubricate very much naturally. Are there any options that you know of besides using egg whites (eewww) as a lubricant, which I've been told might help?

Getting pregnant has not been as easy as I thought. Funny how many years you can spend trying to avoid it, then how many months you can spend taking your temperature, watching your body, etc., with no results! Sex has become a drag. I don't want to add "dry" sex on top of that. Do you have any tips to keep sex fun, after months of carefully monitored frolicking?

Mary in Virginia

Dear Mary,

It's amazing how sex can become such an unpleasant chore when you and your partner start having a menage a trois with a basal thermometer. My wife and I went there for a couple of months and decided to give it up. We became foster parents and eventually adopted.

In researching your question, I am once again reminded of how often the "science" of fertility can also be the voodoo of fertility. For instance, there are all kinds of fertility specialists pontificating about the lube question, often with different answers. One specialist who has written four books on fertility avoids the question altogether by blaming the lubrication problem on the male, saying that any woman can lubricate perfectly well if she has a partner who gives her enough foreplay. I don't think so!

Sperm, like the men who make them, can be finicky little cusses. Sperm start to croak if the pH is less than 7.0 or more than 8.5. They also start to pop if the fluid around them doesn't have enough ions in it, and they shrink like prunes if the surrounding fluid has too many ions. This should make sense if you took biology and remember what osmosis is.

Given that the pH of most store bought sex lubes is so low, a lot of sperm might get fried in an acid bath if you use them. At the other extreme are things like egg whites and mineral oil, which are too alkaline. This brings me a certain amount of relief, because I feared if you used egg whites your child might come out of the womb clucking instead of crying.

As for osmosis, sperm thrive in an environment of 360 mOsm/kg. Most sex lubes have an osmolarity of 1000 mOsm/kg or more, which makes for dehydrated sperm. And while saliva has an optimal pH, its osmolarity tubes out at 151 mOsm/kg, which might cause sperm to explode. (Saliva is a great all around sex lube, except if you are trying to get pregnant.)

So here's what I'd suggest: a special sex lube called Pre-Seed that was formulated by a very reputable andrologist (sperm doctor). It has a pH of 7.3, and an osmolarity of 314 mOsm/kg. You can find it at www.ingfertility.com.

Next, you ask how to make conception-driven sex more fun. This is more important than you think, for a couple of different reasons.

It seems that stress makes the quality of a guy's ejaculation go down. In fact, they've found that men launch a bigger and better load during intercourse than when masturbating in a cup in the bathroom of a doctor's office. If a guy is having a sperm analysis, the quality of his wad will be 2 to 3 times better if his sperm is collected from a condom (non-latex) following intercourse than from his jerking off. And here's something even more important from Dr. Joanna Ellington, who is a leading andrologist:

"Some studies have actually shown better conception rates for couples having untimed regular intercourse as compared to couples using detailed methods to time things." She suggests intercourse 2 to 3 times a week, but with you doing it when you feel loving and horny as opposed to having a calendar and stop watch in hand.

Another study has shown that women who have a regular amount of intercourse every week of the month ovulate more reliably than those who don't. So having fun in bed during your non-fertile weeks could be just as important to the big picture as doing it during your most fertile nanosecond.

So why not leave Mr. Basal in the medicine cabinet and get back to enjoying your lovemaking? Forget trying to engineer a Moonie-like march of sperm toward Fallopia. Your love for each other needs to be respected and enjoyed as much as the love you might have for any child that you may or may not be creating. Couples who are desperate to get pregnant sometimes forget the importance of this.

If you are having trouble getting pregnant, a trusted resource should be Dr. Ellington at www.ingfertility.com. I'd also keep an eye out for anything written about fertility with the name "Sandra Leiblum" attached.

CHAPTER
61
Sex during Pregnancy

If you hadn't noticed by now, each woman has her own unique way of looking at the world and you can't really predict how she will react to the man who knocked her up. Some pregnant women will want more intimacy than ever before, while others will want space—sometimes huge amounts of space. This can be confusing for a dad-to-be, as he is never quite sure if the love of his life wants to snuggle or pluck his eyes out. Also, don't think that the dad-to-be isn't experiencing his own set of pregnancy-related emotions. These may cause him to hesitate sexually while his child-to-be is turning somersaults half a penis-length away. The mom-to-be might be wanting to rip his clothes off, and he's suddenly prim and proper.

This chapter is about sex during pregnancy, from orgasm-related uterine contractions to swelling vulvas and fetal brain development. For most couples, anything that felt good before conception is perfectly okay after, including oral sex, anal sex, bondage, vibrator play and good old fashioned vanilla lovemaking. But no matter what you read in this chapter or anywhere else, please discuss sex during your pregnancy with your healthcare provider. There might be situations where it is prudent to alter some of the more outrageous ways that you and your partner enjoy sex.

Talking to Your Healthcare Professional about Sex

Think about this for a moment: you go to a physician, get totally naked, spread your legs wide apart and let your doctor put her fingers in places where even the IRS doesn't. Yet many of us are nearly paralyzed by asking the simple question "Is it OK for me to have sex while I'm pregnant?"

Plenty of physicians encourage couples to have sex during pregnancy. And obstetricians rely on people having healthy sex lives in order to keep from going broke. So do pediatricians, gynecologists, Lamaze instructors and everyone else in the healthcare industry. There is no way your physician wants you getting out of practice with intercourse as long as the possibility exists that you might have more kids. So don't be afraid to ask.

If your healthcare provider says it's OK to have sex, go to it. If the answer is "No, it's not OK to be having sex," then it is important to ask more questions. The first is "Pork hay?" which is Spanish for "Why not?"

If your healthcare provider is one of the few remaining dinosaurs who doesn't believe that pregnant women should be having sex, get a second opinion. Most physicians feel that having sex during pregnancy is completely normal, unless there are specific reasons such as a prior history of miscarriages or premature labors, the placenta is attached near the cervix (placenta previa), your water has broken or there is bleeding of unknown origin.

If your physician gives a specific reason for why you shouldn't have sex, ask two more questions:

1. "How long should we not have sex—for the next few weeks, months, or for the entire pregnancy?" All too often, when a physician says, "No sex," the couple assumes this means for the entire pregnancy, when the intent was "No sex for the next couple of weeks." If you were to ask the same question in a month, the physician might say, "It was just a precaution. Based on how well you are doing now, I see no reason why you shouldn't have sex."

2. "Does 'no sex' just mean intercourse, or does it include all sexual contact?" For instance, intercourse might pose a concern, but it's fine to have orgasms orally or by masturbating. If all orgasms are a potential problem, ask if you can still have intercourse as long as you don't have an orgasm. For some women, this would be a cruel compromise, while others might welcome the extra intimacy that intercourse allows, orgasm or not.

Urge Surge—The Mood Swing

Some women stay pretty even throughout their pregnancies, while others push the mental envelope. A feature of pregnancy-related moodiness can be the intensity of the mood and the amplitude of its swing. Some pregnant women who are horny feel so intensely horny that they find it hard to think about much but sex. They pounce on the dad-to-be the second he walks through the door. The intensity can be so great that some men feel a little used, while others seize the moment. Other pregnant women don't feel like having sex at all, and some might feel horny one moment and weepy the next. Also, a pregnant woman has the potential to feel hurt by comments that few women in their nonpregnant right minds would find offensive.

For the woman whose moods fluctuate, there might be moments when she blames her man for her condition and other times when she feels elated about being pregnant and is ecstatic to know and love the guy who got her that way. Also, it is normal for a pregnant woman to feel moments of depression alternating with feelings of elation, and to have dreams of her child being a perfect baby as well as fears of it being handicapped.

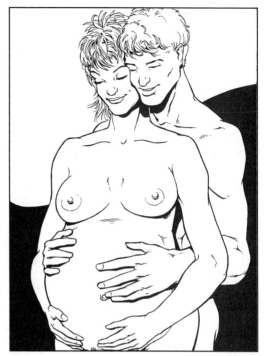

Much has been said about the disruptive effects of hormonal changes on a pregnant woman's mood, and this might be true. On the other hand, oxytocin levels rise throughout pregnancy, and oxytocin is said to make for better moods. It also causes contractions of the uterus which may help to prepare the woman's body for labor. It is thought to be involved in a woman's orgasms whether she is pregnant or not.

Beautiful or Gross?

How you feel about yourself can be an important factor in determining whether you want to have sex. Some pregnant women look in the mirror and feel fat. Others feel they have never been more beautiful. Most women who are pregnant fall somewhere in the middle of these two extremes.

No matter how a woman feels about her pregnant self, it never hurts for her to receive loving reassurance from her partner. While a hard penis and a willing heart might be physical evidence that a man finds the mother of his child to be desirable, loving words and romantic gestures speak to a different part of her soul. Do your best to always be available if not always near.

One of the common disconnects between partners during pregnancy occurs when the dad won't ask the woman for sex—not because he doesn't find her attractive, but because he doesn't want to make her feel like she has to say yes. She, on the other hand, interprets his lack of asking for sex as an indication that he doesn't find her to be sexy or attractive.

One of the better ways to handle this is for the couple to have an agreement that she will be perfectly comfortable telling him no if she doesn't feel like it. That will give him permission to plead and beg for sex as usual without having to worry that he is imposing on her—no harm, no foul.

The Fearless Factor

One of the nice things about being pregnant is not having to worry about getting pregnant. You can put the diaphragm in the deep freeze, keep the condoms in the bottom drawer or forget about taking pills each morning. This can make sex during pregnancy more relaxed and easy to enjoy. If pregnancy is what you wanted, there's no more "We have to do it now because my most fertile three-and-a-half minutes during the next quarter of a century is about to pass." Even if you didn't plan on getting pregnant, the fact that you can't get pregnant again for nine more months allows some couples to relax and enjoy sex in ways that they might not when consequences are a concern.

Genital Swelling—Slip & Slide

Around the fourth month of pregnancy, most women's genitals begin to swell. And swell. And swell. This swelling can lead to full-time lubrication and can make some pregnant women feel very horny. The increased swelling is due to the growing vascular capacity in the pregnant woman's pelvis. As a result, her vulva often becomes a deeper color and her labia thicken.

Couples find that the added swelling may lead to a delightfully snug feeling during intercourse. Genital swelling during pregnancy can also up the intensity of the woman's orgasm. More on this in the pages that follow.

Orgasms during Pregnancy

Some women have no interest in sex or orgasms when they are pregnant. Others not only want orgasms, but report coming in awe-inspiring bursts that are more intense than their most memorable pre-pregnant efforts. Sex during pregnancy can also present a slight contradiction: even if she is more easily aroused and her orgasms are more intense, she might take longer to reach orgasm. The payoff is usually worth the extra effort.

One reason for having whopper orgasms during pregnancy might be the increased level of engorgement in the abdomen. With all the extra blood, her uterus stays hard for a few minutes after orgasm. As a result, a woman who had single orgasms before pregnancy may experience two or more at a time while pregnant. But by the end of the pregnancy, some women find that the swelling in their genitals causes a congested feeling that makes coming feel more frustrating than relieving. Uterine contractions might also be contributing to the discomfort.

Male ejaculate contains prostaglandins, and some types of prostaglandins cause uterine contractions. However, studies show that neither intercourse nor male ejaculate induce labor. There is nothing about intercourse, oral sex or male ejaculate that will move your date up or cause you to go into labor. If you have concerns, be sure to consult your healthcare provider.

It is normal for a pregnant woman to have cramps or Braxton-Hicks contractions either before or after orgasm. These cramps can last for a half-hour or more. Some healthcare professionals believe that these cramps help improve the muscle tone in a pregnant woman's uterus. If the cramping becomes too uncomfortable, you can eliminate one possible cause by using a condom during intercourse or by having the man pull out before he is about to come. See if this makes any difference over a couple of weeks. Another approach that may help relieve cramping is for the woman's partner to give her a loving foot massage or back rub.

Another unexpected source of orgasms during pregnancy may be the prolific array of sex dreams that some women report having: "Never had one before, never had one after, but had a large number of sexual dreams during."

Breasts: Tenderness, Expansion & Leakage

Breast tenderness can happen in any phase of the pregnancy, especially during the first trimester. Breasts which used to cherish firm handling might suddenly prefer a light kiss, caress, or no direct stimulation at all. Some breasts that are painfully tender during the first trimester morph into pleasure zones during the second trimester. Changes like these make it important for pregnant couples to have frequent discussions about "what feels good this week."

It is normal for the breasts of a nonpregnant woman to swell when she is sexually aroused. However, when a woman becomes pregnant, her breasts may remain swollen all the time. As a result, she may get swelling on top of swelling when she is sexually excited. This might feel painful, or it may feel wonderfully, depending on the woman and the stage of her pregnancy. Also, dietary salt might contribute to the swelling.

For some couples, breast tenderness will make the missionary position a thing of the past long before expansion of the abdomen does. Another problem or delight, depending on your point of view, might occur if the woman's breasts start to leak during the latter part of pregnancy. This is perfectly natural and is simply a preview of what's to come.

Bladder Matters

One of the biggest concerns that women have about sex during pregnancy and for up to six months after is about bladder leakage. It's one of the reasons why they don't have sex—because they are afraid of leaking while sexually excited. If this is a concern for you, then it might help to have a conversation with your partner about it, and with your healthcare provider.

Most men won't give a rip if their pregnant partner pees during sex. Most are smart enough to know that they'd be peeing up a storm if they had a baby using their bladder for a trampoline. So the solution for most couples is to put extra towels down and to get a pee-proof mattress-pad cover. Unlike the loud crinkly covers of old, you can't even tell the new ones are there.

What's unexpected for many women is when their bladders continue to leak after delivery. This is not unusual, and it's important to talk to your healthcare provider about it. That's because things can usually be done to help. Again, most guys are smart enough to understand that having a baby inside of your body for all those months can require some substantial recovery time. They're not going to begrudge you some pee when they are relieved it was your abdomen and not theirs that was Junior's rumpus room for nearly ten months. A leaky bladder is no reason to avoid having sex.

Intercourse Concerns Part 1—Fetal Concussions

It is not uncommon for couples to worry that the head of dad's thrusting penis is going to bop junior on the fetal brain and knock him senseless. While it might be nice for dad to think his penis is that powerful, the fetus sits in a sac filled with a fluid that absorbs shocks and provides superb protection. To make it even that far, dad's penis would have to get through mom's cervix and uterine walls.

The most important consideration during intercourse is to find positions and thrusting styles that feel good for mom and her swollen reproductive organs. If it feels good for mom, chances are that the baby will do just fine.

As for questions about squirting junior in the eye with dad's ejaculate, the uterus is sealed off by a mucus plug that is a bit like the cork in a bottle of wine. The amniotic sac provides a secondary barrier that helps keep the ejaculate at bay.

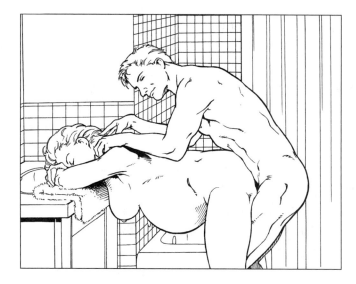

Intercourse Concerns Part 2—"The Baby Will See Us"

The human fetus is not taking notes and won't be emotionally scarred by the things you feel or do during pregnancy, even if you listen to—gulp—rock'n'roll instead of classical music. Exceptions are excessive drinking, smoking, or doing drugs that compromise the infant's developing brain.

The fetal brain is not a miniature of the adult brain. Its memory units (neurons) are hardly functional at birth. There is not enough developed brain structure for the fetus to say, "Oh my gosh, Mom and Dad are having sex and isn't that disgusting" or on a more positive note, "Mom and Dad are having sex, isn't that wonderful!"

Why Don't They Make Sexy Lingerie for Pregnant Moms?

Sex doesn't stop being an expression of love and intimacy because a baby is on the way. Yet you get the feeling that pregnant moms are supposed to be more interested in what color to paint the baby's room than in being lit up sexually or wondering what the new guy at the office looks like naked. Yes, pregnant moms can feel sexy, and some moms and dads find pregnancy to be sexually exciting. For some pregnant women, nature turned up the horny knob instead of turning it down.

Intercourse

Some pregnant women cherish the feeling of having both the baby and the baby's father inside of them at the same time. Others feel like three's a crowd. Dads, too, have their own issues about sex during pregnancy, some of which are discussed later in this chapter. If you feel like having intercourse while pregnant, important elements are a shared sense of humor and a willingness to explore. Here are some particulars to consider:

Clothes On Some couples who are trying new positions do so first with their clothes on. This helps them focus their collective energies on the engineering feat at hand, and it allows them to appreciate the humor of the situation without having to worry about feelings of urgency or declining erections. There's always time to get naked and actually go for it once the target positions have been mapped out and a strategy is planned.

Penetration Some pregnant women have a desire for penetration that's deep and assertive, while others prefer an approach that is more gentle. Talk it over. And different phases of pregnancy may require different styles of penetration while the proverbial bun is in the oven. Also, the swelling of the cervix and uterus can make certain kinds of intercourse feel uncomfortable. Let the woman control the thrusting depth, and if this cramps your style, be mindful that there are plenty of dads-to-be who aren't getting any at all.

Lubrication Some women seem to lubricate all the time when they are pregnant. However, there are plenty of exceptions. If that's the case for you, try adding lube.

Dizziness Some pregnant women experience dizziness or indigestion in certain positions or during certain phases of the pregnancy. This can be particularly true when a woman is on her back. Doing it on her side, on all fours, or while on top might suit her better.

Romancing the Cervix The cervix of a pregnant woman often swells due to the extra blood flow into the uterus. It becomes soft, and can sometimes bleed with deep penetration. Try shallower thrusting or use positions where the head of the penis romances the cervix more gently. This may be especially wise during the later months of pregnancy, when the cervix starts to ripen. If you have questions or if there is any bleeding, consult with your physician.

Third-Trimester Stretch By the third trimester, the cartilage in the pelvic region has had months of pregnancy-related hormones thrown at it. It becomes softer as a result, as part of nature's conspiracy–uh, plan–to ready the pelvic floor for the joys of childbirth. As a result, a woman may find that pressure on her pubic bone feels a little weird. Couples need to be creative in their search for comfortable intercourse positions.

Too Much Swelling For some women, genital swelling may increase to a point where intercourse feels uncomfortable, while for others the desire for intercourse never wanes. Experimenting with positions where the woman has her legs apart might help.

Backaches & All Fours With the muscles between her ribs being slowly pried apart and her pelvic floor feeling trampled on, the pregnant female has been known to suffer an occasional backache. Some women find the rocking motion of intercourse, while on all fours, can help soothe pregnancy-related backaches. It can also soothe the throbbing between her partner's legs.

The Penile Vice (OK—Vise) Grip

Some healthcare professionals think it's good for a pregnant woman to tone and exercise the muscles in her pelvic floor by doing Kegel exercises. What better way to accomplish this than by having a man insert his penis into your vagina, keeping it stationary, while you squeeze it with your pelvic muscles? Most guys would be more than happy to lend a helping penis. This is an exercise that you might keep doing after the baby is born.

When to Stop

Most physicians in this day and age say it's okay to keep having intercourse until your water breaks. Some couples have intercourse until labor itself begins. There are at least four factors which should influence you on when to stop having intercourse: 1. It doesn't feel good any longer. 2. Either partner has a genital infection. 3. The woman experiences bleeding or new discharge. 4. Your healthcare provider says to stop.

Oral Sex

The extra lubrication caused by pregnancy can give the vaginal area a stronger taste or smell, which some men notice when giving their pregnant wives oral sex. However, there are no medical reasons to stop giving or receiving oral sex during pregnancy unless the pregnancy is at risk for other reasons.

This is a concern that pregnant women often have, so we repeat, there is nothing about receiving oral sex during pregnancy that will endanger the baby. The one thing a partner shouldn't do is to make a seal around your vulva with his lips and blow into it like it's a balloon. But what kind of moron would do that anyway?

Nipple & Perineal Massage

One of the nice things about being pregnant is that when the dad-to-be is complaining about the things he usually complains about, you have the perfect excuse to say, "Shut up and rub my nipples!" That's because as the final months of pregnancy approach, it might be helpful for a woman to have two areas on her body massaged, or three areas if you count each nipple as having its own private domain. Put lotion on each nipple and massage and knead it, assuming it isn't too painful. This will help condition the nipples for nursing, and it may also help release extra oxytocin into the system, which seems to be a good thing as the due date approaches. The other area that massage might help is the perineum, which is the real estate between a woman's vagina and rectum. Some pregnancy aficionados believe that massaging this area helps to make it more pliable and reduce the need for an episiotomy.

Bleeding

During the first couple of months of pregnancy, bleeding may occur during the time when you would normally have your period. This is usually less reason for concern than bleeding that is random. Check with your physician when there is any bleeding, just to be on the safe side.

Touch vs. Sex

Some women may experience a decreased desire for sex during pregnancy, but an increased need for touch and cuddling. This can be difficult for the dad-to-be, because all of the cuddling and touching might make him feel extremely horny. To help him make it through these lean times sexually, his pregnant partner can cuddle beside him and caress his thighs, chest or testicles while he does himself by hand. Or he can do what guys do—jerk off in the shower.

Besides being an important time for holding and touching, pregnancy is a time for partners to reassure one another about their feelings of love and attraction, hopefully for each other.

Fears That Bubble Up from The Deep Dark Recesses of the Human Psyche

Contrary to how you think you should be feeling, it is not uncommon for perfectly good parents-to-be to have mixed feelings about the baby-to-be. For instance, you may have planned for years to have this baby and wanted it with the deepest of convictions, but then suddenly start feeling, "Oh my God, what have we done?" Feelings like these can be fleeting or last for weeks.

One reader says that both he and his wife were shocked to discover such feelings, given that their pregnancy was better planned than the average moon walk. Fortunately, they did not experience their bummer moods at the same time. The one who was feeling good about the pregnancy was able to comfort the one who was feeling tragic.

It is perfectly normal for humans to be overwhelmed by inner conflicts. The same is true for livestock, but we are less inclined to attribute such feelings to things we eat. (This edition of *The Guide* nearly missed going to press when the author needed to take a dehydrated two-day old calf from his mom. Anyone who thinks maternal feelings don't cut across species should have seen the look of murder in that cow's eyes.)

Feelings can be especially intense during pregnancy and just after, when so many new demands are placed on you. These are not the sort of feelings that make us want to have sex. It can be very helpful to talk over these conflicts with a friend, partner or even a counselor if you are feeling particularly jammed by them. One reader adds: "Worries about child care, job security, and having to go back to work after only six weeks can be overwhelming."

Recognizing Dad's Role

During pregnancy, all attention usually focuses on the mom-to-be, which is as it should be. But this is also an important time for the pregnant woman to acknowledge the dad-to-be's role. Potential problems can occur when the woman feels that the baby is her creation alone. This can lead to problems in the relationship between father and child, as well as between the parents.

Dad's Emotional & Sexual Issues during Pregnancy

There are plenty of books devoted to the feelings that pregnant moms experience. Yet dads-to-be experience their own pregnancy-related emotions. According to researcher James Herzog, dads-to-be tend to fall into two groups: *more attuned* and *less attuned*. The pregnancy spurs the first group of dads onto a path of personal growth, while the latter group feels threatened by the pregnancy and is not particularly fortified by it.

One factor that impacts how a man responds to his wife's pregnancy is the influence of his own father or father substitutes. Herzog noticed that during the second and third trimesters of pregnancy, a number of pregnant dads turned toward their own fathers in an attempt to reconnect with them. They felt that reconnecting with the "good dad" from their early childhood would help them be better dads to their own children. Men in the less-attuned group tended to experience a high degree of "father hunger"—growing up without an involved and caring father figure. These men tended to act in unsupportive ways, such as becoming competitive with their wives or being sexually promiscuous; some had sexual relations with other men. If you find yourself feeling unsupportive or disconnected from your pregnant wife, it might be a great idea to spend extra time with a friend or acquaintance whose fathering skills you admire. Tell him you are feeling on shaky ground; ask him how he manages as a dad when he's feeling uncertain or overwhelmed.

Other things that Herzog found about pregnant dads:

The Right Stuff Upon learning of the pregnancy, a number of dads-to-be feel good about themselves in a masculine and sexual way. The fact of the pregnancy may help allay fears that they didn't have the right stuff to make a pregnancy happen. With the excitement of being pregnant, a number of couples enjoy sex that is particularly intense and intimate, as though sex now has a different meaning.

Nourishment As the pregnancy progresses, some men feel as if they are nourishing or symbolically feeding their wives during intercourse, especially when they come inside of them. On some level, the dad-to-be might view his semen as a kind of milk that will help nurture both mother and infant.

Coming Harder Some men report feeling more depth to their orgasms when their partners are pregnant, with more physical and emotional awareness both before and after ejaculation. At the same time, the dad-to-be might be rethinking who he is; he is man whose personal identity is expanding. At times, this can be exhilarating, at other times, a frightening burden.

Dreams etc. There are plenty of ways that dads unconsciously identify with a pregnant spouse or wonder about what's going on inside of her. By mid-pregnancy, some fathers experience dreams or fantasies about being penetrated as well as being the one who penetrates. Some start to wonder more about their own inner body parts. Some put on extra weight or feel a kind of gastric fullness or upset. Some men have toothaches during this time that land them in the dentist's office. When a man has a toothache of an undetermined origin, wise dentists know to inquire if the man's wife is pregnant.

Character Evolution Being a dad-to-be can help a man shed unwanted or outdated parts of his character. The pregnancy becomes an excuse and a stimulus to mature and become more responsible. Unfortunately, not all men use pregnancy in such a constructive way, nor do all women.

Sex after Giving Birth

Some parents experience the first three to six months after the child's birth as being the most demanding and difficult time of their lives. They might not feel like having sex, or if they do, they might be too exhausted to actually do it. Other couples enjoy sneaking in quickies while the baby sleeps.

There are hugely important considerations that affect the frequency of sex among new parents, like whether dad does his fair share of the work around the house and with the baby, and whether mom welcomes his help or is nervous and critical whenever he gets near the baby. If one parent is an obvious klutz with the baby, there are plenty of ways that he or she can be helpful other than with actual hands-on baby care. In a few months, the baby may have grown enough that you feel more comfortable handling it.

Even with the best intention and desire, there will be plenty of times when new moms and dads are way too exhausted for sex, especially if there are other children in the family besides the baby. Keep in mind that many couples struggle when it comes to adapting to their new roles as parents and sexual partners.

Body Image & Sexual Desire

A major concern that a lot of women report during the first six months after pregnancy is feeling bad about how their body looks. Along with bladder control issues, this is one of the major reasons why some women don't want to have sex after the baby is born.

Hopefully, both partners will talk about this, and hopefully a male partner's reassurance will be enough to make it a non-issue.

Hormones & Libido

Some women don't feel like having sex after pregnancy due to certain hormones that might be surging through their veins. And women who are nursing are said to produce more anti-horny hormones than women who are bottle feeding, yet statistics show that nursing mothers want sex more often than those who don't nurse. Go figure.

Talking about Sex Before the Baby Is Born

Some of the best advice this book has to offer is that you talk about sex before the baby is actually born. For instance, "I've heard some new parents don't feel like having sex for a few months after giving birth—what are some of the ways we might handle that if it happens to one or both of us?" Or "What do we do if you've got a raging hard-on and I want to be held and cuddled but don't want to have intercourse?" Or "What if I want sex but you start seeing me as a mother type and don't find me exciting?"

One of the worst things you can do about sex after pregnancy is to pretend it is not a problem if it actually is. Nothing is to be gained by rolling over and pretending you are asleep to avoid having sex, by getting defensive, or by feeling attacked. As with other aspects of your relationship, this is a time to redefine and put things in a new perspective. Where sex was once taken for granted, it now needs to be planned or scheduled. There will be many times when sexual desire is a casualty to exhaustion. For a while, you will end up masturbating more often to help fill the gap in partner sex.

When Can We Start Having Intercourse?

After the placenta comes out, it takes time for the place where it was attached to heal. The woman is going to be vulnerable to infections. This is why it might not be such a good idea for male ejaculate and store-bought lube to be working their way up there. Also, it might take a couple of weeks for the vagina to heal after it's been stretched from here to China. Some physicians worry that intercourse before the vagina is healed can cause scar tissue to build. This is why many physicians feel it is wise to wait at least a few weeks after birth before you start doing the nasty. This is particularly true if the woman had an episiotomy, with stitches that need to heal. Don't even think about intercourse after a C-section until the doctor waves the checkered flag.

Birth Control

Be sure to stock up on birth-control products before the baby is born. Do not leave this important detail for after the birth, as you will have your hands full dealing with other things and are likely to let it slip. It is not fair to you or the new baby to have a repeat pregnancy sooner than you want. Also, don't for a moment believe that moms who are nursing are unable to get pregnant. Nursing moms get pregnant all the time. Ditto for couples who have unprotected sex during mom's period.

Lubricated condoms and condoms with contraceptive chemicals can irritate tender vaginal tissues, but your own saliva should be fine. If dryness or irritation are problems, check with your obstetrician's office for advice.

Designated Night Out

Once the baby is three months old, you might be wise to plan at least one evening a week where you and your spouse go out together, without junior in tow, for at least a couple of hours. There are a couple of ways to engineer this, with willing grandparents being top on the list. Every Wednesday night they get the baby and you get each other. If grandparents aren't an option and a baby-sitter is either too hard to find or too expensive, call couples from your Lamaze class or find other parents with young babies and arrange to co-op the baby-sitting. For instance, they take yours every Tuesday, and you take theirs every Thursday.

Children know when something important is missing in their parents' relationship. If there is a lack of intimacy or unity among their parents, they can suffer almost as much as the parents. Do not make the mistake of focusing all your energy on being parents and no energy on being lovers. By the time you notice that something is wrong with your relationship, it may be difficult to repair.

Painful Intercourse?

You may need to work your way up to intercourse. If time permits, you might try taking showers or baths together and sharing a beer or glass of wine beforehand. It never hurts to have an extra tube of lube on the night stand. Some women who have never had a problem getting wet need an assist after giving birth. For other women, it can be just the opposite.

Beware the "Husband's Stitch"

Physicians sometimes do a "husband's stitch" when sewing a woman up after delivery if she had tearing or an episiotomy. This is essentially a little tuck that's done at the opening of the vagina. The physician assumes it will make intercourse feel better for the husband. While the sentiment is nice, the "husband's stitch" is better used in upholstery shops than on women's genitals. Tightening the entrance to the vagina just makes the opening smaller and is liable to make intercourse feel painful for the woman. If a woman is concerned about vaginal tone following pregnancy, she would do much better to practice Kegel exercises, which help to tighten the entire vagina rather than making the opening more difficult to get into. It never hurts to discuss this with your healthcare provider.

Readers' Comments

"I had no sexual desire at all." *female age 36*

"I wanted sex more, and felt more free." *female age 44*

"I was extremely horny during my pregnancy and I felt very sexy until the last month or two." *female age 26*

"I was constantly horny when I wasn't nauseous." *female age 35*

"I viewed her expanding body as just more to love, hold and caress."
male age 41

"Intercourse can hurt toward 39-40 weeks when the baby's head is lower. Sometimes foreplay was just as satisfying." *female age 25*

"I was more horny than anything. Because of the pregnancy, we needed to start using new positions. Some worked so well that we are still using them today." *female age 25*

"We didn't do anything different, except we didn't have to use rubbers. Yea!" *female age 38*

"For intercourse, I was pretty much always on top." *female age 45*

"Don't worry about the baby. If it is firmly implanted, no orgasm will dislodge it." *female age 35*

"If anything, I admired her more for being able to 'do' a pregnancy. It's a real turn-on to feel an essential part of one." *male age 43*

"Sex felt extremely good and multiple orgasms happened all the time. They would sneak up on me. Things would be feeling good and if I concentrated hard I could have another and another." *female age 26*

"My wife seemed to be more lubricated, which was great. She seemed more relaxed also." *male age 38*

"Be gentle, be considerate, encourage her to lead. As for sex after the baby's born, that depends on whether she's in a private room or not."
male age 40

Sex after the kids are born?

"Sex after the kids are born? Baby-sitters, movies for kids, grandmother's house and motel rooms...." *male age 44*

"Lock the door, turn the music up, and put on *The Lion King*." *male age 39*

"When you've got kids, bedtime is the most convenient time for sex, but it's not always the most exciting time for me. If I wake up early and am horny, I wake my husband up, which is something he loves, to have sex when he's just waking up." *female age 45*

"You have to make it clear they can't interrupt. Sometimes I'm just very up front with what we are doing and she knows not to come in." *fem 25*

A PREGNANT THANKS: to Rachel Pauls, MD, FACOG, Urogynecologist and Director, Center for Female Sexual Health at Good Sam in Cincinnati.

CHAPTER

62

The Pill and Your Sex Drive

" I have noticed a big decrease in my sex drive since I started taking the pill. I used to have the biggest libido and wanted to have sex at least once a day but now it just takes a lot more for me to be in the mood. I am not just randomly horny anymore and I used to be all the time. I have less sex on the pill." *female age 20*

"After a not-so-great experience with the first brand I tried, I have switched to a low-dose birth-control pill. I like it. I have no side effects at all. My sex drive is most certainly back, which is great!"

female age 19

"I used the pill and saw no effect on my sex drive whatsoever. However, my twin sister took the pill and saw a marked decrease in her sex drive. It just goes to show that everyone reacts differently— even identical twins." *female age 21*

Very little research has been done on the impact that birth control pills have on a woman's sex drive and mood. Modern medicine seems content to give women hormones without concern. After all, the perception is that women are pretty hormonal to begin with–what's the big deal with topping off the tank?

This chapter looks at what we do and don't know about birth control pills and your sex drive. It also includes a list of questions you might ask yourself before using hormonal birth control. That way, you can have something to refer back to after you've been on the pill for a couple of months.

Fortunately, there are many different formulas of birth-control pills, and having specific questions to ask yourself might come in handy when evaluating which formula works best for you. Trying another formula or type of hormonal birth control might be a better option than quitting altogether.

NOTE: It used to be that the only hormonal method of birth control was the pill. But different delivery systems have emerged, including the Nuva-Ring, the Minera IUD, the patch and the Depo shot. For simplicity's sake, this chapter will refer to all of these as "the pill," unless otherwise specified.

Less Than 5% or More Than 25%?

> "We used to use condoms until six months ago when I started taking the pill. I love the pill! I have noticed no change in my desire for sex since starting it. I was incredibly horny before the pill, and am still incredibly horny now!" *female age 19*

> "I used to take the pill but stopped because it gave me horrible side effects (no sex drive even though I was a newlywed, depression, paranoia, panic attacks, weight gain, and heart burn). I took it for five months before going off of it. Now that I'm off hormones my sex drive is a whole lot better." *female age 21*

A recent study suggests that sexual side effects occur in approximately 25% of the women who try the pill. Still, healthcare providers are often quoted as saying that less than 5% of women stop taking the pill due to sexual side effects. Why the fivefold disparity?

Until recently, the few studies that did inquire about sexual side effects tended to be studies of women who had been taking the pill for five years or more. But we now know that women who experience a drop in sexual desire often stop taking the pill within the first year. So most women who did experience sexual side effects would not be represented in a study of women who had been taking it for five years.

Other problems in getting consistent results have to do with the kind of questionnaires that are used (do they actually measure what the study says it is measuring?), how the data is collected, the length of the study period, if it is double blind and has controls, and how testosterone and other androgens are measured.

It's easy to manipulate just a few of these variables to get the results you are looking for which is why it's also important to know who is funding a particular study.

Are Women Too Suggestible to Deserve Adequate Warnings?

> "This is the third brand I have been on. The first was a three-month kind, which left me spotting for weeks, made me frustrated and took away my sex drive. The second made me very depressed with a sex drive that rose and fell like crazy. This third one has leveled out my emotions and might be making my sex drive a little stronger than before." *female age 20*

"My doctor never told me that I could have any of those side effects. Sure, I was expecting weight gain and such, but not depression and NO sex drive." *female age 21*

As long as healthcare providers are convinced that less than 5% of women who take the pill have undesired sexual side effects, they don't necessarily give warnings about possible sexual side effects. And some healthcare providers feel that to give a warning would plant the idea in a woman's mind. The trouble is, any warning can become a self-fulfilling prophecy. So why warn any patient about anything?

If women know from the start that there can be problems, but that there are as many different types of pills as there are lipstick and nail-polish colors, they might be more willing to make adjustments. With the help of an astute healthcare provider, a woman might find another pill, or a different delivery system such as the NuvaRing, that could work really well for her.

So What's Going On?

"No change whatsoever... Still horny as a dog." *female age 21*

"The pill has totally suppressed my sex drive. I have hardly any desire." *female age 22*

"I definitely enjoy sex way more knowing that I won't get pregnant if the condom breaks or slips off." *female age 24*

One of the big crazes in drug research has been to find a pill for women who have low sexual desire, as if low sexual desire is usually a medical problem. Researchers had hoped that the answer would be Viagra, but it didn't work. It seems that women's sexual interest isn't suddenly switched on by a pill that creates the girl-version of a boner.

Since Viagra was a bust, researchers started focusing on testosterone. While testosterone tends to be associated with male arousal, having a small amount of it pulsing in a woman's veins is often necessary before she will look at a guy and think sexy things.

The reason for discussing this is because birth-control pills lower the amount of testosterone in most women. In other words, if there were a direct connection between lowered testosterone and sex drive, the pill might be a train wreck for a lot of women.

To confuse matters totally, the sexual desire of some women has either gone up or remained constant even though the pill caused their testosterone level to go down substantially. Other women's sexual desire has hit the skids with only a small drop in testosterone. So at this time, it's simply not possible to look at the testosterone level of a woman and predict whether she's having sexual problems or not.

In trying to make sense of all of this, a theory has emerged that each woman has a threshold of testosterone that is necessary for her to experience her normal sex drive. This threshold can be different for different women, and it could be that a woman won't start to experience sexual problems until her testosterone falls below her threshold.

This might explain why one woman can handle a big drop in testosterone with no adverse effects, while another woman might want to curl up with a book instead of her lover after only a small drop in testosterone.

There is also an idea that some women's sexuality is more testosterone dependent–like the male sex drive might be–while other women's sexuality depends more on relationships. So the pill-related drop in testosterone might be more of a turn-off for women whose sexuality is testosterone-driven.

Another interesting finding about testosterone is that even when women report a drop in desire, they usually don't experience a decrease in sexual satisfaction when having sex with a partner. That's because testosterone only impacts the desire to have sex, but not the ability to enjoy sex once the physical part of it begins. They just don't want to have sex very often.

Expectations & Our Own Sex Survey

Another factor that might influence a woman's sexual desire while taking the pill might have to do with her expectations about sex. For instance, researchers found that women reported fewer concerns about the pill in a country where they didn't expect to enjoy sex as much as women in other countries. So it's not like they went into mourning when they started taking the pill and felt less horny.

However, in our online sex survey, the percent of women reporting sexual side effects from taking hormonal methods of birth control has been nearly 50%—except for those using the NuvaRing (see reader's comments at the end of this chapter). While there is nothing scientific about Internet surveys, we were surprised by the high number of sex-related complaints.

The women who take our sex survey tend to be in the 18- to 28-year age range, with most reporting that they enjoy sex and are sexually active.

Perhaps the women who go to www.GoofyFootPress.com expect more from sex than other women. Maybe they find the pill's sexual side effects to be less tolerable than women who aren't quite as amped about sex to begin with.

The Importance of Smell

If you are a woman, does the way your partner smells register in a sexual way? Do you cherish wearing a lover's shirt that has his scent all over it?

Research is showing that a woman's ability to smell a guy's pheromones, can be inversely impacted by the pill. If smell is an important turn-on for a woman and the pill is impacting her ability to sense her partner's smell, then this might contribute to her negative feelings about the pill.

On the other hand, if there were something about a man's pheromones that didn't make her toes curl, it could be that a pill-related decrease in her sniffer's pheromone detector might make sex with him feel better.

Pill Related Benefits

So far, this discussion has explained why taking the pill might lower your sex drive, but it doesn't explain why it might help increase it.

For starters, what about not having to worry about an unwanted pregnancy? It could also be that certain pills help even out premenstrual mood issues for some women, and can help decrease bleeding and cramping. This might explain why some women prefer pills that pack a higher dose of hormones: because they might result in a greater decrease in bleeding, cramping, and premenstrual mood fluctuation.

The zit relief might be enough for some women to help them feel more sexually attractive. And it could also be that certain types of progesterone in some pills can actually create an increase in sexual desire.

The low-estrogen NuvaRing is reported to help some women get wetter, which many find to be an excellent side effect.

A Pre-Pill Inventory

"My sex drive is up, but I'm a little moody." *female age 19*

"On the pill, it's harder to maintain your weight and tone even when you are eating right and exercising regularly. It fluctuates your hormones which fluctuates your water weight and feeling of attractiveness which can affect your desire for sex." *female age 22*

"I'm on the combined pill. My sex drive has dipped a bit, but that may be because we have been together for six months and the initial lust-driven 'we must have sex every night' has died down a little. Of course, staying at his parents house for two months didn't help." *female 21*

You might ask yourself some of these questions before taking the pill. This kind of record can be especially helpful in six months or so, in case you're thinking something has changed but can't quite put a finger on what.

 About how many times a month are you masturbating? Masturbation reflects sexual interest that is generated from within your body and mind so it might be helpful to see if the pill has an impact on that.

 Life events can have a big impact on how you feel about sex. So jot down a few things about how your life is going besides love and sex. How are things at school, at work, with your friends and roommates? How do you feel about yourself? Do you like yourself?

 Take a screenshot of your Facebook, Myspace or Whatever.com pages. This might help you recall your mood before you started taking the pill.

 For a lot of women, the state of your relationship could be the biggest single factor in determining how much you want to jump a guy's bone. So if you are hitched, take a pre-pill inventory of your relationship, including what's going right, and what's not.

 If you have a partner, are you aware of his scent? Is it a turn-on, neutral, or a turn-off?

 If you've been having sex, write down how many times a month and how satisfying it is or isn't.

 Are there times of the month when you feel especially horny? See if it changes after you start taking the pill.

Keep in mind that it's perfectly normal for couples to feel less horny over time, which has nothing to do with the pill.

Different Formulas for Different Feelings?

There are many different pill formulations. There are triphasic pills, diphasic, and monophasic pills. This refers to whether they have progesterone and estrogen, or just progesterone. There are also different kinds of estrogen and different kinds of progesterone, Some researchers feel that certain kinds of progesterone might make some women more horny rather than less.

Just because the first one might not be the answer to your birth-control prayers, there are plenty of others to try.

More Reader Comments

"No hormonal birth control for me, not after a test run." *female age 21*

"I was on the shot, the ring and the pill. The shot made me bleed for 6 months straight, the ring gave me headaches so bad that I threw up, and the pill made me cry all the time. I noticed a decrease in sexual desire. My next adventure in birth control will be the diaphragm." *female age 26*

"These days I am so horny, that I don't think it's affected me!" *female age 33*

"I think my sex drive is lower. But it is something that happens gradually, so it is hard to be sure. It definitely makes my discharge thicker, which sometimes makes it a little harder to have sex. I am not as wet and we have to use lube sometimes. I used to be on Ortho Tri-Cyclin Lo, and that had a huge effect on my sex drive. I was extremely depressed and did not want sex at all." *fem. 26*

"I was on Mirena for 3 years, and I sunk into a period of low sexual drive. Also, in my 3rd year, it made me have my period every week for 3 weeks at a time. Now that I am on Ortho Tri-Cyclin Lo, I have increased sexual energy, and less problems." *female age 28*

"We noticed less physical arousal after she went on the pill." *male age 19*

"I used to be on the pill. I feel like I have tried them all and I hate the pill. Makes me a total bitch." *female age 25*

"I used the pill in college—went through three different brands and had so many side effects. I had very little desire for sex for the most part when I was on the pill. Now I just use condoms and feel like my horny self again. *fem.25*

"When I was on the pill, both combined and pop, I found that my desire definitely waned." *female age 40*

"The pill has totally suppressed my sex drive. I have hardly any desire." *fem. 22*

*Readers who use the NuvaRing have reported fewer side effects
and a more positive experience than readers who take the pill.*

"I use the NuvaRing. I think my sex drive has increased, but I am not sure if it is because of the birth control or if it is environment and situations." *fem. 20*

"I used to be on the Depo shot. And that would cause a great decline in my sex drive. I'm on the NuvaRing now and it seems a lot better. It's not as good when I'm not on anything but it's better." *female age 24*

"I use the NuvaRing, and I love it. I haven't noticed a change in sex drive, but I have noticed that I seem to be constantly wet. I suspect that it's a side effect of the Ring, but I'm not completely sure." *female age 19*

"I use the NuvaRing. I absolutely love it! I no longer forget to take pills, it is more reliable, and my partner doesn't feel it. I'm pretty paranoid, so I still use condoms, but if we're in the shower or something, I feel pretty safe having condom-less sex. It's a pretty new sensation for me!" *female age 21*

"I'm not currently on hormonal birth control, but when I was I used the Nuva-Ring. I found it to be very comfortable and easy to use. The only downside was a slight nausea the first day or two of a new ring." *female age 23*

"I use condoms now, sometimes the Today Sponge. In my last long-term relationship I used the NuvaRing. I had no change in desire while I was on. The only side effect I noticed were the awesome ones: less acne and shorter, lighter periods. The NuvaRing is the BEST BIRTH CONTROL EVER. As soon as I am in a stable relationship again I am getting it so fast." *female age 24*

"I used the NuvaRing for three months and then discontinued. Now I use condoms. I'd rather play the game without altering my body chemistry." *fem. 25*

NOTE: While not a direct cause of lower sex drive, "there is strong evidence that oral contraceptive pill use strongly increases the risk of developing vestibulodynia" [Journal of Sexual Medicine 2008;5:5-15]. Vestibulodynia is chronic pain in the crotch.

Thanks to Cynthia Graham and John Bancroft for their fine research on this subject.

63
Birth Control
Sperm v. Egg

Sharing the responsibility for birth control often increases the sexual trust and enjoyment in a relationship. It's the sort of thing that people do when they care about each other, rather than just making it the responsibility of the woman or ignoring the need altogether. Making birth control a mutual project could be the ante for having better sex.

This chapter looks at several ways of keeping a guy's wad from sliming a girl's egg. Keep in mind that one of the factors in choosing a birth-control method is whether or not you are at risk for getting a sexually transmitted infection. Also, please contact your healthcare provider or local Planned Parenthood office for complete information about birth control. Your best bet is to speak with someone who works with birth control day in and day out, and who can use his or her practical wisdom to help you select a long-term option that will work best for you.

Self-Esteem and Birth Control

Researcher Meg Gerrard spoke to college students about sex and birth control. Later, she gave follow-up tests over what she had presented. She found that students who felt less comfortable about their own sexuality remembered significantly less about birth control, even if they were "A" students in other subjects. Students who scored the highest on measures of sexual self-esteem were able to remember the most about birth control.

These findings were just as true for men as for women. Gerrard found that while being uncomfortable about sex is not enough to keep a person from having sex, it is enough to keep him or her from using birth control.

One way that people who are ambivalent about sex get around their conflicts about sex is by having sex that isn't planned or discussed ahead of time. That way, they can plead temporary insanity if they have to deal with a harsh conscience, or a real-life mom and dad if they are still living at home.

How Many Pregnancies Are Unplanned?

In the United States, 50% of pregnancies in women under the age of 34 are neither planned nor intended. The number rises to 75% for women over 40. More than 80% of pregnant teens had no desire to be that way. Also, people who use abstinence but get swept away in the moment are often without even a condom. They can easily become as pregnant as anyone else.

Sexually active people often fall into one of two extremes: those who have intercourse often and those who don't. Believe it or not, the once-in-a-blue-moon group are at high risk for unwanted pregnancies. There are several reasons for this which could fill an entire book. Please take it on faith that if you have intercourse sporadically rather than regularly, you are in a high risk group for getting pregnant.

When it comes to choosing a birth-control method, please check with your physician or family planning center. This book's information may be out of date by the time you read it.

The Pill

There are more than fifty different kinds of birth-control pills. Most are a combination of estrogen and progesterone, although the original birth-control pill was made of progesterone only. Progesterone-only pills are called POPs or mini-pills.

With the birth-control pill, a woman takes an active pill with hormones in it each day for 21 straight days. Then, for the last 7 days, she takes sugar or placebo pills to allow her to have a period. This creates a 28-day cycle.

Women over 35 who smoke or who have certain health risks should not take birth-control pills that contain estrogen. If they want a hormonal method of birth control, they will need one that is progesterone only, such as the Depo-Provera shot.

If you are concerned about the impact of the pill on your sex drive, please see Chapter 62: "The Pill & Your Sex Drive."

Forget to Take a Pill?

If you forget to take your birth-control pill, check with a pharmacist. Also, keep your pill pack info. It will tell you how to make up for a missed pill. Depending on the timing and the circumstances, it is possible that some form of emergency contraception might be helpful. Emergency contraception is discussed at the end of this chapter.

The NuvaRing

The NuvaRing is a hormonal method of birth control that has been available in the US for the past couple of years. Simply put, it is a 2" diameter plastic ring with hormones in it. You put it in your vagina on day 1 of your menstrual cycle and take it out on day 21. It eliminates the need to take a pill every day or to wear a patch. If you are looking for a hormonal method of birth control, you will be hard-pressed to find one that is more user-friendly.

Because the hormones absorb directly into the blood stream, the dosage of hormones you receive from the NuvaRing is lower than what is in most birth-control pills. The NuvaRing is one of the few hormonal methods of birth control associated with greater vaginal lubrication rather than less. Also, some women report leaving the NuvaRing in all for weeks for period suppression, but please speak to your healthcare provider before trying this.

The NuvaRing sits in the same place as a diaphragm, only you don't have to worry if it's exactly in place because it wasn't designed to be a barrier. If it moves around, that's fine. One size fits all. You might be wondering how the NuvaRing stays put in the back of your vagina. The muscles in your vagina will hold it in place, and most women can't feel it. If for some reason your partner can feel it, you can take it out for up to three hours at a time. If he can't finish doing his business in three hours, send him to the bathroom with a jar of hand cream and a dirty magazine, and pop your NuvaRing back in.

"Ring Tossing" is when your NuvaRing comes out during sex or when you are having a bowel movement.

Birth Control Patch, a.k.a. OrthoEvra

Approved in late 2001, this is another hormone-based contraceptive that eliminates having to take birth-control pills. The patch, sold under the brand name OrthoEvra, is a small 2" square that is applied to the skin. It can be placed on the hips, butt, abdomen, upper arm, or shoulder blade, but not on the breasts or extremities. The patch contains a dose of hormones similar to birth control pills. However, instead of having to swallow them in pill form, the hormones are absorbed through your skin. Once the patch is on, you leave it on for seven days. When the week is up, you take it off and put a new one on. After three consecutive weeks with a new patch, you go patch-free for a week to have a period. They still don't make a "patch grande" for the larger loving lady. So if you weigh in at over 198 pounds, the patch is not for you.

Some studies have shown that the patch does not increase a woman's risk over the pill, others have shown a 2 to 3 fold increase in risk. If you have concerns about the safety of the patch, be sure to discuss them with your healthcare provider.

Depo-Provera —Three Months at a Shot

Depo-Provera is a progesterone-only pill-in-a-shot that lasts for twelve weeks. Women seem to either love it or hate it. But if you end up hating it, you are stuck with it for an entire three months, since there's no way of getting it out of your body once it's inside. A smarter way to approach taking Depo is to first take a progesterone-only pill for two or three cycles. If that works well, then you might try the shot.

One of the main side effects of Depo is irregular bleeding. Some women bleed a lot and some don't bleed at all. Some women find that Depo stops their periods altogether for three months. There has also been concern about bone density loss, so women who are on Depo need to take additional calcium.

There's Nothing New about Seasonale

The idea of stopping menstrual periods for three months at a time is nothing new, although there is a lot of debate about this. Women have been doing it for years by taking certain monophasic birth-control pills for eighty-four straight days. This is often prescribed for women who have serious difficulties with their periods. ("Monophasic" means the dose in each pill is the same.)

With Seasonale, you get 84 monophasic birth-control pills. You take one each day. Then you take seven placebo pills at the end so you can have a period. This makes it a 91-day cycle. There is also a low-dose version of Seasonale called Seasonique, and a new continuous use pill called Lybrel is in the final stages of testing.

If you have trouble remembering to take pills, do not try to eliminate your periods in this way. If you've forgotten to take a couple of pills early on, you might have to wait nearly three months to find out if you are pregnant.

NOTE: If you are using the NuvaRing and want to suppress your periods, you might talk to your healthcare provider about leaving it in all four weeks

IUDs—The Most Reliable & Cost-Effective Birth Control?

IUD stands for "intrauterine device." It is a small T-shaped device that is placed in the uterus to prevent pregnancy. There are two forms of IUD, one that has hormones (the Mirena) and one that doesn't (the ParaGard).

IUDs can be an excellent long-term birth control choice for women, especially those who have been pregnant before. The only part of an IUD that can be felt is two little nylon strings that hang down from it. The strings are there so a woman can reach up and feel them after each period to make sure the IUD didn't slip out. If a man is able to feel the little strings during intercourse, ask your healthcare provider to snip them shorter.

In a recent study of different types of birth control, the IUD was considered to be the most cost-effective and reliable method over a five-year period. However, the initial cost is higher than with other methods such as birth-control pills. While many insurance companies will cover the cost of sterilization, they won't cover the cost of IUDs. Perhaps this is why IUDs are much more popular in Europe than in the United States.

Diaphragm This

The diaphragm is a shallow latex or silicone cup that you put spermicide into and then place over your cervix before you have intercourse. Diaphragms used to be as common as sex itself, but now not many women use them. They require the goop-and-insert routine each and every time. However, the diaphragm has no hormonal side effects. And think of the fine-motor skills you will learn in getting it in and out!

The diaphragm might also be good for a woman who doesn't need to use birth control often, for example, someone who has a long-distance partner where most of the sex is on the phone or by text message. For those of you with latex allergies, they are finally making non-latex diaphragms out of silicone, which is the same material that finer dildos are made from.

Fitting a diaphragm takes a lot more of a healthcare provider's time and effort than prescribing pills for you, so some might hesitate for this reason. Plus, fitting one can be as much art as science. Diaphragms can also cause a feeling of pressure on the bladder. You have to leave it in for eight hours after your last intercourse. If your man is the kind who does a rapid reload and fire, you'll need to squirt in extra spermicide, but you don't need to take the diaphragm out. You need to get a new diaphragm every year or two, which should be accompanied by a refitting.

Cervical Cap

The cervical cap is like a mini version of the diaphragm that fits on your cervix. For some women it feels better than the diaphragm, others don't like the feeling of the cap on the cervix. The only cap currently sold in the US is called the FemCap, and it comes in three sizes which your doctor needs to fit. Instead of putting spermicide on the inside of it, you put it on the outside. After intercourse, you'll need to leave it in place for 8 hours. Effectiveness is an issue, especially if you've already had a baby. Also, not many healthcare professionals know how to fit a cervical cap.

Reality & "Femidon"—Horror Flick Monster from Japan?

Reality is a polyurethane pouch that's inserted into the vagina. It forms a thin, protective barrier between the penis and the walls of the vagina. It is often referred to as "the female condom," and in the UK it is called Femidon. (Femidon–what a hideous name for something they want you to stick into your most private space, not that Reality makes you wet with anticipation.) In spite of early hopes, Reality hasn't made much of a splash. However, it does have some advantages.

Reality is made from polyurethane instead of latex, so it transmits warmth well. Because it sits in the vagina, the man doesn't have to pull out as soon as he comes. It helps women to feel that they have more control in protecting themselves, and some women report that the ring around the outside of the condom stimulates the clitoris during intercourse.

Unfortunately, Reality's birth control properties might be less than optimal and it isn't cheap. It is kind of big and strange, but if you're the type who has already been abducted by aliens and had your genitals probed with interplanetary sex tools, this should be no big deal.

Reality is also being used by some straight and gay couples for anal intercourse, although it's doubtful that the instructions include this small detail.

Spermicides —Sponges, Films, Foams, Suppositories & Jellies

Spermicides are chemicals that are used to kill sperm and hopefully reduce the risk of pregnancy. They come in various forms to be placed inside the vagina before intercourse, including films, foams, sponges, suppositories, and jellies. Most are made with the chemical nonoxynol-9 (N-9). When used by themselves, spermicides can be less effective than other birth control methods, including condoms. If you are using spermicides for protection against pregnancy, it is best to use them along with condoms.

Spermicides can be bought over-the-counter, and they might be a good alternative for women who can't use hormonal methods. However, they can be messy and they taste really nasty. They can also cause irritation in either partner, which increased the chance of getting STIs. Spermicidally-lubricated condoms can cause irritation, as well. They are no more effective for birth control, and provide no benefit over a regular condom.

Natural Family Planning & Fertility Awareness
May the Cervix Be with You

A woman is only fertile for a third or less of every menstrual cycle. Natural methods of birth control are based on trying to accurately calculate when a woman's fertile time is. The couple either uses a condom or diaphragm when she is fertile, or they abstain from intercourse. They can have intercourse without protection the rest of the time.

Until recently, calculating a woman's fertile time has been more of an art than a science. It was called the rhythm or calendar method and it was not particularly effective. But now, natural methods can be as effective as pills or condoms when they are used properly.

Natural methods rely on learning to recognize a woman's physical signs of fertility, and then using these to determine the safest and riskiest times for pregnancy. Women learn to note subtle changes in their bodies, like their waking body temperature, the consistency of their cervical fluid, and the feel of their cervix. These symptoms are put into charts or computer programs that predict whether pregnancy is risky for that day or not.

There are now two styles of natural methods: natural family planning (NFP) and fertility-awareness methods (FAM). NFP is for those with religious concerns. The couple abstains from intercourse during a woman's fertile times. It is very popular worldwide because it is the only birth-control method approved by the Pope, not that he's tried it himself. FAM is the option for people who are fine with using barrier methods of birth control. Instead of abstaining from sex during the risky times, FAM users turn to a back-up method, such as condoms or a diaphragm.

Natural methods can be great because there are little to no costs and no hormonal or medical side effects. In addition to being popular among those with religious concerns, NFP and FAM have also become popular because they utilize a woman's natural cycles. On the flip side, natural planning methods require a couple to change their behavior, which can be difficult for impulsive types. It takes some learning, dedication, and usually a committed and understanding partner to make these methods work.

Highly Recommended: Natural methods are not effective without planning and research. For an excellent, unbiased source on the subject, check out the highly regarded book, *Taking Charge of Your Fertility*, 10th Anniversary Ed. by Toni Weschler, Collins (2006).

Tubal Ligation for Women, Vasectomy for Men

Tubal ligation and vasectomy are permanent forms of birth control. They are highly popular and have a failure rate of 1% or less. Both are done on an out-patient basis. Neither procedure will cause a change in your level of horniness, and many people report they enjoy sex more once they don't have to worry about pregnancy. They are the best form of birth control if you are not interested in having any children or more children.

In tubal ligation, a thin tube-like instrument is passed through a small incision that is slightly below a woman's belly button. The surgeon seals the fallopian tubes with clips, rings, or with electrical current. In order to see the fallopian tubes, a harmless gas is put into the abdomen. The gas is let out once the tubes have been sealed and the eggs from the ovaries can no longer reach the womb. The total procedure takes about 15 to 20 minutes. Tubal ligation does not stop a woman's periods. But it does stop her fears about becoming pregnant again.

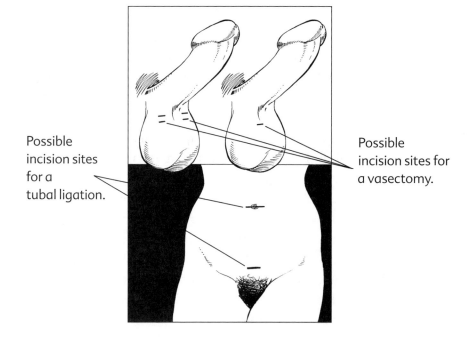

Possible incision sites for a tubal ligation.

Possible incision sites for a vasectomy.

With a vasectomy, a small incision is made in the scrotum. The physician reaches the vas deferens, or sperm-carrying tubes, through the incision with a thin instrument. The tubes are then sealed, so that sperm does not mix with your ejaculate. The procedure should take less than 20 minutes. Since sperm makes up less than 1% of each wad, your ejaculations will have the same volume as before. Neither you nor your partner will notice anything is missing, except for the contraceptives and concerns about pregnancy.

Getting Condoms

Nowadays, rubbers or condoms can be purchased nearly everywhere except for maybe your local post office or Christian Science Reading Room. But you still need to hand them to a cashier before they are yours to wear, unless you get them from a vending machine or receive them by mail.

Hopefully, you will feel good about handing a box of condoms to the cashier. He or she might even feel envious. But for some people, the ability to purchase a condom depends upon who's working the cash register. This is especially true in small towns where there is no such thing as retail anonymity. In some small towns, a person would attract less attention knocking off the local bank than buying a pack of rubbers.

Getting condoms by mail order helps alleviate this problem, but in some households plain unmarked envelopes garner as much attention as a singing telegram. Fortunately, most of you live in cities, and buying condoms shouldn't be a problem for even the shyest of consumers.

Rubber Scoop

After much painstaking research, we have come to the conclusion that what you slop on the outside of a condom is almost as important as what you stuff into it. To help put the slip back in your slide, slop some spit or water-based lubricant on the outside of your condom before you have intercourse. This will help intercourse with a bagged penis feel sweeter.

The extra lubrication also helps to make up for the loss of precum or natural lubrication that normally drips out of the penis. The condom catches the precum, like everything else.

And as long as you've got the lube handy, it never hurts to put a dab on the head of your penis before bagging it. Along with your precum, this will help the head of your penis get an extra ride with each stroke, as it slides against the condom material.

Chronic Condom Busters

Contrary to what you might think, chronic rubber busters aren't usually hung any better than the average guy. The bigger problem is when they don't use condoms correctly.

Using lotions like Nivea, Johnson's Baby Oil, Vaseline Intensive Care, Corn Huskers, or Jergens to lubricate the outside of a condom will instantly rot the latex. Just because hand creams wash off easily doesn't mean they are water-based. The safest lubricants are saliva or water-based lubes like KY, Astroglide or Wet. For more on lubes, see Chapter 11: "Sex Lubes—A New Look."

It seems that a large percentage of college students don't use condoms correctly. The problems included: not pinching air out of the tip before putting the condom on, putting the condom on after they've already started having intercourse and not rolling them all the way down.

A condom won't work for you unless you use it correctly. It also helps to get an extra big condom if your penis is extra big, or a snug one if your penis doesn't cast the widest shadow in town.

If a Condom Doesn't Come Out When You Do

For a condom that doesn't come out with the penis it rode in on, take solace in knowing there's no place for it to go. The condom might play a mean game of hide'n'seek behind the woman's cervix, but that's about it.

The first step in finding an unmoored condom is to wash your hands and make sure your nails are well-trimmed. The woman might try lying on her back with her knees up, like when she's at the gyno's. This is no time for modesty: the farther apart her legs, the better. Explore her vagina with your index finger. If lube is necessary, use just a little. Extra lube might make it difficult to grab the condom. If you don't have lube, try spit.

If female sexual anatomy is one of life's great mysteries for you, see the illustrations in chapter 7. You can see how the cervix is at the far end of the vagina on the roof side. It might feel like the tip of a nose. Try exploring the space in the back of the cervix with your finger. If the condom is there, try to dislodge it and edge it into a more accessible part of her vagina, like where your penis was when it jettisoned the thing.

Once you have a good handle on the condom, you might try inserting two fingers in the hopes of snagging it between them. Condoms are stretchy, so pull it out slowly but firmly. If your partner clamps down when you are

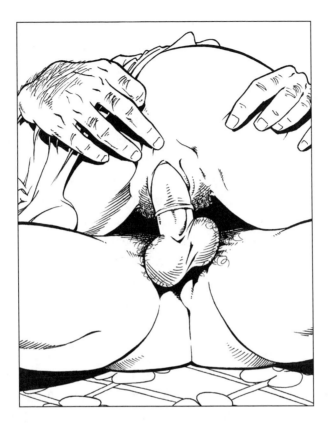

trying to insert two fingers, go slowly and gently. It's not like her vagina is going to suddenly implode if you take an extra ten minutes searching for the buried Trojan treasure.

If you have any questions or concerns, call your healthcare provider or visit an emergency room. If you were using the condom for birth control, the operative words are "Plan B" or "Emergency Contraception." *For condoms that get lost during anal sex, see "lost condom—anal sex" in the index.*

If a Condom Breaks

Nasty, nasty, nasty. If you were using a condom for birth control and discover that it broke while in service, immediately take Plan B (see "emergency contraception"). Plan B is a morning-after pill that is very effective in preventing pregnancy. In the meantime, do not inject birth control foam or jelly into the vagina. The pressure might push the ejaculate up into the cervix. The same is true for douching. Instead, try inserting a contraceptive suppository if you've got one. Wash your external genitals and pee. And for heavens sake, if you honestly think that douching with Pepsi or Coke is going to do anything but prove that you're the world's biggest fool, nothing this book has to say is going to count for much.

Fear of Condoms

If you have deep feelings for your partner and fear that using a condom will ruin your spontaneity or somehow dampen the moment, please read the following to him or her:

"I love you way too much to risk putting our relationship through the strain of having to deal with an unwanted pregnancy. I also love you way too much to risk giving you something that I may have gotten from a toilet seat. (Leave out who you were on the toilet seat with.) So if we are both serious about being together, let's work on a timetable for ditching the condoms. To do this, we need to get tested for sexually transmitted infections, and we have to start using an effective method of birth control. Then we can work on dumping the condoms."

Extra Large Condoms

If you are really lucky and need a bigger size condom than the rest of us, there are several choices on the market. If the reasons you are buying the bigger rubbers is to impress your friends or a partner, the truth is going to come out once your pants are down. So why create an added expectation that you might not be able to fill? Plus, if you get the extra large size and don't need them, they are more likely to slip off during intercourse. However, at least 10% of men really do need the bigger rubbers:

"The one traumatic thing I dealt with my first partner in high school was using a condom. I'm on the larger side. The first time I tried to use a condom, it was so tight I could barely get it on and it felt like a tourniquet at the base of my penis. It was awful and I couldn't keep an erection with one on. Unfortunately, I'd read that the whole "the condom's too small" excuse is not valid because someone once squeezed 17 oranges into a condom so it's silly that a guy can't fit into one. So, of course, I was convinced that something was wrong with me. I kept trying, and once broke two condoms while trying to get them on! I didn't even know that they made large condoms at the time—all I knew was that if I tried to use any condom, sex

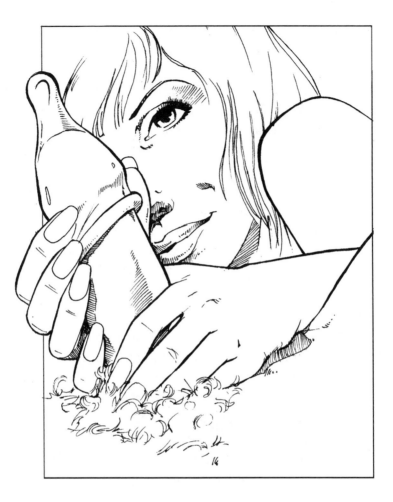

would end in disaster. All they needed to say was, 'Larger condoms
are available for those who need them' and my adolescence would
have been a lot less stressful." *male age 26*

Baggy Rubbers?

Some condom companies are now manufacturing rubbers that are extra-
baggy around the head. They fit snugly around the base of your penis, but the
top inch or two bags out like the pants that the gangbanger wannabes wear.
This lets the head of your penis slosh around inside the rubber, which, believe
it or not, can feel really nice. (Baggy-headed rubbers are different from those
with reservoir tips, which have a little finger-like tip at the end of the rubber that supposedly collects cum.) Baggy-headed brands include the Pleasure

Plus, the Trojan Ultra Pleasure, Lifestyle's Xtra Pleasure and the Inspiral. Each has its own sensation and it is fun to experiment with them.

The one place where rubbers need to fit snugly is around the base of the penis. Otherwise, they might slip off. The penis usually starts shrinking right after ejaculation, so a guy shouldn't keep thrusting after he comes. He also needs to clamp the edge of the rubber against his penis with his fingers when he is pulling out.

So what about all those situations when a man comes before his sweetheart? What about her sexual pleasure if he's supposed to pull out? Why not help her come before intercourse? That's why Father Nature invented vibrators, oral sex and finger fucking. Or once you begin having intercourse, one of you can reach down with your fingers or a vibrator to help her get more stimulation. Another way to increase the stimulation is for the woman to be in a position where she can push her clitoris against her partner's pubic bone.

Reservoir Tips?

Some rubber brands make a big deal about having reservoir tips to hold a guy's ejaculate. There are a couple of problems with this concept. The first is that most reservoir tips hold about 2.9 ml. of ejaculate. While half of all guys produce 2.9 ml. or less, there's still another 50% of guys who produce more than 2.9 ml., which means their tips runneth over.

The other problem with reservoir tips is the assumption that they really do hold the fluid. Reservoir tip or not, leave a half-inch or so of space at the end of the rubber. Be sure to squish the air out of it before rolling it down the shaft of your penis.

Throat Hygiene

With the apparent increase in oral sex, healthcare professionals are seeing more sexually transmitted infections in the back of people's throats. Plus, it is possible to give your partner certain STIs by doing oral sex on them.

To avoid something disgusting like a gonorrhea infection where your tonsils ought to be, consider bagging a penis before sucking on it. The only trouble is, condoms aren't known for their appetizing flavors. Worse yet, a lot of the condoms that call themselves flavored taste truly disgusting.

The flavoring on condoms isn't embedded into the latex, so it comes off quickly. And most condoms are pre-lubed, which means you get to enjoy the bitter taste of the pre-lube.

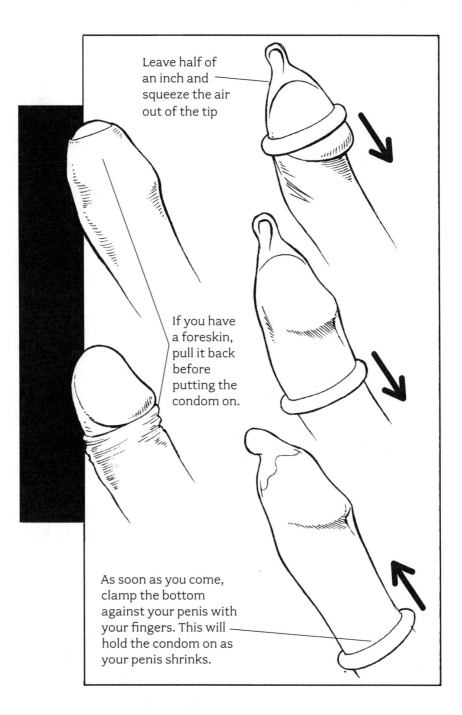

Leave half of an inch and squeeze the air out of the tip

If you have a foreskin, pull it back before putting the condom on.

As soon as you come, clamp the bottom against your penis with your fingers. This will hold the condom on as your penis shrinks.

For the Ride of Your Life!

One brand of flavored condoms that seem to taste OK are those made by Trustex. If you can, find nonlubricated rubbers for blowjobs. If the initial taste of latex bothers you, rinse your mouth out with something like mouthwash, cognac, or toothpaste first, but make sure it's not something that reacts with the latex.

If you don't mind the taste of pre-lube, give the condoms made of polyurethane a try. They transmit warmth better than latex condoms, and one of the really nice things about receiving a blowjob is the warmth.

Other Condom Tips & Trivia

💡If you've never used a condom before, try to get a couple for testing. Pay close attention when you tear open the package. Get a sense of what side of the condom goes over the head of your penis. Practice leaving a half inch at the top of your penis and squeezing the air out of it. Roll it all the way down. Put some water-based lube in your hand. Use your hand like a vagina, thrusting into it. Once you come, pay close attention to the diameter of your penis. Does it deflate? If you are like most guys, it will. This is why you need to clamp your fingers on the part of the condom that is around the base of your penis as soon as you come. Otherwise, you are likely to leave it inside of your partner when you pull out.

💡Some guys tie off the end of a spent rubber before throwing it in the trash. This is similar to tying the end of a balloon, but for slightly different purposes. It keeps the liquid from running out and getting all over the place.

💡Don't recycle your rubbers. Use a new one each time you have intercourse whether you come or not. Don't carry them around in a wallet. Don't put them in the glove compartment of a car. They don't like that kind of heat.

💡In case you bought a stash of condoms at the start of a really long dry spell, be sure to check the expiration date. Condoms can go bad.

💡Do experiment with different brands until you find one that you like best; however, don't use the ones with ribs or nubs if you are having anal sex. The next time you want to have extra fun with your friends, sacrifice a couple of latex rubbers by blowing them up really big. If you have helium, you can fly them to the moon.

Emergency Contraception and Morning-After Pills

Let's say the condom broke, or you were raped or pressured into having intercourse, or your level of passion suddenly overwhelmed your level of sanity and the condom never went on or the diaphragm never went in. Believe it or not, there is a simple, relatively safe way of decreasing your chance of becoming pregnant by 89% or more. It's been known about for 30 years and is called emergency contraception.

It is now called Plan B or "the morning-after pill" which is the right strength for emergency contraception. Even the American College of Obstetrics and Gynecology believes that Plan B should be next to your box of condoms and rolling papers—just in case.

Don't let the "term morning-after pill" fool you. It can work if you take it up to five days after having unprotected intercourse. You will need to take one pill within 120 hours after the sperm train has left the station, and a second pill 12 hours after that. The side effects are minimal and the hassle is almost nonexistent compared to a pregnancy or getting an abortion. It is only approved for over the counter if you are 18 or older. You need a prescription if you are younger. Not all pharmacies stock it, and some won't sell it to men.

Another option for emergency contraception is IUD insertion. It can be inserted as long as 5 to 8 days after unprotected intercourse and can reduce the risk of pregnancy following unprotected intercourse by 99%. It can also be left in place to provide effective contraception for years.

How to Get Emergency Contraception

Plan B emergency contraception is available over-the-counter in the United States. However, some drug stores won't carry it, or you need to ask for it. So if you don't see it, be sure to ask. If you can't find it, try (888)668-2528 or http://not-2-late.com.

A Very Special Thanks to Angela Hoffman, birth control and sex education expert, for help above and beyond the call of duty with this chapter. .

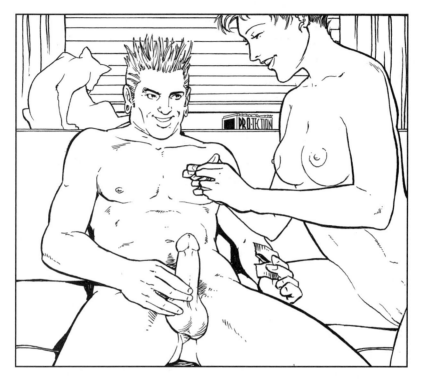

A New Choice in Non-Latex Condoms

The Lifestyles SKYN is a new non-latex condom. Until now, the options for non-latex condoms haven't been too great. The polyurethane Avanti Durex has been taken off the market, which left the Trojan Supra as the only latex alternative until the Skyn. So if you'd like to try a non-latex condom, stick your skin into one of the new SKYNs. They are supposed to feel a bit better than latex, but are NOT for use with oil-based lubes.

CHAPTER

64

Sex in Cyberspace
For Parents

Much of what parents hear regarding their kids and the Internet focuses on pornography and sexual predators. While these are certainly dangers, let's start with what we discovered about the Internet in the earlier chapters on cyberspace:

1. Pornography did not exist before people started using the Internet.

2. Adultery did not exist before people started to find lovers online.

And now, as is relevant to this chapter:

3. Children were never sexually abused before predators found them on the Internet.

4. Kids never saw pornography before they started going online.

This chapter provides specific advice about your kids and the Internet. For those of you who would like to deal with reality, the chances are good that your teenage daughter is at much greater risk of getting into serious trouble from the influence of the 21-year-old fry cook who she works with at her job at Taco Bell than she is from the Internet. And if your child is going to be molested, in 9-out-of-10 cases, it will be done by someone you personally know. You have more to fear from your in-laws, baby sitter, neighbors, or your latest romantic interest if you are dating. In far less than 1-in-100 cases will it happen through a predator on the Internet.

This doesn't mean that you shouldn't be vigilant about what your kids do on the Internet. It just means that if you are concerned about harm reduction, there may be bigger fish to fry in most kid's lives than they are facing online.

In this chapter, we look at what you can realistically do to help your kids negotiate the world of sex online. But blanket prohibitions aren't going to work any better with the Internet than abstinence-only sex education does for the average teenager. Even if you take your kids' computers away, they will get access at a friend's house. So unlike the "Just say no!" philosophy that many people recommend, *The Guide's* advice is, "Say yes some of the time, but don't be dumb about it."

This chapter will focus on two specific situations: 1. You just found that your 12-year-old son has been bookmarking some seriously raunchy porn; and 2. Your 12-year-old daughter's online identity is *sexysuzzie69*.

Junior Inherited His Dad's Appreciation for All Things Sexual

So, you've discovered that your little altar boy has bookmarked some seriously crude websites. Lord knows, the stuff is out there.

The first time the author of this book used a web browser he put the word "erotic" in the search engine. About a zillion sites popped up, so he selected the first site on the list. Moments later, a close-up photo of a smiling, attractive woman with her mouth wide open started to fill the screen. A stream of liquid was flowing into her mouth, and then a penis appeared. What emerged was a close-up of some guy peeing into the mouth of a young woman who could have been the girl next door. The second site on the list showed a close-up of a woman's pelvis with one penis sticking up her rear and another in her vagina. As an experiment, he entered "Beanie Babies" in the search engines. He got a number of sex sites from that.

This is different from what he had seen as a kid. Back then, he was lucky to see a tattered page from *Playboy*. While *Playboy* may not show the most accurate representation of what nature put on the average woman's chest, it is at least an approximation of what you'll get if you are going to have sex. He had no idea that someone would ever want to pee into another person's mouth until he moved to Los Angeles and started meeting people in the entertainment industry.

So the biggest concern isn't that your son is seeing pornography, but that much of the pornography he is seeing is so darned twisted. You wouldn't want anybody's son or daughter to see some of the porn that's out there today. But try as you might, there is no way to keep kids from seeing this stuff. Even if you have the most effective screening program in the world, your kid's friend down the street will have found a way to circumvent it, or they will get on his parents' computer when his mom and dad are at work (from 7 a.m. to 8 p.m.). If they can't access it on the Internet, there are plenty of DVDs floating around that show some of the same things.

And that's where you need to enter the picture. As a parent, you are not going to keep your kid from seeing seriously demented porn. So instead of just ignoring it, or pretending that you can prevent all of it, consider this an opportunity to be the emotional anchor your son needs to develop a healthy and caring sexual self.

One strategy is to let your kids know that it's perfectly normal to be curious about sex, and despite your best efforts, they might see things on the Internet that are weird and way out of the range of normal. If your kids know that you won't suddenly transform into a lunatic when the subject comes up, you might ask them about some of the weird things they've seen on the net. If they have seen sexual sites and are able to tell you about them, your response might vary from "That sounds really strange; you're not describing any sex acts I'd ever want to do" to "I know it's hard to believe, but maybe that's something you'll like to do when you get older."

Tell your kids that there's sometimes a big difference between looking at pictures of people having sex and what happens when two people actually have a good sexual relationship. Sex with a real-life partner is full of tender and caring moments. You rarely see any of this if you are watching sex on the Internet or on a DVD player.

Also, keep in mind that even regular intercourse or oral sex can be scary or disturbing for teenagers. They'll try to dismiss it by saying, "Oh Mom, I know all about that," but they can still be very anxious about it.

Your job is to help your son or daughter digest some of what they will be seeing in the next couple of years—from twisted porn to bizarre and disturbing video collections of people killing themselves or getting wasted in accidents. Through your attitude and willingness to be involved, you can help your son sort through the bizarre and twisted images that he will most likely be seeing.

If your children are spending countless hours on the web, it might be due to loneliness and isolation in addition to normal curiosity. On the other hand, there are whole communities of people on the Internet who can be better friends and a better influence than some of the kids he's probably meeting in school. If it seems like your son is spending hours on sex sites, try to get him involved in extracurricular activities where his time is structured and he is doing things that make him feel good about himself.

Masturbating to porn on the Internet is pretty normal. But if one-handed surfing is his main activity in life, let him know he will have plenty of time for that after he's 18 and living on his own. For now, your job as a parent is to decide what is and isn't good for him, and the hours-on-end stuff has to stop.

There is software that can help keep your kid from watching porn at home, but be aware that he will be seeing it elsewhere.

If he is really isolated and the computer is an emotional lifeline, you might try to get him involved in a computer class. Use it as a bridge.

One Young Man's Experience

The Guide's tech advisor said that when he was a young teen in the mid-90s, his family had the latest Internet set up because his mom was a university professor. Although he assured her he wasn't looking at porn, what else was a healthy young guy with a mouse and browser to do?

Like any of us, he found porn that was seriously twisted, and porn that wasn't. Yet when he started dating and needed to decide what parts of Internet porn were going to influence his relationship with women, it all boiled down to the values his mom had taught him when he was growing up. Porn had nothing to do with it.

His mom clearly got hoodwinked on the smaller issue of porn on the net, but she won the much larger battle, which was to instill in her son moral values that he has taken with him on his journey through life.

When Your 12-Year-Old Is SXYsuzzie69@hotmale.com

You just discovered your 12-year-old daughter is in chatrooms calling herself SXYsuzzie69@hotmale.com. She's never even spoken to you about sex. How do you protect her?"

Protect her? Hmmmm. Let's look at the territory where she might be hanging out. If you look up the term *MySpace Whore* in the glossary at the back of this book, you will find:

> MySpace Whore—A girl who spends way too much time on myspace.com, is obsessed about having hundreds of myspace "friends" and will change her pictures often in an attempt to get even more "'friends." She'll post all kinds of bulletins saying "NEW PICZZZ! OMG, they are sooo hoTTTT. PLZZZZ comment!!! (MySpace whores can be boys, too.)

Kind of a harsh awakening for parents who still think of their daughter as playing for hours on end with her Polly Pockets dolls. On the other hand, it's unlikely that their daughter is meeting a strange guy from Atlanta at the airport who she met online. (Forgive us for not buying into the latest and greatest national hysteria. Bad things happen via the Internet, but how often?)

Yes, there are things parents should be concerned about and steps they should take. We will list them. But today's parents shouldn't fear the technology that their kids are using any more than parents in the 1900 needed to fear how the new technology of the telephone might be ruining their daughters. If ruin is on the way, it's on the way, regardless of the technology.

First and foremost, there are worse things for today's parents to worry about than the Internet. Paul's wife works in the juvenile-justice system with teenagers, and she'll tell you about a problem that is a MILLION times more immediate for most kids. It's when teenage girls go to the beach, river, park, or to some unknown house with boys and drink alcohol. It's where one of the girls maybe knows the cousin of one of the boys. She sees case after case of this, and she says the number of young girls who are in trouble with alcohol has skyrocketed in the past seven years. We're talking girls with straight As from good homes who get into cars with guys who they've never met—online or anywhere else.

So if you are trying to get your harm-reduction priorities straight, drinking and smoking should be at the top of your list.

A big problem with the Internet is when girls with poor self-esteem hook up with local guys after being sweet-talked in a chat situation. This can be a problem for any girl who is desperate for attention. But this is where America's new chatroom hysteria takes us off course. Parents will focus on the Internet when the chances are just as good that bad things will happen with a guy at Starbucks or at a party. Especially bad is the influence of co-workers if she has a job.

If there is a problem, it's not the Internet that is causing it, any more than the girl's cell phone or Starbucks is causing the problem. Does the new technology of the Internet require adjustments? You bet, just as you can't hand a 16-year-old the car keys and say, "See ya' in a couple of days."

If your young daughter is calling herself "SXYsuzzie69," she may have emotional issues that need to be worked with, and that's where her parents need to start. If she has serious issues with self-esteem or judgement, you need to be just as concerned when she says she's spending the night at her friend's house or goes to a party as when she logs on to a computer.

As a general advisory, all parents should help their kids set up their profiles or online identities. If you don't know what that is, ask a teacher, friend or someone you trust to help your kid do it, and do it on all the different sites where she logs on. If you are concerned, you can go on these sites and review what she is saying about herself, although don't assume you will be able to find anything if she is using all kinds of aliases.

The profile or online identity is the information users give about themselves. It is info that anyone can harvest. Also talk with your kids about giving out any personal information, including their real name, address, phone number and credit-card information. This is not the time to become a liberal parent. Strongly emphasize the words "NEVER" and "Give out your phone number or address on the computer, and I'll make sure you don't get your driver's license until you are ninety!" Make sure your children understand that even though they might be alone in their bedroom, there isn't a person in the world who can't see what they are saying on a computer, including you.

If you think it would be helpful, make a contract with your child about what you will and won't tolerate in terms of Internet usage. Review the contract often. Even if your child isn't struggling, you need to be aware that the Internet can be just as good, or just as bad, as any other place where your child might go alone. Determine what your minimum standards are, set clear limits, and do what you can to enforce them. But don't blame the Internet for bad things that might happen in your child's life, anymore than you should blame the mall, Starbucks, or cell phones. These are all a part of the world we live in.

Talking to Your Kids about Sex

If parents don't take the time and effort to instill values in their kids when they are five, it won't suddenly happen because they have decided Junior needs them since he's a teen. And if you didn't start talking to your kid about sex when she was five, it isn't going to suddenly happen now when she's borrowing your tampons.

The next chapter is all about that—talking to your kids about sex.

Note Even the most knee-jerk of Internet alarmists admit that the Internet can be a lifesaver for the isolated gay teen who is growing up in a rural community, and for kids who grow up with no sex education. At least on the Internet they can see that their questions aren't strange. And if they are looking at porn, it's in the safety of their own bedroom.

CHAPTER

65
Explaining Sex to Kids

Let's say that little Billy has gone shopping with his dad for the afternoon and you steal half an hour to lie on your bed with stereo headphones bolted to your ears, eyes closed and fingers massaging a very important place between your legs. You are all alone and the sensations begin to feel wonderful. Next thing you know, the headphones are being yanked off your head by little Billy, who is asking, "Mommy, what color napkins were we supposed to get for the birthday party?"

Or perhaps you assume that little Amber is fast asleep and you begin enjoying an all-too-rare moment of sex when a little hand suddenly taps you on the shoulder and you hear the words, "Daddy, how come Mommy's sucking on your penis?"

The pages that follow don't pretend to have all the answers about children and sex; they are simply a way of getting you to think about the subject before most parents do, which is sometimes too late for an effective response. Topics range from talking about genitals and masturbation to menstruation, sex play and even sex on the internet.

Children's Sexual Development

People often think of sex as something that happens once we become teenagers. Not true. Most of us started having sexual feelings when we were little babies. Each time someone changed our diapers and powdered our private parts we had sexual feelings in the most basic sense—nice physical sensations down where the Pampers go.

As children get a few years older, they often enjoy playing sex games with friends and relatives, same sex or otherwise. Sometimes they just compare and contrast; other times they enjoy doing things that big people do, like sucking on each other's genitals. Occasionally they might explore by sticking fingers, penises and heaven knows what else up each other's front and rear ends. Eventually you might encounter a third-grade child who's sitting there with both hands in his or her pants, happily rubbing away, while claiming how yucky it would be to ever kiss on the lips.

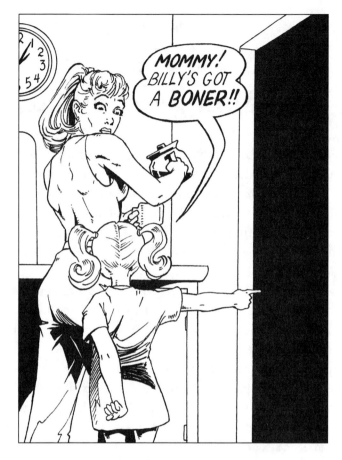

As children's minds grow and become more complex, so does their ability to have sexual fantasies that include others. With time, the thought of making love doesn't seem so "yucky" anymore. Eventually, they might even want to read books like the *Guide to Getting It On!* In the meantime, one parent might wonder if it is normal for her four-year-old boy to be playing with his penis, while another might say, "Thank heavens he's got his penis to play with. It's a never-ending source of pleasure for him!"

Telling Children about Sexual Enjoyment

Parents usually tell their children all there is to know about things like blowing noses and wiping rear ends, but rarely do they mention that genitals can be the source of good feelings. As a result, children learn that it's OK to seek their parents' wisdom on just about everything but sexual feelings. This is unfortunate, because kids need their parents' guidance on sexual feelings as much as they do on wiping their rear ends or learning to drive a car.

Some parents assume that a 3-year-old who is rubbing her genitals has the same intent and fantasies as a 23-year-old. They either try to stop her or simply pretend that nothing is happening. Perhaps it would be helpful for parents to understand that their masturbating 3-year-old isn't thinking about how good Johnnie, her day-care buddy, might be in bed! The child is simply touching her genitals because it feels good. It is perfectly normal for little hands to reach between little legs when a child is happy or excited, at naptime or even when you are reading Dr. Seuss to her. All a parent needs to do is say an occasional, "It feels good when you touch yourself there." This gives mom and dad credibility about such matters and lets the child know it will be safe to talk to the parents about things of a sexual nature.

Also, little boys have erections from a very early age, yet parents seldom explain to them that males get erections when they are having fun with their penis, as well as at other times like when waking up in the morning. Parents tell boys that they have nice eyes, ears or even feet, but they avoid telling a boy about his penis or saying anything nice about it. Nor do they tell a girl positive things about her genitals or let an older girl her know that her vagina will sometimes get wet. Yet girls get wet as often as boys get erections. (Parents who explain such matters to their children may need to distinguish between the sexual kind of wet and the peeing-in-your-pants kind of wet.)

Nanny Interruptus

Everyone these days is worried about nannies shaking their baby to death or kidnapping Junior or being lazy when no one else is around. Few people think to ask the nanny how she responds if she encounters junior playing with his or her genitals. What if you are trying to encourage a healthy attitude about sex, but during the nine hours a day when you are away, Consuela is slapping the kid's hand and warning of a thousand curses if your child ever touches him or herself again?

Ask about this when you are interviewing for a nanny. Otherwise, much of your hard work may be for naught.

Opportunity Knocks, and Knocks, and Knocks

4-year-old girl: Daddy, how come boys have penises?

Dad: I don't know. But I do know that boys and girls are both really lucky to have something between their legs that feels so good when they play with it!

The wonderful thing about explaining sex to kids is that you usually don't have to bring up the subject. It comes up on its own. Whether it's dogs mating in the backyard or your kid rubbing her genitals while you read her a good-night story, opportunities abound to make talking about sex a normal and natural part of growing up.

Unfortunately, parents who explain sex in an open way should be prepared for nasty glares from other adults, because their children won't know it is bad to talk about sex; e.g., "Mr. Johnson, my daddy gets erections. Do you?" or "Sister Mary Elizabeth, does your vulva tingle when you feel excited?"

This kind of embarrassment is nothing compared to what you will feel if the first time you talk about sex is when your 15-year-old daughter informs you she is pregnant. (In Sweden, where children have better access to sexual information and birth control, the rate of teenage pregnancy is one-sixth of what it is in the United States. Also, the kids there don't start having sex any earlier than they do here.)

Playing with Themselves

Since many parents don't talk about masturbation, their children may regard it as a dirty secret. You can explain it to a child by saying, "Masturbation is when you touch yourself between your legs in a way that feels good." Or, if your kid loves to hump her favorite bear or some other object, you can say, "They have a special word for humping things. It's called 'masturbation.'"

If your child asks for details and you feel comfortable about it, you can make a pretend penis with a finger while saying, "This is how boys do it" or point two fingers downward and rub the knuckle part to explain how girls do it. Or you can say, "It's what you've done since you were little and you put your hand between your legs about 50 times every day and rubbed." Also, it might be reassuring for an older boy to hear his father say, "I started masturbating when I was your age" or for a girl to hear her mother say, "I masturbate, too."

Keep in mind that masturbation is very common for kids between the ages of 2 and 11, and it's not unusual for a younger child to hump or rub their genitals up against just about anything that suits their fancy.

Public vs. Private

In doing research for this book, the author met with a class of high-school students to talk about sex. Before he had even introduced himself, one of the boys yelled, "Do you masturbate?" It's not the sort of question he is used to being asked, let alone by a young punk with baggy pants and a strange hair-cut. Embarrassing? You bet, yet to have said anything but "Sure" would have created a serious credibility gap, and it would have been dishonest. Beyond that, it would have been inappropriate for him to have discussed details about his private sex life with the young and restless. Hopefully, parents will keep in mind that it is neither necessary nor advisable to discuss the details of their private sex lives with their children. On the other hand, it is fine for parents to let their children know that sex is a fun and important part of their lives.

Younger children may need constant help in learning the difference between public and private. You may need to remind your 3- or 4-year-old numerous times that they aren't to play with their vulva or penis in the yard. Hopefully, you will never hear them reply, "But you and daddy do!"

Liberal-Parent Alert For super-permissive parents who feel that put-ting limits on children destroys their little spirits, keep in mind that children won't feel safe with their sexuality if it is allowed to explode all over the place. If a child won't stop masturbating or exposing himself or herself in a public place, there is no harm in saying, "I know that feels really good, but the place to do it is in the privacy of your own room and you should consider stopping it right now if you ever want to eat ice cream again as long as you live."

Also, older children who constantly rub their genitals might be dealing with emotional anxieties that have little to do with sex. Before getting too concerned, you need to consider how the kid is doing with the rest of his or her life. Is this one of many things that isn't going right, or is it simply an iso-lated problem that needs caring and firm guidance?

Naming Private Parts

Modern parents usually have no problem telling little boys that they've got a penis and testicles between their legs, although little boys rarely refer to these items by their proper names. For that matter, neither do big boys.

Female sexual anatomy is mislabeled from practically day one. First of all, what you see from the outside is not a vagina, but that has become the generic term for what is nestled between a woman's legs. What you see from the outside is a vulva, which means lips. The vagina doesn't appear until after the vulva is spread open, and even then you only see the outer rim of it. It is also helpful for parents to identify the clitoris.

Parents might do well to inform boys about girls' genitals and visa versa. This way, girls' genitals won't seem like such a mystery. Also, it is through such talks that parents can teach boys to respect and care about girls' genitals. Otherwise, how are boys expected to learn such things? In a locker room?

The Difference between Cum and Pee

When you are ready to explain the concept of ejaculation to an older child, he or she might assume you are talking about pee. After all, that's what comes out of a penis, right? Kids will likely surmise from early talks about the birds and bees that the man pees into the woman to make her pregnant. One way of avoiding this confusion is to explain that there is a big difference between pee and ejaculate. Pee is thin and mostly clear like water and there is a lot of it, while ejaculate is white and thick, and there is only a teaspoon or two of it at a time. It won't hurt to explain that nature was very smart about all of this and made it so that a man can pee when his penis is soft and have an ejaculation when his penis is hard. You can say that when a man has intercourse and his penis is hard, there comes a certain point where his penis feels really good and warm and the ejaculate starts to squirt out. That's the stuff that can get a woman pregnant. Let them know that boys don't start making this fluid until they go through puberty, which happens sometime between the ages of 11 and 16. Also explain that a man can't get a woman pregnant by simply hugging her or kissing her.

Child-Abuse Warnings

Now that our society is so revved up about child abuse, we've got parents and teachers telling young children, "Don't let anyone ever touch you down there!" Think about this.

In this day and age, the first time parents mention sex to children is often through warnings about sexual abuse—complete with those deep, measured parental tones that barely hide mom and dad's fear and concern. Consider how dumb it would be if the first thing parents told kids about bike riding is how many scraped knees, broken bones and fractured skulls they are likely to get. At best, the child would learn to hide his excitement and questions from mom and dad. And if the kid did have a bad encounter on the bike, it is only natural that he or she would try to hide that, too, and perhaps feel horribly guilty.

Why not establish a good rapport about sex with your child from early on? Then your child can take in your eventual warnings about child abuse with intelligence rather than guilt or trepidation.

As for an actual strategy, try giving young children a sense that their bodies belong to them and no one else. Tell them they don't need to give hugs or kisses if they don't want to. If parents respect this in their interactions with the child, then the child will learn from an early age that it's OK to say NO to unwanted physical touching. This is a far better approach to preventing child abuse than the stern fear-based warnings that some parents give.

When your child is older and able to speak with you about sexual matters, you can say, "No one should touch you in a sexual way unless it's what you want." Let your child know that no adults should ever touch their genitals and bottoms or ask to see them undressed unless it's at a doctor's office when mom and dad are present, or it is with a helping teacher whom mom and dad say is OK. If anyone ever touches them anywhere on the body or takes pictures of them and says to keep it a secret, they should tell you anyway. Also encourage them to tell you about any kind of touching that makes them feel strange or uncomfortable. And tell them if a stranger ever asks for their help in finding a lost pet, to come straight home and get you.

Some parents tell their children that there are "good kinds of touch" and "bad kinds of touch." This is too abstract and is seldom helpful, as children often confuse "good touch" and "bad touch." Any child abuser worth his or her salt will be able to turn this around to his or her advantage.

One of the greatest tools you have in combating child abuse is to spend lots of time with your child, being a real and vital part of his or her youth. Children who only get limited amounts of time from their parents (aka "quality time") are far more likely to be interested in the attention that child abusers have to offer. Child abusers are very savvy in their ability to select children who aren't getting enough attention at home or who have lots of unanswered questions about sex. They then become the involved, exciting and understanding adult figure that the child longs for. They end up doing your job for you, and, unfortunately, more.

Children's Questions about Sex

Some parents have the fantasy that children will ask about sex as the need arises. But when parents volunteer information about all things under the sun except sexual feelings, children grow up sensing that questions about sex are off-limits.

What children need to know are the proper names of the things that they can see or touch, and an acknowledgment that touching or rubbing their genitals can feel quite nice. The latter isn't anything that kids don't know, but it gives them a message that it's OK to talk to mom and dad about things that are sexual.

Also, some parents overwhelm young children with biological facts about sex. Folks, a five-year-old can't understand the concept of Fallopian tubes! If a child under the age of five asks, "Where do babies come from?" it's fine to say that the baby grows in mommy's uterus and point to your abdomen. And then they might want to know how the baby gets out. You can explain that there's a another hole between their poop hole and pee hole where the baby comes out.

When you explain sex, try to make it a "we" thing when possible. For instance, if children want to know how sperm gets from daddy's body into mommy's body, try to say, "Mommy and Daddy place Daddy's penis inside of Mommy's vagina," and not "Daddy places his penis inside of Mommy's vagina." For birds-and-bees information, you might find a book with fun illustrations and read it together with your child.

Once a child asks a question about sex, he has often created a scenario or answer to the question in his own mind. So you might ask Junior to tell you what he or she thinks the answer is. That way, you may get more clues about what the child needs. If there is no evidence that he or she is courting a hidden hypothesis, answer the question the best you can.

When it comes to questions about sex, or anything else for that matter, don't be afraid to tell a child that you don't know the answer. Acknowledge that it's a really good question, and say that you will do your best to find the answer. Then ask a friend, find a book or call one of the national sex lines. This way your child will feel that you take his or her questions seriously and will feel free to ask for your opinion in the future.

Keep in mind that you may be asked the same question about sex ten or twenty times. It could be that young children have a profound need for repetition, or maybe they get a secret sense of joy from seeing mom and dad break down in tears after they've been asked the same question so many times. Also be aware that you will be giving a very different answer to a 5-year-old's question about intercourse than you will to the same child when he or she is 10 or 15. Just because you answered a question when your child was five doesn't mean you won't be answering the same question every couple of years, but each time in a slightly different way.

A wonderful and hopefully helpful book on sex for children age 10 and up is *It's Perfectly Normal,* Candlewick Press, (1996).

A Normal Five-Year-Old's Feelings about Sex

> "In second grade, a little boy kept squeezing my vulva and it felt so good and tingly and warm and throbbing that I waited quite a while until I told my teacher!" *female age 23*

As part of his training, the author of this Guide followed the growth of several normal children from birth on, discussing child-development quandaries with their parents as they arose.

One of those children was a 5-year-old girl whose lifelong best friend had been a boy of her own age. The girl's mother was shocked one day to find both kids buck naked with the little boy's fingers on her daughter's vulva. The mom's first thought was to break every bone in the little boy's hand, but her daughter was just as happily involved as he. So she went into the kitchen and forced herself to count to 20. She then decided that the last thing she wanted to do was respond as her own mother would have. Needless to say, your author got a phone call asking for help.

The mom and he discussed how blanket prohibitions about sex often teach children to hide their sexuality from their parents. So rather than being guided by her initial response to protect her daughter, the mother asked the little girl how she felt about the way her friend had been touching her. Realizing that it was safe to answer truthfully, her daughter replied that it felt so wonderful she simply couldn't find a way to say no!

Since then, this little girl has asked her mother questions about who can touch her genitals and how to say no if she doesn't want them to. She asked these questions on her own initiative without being prompted by her parents. Few moms and dads have "perfect" answers for such questions, but just letting your child discuss it with you can be amazingly helpful. It helps the child learn how to use reason when dealing with sex.

It is likely that when this little girl becomes a young woman she will have more respect for her own sexuality than the vast majority of her peers. Her sexual decisions may even be the result of good judgment, instead of the all-too-common adolescent rush to just do it because the opportunity presented itself. Also, it seems that she values herself and won't be agreeing to sleep with a boy out of fear that he will go away if she says no.

Don't for a moment think that this Guide is saying to avoid setting limits on your children's sexual behavior. Parents who set no limits on their children's behavior tend to raise obnoxious brats. Instead, why not think about strategies that might be more effective than simply yelling NO!—although there are times when a contemptuous glare or a straightforward no are fine parental responses. Hopefully, you will encourage your children to think about their sexuality in ways that are constructive, rather than raising kids who are mindless about sex.

When Children See (or Hear) You Having Sex

If a young child walks in when you are having sex, cover up slowly and try not to look like you were doing something bad, because you weren't. One of you should take the child back to his or her own bed and tuck the kid in. It's a good idea to ask the child in a fun voice, "What did you think Mommy and Daddy were doing?" This will help you to know what they saw and how they interpreted it; e.g., "Daddy was hurting you!" Please resist saying, "I'd be a very happy person if daddy hurt me like that more often."

If the child has a negative read on what he or she saw, be sure to disagree with his or her interpretation and give it a positive spin. You might also say in a reassuring voice that you and daddy were having sex which was a lot of fun and you will be happy to talk about it in the morning. Even if the child doesn't ask, try to raise the issue the next day.

Parents who make a fair amount of noise when they are making love should consider telling their young children about it, saying that mom and dad sometimes make noises at night when they are sharing sexual feelings. Explain that these are happy noises which are very different from the noises that mom and dad make when they are fighting. This is an important distinction to make.

The good thing to know about being seen by your kids is that Dr. Paul Abramson and colleagues at UCLA completed an eighteen-year longitudinal study of *Early Exposure to Parental Nudity and Scenes of Parental Sexuality.* 18-year-olds who, as kids, had walked in on mom and dad when they were having sex showed no differences from other 18-year-olds. In fact, young boys who walked in on mom and dad actually seemed to demonstrate a better long-term outcome than those who didn't. Hmmm.

"Why Can't I Watch You and Mommy Have Sex?"

You've worked hard to be an open, honest parent about sex and your child suddenly rewards you with the statement, "I want to watch you and Mommy have sex!" Instead of convulsing with panic, regard this as yet another opportunity to talk about privacy and sex; for instance: "One of the things that makes sex so special for Mommy and Daddy is that it's private, just between the two of us. Since sex between us is private and personal, I wouldn't feel comfortable having anyone else watching." "Well, what about that time I saw you kissing Mommy's vulva. Will you kiss mine?" "Your vulva is very sweet and nice. But I wouldn't feel comfortable kissing your vulva like I kiss Mommy's because it's a private sexual thing that I only do with her."

Nudity at Home

"Nudity was a normal part of bathing, dressing, getting up in the morning or going to bed at night. I think this is ideal. Kids get a lot of reassurance and education from the occasional observation of natural (not contrived) nudity." *female age 35*

"My daughter always felt comfortable walking around the house naked, but my teenage son is so modest that nobody can remember seeing him naked since he was five years old!" *male age 65*

Is nudity around the house good or bad? A retrospective study of college students compared how much nudity they reported when growing up with their current levels of sexual activity. There was no correlation between high levels of nudity at home and sexual promiscuity at college age. Kids who reported higher levels of nudity at home seemed to report more feelings of warmth or security when away at college. Perhaps one reason for this is because it's easier for them to adjust to communal bathroom and shower situations that are so common in college life. It's also possible that they feel better about their bodies.

Parents' Sexual Feelings about Their Children

Our society gives parents little guidance about sexual feelings toward their children, except blanket condemnation. Children of all ages are able to evoke sexual feelings in parents, from a nursing experience that leaves a baby's mother with pleasant genital sensations, to a teenage son whose developing body gives mom an occasional sexual stirring, perhaps reminding her of the excitement she used to feel when seeing the boy's father when he was younger. The problem isn't in having occasional sexual feelings about your children; it's in what to do with the feelings.

For instance, let's say that a dad is playfully wrestling with his young daughter and finds that he is getting an erection. A healthy dad might think to himself, "Oops!," beg out of the roughhousing, and say to his daughter, "Why don't you grab the mitts so we can work on your pitching?" or "How about a game of Scrabble?" A less-healthy dad might keep doing the same activity over and over without adjusting to the reality of the situation.

Upon discovering their own arousal, some very good dads withdraw from physical and sometimes even emotional contact with a child. In these cases, dad's own harsh superego can ruin a very important parent-child relationship. This can be quite sad for both parent and child, if the relationship had been a healthy one to begin with.

As for mother-son feelings, let's say that mom enjoys rubbing her teenage son's back, but finds that she is starting to have a sexual response. Maybe it's time to give Junior a quick hug instead and to realize that it is more appropriate for him to have his back rubbed by girls his own age. Or maybe mom enjoys the way her son's teenage body looks. This is fine, but it starts to cross the line if she ends up in his bedroom whenever he is getting undressed. Particularly troublesome are lonely moms who encourage their sons to share the bed with them, unless such conditions are dictated by abject poverty. The same is true for lonely dads.

Problems sometimes abound in families where the parents' sexual relationship is not a particularly good one. One of the children might decide that it's up to him or her to be a replacement spouse. What's amazing about this kind of mutual seduction is if a therapist suggests that something might be askew, both parent and child may glare at the therapist as though he or she were some sort of twisted pervert. Especially destructive are situations where the parent alternates between being seductive and puritanical.

It's not possible to set specific rules and standards for all households. For instance, nudity in one family might be perfectly healthy, while nudity in another family might be part of a syrupy, seductive mess. And while it might be best for parents to put boundaries on one child's sexual expression, another child might do well with the opposite kind of response. For instance, a teenager who is an exhibitionist with his or her naked body can clearly use some limit-setting, while a highly-inhibited child who is embarrassed about his or her body might find it helpful to hear that it's OK to be naked. Another example involves a young child who enjoys masturbating before naps or when tucked into bed as mom or dad are reading a favorite story. This is perfectly normal. However, another child who rocks and masturbates anxiously throughout the day needs help.

It would be nice to say that common sense should prevail, but when it comes to sexual development within the family, there doesn't seem to be an abundance of collective common sense in our culture.

Explaining Puberty

"When I got my first period I was excited, but then my mother wouldn't let me climb trees or play with the guys anymore."

female age 55

"My mom had always been really open with me, so I was prepared when my body started changing. I was even glad to get my period.

female age 19

"I started growing awfully fast and none of my clothes fit anymore. I'd consume everything in the refrigerator and would still feel hungry. My armpits had never perspired or smelled. Suddenly, it was like someone had turned on a faucet under each one. I dreaded being called on in morning classes, because I'd often have a raging hard-on. My beard was really strange, mostly boyhood fuzz with man hairs growing through it. So I appropriated one of my dad's razors and started shaving. I didn't know why I was suddenly having wet dreams, and I used to hide my underwear and wash them myself so my mom wouldn't see the stains. I was sure I was damaging myself by masturbating once a day, but couldn't stop to save my life. Hair started growing from my neck down. And suddenly there were zits. That's what I remember of puberty. It would have been nice if a parent or some adult had taken a moment to explain some of these things to me." *male age 44*

It never hurts to let your children know that their bodies will change as they get older. Of course, you will need to address the issue in different ways depending on the child's age. For instance, you can tell your 7-year-old that puberty is what happens when you stop looking like a kid and start look-

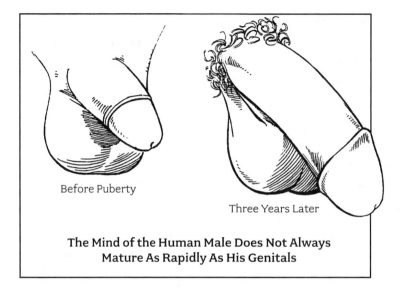

Before Puberty

Three Years Later

The Mind of the Human Male Does Not Always Mature As Rapidly As His Genitals

ing like an adult—that boys get taller, their voices deepen, they start getting hair under their armpits and around their genitals. You can also say that girls' hips start to get wider, they grow breasts, and their armpits and genitals get hair too. For more about teenage boys and their unwanted erections, see Chapter 5 "On The Penis."

When your child is a few years older, you can explain that puberty is a process that takes a couple of years to complete and that it usually starts to happen for girls when they turn 10 or 11 and for boys when they turn 12 or 13. Let them know that puberty is a little like the repair people from the phone company: sometimes they arrive when they're supposed to, sometimes they are late, and occasionally they get there before you expected. You can mention that puberty is the time when girls start to menstruate and boys start to ejaculate when they have orgasms, and that everyone's genitals start to look more adult-like (bigger and hairier).

Kids can be awfully cruel toward other kids who are in the throes of puberty. Let your child know that you will ring his or her neck if they ever make fun of another kid whose body starts to change sooner than theirs, or if they taunt a kid who is really late.

Menstrual Bleeding

"Puberty was not a really big deal for me. I read *Are You There God, It's Me Margaret*, so I knew what my period was when I got it, although my mom never bothered to tell me." *female age 25*

"I was afraid that I would just start bleeding sometime and that it might go through my clothes and I would be embarrassed."

female age 49

"My first period was a celebration. I was at my friend's house and I noticed bleeding between my legs. I rushed home to tell my mother, fully aware I was having my period. She was thrilled, and we went out to dinner to celebrate." *female age 18*

The only time when many parents mention sex to their daughters is while explaining menstruation. What an unfortunate association, bleeding and sex. Now it's even worse, as the first thing young girls often hear about sex from their parents is a warning of sexual abuse.

As children, we learn that blood is a sign of bodily injury. We are never told that some bleeding is good for us. So when girls start menstruating, the blood that drips from their vulvas is often equated by the unconscious mind with injury or internal damage. When explaining menstruation, girls should be informed that the bleeding which comes during their menstrual periods is a good thing, and that menstruation is the body's way of keeping the walls of their reproductive organs clean and fresh.

Girls are now menstruating at ages 12 or 13; their grandmothers started menstruating when they were three to four years older. The bodies of these young girls are more developed than their grandmothers' were at the same ages, but their emotional development is about the same. This means they will need plenty of encouragement and support from their parents in negotiating the puberty process, especially if they begin menstruating earlier or later than most of their friends.

Growing Girls

Young girls tend to be very self-conscious about physical changes, especially around fathers and brothers, so don't be talking about tampons and training bras when the guys are around. If they mature earlier than their friends, you'll need to be aware that other girls might shun them and boys might tease them. Keep reminding them that things will be fine in a couple of years when everybody else has started to mature. Make sure they are involved in activities like sports, science, 4-H—anything where value is placed on their achievements and abilities.

If your child is comparing herself in negative ways to actresses on TV, let her know that many of the allegedly "perfect" girls on TV are, for the most part, self-absorbed lunatics who think nothing of barfing up a perfectly good meal so they won't get "fat." These are people who have more surgery than a BMW in a Tijuana chop shop, and in spite of the stories that their publicists send to *People Magazine,* few have off-screen lives that are particularly happy. Double ditto for models who are in magazines like *Seventeen* and *Cosmo.*

Teenagers & Sex

"I used to pretend my friend Heather was another boy that I liked in school in fifth grade and we would touch each other's vulvas and breasts and have a lot of fun until my Mom found out and sent me to a psychiatrist for being a lesbian!" *female age 24*

If you ask a group of 16-year-olds if they are emotionally ready to have sex, most will say yes. If you ask their parents whether their 16-year-olds are emotionally ready to have sex, most will say no. Chances are your teenagers do not view sex the way you wish they would.

As a parent, you can't expect a teenager to be verbal about sex just because you have suddenly decided to offer wise counsel. Having an open dialogue about sex is an option that some parents lost when the child was 3 to 5 years old. If mom and dad ignored the existence of sexual feelings back then, it might be very uncomfortable for the child who is now a teenager to suddenly start talking about sex. If there is tension between you and your teen, or if the kid is engaged in reckless acting-out behavior, you might do better to solicit the help of a favorite aunt, uncle, teacher or therapist to whom the teen is more apt to open up to. And if there are problems, you will need to become more involved in their lives than you might currently be.

When Teenagers Ask on Their Own

Let's say your teenager asks you a question about sex: "How do you know if you're gay?" or "What if you get so nervous before having sex that you feel like throwing up?" or "Would I have to leave home if I got pregnant?" Don't assume that she or he is thinking about being gay, is about to have sex or is pregnant. Maybe your kid heard something on the TV or radio and is putting him or herself in the other person's place.

Try to respond by saying things that will help expand the question into a discussion, such as "What are your thoughts about that?" or "I'll be able to give you a better answer if you could tell me more about your question." This buys you precious time, which parents can never have enough of when being asked

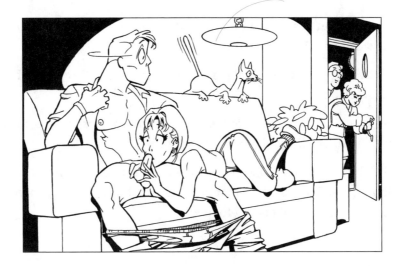

questions about sex, and it helps you squelch any potential screams that are about to explode from the depths of your parental craw.

You might take solace from the following words by one of the top sex educators in the country, Debra Haffner: "Like most parents, I have found myself at a loss for words when a question I never expected popped up. There have been times when I have responded in ways that I later regretted. I struggled with how to respond to my daughter when she asked about the Bobbit case, and then about Michael Jackson, and Monica Lewinsky."

Don't think that you need to come up with perfect answers. The most important thing is to provide an atmosphere where the child can ask questions and know that it's OK to think out loud about sex.

Wouldn't It Be Nice If...

Perhaps these questions can act as guides in helping your child think about what they might want from sex.

🔅Why does this person want to have sex with me? Is it fun, romance, a personal quest?

🔅Does having sex mean something different to him or her than it does to me?

🔅Do I know what it feels like in my body to be sexually excited?

🔅Do I want to have sex because I am physically excited about it, or is it just to please a partner or to keep him or her interested in me?

💡What kind of stimulation does a woman need before intercourse so it feels good?

💡Are there ways we could please each other sexually without having intercourse?

💡How do I say no to someone who is pestering me for a date, or no to sex without feeling like a coward or geek?

💡If we do have sex, how do I get genuine feedback from my partner about what felt good and what didn't? How do I tell him or her what feels good and what doesn't for me?

💡Will I feel good about myself the next day?

💡Who sticks what into where when we have intercourse, and how can we do it in ways that will make it feel better?

💡What would we do if we had intercourse and became pregnant? To whom would we turn? How would we tell our parents? Would we face it together? Am I ready to be a parent? No kid should begin dating without seriously discussing questions about pregnancy with his or her parents.

Toward Higher Expectations

The mere thought of asking an 11-year-old what qualities she would want in a sexual partner would send most American parents racing to the bathroom for a hit of Tagamet or Imodium. But let's think about it. If you as a parent don't introduce the notions of chivalry and respect in sex, where else are your children going to learn them? From MTV?

There is nothing wrong with talking to your child about the difference between a partner who's just trying to get laid and one who is going to be a caring and loving sexual companion. For instance, does a partner who is going to be a respectful lover say, "I won't go out with you anymore if we can't have intercourse?" Is he or she responsible and caring toward family and friends? Are his or her friends good people? Do they drink or get loaded a lot? And what about introducing the expectation that a truly desirable partner is one who is trustworthy and dependable and says things such as, "I'd really like to please you. What can I do?"

Of course, none of this is going to stop your kid from shacking up with one of the local Hell's Angels, but it does kick into motion the idea that an important part of self-respect means choosing your sexual partners carefully. With enough intelligent concern and involvement on your part, your kid may even search out a sexual partner who has some of the characteristics and values that you do. Hopefully that's a good thing.

Condom Advice — For Teenage Boys

Give your teenage boy a couple of condoms and a tube of lube, saying that these are for him to put on when he's alone to see what it feels like. If you have a straightforward relationship with him, you might suggest that he try masturbating with a condom on, which is the condom equivalent of taking a test drive. Tell him to pay attention to how long it takes after he ejaculates before his penis starts to shrink and the condom gets baggy. That's how much time he has to pull out; otherwise the condom might stay in his partner's vagina. Tell him that the shrinking-penis factor is why he needs to clasp the condom around the base of his penis as he is pulling out. Maybe you could try reading the instructions together. Let him know that the lube is to put on the outside of the condom to help it slip and slide better when he is having intercourse.

Condom Advice — For Teenage Girls

Give your daughter a couple of condoms, a tube of lube and a penis-sized banana. Tell her that one of the condoms is for her to practice putting on the banana; the others are for whatever she wants to do with them. If you have an open relationship with her, try putting the condom on the banana together. This should result in a number of giggles and laughs. If it doesn't, you're being way too serious. Explain that she needs to leave an extra half inch at the tip of the penis so it can fill with ejaculate when the guy comes. Also explain that as soon as a guy ejaculates, his penis starts to shrink. This means that she should clasp the condom with her fingers and push it against the base of his penis as he withdraws so he won't leave it inside her. Let her know that it never hurts to put a little lube on the outside of the condom before having intercourse. This will help it slip and slide better. Maybe you can try reading the condom instructions together.

You should be sure that she has a prescription for morning-after birth control pills, and that you and she have discussed that this is important to take right away if something strange happened with the condom, or if she is worried that it didn't work right. Seem more in the chapter on birth control.

By the way, teenage girls who know what kind of birth control their mother uses are more likely to use birth control themselves.

Odds'N'Ends

💡 If you have a son, make sure he's got a big box of Kleenex next to his bed, and when it's all used up in three days don't make smart remarks like "I didn't know you had such a bad cold." Better you have to stock up on Kleenex than he is out knocking up some young thing.

💡 If your child begins to wash his or her own underwear or pajamas, be sure they have proper information about menstruation, masturbation and wet dreams. While most of us know what happens when boys ejaculate, we forget that some teenage girls get major wet spots in their underwear when they become sexually excited.

💡 Abstinence-only programs do not significantly delay the onset of intercourse. Unfortunately, the entire "just say no" approach had no significant impact on drug use, and it works about as well on teenagers as it does on adults. If you don't want them to be doing this or that, get them involved in activities that will fill their time.

💡 Let your kids know that it's fine to wait until they are older before having sex with a partner and that masturbation is what you do in the meantime, which is why we humans have two more fingers than ET.

💡 Inform them that what they see on TV about sex is usually pretty twisted, exaggerated and outright incorrect, unless they're watching reruns of *Married With Children*.

A Final Word about Boundaries

If you think your younger teenagers would do better to wait a couple of years before sharing sex with partners, then you might do something other than tempt the fates.

One thing is to talk to your kids about sex and encourage them to talk to you. That way, if they're going to become sexually active, it won't be just to get back at a prudish parent. Another thing that helps delay sexual activity is getting teenagers involved in activities that challenge their minds and bodies, we're talking about things like science fairs and playing soccer or building things. You're thinking, "Isn't that about the tenth time they said that?"

Understand that good kids do not always make good decisions. If you give them enough rope to hang themselves, most will. On the other hand, no kid ever lost a friend because their parents insisted on knowing where they were and with whom. No teenager ever died because his or her parents set a curfew on weekends. No kid ever shriveled up and blew away because one parent called another parent to make sure that an adult would be home when their kid was sleeping over.

Your kids will have plenty of time to do what they want once they are adults. Until then, it is your job as parents to get them there safe and sound.

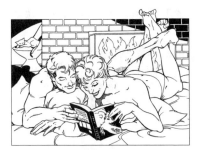

Dear Paul,

I am 14 and my mom, who is totally cool, just got me birth-control pills. My boyfriend and I are totally committed to each other. Do we still need to use a condom?

Shelby from Shafter

Dear Shelby

I am not 14, but I am a fairly liberal guy and have produced one of the more liberal books on sex ever written. I want to disagree with your first statement. I don't think your mom is totally cool because she got her 14-year-old daughter birth-control pills. Maybe she did it because she knows she doesn't have any control over her daughter, or maybe she doesn't want to have any control over her daughter. After all, it takes a lot of effort and involvement to guide a child through the teenage years.

You're not going to like this, but I don't think 14-year-olds should be having intercourse. You might feel I am being hypocritical, given how I encourage parents to speak with their children about everything from masturbation and orgasms to ways of telling a partner what you like in bed. But this assumes that talking about sex encourages kids to do it sooner. I don't think so.

One reason why I feel 14-year-olds should wait is because our minds handle abstract concepts better at age 17 or 18 than at 14. And believe it or not, there's a lot of abstract stuff to cope with when you are in a relationship and having sex. You might be the most mature and responsible person in your entire class, and I think it's great that you are thinking about birth control and condoms, but I also think you'll appreciate sex a lot more when your mental equipment catches up with your physical equipment, which doesn't happen for a few more years yet.

In the meantime, your mom should help you get something under your belt other than your boyfriend's penis. Perhaps she could help you get involved in activities like volunteering at an old folks' home or at an animal shelter.

This is just one man's opinion, but I feel it's important for someone your age to channel your sexual energy into expanding your mind and creativity. Then, when you are a few years older, the sex you have will complement who you are as a person rather than define it, as is often the case when 14-year-olds are having intercourse. I am concerned that it's just too big, too soon right now.

And yes, Shelby, if you do have intercourse, it's a good idea to use a condom in addition to taking the pill. Once you are in a time-tested, true-blue relationship, you can ditch the condom.

Special thanks to Bill Taverner, co-editor of the *American Journal of Sex Education*. Also, to *Not with My Child*, United Youth Security (1999), for insight into how child abusers think. And to Debra Hafner's *From Diapers to Dating: A Parent's Guide To Raising Sexually Healthy Children*, Newmarket Press (1999), for a reminder about nannies and other things mentioned in this chapter.

66

Love Dreams, Sex Dreams, Sweet Dreams

Some people have dreams of misty-eyed romance, the kind of dreams that leave you floating in the clouds. Some people have dreams that include sex. These are the dreams that this chapter is about. And some people have dreams that combine sex and romance. These are the dreams that we dream about dreaming — the rocket-fuel variety of dream that fills the soul and tugs at the edges of who we are.

Sex-Dream Statistics

Less than 10% of American parents inform their children about sex dreams, yet the majority of young adults at one time or another have them. More than 50% of women have sex dreams, yet many women don't start having their sex dreams until they are in their twenties. With the male of the species it is different. Males often experience sex dreams as teenagers, with the frequency tending to decrease as they get older.

Sex-Dream History

In the mid-1800s, it was believed that sex dreams were caused by immoral thoughts. Some of the more fanatical experts of the day proposed bizarre operations for the penises of men who had wet dreams, and all sorts of devices were patented for a man to wear on his penis at night to prevent him from having erections and the dreaded sex dreams that were thought to follow. One device was designed to wake him up by pulling on his pubic hair when he got an erection. Another machine poured cold water on him whenever he became erect during his sleep.

Dreamtime Sex Cinema—Pass the Kleenex, or Not?

During an average night of sleep, human genitals get hard or wet several times. This usually happens whenever you are dreaming, regardless of the dream's content, even if the dream is about your grandmother or someplace you once visited. A "wet dream" happens when you are actually dreaming about sex and have an orgasm.

A lot of "wet dream" orgasms are actually dry and don't include ejaculation, which makes the term "wet dream" a bit of a misnomer when it is used to describe men's sex dreams. While having an orgasm in your sleep isn't much of a problem for a woman, it sometimes leaves a guy with a sticky mess. In a more understanding world, a male wouldn't have to feel embarrassed about wet-dream stains. But wet dreams often leave a splotch on the sheets or in your underwear, and what's a boy to say? Since there is no way of predicting when you will have a sex dream, packing your shorts with Kleenex at bedtime isn't going to help.

Sex Dreams vs. Masturbation

Talk about difficult bedtime decisions. Some people assume they will be more likely to have a wet dream if they don't masturbate. They might hold out, trying not to masturbate for as many days as possible in order to force a wet dream. This usually doesn't work. Sometimes a person can have a wet dream the same night that he or she masturbates or has sex, but not masturbating doesn't seem to increase your chances by one little drip.

There is simply no way to will yourself a wet dream, unless you are good at lucid-dream enhancement, or whatever the people at Stanford are calling it these days. A seminal book on the subject of lucid dreaming is *Lucid Dreaming* by Stephen LeBerge, Ballantine. Another helpful book (except for its dumb title) is *Lucid Dreams in 30 Days* by Keith Harary and Pamela Weintraub.

Sex-Dream Complications

Not only are sex dreams a sign that you are growing up, but they are a great way of having sex when it is not readily available. Some people even have their first orgasms while asleep and dreaming. Still, other people feel upset by their sex dreams. For instance, you might have a sex dream that includes someone you know, maybe a friend, boss or teacher. This might make you feel a bit sheepish when you see that person in real life. This book's suggestion is to scope out the person from head to toe. Check everything from subtle mannerisms to what kind of clothes he or she is wearing. Then ask yourself: "Is he or she as good (or bad) in real life as he or she was in my dream?"

There can also be wet-dream downers. Wet dreams can leave you feeling frustrated when the love of your dreams doesn't want anything to do with you in waking life. This can be particularly bittersweet when the person is a former lover and is now with someone else or is no longer living. Also, it is not unusual for heterosexuals to dream about having sex with members of the same sex, and gay people have occasional "straight" sex in their dreams with members of the opposite sex. Gay men call these nightmares.

The Family That Dreams Together...

People sometimes have sex dreams that include members of the family. This doesn't necessarily indicate a problem. Actions that transpire in dreams are often symbols for something very different than what meets the eye, so you can't assume that the sexual partners or the sexual activity in a dream reflects what the dream is really about. Psychologists might refer to this as the manifest content versus the latent content of the dream. If, however, disturbing dreams happen on a regular basis and you are bothered by them, consider seeking the help of a trained mental- health professional.

Another reason to get outside help is if you usually end up frustrated, hurt, frightened or angry in your dreams. You don't have to be Sigmund Freud to realize that repeated dreams of a disturbing nature reflect an inner struggle of major proportion. The exception is with children, since bad dreams are quite common during the younger years. It is not unusual for children who are happy and whose emotional development is normal to have bad dreams two to four times a week. If, on the other hand, the child is also struggling during the waking hours, it might be prudent to seek a professional assist.

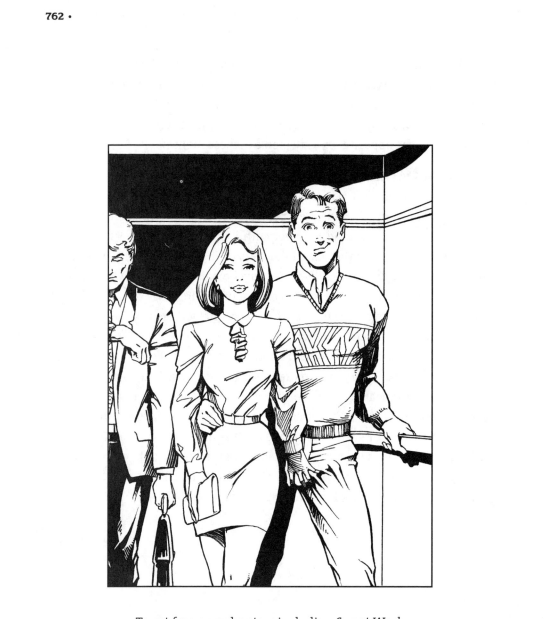

To get free new chapters including *Sex at Work,*
which covers the ins and outs of dating a co-worker or client,
and *Sex with a Single Parent*—plus the author's latest
podcast on what's new in sex, science
and medicine—please visit

www.GuideToGettingItOn.com

67
Hooking-Up-Sex

66 There's a sort of thrill when it's someone you don't know. It's like your first roller-coaster ride except there's no safety bar. You don't know anything about this guy but that you both want that contact. On the other hand, me and my boyfriend's sex has always been amazing because we know what each other likes and what buttons to push. Plus there's always the comfort afterward whereas with a stranger it's kind of awkward afterward." *female, 23*

"When I was involved in my hook-up relationship I would never call him up for a sober booty call. It was always when I was drunk and wanted sex. That is also how I knew there was no emotional attachment because I wasn't even interested in hanging out with the guy unless I had been drinking. He wasn't really my type. He just wasn't someone that I wanted to be in a relationship with. We didn't have a lot in common other than the sex." *female age 22*

"The hook-up guy never, ever asked me how it was for me. He always quit after he finished, and there was rarely foreplay. You could tell it was strictly sex. My boyfriend always asks how it was for me; he is always worried that he is not doing it good enough." *female age 22*

"I think relationships are still the goal. It's just more relaxed on how we get to that point." *female age 23*

From a survey of fourteen college-age women who know a thing or three about hooking-up sex.

You might wonder why the longest chapter in a book like this would be on sex in the 1800s, and why we would mention the 1800s at the start of a chapter on hooking-up sex. Couldn't the space have been better used for more intercourse-position illustrations, or maybe astrological charts to help you find your best days for getting oral sex?

The fascinating thing about the chapter on sex in the 1800s is that it's about how we got from there to almost here—how dating and relating evolved and took much of its current shape. One of the neat things about hooking-up sex is that it marks another change in how we date and relate. It's a radical departure that mostly impacts people under the age of 25, but ripple it does and ripple it will.

It's much easier to look at how sex and dating came to be since the 1800s and go "WOW!" That's because we can look at it from so many different angles and connect 100 years of dots. For those of you who did the *stride of pride* or made the *walk of shame* this morning, it's still too soon to have a sense of perspective on hooking-up sex. And hooking-up sex is still too sensational for the media to give it much depth given how their ratings go up when they can stir the pots of moral panic.

Unlike the way that hooking-up sex has been portrayed for the viewing public, it didn't just sprout up or suddenly arrive like the aliens in War of the Worlds. Hooking-up sex evolved and it continues to evolve. How many people are actually doing it or for how long isn't the point and doesn't matter.

In this chapter, we try to describe what hooking-up sex is, and we try to look at the fascinating story of how came to be.

Note: The terms *hooking-up, hooking-up sex* and *hook-up sex* are often interchangeable, although the context matters. We mostly use *hooking-up sex* in this chapter for consistency and so the book's copy editor doesn't have a coronary.

So What Is It?

While hooking-up sex has its own little universe of problems, one of the things about it that's so cool is how it totally blows the premise of books like this one out of the water. It's Top-Ramen noodles and Pizza Pockets compared to the bloated meal that we've proclaimed sex should be. It's popping one out without telling each other what feels good or cluing your partner in to how a well-timed kiss or caress here or there is what you need to help push you over the edge. It annihilates our idea that what makes sex special is having sex with someone who is special. And for most people, it seems to work.

Is hooking-up what they want sex to be for the rest of their life? Of course not—or not until they are married and have kids and are looking back on the good old days.

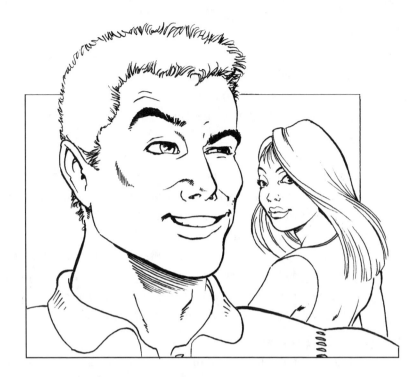

Unlike traditional dating, hooking-up sex is mostly about sex. Its most distinguishing factor is that it puts the gender roles totally in the toilet. There's no expectation that this might lead to something else, or at least it's understood that you leave your expectations at the door.

For hooking-up sex to become possible, traditional gender roles had to become irrelevant, and it's women who had to make them irrelevant. That's because for years, we've had this sex paradigm in which young men are supposed to be the ones who are pawing to get between a woman's legs, and she's the one who is supposed to keep them together until certain conditions were met—including whether a relationship might be coming out of this. It was his wad vs. her future.

Now, with hooking-up sex, women have decided they aren't playing the gate-keeper role anymore. Women who are having hooking-up sex are just as likely to dive into a man's pants as a guy is into theirs. If a relationship happens, it happens, but that's not the reason they are hooking up. The fact that a relationship is not part of the mix can make hooking-up sex particularly appealing to a lot of women and men who don't want to be part of a couple at their particular stage in life. And if attachments do happen, the chances are good they will be one-sided, and it's just as likely to be the guy who ends up getting hurt or feeling jealous.

As for what happens in hooking-up sex, it might be making out for an hour with a total stranger, it might be oral sex, or it might be intercourse. A key element is that it's about excitement rather than emotions, it's about being horny and wanting sex, plain and simple, same for girls as it is for boys. It's about wanting more comfort than you can get when you masturbate, and that seems to be a possibility if you aren't expecting the stars and the moon. Of course, there might be the occasional cross purpose, like indiscriminately fucking a rival's boyfriend or rubbing it in an ex's face, but that's been a part of sex since the beginning of time.

ORAL NOTE: As for the idea that oral sex is casual and women are indiscriminately sucking dicks as a part of hooking-up sex, we don't buy it. While this might be true for some, for a lot of other people oral sex is a pretty intimate act and doesn't just happen without some feelings of closeness.

Dating vs. Hooking-Up Sex

If you look at the media, you might think that hooking-up sex is defining young adults today and that everyone's having it. That's not our take. For some people it only happens once or twice; for plenty of others, never.

Dating still happens, and it is still important, especially after you've sewn your hooking-up oats and are getting near the dangerously ancient age of 25. There tends to be a turn toward dating once people reach their last years of college, or get their first full-time job or become more established in the working world.

But dating is seldom as formal as it used to be, nor is it necessarily the major social event that it once was. Whether it's having coffee together or going to see a movie, dating is what you do if you are exploring the possibility that you and your date might become friends or lovers. It's different from hooking-up sex in that there's expectations for more than just sex. There are still rules and male-female roles in dating, although they don't exactly scream at you like they used to.

One of the reasons why dating is no longer the cornerstone of male-female relations is because males and females socialize or hang out more in groups than they used to.

When people used to say "peer group," it was assumed they were talking about groups of males or groups of females. Now that peer groups are more mixed, men and women don't have to go on a formal date to get to know each other better.

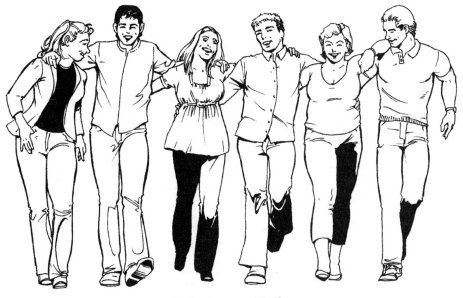

Peer Groups Today

There's also the Facebook factor. You can learn about another person today without having to ask.

Dating Adjacent

At the start of this chapter we talked about the ripple-down effect of hooking-up sex. "Dating adjacent" is an example of just that.

"Dating adjacent" is a hazy area between dating and hooking-up sex. It's where two people are checking each other out as possible relationship material, but the threshold for having sex isn't particularly high. So the sex might happen right away as a means of exploring whether things could evolve into something that's more long-term, as in a "relationship."

A number of relationships started out as hooking-up sex, with little expectation that anything more would come of it. The fact is, the divide between hooking-up sex and dating isn't clearly defined.

Alcohol & Awkward, Horny & Excited

This chapter includes the observations of fourteen women between the ages of 19 and 23 who are familiar with hooking-up sex. No males who are involved in hooking-up sex took the survey, which is why the comments are all from women. Hopefully that will change.

Two of the most frequent words that these women used in describing hooking-up sex were *alcohol* and *awkward,* but *horny* and *excited* were up there as well. In more than 25 pages of transcripts, *love* was used twice only, and that was regarding current boyfriends as opposed to former hooking-up partners. *Comfort, comforting* and *uncomfortable* were used often. *Abusive, unhappy,* and *pain* were not used at all. In fact, the women were quite articulate about it: When it comes to hooking-up sex, the kind of emotions that we value in a long-term relationship are usually not a big part of it—nor are the ones we usually dread.

> "When you are not in a relationship, and you want sex, you have hook-up sex. At times it can be satisfying sexually, but not emotionally. To have just hook-up sex you need to be able to separate the emotions. When I was involved in hook-up sex it was with the same guy, but there were no attachments. If one of us hooked up with someone else then the arrangement would be over. Now that I am in a committed relationship, I think that the sex with someone you know and are emotionally invested in is so much better. Knowing the person cares about you makes sex a lot more worthwhile." *female age 22*

While much of the media coverage of hook-up sex ends with poignant accounts of how empty it can be and how hurt at least one of the partners ends up being, that's not what the women who took our survey focused on.

> "He just wasn't really my type. He was a football player and just wasn't someone that I wanted to be in a relationship with. We didn't have a lot in common other than the sex. Most people didn't even know we were hooking up." *female age 22*

By far the most fascinating part of hooking-up sex has to do with alcohol. Almost all of the women said that alcohol was their gasoline for hooking-up sex, but they didn't seem particularly concerned about it.

> "I definitely think random hook-ups have more to do with alcohol than what is believed in the media." *female age 22*

> "Alcohol plays a big role in hooking up. Many (including myself) have used the excuse 'I was drunk.' It's almost like a free pass." *female, 22*

> "Alcohol is a huge influence on hooking up, especially for girls! I don't think I would ever hook up with a guy I didn't know unless I have the comfort of saying I was drunk at the time so I had an excuse in the morning." *female age 21*

"When I drink I want sex, so then I knew I could get it from him. Drinking just makes sex more interesting to me because I am more open to trying things, and I am not worried about what I look like or how I am doing. I am more worried about my receiving sexual pleasure than anything else." *female age 22*

"You may think this person was attractive when drunk, but when you wake up the next morning and see him, you are like 'Whoa... I'm out of here.'" *female age 23*

"I see hook-up sex more when alcohol or substances are being used, especially in college. People don't think about what they are doing until the next morning when guilt settles in. I know this because, unfortunately it has happened to me and a lot of my friends." *fem 23*

"Alcohol is more of an excuse than a reason sex happens. When I drink I act on my sexual needs more than when I am sober." *fem. 22*

"Alcohol has a huge impact on my sexual activities. If I drink enough I have no moral rules with myself anymore. The next day I can wake up and make it okay by just saying, 'I was drunk.'" *female age 21*

Alcohol certainly helps with the inhibitions. It also helps make it possible to have sex with a guy you don't particularly like except for the sex.

If these same women had heard about someone who was not an alcoholic but who needed to drink before he went to work each day, most would say he had a really bad job, it was too stressful, or his boss must be evil. They would tell him to quit and find another job, or maybe see a therapist.

But when it comes to hooking-up sex, getting drunk allows women to act more like men. It's a testosterone patch in a can. It's still not a level playing field between men and women when it comes to sex. It's hard for a girl to grow up feeling good about her body in our supermodel-gawking society. While guys usually know what a penis and testicles are from early on, women still grow up referring to their genitals as "down there" instead.

When we asked the women if they needed to hammer down a few Stolis before having sex with a boyfriend as opposed to someone they were hooking up with, you could hear the "hell no!" all the way across the country.

While plenty of women (and men) feel less inhibited by having sex after a drink or six, alcohol is not the ante for having sex with a boyfriend.

However, being sober is often a deal-breaker when it comes to hooking-up sex with Mr. Unknown.

Alcohol could be what's needed for these women to allow their knees to swing as wide open as guys' do when they are having casual sex.

Causing the Boots of Old Berkeley Feminists to Spin

It's clear that a lot of women who are having hooking-up sex see it as a sign of liberation. However, the old warhorse front-line feminists at Berkeley during the dawn of the second wave of feminism might have had some misgivings about this. It's not the lack of commitment that would bother them, or needing a drink before having sex with a guy. They would have sympathized and perhaps suggested you ditch the dick altogether for a little muff. But to intentionally get drunk so you could hook up with some guy who you don't know how he voted in the last election?

What these women might have asked is if you are sure you aren't giving more than you are getting. Not only are you the one who is running the risk of getting pregnant and getting a sexually transmitted infection that might result in cervical cancer, but women still have to pay a higher social cost for casual sex than men.

As for sexual freedom, being liberated meant being able to make choices you were pleased with when you were sober, not ones you needed to make while drunk.

Double Standard: Without Sluts, There Would Be No Studs

"We expect to hear a guy say, 'Oh I'm gonna go get me some ass tonight,' but rarely hear a woman say the same thing, as she would be considered sexually promiscuous, a slut, too open with her sexuality, unladylike, etc." *female age 21*

"How many are too many? How much is too much? How assertive is too assertive? What is experimental vs. promiscuous? All of these questions are always there in the back of women's heads, and I don't think a lot of men realize that, or maybe they do and just don't care." *female age 22*

"The double standard still exists. If a guy sleeps with a lot of girls then all his friends think he's a player, but if a girl sleeps with too many guys she's a whore and no one wants to be her friend. I think of course girls have a lot more freedom sexually, but that doesn't mean that times have changed as much as to have the girl starting making every first move. I am kind of weird on this topic; I would never sleep with a guy who's had an outrageous number of women, but I also would not sleep with a guy who hasn't ever been with someone, not because of how they would be in bed but I just don't want to be someone's first because then they have to remember me forever." *female age 23*

"I hear my guy friends saying, 'I hooked up with this girl last night' and then add a number to it. However, when a guy asks me how many people I have slept with, I am ashamed to say eight. I feel like it is so high. However, then when you ask a guy he will proudly say twenty." *female age 21*

It's not necessary to say much more than these women have said. The biggest difference between the double standard today and how it was a few generations ago is in how many guys a girl can sleep with before she's slept with too many.

Of course, double standards work both ways:

"Women who sleep around are very much put down by other women and men, but mostly put down by women. Men, on the other hand, are pressured and encouraged to sleep around." *fem, 21*

"Girls want to be on the same playing field as the boys, but when it comes to paying, asking out, approaching, calling and everything like that, a lot of girls still want the boys to be the initiator." *fem, 22*

"Girls are also calling girls sluts. We don't like to be called it ourselves, but yet we use it to put down other women. It's just a vicious cycle." *female age 22*

Our Changing Sexual Patterns

While plenty of people in their twenties still hope to have a relationship, they aren't as disposed to sit at home and masturbate until a relationship comes calling. Not all of them see sex and relationships as being joined at the hip, and for the first time that anyone can remember, it is okay for women to have sex that's totally disconnected from love or romance.

Strangely enough, this latest revolution in sex has raised the hackles of some of the people who championed the last revolution way back when. But if you really think about it, the current changes have been a reflection of the way those very people raised their children, especially their daughters, who are now of college age.

Today's young women were told by their parents they could be anything they want to be. They were raised playing baseball, basketball and soccer. They were encouraged not to feel like second-class citizens in what had been a man's world.

They were also told there's no point in burdening themselves with kids and marriages too soon.

And there were the powerful messages about sex, if not from parents, but from the media and from books like this. Those messages helped do for women in the bedroom what Title IX did for them on the playing field. What they were reading in *Cosmo* and seeing on TV since they were ten years old was that young women get just as horny as guys do and they want and deserve sex just as much. No other generation of women has been told so clearly that they should be proactive rather than passive when it comes to receiving sexual pleasure.

So we've taken away the old rules about relationships and marriage, and we've raised girls with the belief that they can do anything boys can. But when the young women take it to heart and start looking to satisfy their own sexual needs rather than being the regulators of who has sex and when, people from older generations get all pissy. Instead, they should look at how their child-rearing messages helped change the landscape of sex and dating.

A Less Significant Factor—Technology

Anticipation is often an important part of getting yourself worked up sexually. Back when your great, great, great grandparents were young and they were horny, they didn't have iPhones and they couldn't check out someone's Facebook page. They didn't even have wall phones. But that doesn't mean they didn't wait with hearts beating and in intense anticipation. But what they were waiting for wasn't a text message or a phone call. It was a letter. A letter that would often arrive by Pony Express.

Today, people wait with as much anticipation. But as technology has changed, so have our expectations. Where the window of anticipation might

have been two weeks in the days of Pony Express, it might be only two minutes or two hours in the day of Tweets. We're probably talking the same
amount of sexual tension, but highly compressed due to the change in anticipation. (Imagine waiting two weeks for someone to return a text message?)

And what about the hooking-up that goes on via Craigslist> Personals>
NSA? Pretty much the express highway to booty heaven if you are a woman,
although at least at a bar WYSIWYG.

Technology also comes into play when you are checking out potential
hook-ups at a crowded place. You can snap a picture of them with your cell-
phone as you give them your contact info. That way, if you get a booty call
four hours later, or the next week, you'll at least know what the person looks
like if there are a bunch of people in the room when you arrive!

What This Chapter Has Left Out

This chapter did not explore drinking among people who hook up for
sex in a greater context than just the sex. But this comment from one of the
women who took our survey suggests there is more to it:

> "Alcohol is a big part of my life as a college student. I know it sounds
> like a crutch, but on the weekends, everyone I know is drinking."
>
> *female age 21*

While not outright avoiding it, this chapter has not exactly stared the
deeper motivations of people who are hooking-up in the eye. For the guys,
there appears to be a combination of motivators. There's the fact that a warm
and wet vagina feels a lot better on your penis than your cold rough hand.
There's also the little problem that if they don't have sex, their friends might
wonder if they are gay. And there also seems to be a sport-fucking culture
that's not unlike the men's sporting culture in the middle of the 1800s when
there were whorehouses on every corner.

There's also the fact that guys get just as lonely as girls do, and they need
to be held and touched. But it's not always easy to admit that, and hooking-
up sex is a way for it to happen without feeling too vulnerable or trapped.
This is just speculation, and hopefully by the time the next edition is ready
we'll have heard from young men who are having hooking-up sex.

As for women, the changes that are represented by hooking-up sex are
far greater than for men. It's hard to think of a time that was similar in our

country's history, when a woman could pick up a guy in a bar for sex for her own gratification.

What are women's motivations? Are they afraid of being trapped in a suffocating relationship? Does hooking-up sex give a sense of being desirable and powerful? Does it have something to do with their culture of friends? (The appeal of "Sex & The City" was always the relationship between the women, rather than their hook-ups with men. But the hook-ups with men always gave them something to talk about.)

And maybe it's a normal form of curiosity for a woman to want to feel what different guys are like in bed—one that most women have not been allowed free rein to act upon until now.

Will the next generation of young women need to be drunk before having hooking-up sex? Or will whatever stigma and inner voices that they need to quiet with alcohol be long gone, the result of having been raised by mothers who were hooking-up themselves and had a better understanding of the experience. Will the sexual playing field between men and women be even more level in twenty more years?

Hooking-Up Babies and Birth Control

A college instructor who uses *The Guide* in her sex-ed course recently sent in the following regarding what she's heard from her students:

> "I don't know if you are currently engaged in any work regarding the use of the morning-after pill and abortions as birth-control measures... The young women often hook up with guys they know and have unprotected sex. Their doctors prescribe them three months' worth of morning-after pills. Some of the young women use the pills as many as three times in a month. I am not certain what impact this type of use may have on their bodies. Additionally, some of the girls admitted to psychological challenges following the abortions."

It's one thing to blame what you did last night on alcohol, but it's quite another to be having hooking-up sex and not have sound birth-control strategy in place.

While men and women should both be responsible for birth control, we do know of at least two hooking-up-sex babies whose hooking-up dads are paying child support and will continue to for the next 18 years.

Today's women might not be birth-control fanatics, but few are going to bear the burden of raising a baby for the next 18 years and not go after the father for child support—which is not a difficult thing to prove with a simple DNA test.

Absorption and Assimilation

As you will see in the chapter on *Sex in the 1800s*, what people today refer to as "traditional dating" was not always traditional. Dating as we know it took shape as America took shape. It molded itself around the social changes that coincided with industrialization and leaps in technology.

Like the *sporting culture* of the 1800s, the *flappers* of the 1920s and the *sexual revolution* of the 1960s, hooking-up sex won't be sensational for long. But it won't go away either. It is helping to change sex and dating.

More Responses From Our Female Survey Takers

"For me hook-up sex is not as great as sex in a relationship. Hook-up sex can be somewhat uncomfortable or awkward. You don't know what to expect with this person, what they expect, or if the sex was bad. There is some excitement and adrenaline rush in hook-up sex, but there is a great amount of excitement in a relationship. You know what the person likes, or what they are willingly to try, and you know their comfort levels."

"If you go into it knowing that it is just going to be a one-night stand then it is satisfying. If there was supposed to be more and there ends up not being anything else, then it is disappointing."

"I absolutely still see relationships as a goal, but if you aren't getting anywhere near finding someone to meet your goal it becomes repetitious and you get bored, so why not have fun until you find your goal?"

"I think that guys look at girls who sleep with them early in the relationship as slutty. If you sleep with a guy before you really know him he assumes that you do this with everyone. He is not considered unfit because of the double standard. It doesn't matter how many girls a guy has slept with but it does matter how many guys a girl has slept with."

"Hook-up sex cannot be with a guy you are wanting a relationship with. It has to be just for the sex."

"I haven't met many men who don't want sex right away."

"If I am at a party and meet a guy and I really like him and we start fooling around and he calls the next day well then great, let's hang out, but not because we fucked, but because I liked hanging out with him. It's always a scary possibility that you get into a relationship and not have sex in the beginning and when you finally do, your lover is horrible, when then you're stuck in a bad-sex relationship and if we're being honest, sex is a huge part. For me, I like to meet the guy first, enjoy being with him and then sleep together, as scary as that is, because I don't really like to sleep with people without knowing them if I am trying to invest time and a relationship in them."

"To me hooking up/one nighters are just that... one nighters. Generally there are no feelings towards the other person. If you're horny one night then you call them up and have sex and that's about it. Alcohol is a huge factor in having sex with no strings attached. More than likely we will both be drinking with the same people at the same bar and then one thing leads to another and we are having sex."

"I know people that were friends with their significant other and then started having sex. I also know people who have sex and then a relationship happens. I have tried both. I can't tell you which one is better. They both worked for me. I think it depends on the chemistry and how the two of you are."

A Very Special Thanks to Dr. Dennis Waskul and his students at Minnesota State University, Mankato, to Heather Flores, M.S., Madera and Clovis Community College Centers, California, and to Abigail Nitzel and Dr. Joan Chrisler of Connecticut College for some of the most thoughtful and clearly best research done on Hooking-Up ("Hooking-Up versus Dating").

CHAPTER

68
Dirty Word Chapter

You might be wondering why a chapter on dirty words would be in such a fine and upstanding book. Perhaps there is more to this chapter than just dirty words. Whether you agree with these observations about sexual slang is not the point. This chapter, like all of the others in this book, was written to encourage you to think.

Hans, Sven & Yellow Snow

We at Goofy Foot Press probably use the word "fuck" more times each day than the Pope says Amen. The sad thing is, we mainly use our fucks to express anger or frustration. Seldom do we use them in the fun way. This is often the case with sexual slang here in America, where swear words and sex words are often the same.

"Fuck" as an expression of anger or despair is such an integral part of our language that we have created more acceptable ways of saying it, such as "friggin'" or "frackin'" (as is used on TV's *Battlestar Gallactica*).

While people who use fuck-slang aren't always aware of the sexual connection, there's no way a phrase like "Oh no, we just entered a frackin' Cylon Battle Zone!" has any power without its connection to sex.

In Sweden, a culture that is more sex-friendly than our own, sexual slang is not usually used to express anger or frustration. If Sven or Hans are really annoyed, they are more likely to yell something about yellow snow than sex. Even our own Pueblo Indians had no history of using sexual slang for hurling insults. If a Pueblo Indian was really bent out of shape, he or she might have implied that the offending party was a lousy farmer or kept a sloppy wigwam. But then again, the Pueblos had a less repressive attitude about sex than some of our forefathers.

Calling People by the Female Genitals

Back when he was a kid, the worst thing your author knew to call another person was a "cunt." He never could bring himself to use the word, but then again, he had yet to work with anyone in the entertainment industry.

Another slang word that kids often use is "pussy." While pussy is a term that refers to the female genitals, it is also an expression that boys use to taunt other boys who are being wimps, cowards or who are using good sense.

Why does our culture associate cowardice with being a woman or having a woman's genitals? And why would we want to discredit the very female genitals that so many of us craved (and still crave) to touch and know more about? What kind of number is our culture doing on us, anyway?

Mother-Fucking, Titty-Sucking, Blue-Balled What?

A researcher by the name of Warren Johnson studied how normal eight-year-old boys and girls use slang. According to Johnson, the children's favorite expression when out of parental earshot was "mother-fucking, titty-sucking, blue-balled bitch." Johnson hadn't expected to find America's eight-year-old children capable of outswearing his former Marine troop.

Of particular interest is Johnson's observation of an eight-year-old girl yelling "Suck my dick!" to another child who was annoying her. As long as she was going to use sexual slang for swearing, why didn't the little girl yell the more anatomically correct "Eat my pussy!"? Perhaps even an eight-year-old child knows that the way to insult someone in our society is to tell them to take the woman's place in a sexual act, with terms such as "You cocksucker!" and "Screw you!" being crude ways of saying, "You're the woman in sex!"

It is difficult to understand how something as sweet and delicious as sex could be linked to anger or frustration, unless you haven't gotten any in a coon's age. It is equally difficult to understand why being the woman in sex is a put-down. Yet these are the premises about sex that we Norte del Americanos grow up with.

When Eight Turns Eighteen

What's going to happen when the little girl who yelled "suck my dick" gets older and wants to share sex with a boy? How is she supposed to enjoy performing the very insults that our society has taught her to hurl at others? Is she going to require the young man to swear undying adoration before she blows him? Will she use sex as a commodity, weapon, or way of achieving security? Will she turn men into sex objects? Worst of all, will she pretend that giving a blowjob isn't really sex?

Equally disconcerting is what this attitude does to boys. The message is that you either screw or get screwed, the former being associated with winning, the latter with losing. This turns sex into a performance or competition.

Sluts, Whores, Virginity & Sewers

Western religions have never done well with the notion of women and sexuality. For instance, early Christians taught that a virgin daughter occupied a higher place in heaven than her mother, since the mother had sex for the daughter to have been born. And around 400 A.D., Christianity's St. Jerome wrote, "Though God can do all things, He cannot raise a virgin after she has fallen" (Epistles 22). Not even God can help you when you lose your virginity, if you are a woman anyway. It's never been a problem for men, but then again, men are the ones who wrote the scriptures. (You don't have to be religious to know that when a boy has intercourse for the first time, he becomes a man. Yet a girl who has intercourse loses her virginity and is no longer pure as the driven snow, assuming she was in the first place.)

Rigid as St. Jerome may have been about women's virginity, he was quite the feminist compared to some of his Christian and Jewish predecessors. For instance, one early church father described woman as "a temple built over a sewer," with sewer referring to her genitals. Men who made statements like these were later declared saints.

Perhaps it's no coincidence that many women who are unable to have orgasms were raised in households where the temple/sewer notion still holds sway.

To this day people still equate a woman's personal reputation with her appetite for sex: if her sex drive is too low, she is cold or frigid; too high and the sewer floods the temple, and she is easy, a slut, whore, ho, or nympho. While young men are free to strut their sexuality, young women learn to carefully regulate theirs. Otherwise, they risk being called dirty words.

Note Contrary to what makes sense, women are often the first to accuse other women of being sluts or whores. Men may have been the bozos who wrote the anti-woman theology, but women can be its cruelest enforcers. Also, scripture tells us that the man from Nazareth was loving and respectful to women. Why did the church fathers who followed him have so many problems with this? If the human body was made in the image and likeness of God, as scripture says, why were church leaders so rejecting of women's genitals and sexuality? Had God been drinking the day He crafted the clitoris and vagina?

Dicks, Pricks & Morons

Why do we refer to a person who is being a total jerk as a "dick" or "prick"? A dick should be someone who brings pleasure, but that is not what our culture teaches us.

For instance, adults will praise a young boy for his latest drawing or for making it to the toilet on time, but if he proudly displays his pint-sized boner, throats get cleared. Boys in our society are encouraged to spend eons learning how to make a baseline jump shot or to hit an A-minor flat nine on a guitar, yet they are taught to ignore their own sexuality in hopes that it will simply go away until they get older. Maybe that's why many of us grow up having more sensitivity for what happens in music, art, or sports than for what happens in bed.

Power-Booting & Name-Calling at Dartmouth

While our culture encourages its straight men to strut their sexuality, this doesn't mean we always do. For instance, the following story tells of how the term "faggot" is used by straight guys to deride other straight guys for preferring women to beer. It is from Regina Barreca's *They Used to Call Me Snow White But Then I Drifted,* Viking/Penguin:

> "When I started my first year as a student at Dartmouth College, there were four men for every woman. I thought I had it made. Dartmouth had only recently admitted women, and the administration thought it best to get the alumni accustomed to the idea by sneaking us in a few at a time. With such terrific odds in my favor socially, how could I lose? I'd dated in high school and although I wasn't exactly Miss Budweiser, I figured I'd have no problem getting a date every Saturday night. But I noticed an unnerving pattern. I'd meet a cute guy at a party and talk for a while. We would then be interrupted by some buddy of his who would drag him off to another room to watch a friend of theirs "power-boot" (the local vernacular for 'projectile vomiting'), and I realized that the social situation was not what I had expected.

Then somebody explained to me that on the Dartmouth campus they think you're a faggot if you like women more than beer. This statement indicated by its very vocabulary the advanced nature of the sentiment behind it. If a guy said he wanted to spend the weekend with his girl-friend, for example, he'd be taunted by his pals, who would yell in beery bass voices 'Whatsa matter with you, Skip? We're gonna get plowed, absolutely blind this weekend, then we're all gonna power-boot. And you wanna see that broad again? Whaddayou, a faggot or something?'"

While many boys who end up at colleges like Dartmouth have inter-course by the age of 16, a fair number remain crude in their ability to respect their sexual partners or see them as friends. While they may be coordinated enough to guide a penis into a vagina, on an emotional level some still belong in the arms of their drinking buddies. Equally puzzling are the young women who agree to have sex with these emotional giants.

Sexuality here in America remains a confusing entity. A "just say no" mentality thrives in a culture that uses sex to advertise and sell everything from soap to beer. As a result, there are times when we flaunt our sexuality, and other times when we deny it completely.

Bitch vs. Faggot

While the dirty words aimed at women often speak to how they regu-late the space between their legs, it's almost always assumed that women are heterosexual. A woman is more often called a "bitch" than a "dyke."

Insults at men are aimed at a different level. Guys are forever needing to demonstrate manliness. If we slip up, we're called a faggot or queer, even if the only dick we've ever held is our own. This is particularly true among teenagers. A knee-jerk response that teenage boys have whenever another boy steps outside of the fragile notion of what's considered masculine is to call him a "fag."

On the surface, the insults for men and women have the same premise: each likes dick too much. But a woman who is being insulted is usually al-lowed to remain heterosexual, albeit a slutty one. The guy, however, has his sexual identity called into question.

A woman is usually considered to be heterosexual to the core, while a man's heterosexual status is something that knows no rest. It has to be earned and re-earned or he risks falling off the stilts that define him as straight.

Origin of the Bimbo & the Stud

"Bimbo" and "stud" aren't dirty words *per se*. But they achieve dirty-word status when you consider the following observation made by a female friend of the author who was sitting on the beach:

> A father was standing a few feet into the surf with a young boy on his right side and a young girl on his left. The children were the same size. Whenever a wave came in the father would keep his right arm rigid. This helped the boy brave the oncoming splash. At the same time, the father would lift his left arm, pulling the girl into the air so she could avoid the splash. The little boy was being taught how to face the wave; the little girl was being taught to expect a man to rescue her.

Bimbo training starts early in our country. All too often, the first step is getting little girls to believe that they are more fragile than boys. Then, ads in women's magazines spawn the belief that there is something unsexy about the female body unless it's plugged with a scented tampon and accessorized with perfume, high heels and fake boobs.

Seldom does our society encourage boys and girls to value and respect each other for their strength. More often, boys are taught to protect girls because the latter are supposed to be weak, while many girls still believe that their worth is determined by the desirability of the boys they date.

Blowjobs & Bounced Checks

Consider the following words of a modern American wife:

> "My husband's going to be furious when he finds out about the check I bounced, so I better give him a really good blowjob tonight."

As you will discover in the chapters that follow, this book has no problem with really good blowjobs, but not when they are motivated by fear, lack of power, or crass manipulation.

Note After this was first published, protests from female readers flooded in, e.g. trading blowjobs for money is one of the few ways that women have had throughout the ages to even the score economically; trading sex for money brings far more joy into the world and is less destructive than the ways that many men earn their paychecks; and what about the possibility that the above-mentioned housewife finds the situation to be a sexual turn-on and might totally enjoy giving the payback blowjob?

Rearranging the Bed Sheets on the Titanic with "Foreplay"

The term "foreplay" was invented by people who write books on sex. Foreplay is what you are supposed to do to get a woman wet enough so the two of you can have intercourse. It may seem strange that this book considers foreplay to be a dirty word, since caring guys are usually encouraged to embrace the concept. Yet there is nothing caring about the underlying premise of foreplay: that women are somehow a little retarded and need to be warmed up before they want to become sexual. Shoot, you have to warm up the old Ford on cold days, so why not the woman you love?

Most sex books forget to mention that a woman who is masturbating can get herself off just as fast or slow as a man. Perhaps the problem isn't that women have a slower warm-up time, as the notion of foreplay seems to imply. Perhaps the real problem is our culture's concept of sexuality, where being a woman (e.g. getting fucked) is a common insult, where "scoring" makes a boy feel like a man, and where respect, friendship and caring are not necessary conditions for sex.

The concept of foreplay implies that tenderness is little more than a tollbooth on the highway to intercourse. Hopefully you will appreciate that tender kisses and caresses do not need to be trailed by intercourse to justify their importance or necessity. They are as important as intercourse, if not more so.

If you can't get past the notion of foreplay, try to think of it as everything that's happened between you and your partner since the last time you had sex. How you treat each other with your clothes on has more impact on what happens in bed than carefully planted kisses minutes before intercourse. This is just as true for the way that women treat men as for how men treat women.

Why Even Care?

Studs, bimbos, bounced checks—why even care? How can you not care? These are the myths about each other that we take to bed with us. They're what gets in the way.

Notes Regarding the wigwam comment at the start of the chapter, Pueblo Indians don't really live in wigwams. Their homes are either adobe/stone pueblos or caves. Unfortunately, life on the reservation has not been good to the sexual habits of the Pueblo, and incidents of rape are now being reported. • There are certainly times when fuck-slang is used in a positive sense, as in "fuckin' wonderful" or "fuckin' amazing." But when the word is used this way it tends to be role-neutral and refers to the act of intercourse rather than the woman's role in it. When it takes its more usual form of "We're totally fucked now!" it's got "girl" all over it. As for the idea that the insult gets its grit from the homosexual implication, we have plenty of insults in our culture for that and few people hesitate to use them when that's what they mean to say. • Did the little girl mentioned earlier in this chapter actually understand the premise of the slang phrase "suck my dick" or was she simply mimicking the correct social usage? Does it matter? Is there any difference in the long run?

Special thanks to the writings of Ira Reiss, Paul Evdokimov, David Schnarch, Regina Barreca, Carol Tavris, the late Bob Stoller, and many others for inspiring concepts used in this chapter. Thanks also to Paul Kroskrity, anthropology professor at UCLA, for the information about the Pueblos. And finally, thanks to the famous sex researchers who originally suggested that people should think of foreplay as everything that happened since the last time you had sex. Perhaps giving foreplay a name was an improvement over what had come before, or so it is said.

69
Barbie the Icon

This chapter is about Barbie. You might be wondering what a cultural icon like Barbie is doing in a book on sex. Perhaps the following statements by our female readers will help explain:

When you were a little girl, did your Barbie doll ever have sex?

"I had lots of Barbies. She and my giant panda bear got naked and 'did it,' and my sister and I dressed her up in Ken's clothes. Unfortunately, you can't dress up Ken in Barbie's clothes. We tried." *female age 18*

"My basement was a temple to Barbie and all her relatives. Barbie lived in a soap opera complete with abortions, sex changes, and adultery. She and Ken frequently got naked in their Laura Ashley canopy bed." *female age 24*

"Barbie and Ken had a very active relationship and 'sex' life. It's hard to say it was a sex life without any genitalia. I guess I used them to emulate the adults around me. Barbie and Ken often went skinny dipping at the ocean, and slept nude most times." *female age 35*

"My Barbie had Ken on her ALL the time. If I knew then what I know now, Barbie would have been on top more often." *female age 44*

"My friend had a Ken and we used to make them have sex by making their little plastic bodies rub against each other when they were lying in Barbie's little nylon bed. We were about ten and were disappointed that Ken's underwear was glued on." *female age 22*

"You know those parts in movies that parents were always trying to hide from younger children? I got a slight peek one day, but all I saw were sheets moving. After I saw that, Barbie and Ken made those sounds and simulated those actions. But I wasn't sure what they were really doing." *female age 22*

"She had kinky fantasies and a lot of BDSM. Barbie was a fun girl."
female age 18

"Not Barbies but definitely with my Lego men. Don't ask me why, but those spacemen certainly had interesting encounters when I sent them on missions. I was pretty inventive for a 7-year-old."

female age 19

While these women's experiences by no means represent that of most girls, it is likely they represent a significant number. (See more reader comments on their Barbie's sex life at the end of the chapter.)

Eleven Inches of Attitude

The year was 1959. The place was the Toy Fair in New York that's held every February. Mattel's new toy named Barbie was falling flat on her face, or would have if such a thing had been anatomically possible.

Since the beginning of time, toy buyers in America have placed orders for their Christmas inventory at the annual Toy Fair. It is the moment that determines which toys make it to toy-store shelves the following Christmas, and Barbie was getting the cold shoulder.

This was nearly fifty years ago, and the radical new doll named Barbie was shattering everyone's idea of what a child's toy should be. The price she paid for her uniqueness was to be ignored by toy buyers. Buyers for toy stores in 1959 were placing orders for dolls that were soft and huggable, dolls whose souls were made from rags.

Believe it or not, Barbie was cloned from a mother doll named Lilli who was made in Germany. In the late 1950s, Lilli caught the eye of Ruth Handler, co-founder of the Mattel toy company. Lilli was a sexpot of a doll who was marketed to horny German males. She looked like a German streetwalker. Lilli had been adapted from an adult comic strip where she had been a comical gold-digger and barfly.

Both Barbie and Lilli were 11 inches tall. The apples did not fall far from the tree when it came to looks, but Ms. Handler made sure that Barbie was born into an entirely different social class. Lilli was more like Anna Nicole Smith, while Barbie was Jackie Kennedy. Interestingly, Barbie's place of birth (at least the address of Mattel) was Hawthorne, California, the same city where America's other sex idol, Marilyn Monroe, was born.

Large Breasts and No Panties

In 1959, toy-store buyers wanted what they knew—dolls that reflected our society's idea of what a good girl should be and what she would hopefully become: a selfless mother, teacher, housewife, or nurse. They didn't get it when they saw Barbie, a doll who has been described by author Christopher Varaste as:

> "An 11½ inch glamour queen with exotic features in a striking black and white swimsuit. She was everyone and defiantly no one. She seemed ageless, though she was supposed to be a teenager. She was beguiling, mysterious, and yet innocent. She was a symbol of a culture struggling to find a suitable identity. As a toy for young girls, her rather severe look took some getting used to. Her Asian eyes, curly bangs, and big red lips could have belonged to a wide range of ethnic backgrounds. She was, in a word, peculiar." (From Christopher Varaste's incredible book of Barbie photographs *Face of the American Dream–Barbie Doll, 1959 - 1971*)

If it hadn't been for a stroke of marketing genius, Barbie would have gone down in flames. But Mattel's strategy for selling Barbie to the American public was as unique as their product. They were one of the first companies in history to make TV commercials that were aimed at children viewers.

From the very first commercial, Barbie was portrayed as a human with a glamorous and adventurous life. She was never described as a doll and she was never burdened with trivial limitations such as parents or a husband.

Mattel aired their first Barbie commercial during the wildly popular *Mickey Mouse Club* TV show. If parents didn't know what to make of Barbie, their American daughters certainly did. Once the summer of 1959 started, every Barbie in every toy store was bought as quickly as it arrived.

Barbie's official name was Barbie Millicent Roberts. When Ken was created a few years later, his name was Ken Carson. It is fitting and telling that Barbie and Ken's namesake was Carson/Roberts. Carson/Roberts was the advertising company that played such a dramatic role in Barbie's success.

Not Your Normal Housewife

Barbie's persona was created by two women who had both violated the housewife norm of the 1950s. One had co-founded a large corporation, the other was a tall, striking, unmarried veteran of the fashion industry. Unlike any doll before her, Barbie was created as a young woman whose life didn't revolve around a husband and a family. Her limitations were as thin as her waist and her possibilities as large as her breasts.

Early in Barbie's evolution, someone wanted to make a miniature vacuum cleaner that Barbie could use to vacuum the house. But Ruth Handler, Mattel's co-founder, refused to allow this. During the era when Barbie was born, it was automatically assumed that a woman's role was to be a housewife and raise babies. Keeping Barbie vacuum-cleaner-free was an important statement to little girls. It was a signal that they could exceed the boundaries that our culture had traditionally placed on them.

Barbie Is Nobody's Wife

Islamic leaders in Iran have described Barbie as being Satanic. They have expressed concerns that "the unwholesome flexibility of these dolls, their destructive beauty, and their semi-nudity have an effect on the minds and morality of young children." Plenty of American parents have felt the same.

However, if you read Mattel's press releases for Barbie, you'll see that when she dresses to the nines, it's not to capture the gaze of a guy or even a girl. Mattel's Barbie dresses for Barbie. She has no need to please anyone but herself. This is one of the many Barbie qualities that throws feminists for a loop: they detest the emphasis on glamour, yet no one can ever accuse Barbie of coddling to the whims of a man. The Barbie that Ruth Handler created doesn't care if she goes home alone and she doesn't need the approval of a male to make her feel good about herself. That's been as much a part of her message to little girls as the big boobs and tiny waist.

Here's another part of the Barbie mystique that upsets feminists: Barbie succeeds and succeeds well in traditional male professions. But whether she's being a firefighter or a physician, an astronaut or a police detective, Barbie always pulls it off with her femininity fully intact. Some women have said this sets an impossible standard for little girls, but it also tells little girls that you don't have to grow balls to have balls. Barbie has shown little girls that they don't have to surrender the things that they like about their femininity to compete in a man's world. Barbie has provided a way for little girls to experiment with the positive messages their parents and teachers are hopefully giving them. She also provides a way for little girls to be selfish and mean, as all children can be.

Mattel's Barbie has come with so few of the traditional limitations that any little girl can make her do and be anything she wants.

Less Fighting, Better Play?

Researchers have studied what types of play lead to more bickering and what kinds lead to less. One thing they didn't expect to find was that girls who are playing with Barbie dolls tend to fight less and display more advanced levels of play than girls who are playing with traditional dolls. The range of activities that Barbie play provides is much greater than a doll that you simply hold, feed, and change. Barbie has friends, activities, and a whole life that's as expansive as her different outfits and hairstyles. In addition, Barbie's presence invites the involvement of mothers, aunts, gay uncles, and even grandmothers who had their own Barbies when they were growing up.

Barbie was never intended to be the *Leap Frog* or *Hooked On Phonics* of children's play. The fact that Barbie inspires a high quality of play and better language development was not Mattel's goal. Mattel's emphasis has been for people to buy more Barbies and especially more Barbie accessories, perhaps in the same way that companies who make computer printers hope to nail you for the cost of the pricey replacement ink cartridges. It is fascinating how Mattel has managed to achieve this goal without limiting the persona of Barbie.

For instance, Mattel has never married off Barbie. Yet Mattel has sold millions of Barbie wedding dresses and thousands of Dream-Bride Barbies or Wedding-Fantasy Barbies. The hitch has been that the wedding idea is all just a big Barbie dream or fantasy. Keeping Barbie from really being married allows little girls to marry and unmarry her as often as they desire. Being perpetually single keeps Barbie footloose and fancy-free.

Mattel never wanted Barbie to be pregnant, but plenty of children wanted her to have a baby. So they devised a "Barbie Baby-Sits" kit which contained an infant and other childcare objects.

As much as Barbie has been associated with fashion and glamour, Barbie has never defined fashion nor been at the cutting edge. She has always been a year or two behind, like most women who can't afford this year's originals.

Keeping Barbie a Moving Target

Few people will dispute that Barbie has become an American icon. Given her iconic status, you would think she would appear the same today as she was in 1959. But since the very beginning, Mattel has made Barbie change and evolve. Some of these changes have been technological, like using different vinyls, skin tones, and hair. Other changes have been purely stylistic.

Barbie's face has changed as well. The first Barbie's face was a combination of her harsh-looking German mother and the Geishas of Japan, the country that first manufactured and helped to refine her. You can also see how the vinyl used in the #5 Ponytail Barbie of 1961 contained an oily compound that makes her look like she has a greasy face or is perspiring. Unfortunately, the more recent Barbies have been given a bubbly, wide-eyed generic smile rather than the more intriguing streetwalker-Geisha expression of the early years. The faces on the early Barbies were all hand-painted in Japan, while the latter ones are machine stenciled.

Barbie Torture Sessions

A study by Tara Kuther of Western Connecticut State titled "Early Adolescents' experiences with, and Views of, Barbie" clearly echoes our own readers' experiences with Barbie. When Kuther interviewed 10 to 13 year old children about Barbie, she found reports of frequent Barbie torture sessions. These included seeing if Barbie can successfully fly out of a second-story window, cutting Barbie's hair off and burning her clothes because she talked too much, making her dress up as a GI Joe, tearing off her head, drowning her at sea, melting her in a microwave, burning her at the stake upside down and attaching explosives to her.

We welcome these enterprising middle schoolers as future readers of the *Guide To Getting It On!*

A Cock-Ring Ken?

Ken was an afterthought to Barbie. He was released in answer to the demand for a Barbie boyfriend, but he was always expendable.

When Ken was being conceived, the two women who had created the persona of Barbie wanted him to have a bulge between his legs. The male executives at Mattel were horrified and embarrassed at the suggestion. They wanted Ken to have the same crotch as Barbie. The women held out and Ken got a compromise bulge, although no one would ever accuse him of holding a candle to a doll with the masculine persona of GI Joe.

In the mid-1960s, Mattel released a "Ken a Go Go" doll, where Ken played the ukulele. Not long after that, Ken was euthanized. He reappeared in 1969 with an extreme makeover that Mattel hoped would revive his dismal sales. Then, in 1993, Mattel released the truly amazing "Earring Magic Ken." This Ken was literally swept off the shelves by a stampede of adult gay males.

"Earring Magic Ken," also known as "Cock Ring Ken," was dressed in a lavender vest and had a necklace around his neck with a cock ring on it. The cock ring was not only the spitting image of the cock rings that men at gay male rages were wearing around their necks, but it was scaled to the exact dimensions as well. (It seems that someone in the design department at Mattel got one by the corporate brass.)

The more recent Kens have actually appeared as if they might be straight and even have a bit of a hunk factor. If Ken really is up for servicing Barbie, Mattel should consider making a Viagra Ken. That's because the average Ken has at least eight Barbies that he needs to put out for.

Late Breaking News—Does Ken Have Alzheimer's? Is Barbie Doing a Hunk Who Is 40 Years Younger?

At the 2004 Toy Fair, Mattel executives announced that after forty-three years together, Barbie was dumping Ken. Poor Ken: Mattel put him into assisted living. Mattel was pushing one of their newer boytoys named Blaine. Blaine looked like a Southern California mall-rat druggie. As for how well Blaine might have been equipped, in one of his earlier packagings he was holding an electric guitar with a neck that was so long it was at least the equivalent of a nine-inch penis. Blaine came out like a lion, racking up respectable sales, but he had absolutely no staying power. You will be hard pressed to find him anymore.

By 2007, Mattel announced they were bringing Ken out of retirement. What the heck, with Viagra and all... The new Ken had obviously received a great deal of reparative therapy, as he had a radical new hairdo, a more manly face, and he screamed "I'm straight." But as of early 2009, you'd be hard-pressed to find the new Ken anywhere. While you could pick up a "Fashion Fever Ken" as late as August of 2008 at Target, he was no where to be found as of presstime. Is it possible that Ken had a reparative-therapy relapse, and he and Blaine hooked-up?

Note: Just as Barbie's boys have been seriously fey, their accessories have often been quite phallic. Ken's cookout set has a long fork that is skewering a big pink weenie, his hunting outfit has a massive rifle, and his baseball outfit includes a really long bat.

Mattel Misses the Muslim Market, But Nails India

With the highly successful release of Fulla, a Middle East knockoff of Barbie, it's clear that Mattel missed what could have been a lucrative opportunity in the Muslim world. Fulla is a fine Muslim doll of Barbie proportions who comes in a bright pink box with her own prayer mat and a black abaya and headscarf. Fulla is selling like gangbusters in the Middle East.

We at Goofy Foot Press are, however, the proud owners of a Barbie in India doll. The Indian Barbie comes wearing a colorful saree and ethnic jewelry. Better yet, she has a bindi, which is the traditional red spot between her eyes. We haven't undressed her to she if she might have a bindi between her gravity-defying breasts as well, but we're sure millions of Indian kids have.

Parents & Barbie

What follows is the ultimate discussion of Barbie by the parents of a young girl. It is from Margaret Atwood's piece *The Female Body:*

> He said, I won't have one of those things around the house. It gives a young girl a false notion of beauty, not to mention anatomy. If a real woman was built like that, she'd fall flat on her face.

> She said, If we don't let her have one like all the other girls she'll feel singled out. It'll become an issue. She'll long for one and she'll long to turn into one. Repression breeds sublimation. You know that.

> He said, It's not just the pointy plastic tits, it's the wardrobes. The wardrobes and that stupid male doll, what's his name, the one with the underwear glued on.

> She said, Better to get it over with when she's young.

> He said, All right, but don't let me see it.

> She came whizzing down the stairs, thrown like a dart. She was stark naked. Her hair had been chopped off, her head was turned back to front, she was missing some toes, and she'd been tattooed all over her body with purple ink, in a scrollwork design. She hit the potted azalea, trembled there for a moment like a botched angel, and fell.

> He said, I guess we're safe.

> *The Female Body* by Margaret Atwood, originally printed in Vol. XXIX, No. 4, Fall 1990 issue of *Michigan Quarterly Review*, edited by Laurence Goldstein.

Excellent Resources: This discussion of Barbie has provided only a small sketch of the truly rich and fascinating history of this cultural icon. If it has piqued your interest, you are strongly encouraged to check out at least two excellent books on the subject. One is M.G. Lord's *Forever Barbie—The Unauthorized Biography of a Real Doll, 1994/1995,* Avon Books. One of Lord's many fine observations can be found in her discussion of Barbie's friend, Midge: "If plastic dolls could kill themselves, I'm sure Midge would have tried." Talk about having to spend your entire life playing second fiddle!

Regarding the second highly recommended book, *Face of the American Dream, Barbie Doll (1959-1971)* by Christopher Varaste, Hobby House Press, (1999), who knew that photos of the early Barbie could be so fascinating and compelling? Barbie's face and expression during this period was much more interesting than now, and Varaste does an exceptional job of capturing it.

Reader's Comments

"Ways Barbie impacted my femininity? She made me hate clothes."
female age 21

"Ways Barbie impacted my femininity? I dress better now."
female age 20

"My sister and I were a little obsessed with Barbie. We turned old dressers and coffee tables into Barbie mansions. I played with Barbie from the time I was 4 until I was 11 or 12. I'm not sure when Barbie and Ken started having sex (they weren't just sleeping in the same bed), maybe when I was 7, that's when I learned what intercourse involved. Mostly, I got the dolls undressed, put them in bed and twisted their bodies back and forth. They couldn't really do anything since Barbie didn't have a vagina and Ken didn't have a penis. However, once Barbie and Ken started having sex, they never stopped. Every night. That's how I thought it was done, only at night, only in bed. Several Barbies went through a sex change. I got her ready for the operation (remember Dr. Barbie?), wheeled her into the operating room, and when she came out, she'd been replaced with a Ken doll. All of Barbie's friends talked about her behind her back when she got the change–her mother (grandma Barbie) had a hard time coping. I'm being glib, but I did act all of this out. My Barbies had detailed conversations, had intimate family lives, detailed jobs, etc. There was a lot of adultery in Barbie's world which resulted in divorces, private investigators, and alcoholism. All the adultery was acted out in full detail, from Ken coming on to his secretary at work to the act itself to Barbie throwing all of Ken's clothes out the window... Barbie helped me act out my own questions about being an adult. I'm a feminist now, I have a healthy relationship, earn more than my spouse, don't wear make-up or high-heeled shoes, and my husband helps with all the housework. It's okay to let little girls play with Barbie." *female age 24*

"Ways Barbie impacted your femininity and/or sexuality: There was one summer when I was fairly obsessed with the fact that Ken had no dick. Beach Ken had a totally inaccurately placed suggestion of one, but no balls." *female age 21*

"My cousin and I were addicted to our Barbies, from as early as I can remember. I think I was 7 or 8 when our Barbies started having all sorts of high-drama romances, and there were ALL SORTS of different sexual experiences going on. My cousin and I were very creative with our Barbies' sexual escapades. I remember mine even having some homosexual experiences, which my cousin thought was weird. I actually think that my Barbies were a big outlet for my sexual curiosity growing up. When I was a teenager and no longer played with Barbies, I wondered if maybe it was odd that I made my Barbies have all sorts of sexual experiences when I was so young. But as I've gotten older, I've realized that sexually, I'm a very open and curious person, and I think it's just that I've always been that way. When I played with Barbies with my cousin though, I almost always had to play Ken. I find myself now very comfortable filling a lot of traditionally masculine roles in my relationships. The two may or may not be related." *female age 22*

"Ugh, as much as I hate to admit it, yes, my Barbies had sex. And since I also had a twelve-inch Luke Skywalker doll, they did it A LOT. I also played with a girlfriend at the time. We did sex play with our dolls."
female age 34

CHAPTER

70
The Historical Breast & Bra

An early reader of this chapter said, "I'd rather be flogged with my Wonderbra than do a boring chapter on bras and breasts. I'm going straight to Chapter 19 where I can learn how to give a better blow-job." Imagine that, a woman who takes her Wonderbra for granted! Before the 1920s, women were skeptical about bras. They preferred to wear corsets. As for bras being thought of as cute or sexy, that wouldn't happen until World War II.

There's hardly a woman in Western culture who doesn't have a bunch of bras, including a favorite one or two that she wears when she wants to feel extra sexy. She can also make a sexual statement by not wearing a bra. And what teenage boy doesn't equate success in dating with whether a girl let him put his hand under her bra?

This chapter looks at breasts and the bras that hold them up. It begins with a peek at breasts in different times and different places. It then focuses on the fascinating evolution of the bra: how it came to be in 1860, and how it eventually came to have a sexual edge.

The Ups and Downs of the French Breast

In the time of Renaissance France, it was believed that breast milk was made from blood that flowed from the vagina. This notion was handed down from the ancient Greeks, with Leonardo DiVinci eventually making a diagram of it (as shown here by our own Daerick DiVinci). Since it was assumed that breast milk rose up from the vagina, intercourse was thought

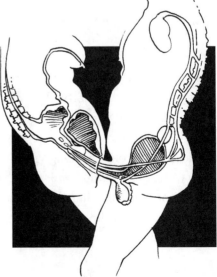

to curdle the breast-milk supply. Perhaps the French believed that a penis going in and out of a vagina was like a paddle churning buttermilk. Women who were nursing babies were not supposed to have intercourse.

Given that upper-class French women would rather have sex than nurse babies, the nursing job was pawned off on the women of the lower class. This caused there to be a distinction between the breasts of the lower class and those of the upper class. Breasts of the lower class were expected to be large and lactating, while upper-class breasts were expected to be small and perky. (They must have assumed that poor women didn't like sex, so their supply of milk was safe.)

Before the revolution, women used the same kind of makeup on their breasts as they used on their faces. The goal was to make their breasts look exceptionally white. Older women would paint blue veins on their breasts to make them look like the more transparent skin of the younger girls. Unfortunately, the makeup they used on their faces and breasts was a compound that contained lead. Not only did it corrode the skin but it contributed to cases of lead poisoning. Not to be outdone by their sisters from the past, today's runway models sometimes paint nail polish on their erect nipples as a way of keeping them erect.

In time and with the coming of the French Revolution, the heads of many upper-class French women became separated from their perky breasts. Eventually it became not only fashionable but a sign of patriotism for all French women to nurse their babies.

Saggy and Happy in Papua

In Papua, New Guinea, grown women parade their saggy breasts with pride. It's considered a sign of childishness or immaturity for a woman in Papua to have the kind of breasts that Americans value. In fact, when ladies in Papua are getting catty, they might accuse someone of having the taut round breasts of a younger woman.

To the traditional Papuan male, the surgically stuffed breasts of American actresses would be a big waste of time and money. And the traditional Papuan woman would think to herself, "Why would a woman want to do something crazy like that to her breasts just when they were starting to sag?"

In our culture, breasts have been often been regarded as the crown jewels of feminine appeal. For whatever reason, American breasts are covered in public. But in Africa and the South Pacific, women have walked around for centuries with their breasts bare. The men in those cultures don't get much of a rise from women's breasts. Instead, it's the parts that are covered up, namely the buttocks, that the men tend to find erotic.

Imagine what a dent it would have put in the lingerie, porn and plastic-surgery businesses if women in America were always topless and breasts weren't considered sexy? The entire *Playboy* empire would have never been, and Victoria's Secret would have started with thongs instead of bras.

War Bonds and Liberty's Breasts

To see how breasts were starting to be sexualized in America, consider World War I "Liberty Bonds" posters featuring Lady Liberty.

In the first poster, Liberty is a sturdy woman with the sexual appeal of a truck driver. The only way you can tell she is a woman is by the endless yards of drapes that are covering every inch of her body except for her manly, muscled arms and her stern, angular face. After the release of this poster, bond sales continued to sag.

Months later, the next poster was released. Liberty had become less manly and she was even a bit sensual. A year later, by the time the fifth "Buy Bonds" poster was out, Liberty was quite feminine and scantily clad. She looked like she had been dressed by the people at Trashy Lingerie instead of being outfitted in a drapery shop. While her breasts were by no means large, they were taut and had an erotic edge. You actually had to look twice to see if any material from her nearly see-through gown was covering them. By the end of World War I, Uncle Sam was learning what it takes to sell bonds.

Twenty years later, during the second World War, American soldiers consumed six million copies of *Esquire Magazine*. Perhaps this is because it showcased Vargas girls with their massive, gravity-defying bosoms. It was during World War II that pinup girls became famous. The women who prepared the pinup models for the photography shoots would stuff the models' bras with layer after layer of felt pads. They felt this would help lift the soldiers' morale, among other things.

Birth of the Bra

For several centuries, the corset was the undergarment that supported the weight of women's breasts. The first brassiere wasn't patented until the time of the Civil War and it didn't appear in the marketplace until the late

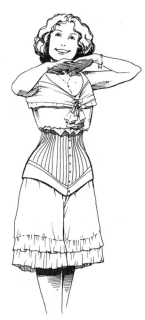

The corset has a rich and interesting history. Contrary to what you often hear, very few women who wore corsets did a practice known as "tight-lacing." Tight-lacing is a fetish where the person wearing the corset laces it up so tight that his or her waist becomes unnaturally small. Many women in the early 1900s were hesitant to give up wearing corsets. Switching to a bra or "bosom supporter" might have been like a woman today going from panties to a thong.

1800s. It would be another twenty years after the end of the century before the brassiere would win widespread acceptance among American women. Several elements needed to converge for the bra to knock out the corset.

According to Jane Farrell-Beck and Colleen Gau in their excellent book *Uplift—The Bra in America,* here are some of the changes that needed to occur in women's lives for the bra to become popular:

💡A large increase in the number of women involved in physical activities such as bicycle riding, golf, tennis, and swimming. It is difficult to do these things while wearing a corset.

💡A major increase in the number of women in the workforce. For instance, there were virtually no female telephone operators in the 1880s. By the 1920s, with the explosion of telephones, there were huge numbers of female operators. These operators needed to reach across large switchboards to plug in cords to complete each call. This would have been difficult to do while wearing a corset with bones sewn into it.

💡The materials and design of the bra had to improve. Bras needed to fit better, have adjustable straps, be able to fasten easily, and they needed to have soft cups with underwiring to help lift and separate the breasts. The latter, when first introduced in 1910 by brassiere visionary Madeleine Gabeau, seriously clashed with the monobosom or monobreast look of the day. The monobosom look made women appear as though they had no defined breasts or cleavage. It was the bodice equivalent of wrap-around sunglasses. Needless to say, there needed to be significant changes in women's fashion for the bra to nose out the corset.

💡Women would need to start wearing ready-made clothing rather than having clothes custom made, and the price of the bra had to come down to fit the budget of the "new" working woman.

💡A further stumbling block to acceptance of the bra was the lack of a universal sizing code. It wasn't until 1933 that a bra manufacturer proposed sizing bras according to cup sizes A, B, C and D.

World War II—Bad for Adolf, a Boon for the Bra

Before World War II, many American women had never worn pants. But once women began manning America's War Machine, pants are what they wore. Most women were not prepared for this. Articles began appearing in women's magazines giving tips and suggestions for how to wear pants. With the changes brought about by World War II, American women weren't just wearing pants and bras, they were punishing them.

This is the first time in history that welders, riveters, and ship builders wore bras, or admitted to it anyway. Bra design needed to seriously evolve to accommodate the range of motion of the new female workforce. Yet the supply of bra-making materials such as rubber, cotton, metal, and rayon was now rationed and in short supply.

It required 1,000 pounds of rubber to build an airplane, 1,750 pounds of rubber to build a tank, and 150,000 pounds of rubber to build a battleship. Yet America's main supply for rubber had been through Asia—a trade route that evaporated with the beginning of hostilities. Without rubber there was little elastic with which to make bras. It was not easy for bra manufacturers to make it through the war!

Not only were bras keeping Rosie the Riveter's breasts from flopping, one bra manufacturer was given a secret contract by the government to produce special vests that carrier pigeons could wear. The vests, which employed much of Maidenform's bra technology, allowed paratroopers to parachute while holding carrier pigeons. The pigeons were used for communications when radio silence was essential, such as right before D-Day.

Along with making pants a part of women's wardrobes, World War II also gave the bra, with its increasingly pointed cups, a new name: the Torpedo.

Foundations Start to Shake & Bras Become Sexy

By the end of World War II, actresses started sprouting seriously pointed breasts. It was as if the sultry Vargas Girl drawings were suddenly hopping off the pages of *Esquire* and coming to life. Books like *Peyton Place* were bringing small-town sleaze into the public eye, and the Kinsey reports on the sexuality of Americans shocked and intrigued the masses. Sex was in the air!

Shortly after World War II, the Sweater Girl started to appear. When viewed from the side, Sweater Girl actress Lana Turner's breasts came out at a 90 degree angle. This was achieved by a bra which was the latex equivalent of the Golden Gate Bridge. A similar two-cupped engineering marvel called the "Bullet Bra" sold in the millions.

1947 was the year when Frederick Mellinger opened the first Frederick's of Hollywood. Millions of Americans were seeing his sexy magazine ads and receiving his Frederick's catalogue. Frederick's teased and titillated customers with their Peek-A-Boo brassiere and half-moon stick-on brassiere.

By 1949, Maidenform had begun its Dream campaign, which showed women wearing bras and flowing skirts saying things like, "I dreamed I danced all night in my Maidenform Bra" or "I dreamed I won the election in my Maidenform Bra." One of the Maidenform ads from 1962 showed a sexy young woman wearing only a bra with a bare midriff, a long tight skirt, and elbow-length gloves. She was standing next to a large bull with one hand sensuously stroking one of the bull's big horns. The caption read, "I dreamed I took the bull by the horns in my Maidenform Bra." Only a blind person would have missed the sexual innuendo of the ad. Many of today's feminists would have concerns about this notion, saying that it implied women's power was dependent on their sexuality or sexual allure. Nonetheless, like their gutsy mothers who built our planes and tanks in World War II, women in the 1960s, with their Maidenform bras, were as much of a force to be reckoned with.

The 1950s also gave birth to the inflatable bra, which gave a woman the option of pulling a tube out of each breast cup and filling it up to the desired level of allure. This was also helpful if the woman was flying in a plane and it went down over the ocean.

In 1970, Victoria's Secret emerged to grab the sexy-bra baton from Frederick's of Hollywood. Frederick's had acquired a sleazy edge, while Victoria's Secret screamed "classy and elegant." Victoria's Secret suddenly worked its way under women's blouses and into their pants. American women no lon-

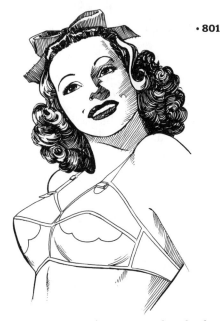

This is our illustrator's interpretation of a 1950s bra ad. The ad copy read:

"Perma•Lift, the lift that never lets you down! New, exciting, exquisite. Secretly processed Perma•Lift cushioned insets. Achieve the permanent uplift."

Sounds like an ad for car tires!

ger needed to blush or make excuses to enter a Victoria's Secret as they had in the later Frederick's years. And if the thousand-or-so Victoria's Secret stores weren't enough, millions upon millions of Victoria's Secret catalogues have been read by American women and men from coast to coast. Unfortunately, there has been a price to be paid for the new elegance and sexual allure—a bra from Victoria's Secret often costs two or three times as much as a similar design from Sears or Target.

The bra is the final outpost that separates the outside world from the sensuous breast. Because of what it covers, the bra has achieved a kind of fetish quality for both men and women. That fetish quality has reached new heights in the last few decades when rock icons like Madonna started wearing designer underwear on the outside rather than on the inside. Foundations were shifting once more.

Crossing Your Heart from 1920 to Today

Bra and breast fashion has yo-yo'ed over the years, going from boy-like breasts to the Torpedo, and back again. In the 1920s, the flat-chested look was in fashion. By the 1930s, the full-busted look was back. By the 1940s, women started calling the brassiere a "bra." Bras and panties were populating underwear drawers nationwide.

During the first wave of 1960s feminism, the popular saying *Burn Your Bra* came into being, as if bras were a ball and chain placed on women's chests by male jailers. Yet women hold almost half of the bra patents that have been awarded, and women have owned a number of bra-manufacturing plants.

There's never been a glass ceiling holding women back from the higher ranks of corporate bradom.

Far from holding women back, the bra was designed to hold parts of them up. It was made to help women deal with the discomforting pull of gravity. Of course, considering that breasts weigh from eight ounces to ten pounds, gravity has meant different things to different women.

Since the 1970s, some women have been trading in their natural breasts for surgically-enhanced models where the Torpedo Bra of the 1940s seems to be sewn into their chests.

The First Falsies

In case you think that insecurity about the size of body parts is a newly-acquired disease in America, some of the first falsies could be ordered through

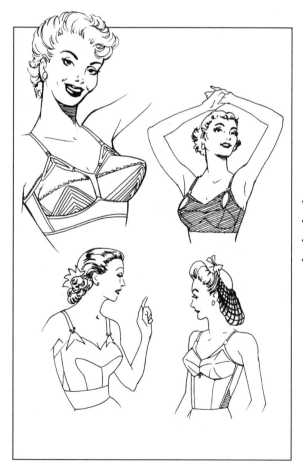

Our drawing of a 1950s WonderBra ad. The copy reads:

"She's Adorable."
"She's Bewitching."
"She's Delightfully Deceiving."
"She's Exclusively Elegant."

With the way the ad is written, it is hard to tell if it is referring to the women, their breasts or their bras. But that was the point. If you bought the bra, you got it all!

the Sears Catalogue in the late 1890s. They were called "bust pads" and were described as helping to "plump up the bosom." The same Sears, Roebuck & Co. catalogue with the bust pads also sold "The Princess Bust Developer, a New Scientific Help To Nature, If Nature Has Not Favored You." The Princess Bust Developer promised to enlarge and shape the bosom. It included a cream that was called "Bust Cream or Food, Unrivaled for Enlargement of the Bust," and a pump that looked like a toilet plunger. This sort of thing is still being advertised in magazines and on late-night TV!

For those of you who think that body-part insecurity only belonged to women, dozens of ads from the *Police Gazette* in the 1890s promised solutions for enlarging the penis.

No Room for Misfits

It is estimated that 80% of women aren't wearing the right bra. It's not like they accidently put on someone else's bra, but they might as well have. It takes a real effort to get the right bra size. Bra cup sizes can range from A to H, with stops in between at B, C, D, DD, E, F, FF, G and GG. There are also a large number of options for rib cage and back sizes.

If you compare the chests of two women who wear 36-C bras, their breasts can be shaped very differently. One woman's breasts might be shaped like eggplants, another's like cones.

Many women ignore that their breasts change size and shape over time. Just because you were a 36-B two years ago doesn't mean you are a 36-B today. Some breasts undergo significant changes in tenderness and size during the menstrual cycle. A bra that might have been just fine on day one might be uncomfortable on day 27. Also keep in mind that your breast size can increase if you go on the birth-control pill, and might decrease if you go off of it.

Bra shopping is not the sort of thing you should do by mail order, and you would be well-served to seek out a lingerie shop where the sales help has been fitting bras since the beginning of time. Avoid the sales clerk who is chewing gum and hasn't finished high school. Also avoid bras where there are bulges in the armpits or if the bra makes your breasts go out to the side. Your breasts shouldn't bulge along the top of the cups. And keep in mind that one company's 40-DD might be another company's 38-E.

Not only do you want a bra that fits and feels great through a full range of body motions, but you want one that holds up to repeated washings. It needs to support you in a way that keeps the ligaments in your breasts from stretching. Otherwise, there's not much point in wearing one.

Purchasing a bra isn't something a woman should do on the fly, and she shouldn't try to do it with two small children in tow. A caring partner will make sure that a woman has plenty of time to try on every bra in the store if she needs to.

Whether breasts are large or small, they are attached to the chest by suspensory ligaments. These ligaments are not elastic. Once they stretch they don't snap back. In her *Breast Book*, Dr. Miriam Stoppard recommends that young girls be given good supporting bras to wear, and that a woman should not go braless for long if she does not want her breasts to sag. (This would be a hard sell in places like Papua.)

NOTE: An April, 2008 Consumer Reports test compared a $127 LaPerla Vintage bra, a $45 Victoria's Secret Ipex demi bra, and a $11 Gilligan & O'Malley padded demi bra from Target. Of the three, the $11 bra from Target had better cup molding, more comfortable underwiring, fit well and held up better after three washings.

Highest Recommendation You will be hard-pressed to find a more interesting book on the bra than *Uplift–The Bra in America* by Jane Farrell-Beck and Colleen Gau, University of Pennsylvania Press, (2002). This book is the kind of marvel that should be—but seldom is—the staple of America's university presses. It is better researched than most of the other books on women's foundations, but it doesn't insult the reader with poor editing or incomprehensible sentences. In addition to exploring changes in fashion, *Uplift* shows the evolution of the bra within different social and economic contexts. If you want a good read about a fascinating subject, *Uplift* is a great choice.

If you are interested in more about corsets, consider the highly intelligent writings of Valerie Steele. Ms. Steele has managed to anger male corset enthusiasts because she calls their practice of wearing women's corsets a fetish. (Where would she ever get a silly idea like that?) Men who are strapping themselves into women's corsets are concerned that Ms. Steele is giving them an undeserved stigma. She's also managed to anger some academic feminists, because she has discussed how wearing corsets has had erotic associations and how the dangers have been blown out of proportion. They see her as being an apologist for the "corset torture" of women.

CHAPTER

71
Men's Underwear
The Fruit in Your Loom

What would you think if a guy phoned his partner and said, "God, honey, I start to get hard when I think about the new briefs I'm wearing." Contrast this with a woman who calls her partner and says, "God, honey, my nipples start to get hard when I think about the new bra that I'm wearing."

In our culture, it's cool for a girl to get excited about her lingerie, but we would consider a man who talked this way about his own briefs to be strange. Of course, if he just spent $20 for a single pair of tightie-whities with a fancy name on the waistband, we'd hope the things would give him a rise.

Calvin Klein—The Pricey Jockey[1] in Your Underwear Drawer

In the early 1980s, manufacturers like Calvin Klein teamed up with famed homoerotic photographers like Bruce Weber to help make men look sexy in their traditional white briefs. Needless to say, the men they used in their photo shoots would have looked sexy wearing a loincloth of cornhusks. Some people might say that the real emphasis of these ads boiled down to the bulge in the crotch—with all visual roads in those huge billboard ads drawing your eye to the sausage behind the fly.

The Calvin ads had two primary targets—gay men and straight women who buy underwear for their husbands and boyfriends. Nail these two groups, and straight guys are putty in the corporate hand.

In these underwear ads, the hazy image of a penis behind the fly was sexier than if the guy had been naked or if his penis had been hanging out. With his penis behind a white cotton veil, the model was able to give attitude in a way that a man who is buck naked can't. The combination of attitude and

---

[1] We think of the "jock" in *jock strap* as referring to athletes. But it comes from "bicycle jockeys" who the supporters were invented for in 1874 by the Bike Web Company. Bicycle jockeys were bike-riding messenger boys who rode over the cobblestone streets of Boston. The cobblestones made their testicles jiggle furiously.

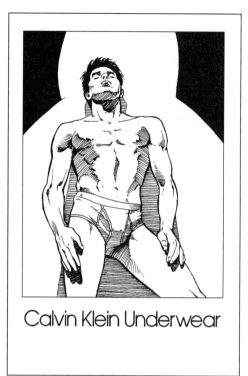

Calvin Klein Underwear

mystery about what's inside the briefs was fuel for many a fantasy. So while all roads led to the bulge in the briefs, it wouldn't have worked if the briefs had been pulled down to the hunk's knees. Women were being exposed to the same kind of "babe-in-a-lacy-bra" eye candy that's stimulated men over the ages, only with an urban contemporary edge.

Subliminal Messages?

Wouldn't it be something if a woman could buy a pair of Calvin briefs for her man and have him suddenly look like the models in the Calvin ads? And wouldn't it be amazing if a man could slip on his Calvin briefs and suddenly feel like the Calvin-Klein-version of the Marlboro Man, minus the horse and the lung cancer?

Naturally, if one of the models in the early Calvin ads walked into a room full of straight women, he would have no trouble finding a place to spend the night, even if his day job was collecting trash and he wore $2 briefs from Wal-Mart.

Contemporary Girl Underwear—Finally, a Fly for Your Clitoris!

There have been a few interesting changes in the underwear scene in the past two decades. For one, manufacturers have started making men's underwear for women. This has been perceived as massively cool. The boybrief as worn by women even has a fly or the suggestion of a fly in the front.

If you are in gender studies, you might assume that girls enjoy wearing boybriefs because it's a girl's way of taking the patriarchy's pecker and making it her own. Wearing boybriefs with a fly in the front makes the message even clearer. It also helps with pantylines.

But something more practical is involved. Women in our culture receive far more encouragement to explore and experiment with fashion than men do. For many women, fashion is a great adventure, and they have adopted zillions of styles throughout the ages—from some that were simply hideous to those that were elegant. Few of these had anything to do with trying to assume dimensions of masculinity. Quite to the contrary, much of women's fashion is designed to win the awe and delight of a girl's female friends.

As you will see in the next section, the road to making men's underwear cool for women to wear is much different from the road to making women's underwear safe for men to wear.

Men with Bikini Briefs, Trimmed Pubes, and Waxed Backs

Over the last decade, males in university settings have started teaching courses on men's studies. Of the many things these men worry about, trying to define masculinity is near the top of their list. They often say that a defining hallmark of masculinity is that it tries to be the opposite of anything that's feminine.

Perhaps these scholars haven't noticed that straight guys have been doing a lot of girly things as of late, such as wearing earrings, and having the hair on their entire upper body waxed or zapped with lasers. Some even shave their legs, and plenty have taken to trimming their pubes and wearing underwear that's like a woman's bikini bottom or even a thong.

Since this chapter is about underwear, we'll save the earrings and shaved scrotums for another day. For now, let's look at some of the factors that have made it safe for men to wear women's bikini bottoms.

The Speedo Coefficient We have had generations of incredible-looking Olympic male swimmers and water-polo players who wear nothing but Speedos, which are basically G-strings on steroids.[1] Hard as you might try to keep looking straight ahead, Speedos have a built-in device that forces your eyes to stare at the guy's crotch and butt, even if this would be followed by a scream of horror if the man in the Speedo were 60 years old and 90 pounds overweight. Clearly, there is a precedent for a straight guy to wear girls' bikini bottoms for underwear. It's called the *Speedo Coefficient*.

---

[1] **Competitive Swimming's Darkest Hour:** As a spectator sport, swimming at the Olympics recently took it in the shorts when the traditional men's Speedos were replaced by a cross between bicycle shorts and a wetsuit. Forget steroids, the women of Goofy Foot Press want the new suits banned.

Men-With-Pro-Balls Effect It didn't hurt the cause of the male bikini when professional male athletes in bikini briefs were hired to be in magazine ads and on posters. These half-naked athletes had women swooning, and they reassured men that they wouldn't risk being seen as gay if they wore women's bikini bottoms.

The "Honey Do" Influence A guy would have less resistance to wearing girls' bikini bottoms if his wife said, "Honey, I think you'll look sexy in these." This fact wasn't lost on the underwear manufacturers, as the ads with the male athletes in their bikini briefs were clearly aimed at women.

Penis-Over-The-Top Factor The transition to bikini underwear for men had a good deal of practical significance. That's because when we pee, a lot of us don't pull the penis through the fly in men's briefs or boxers. Instead, we yank the elastic waistband down and plop the penis over the top. So the fly is totally useless for a lot of men and having the lower waistband makes the process of peeing easier.

Briefs and Bras in Perspective

Publications in gender studies tend to focus on subjects like violence, rape, and the truly awful things that some people do to others. They would consider our look at men's and women's underwear superficial. However, "superficial" means "on the outside." In the last two chapters, we took your blouses off and pulled your pants down.

If we had a gender studies course at Goofy Foot University (a.k.a. G F-U!), students would spend the first week playing with Barbie, GI Joe, Legos, and Matchbox Cars. They would then be asked to consider the relationships between play and gender identification. The next week, they would have to strip down to their undies and free-associate about what's masculine and feminine. Hopefully, one of the women would be wearing a Granny Bra.

The most important lesson, however, is that a hundred years ago, no one would have been able to predict that the bra would ever be sexy. And as little as fifty years ago, no one would have been able to predict that men would feel manly wearing women's bikini bottoms. Look at all of the effort that went into weaving these pieces of cloth into the sexual fabric of our culture.

A Note on Different Water Cultures Most male surfers wouldn't be caught dead in Speedos. The only commonality between many male swimmers and surfers seems to be water, and the water of the former smells like chlorine while the water of the latter tastes like salt.

CHAPTER
72
What's Masculine, Feminine & Erotic?

The thinking in some academic circles is that masculinity and femininity are constructed by society in the same way that a beer commercial or Victoria's Secret lingerie commercial might be. And once you start chipping away at what's masculine and what's feminine in different cultures, you can't help but agree, at least a little. Men and women may arrive at things like sexual orientation in different ways, and our brains might even process certain aspects of sexuality differently, but culture plays a big role in determining our sex roles. This chapter takes a brief look at matters that can be incredibly complex.

Masculinity, Then and Now

A little more than a hundred years ago, men who didn't have much money worked in jobs that required a good deal of physical labor. Unlike today, a lean, buff man with sexy muscles did not get that way from working out at a gym. His well-defined, masculine muscles were usually the result of a low-paying job. As a result, a well-dressed man with a pot belly was a better catch for an attractive young woman in the year 1900. The big belly and nice clothes meant being able to protect your wife and children from an economy that suffered frequent and wicked downturns. They meant a woman wouldn't have to work outside the home, which was significant when the best jobs most women could get in 1900 were to be a domestic or a seamstress, working long hours at very low pay. To earn more, she might need to become a prostitute.

Have things changed just a bit? Well, not with the economy, but with the muscles. Nowadays we assume that most men with buff muscles have enough leisure time to spend hours at the gym. It's unlikely that someone who is working two jobs as a janitor will be able to work out as well. A guy who has a job as computer programmer may work out at the gym in an attempt to hide the fact that his biggest physical challenge at work is opening up his laptop. And the young woman of olde who may have viewed Mr. Portly as a good catch might very well be working out at the gym today with Mr. Buff and making as much money as he is. Such an independent woman would not have been considered "feminine" as she might be today. People would have wondered what was wrong her. In 1900, feigning frailty was an important element of femininity, even if most women weren't frail.

What Different Societies Have to Say

Each culture has its own definition of what's masculine, feminine and erotic. Here are some examples of how these definitions differ from culture to culture, year to year:

💡Women in Muslim cultures cover themselves from head to toe when appearing in public. Women in Hollywood show up wearing a few molecules of fabric, designed to tease rather than cover. The women in Hollywood claim that their Muslim counterparts are sexual prisoners. The Muslim women say the real prisoners are the females in Hollywood. A neutral observer might call it a toss-up. One female reader says that neither women are sexual prisoners, since they both use sex to control the people around them!

💡In Japan, it's a common practice for people to strip naked and bathe together. Nobody finds this kind of public nudity to be erotic or shameful, but Lord help two Japanese who kiss in public, at least until recently. In our society, it's nearly the opposite, with kissing being fine and nudity an offense.

💡Kim Edwards is a woman who taught English in a rigid Islamic country for two years and then moved to Japan. In the Islamic country, an exposed female body is considered to be the tool of the devil, and women cover it from head to toe to save the souls of men. After a few years in a rigid Islamic country, Ms. Edwards literally started hating her own body. When she moved to Japan, she was shocked to find herself treated as a normal person no matter what she wore. She could even bathe naked in public bathhouses, while she could have been stoned to death for doing this in an Islamic country.

💡During the Summer Olympics, male gymnasts from the Russian team often celebrated good performances by kissing other male team members on the lips. Our U.S. male gymnasts wouldn't be caught dead doing that, not in public anyway.

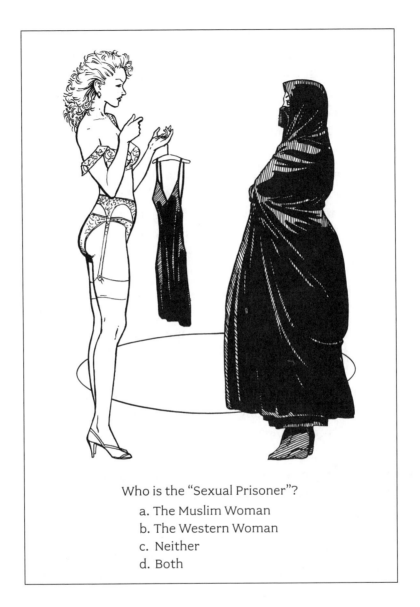

Who is the "Sexual Prisoner"?
a. The Muslim Woman
b. The Western Woman
c. Neither
d. Both

💡In America, many straight women now wear their hair short, and many straight men wear their hair long. Fifty years ago, this meant that you were homosexual. And think of the public outcry if a 1950s professional baseball player appeared in billboard ads wearing a pair of red bikini briefs; or if his 1950s beehive-coiffed girlfriend went to the grocery store wearing Doc Martens and male boxers. Or what if a straight American male wore a pierced earring before the 1980s, or trimmed or shaved his pubic hair?

💡In America, there is nothing unusual about an unmarried 18-year-old woman having sex; but among more traditional Arab-Muslims, Christians, Druze, and Israelis in places like the Gaza Strip and the West Bank, such a woman risks harming the honor of her family. In rural villages, she might be murdered by her own mother and sisters in what is known as an "honor killing" to protect the family name, although the practice is not as common as it was a few decades ago.

💡Less than a decade ago, a consultant to *The Guide* was invited to India to speak on "Alternatives to Wife Burning." Seems that if a husband and his mother are unhappy with his wife, fatal "kitchen accidents" are apt to happen with few legal consequences. What surprised the consultant the most was that it was the men at this meeting, rather than the women, who welcomed the alternatives.

💡In Africa, millions of women have their clitorises and inner labia crudely cut out of their bodies as children. This type of "surgery" has been considered an important passage to womanhood which many African mothers have done to their young daughters. In the West, a mother who did such a thing to her daughters would be put in prison. Of course, African women might claim that the clitoridectomy is just as cosmetic and feminine as our Western penchant for mutilating female bodies with breast implants. Who knows what an African woman might say about liposuction or labioplasty.

💡Historically, in the Latino culture of East Los Angeles, males didn't feel masculine until they had made a woman pregnant ("given her a child"). Likewise, some Latino teenage girls didn't feel good about themselves as women until they had borne children. Twenty miles to the west, in Pacific Palisades and Malibu, the last thing a teenage couple wanted to do was get pregnant. They often sought an abortion if it happened, and pregnant girls worried about losing their hard-earned anorexic shape. These stereotypes are quickly breaking down, at least in East L.A.

💡In the early 1800s, Americans believed that a woman's sexual pleasure was as important as men's pleasure. Then, from the late 1800s until the 1960s, it was considered unfeminine for women in our society to enjoy sex as much as men. Valuing sex became a masculine trait, and some women even believed that it was unladylike to have orgasms.

💡In North America and Europe, we view a woman's sexual wetness as a good thing—the wetter, the better. Vaginal wetness is the female equiva-

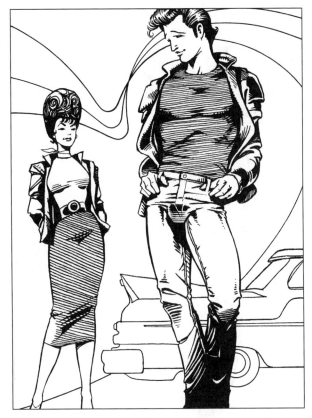

Sex roles, anyone?

lent of an erect penis, a sign that a woman is turned on and ready to romp. But in Zimbabawe and Zaire, women traditionally worked at drying out their vaginas before a penis went in. In these countries, a wet vagina was traditionally viewed as dirty, smelly and possibly infected. It also causes embarrassing sounds during intercourse and risks being seen as a sign of infidelity. Here we use one of many brands of sex lube if a vagina isn't wet enough.

Masculinity & Femininity

For many of us, masculinity and femininity are concepts that make all the sense in the world as long as you don't try to define them.

For example, people in this country think of masculine as being rough-and-tumble and feminine as being dainty and nurturing. Yet this isn't nearly as true in preschools that require little girls to wear the same kind of clothes as little boys. Once freed from wearing dainty outfits, a lot of little girls get rough-and-tumble too. Likewise, if little boys had to wear outfits that needed to be kept clean, at least some of them might act more daintily.

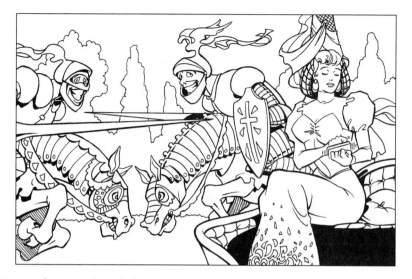

Men and women have behaved differently over the ages, but how much of the difference has been due to biology, and how much to culture and custom?

Equally puzzling are rough-and-tumble men who become extremely nurturing and maternal when it is time to feed the baby. Do their aggressive male hormones suddenly dry up at dinner time? Do the structures inside of their brains change shape? And if you assume that women are less aggressive or are the more nurturing sex, try talking to a random group of female lawyers, advertising execs or women in entertainment.

While hormones may have some impact in determining male and female behaviors, what we learn from culture about our respective sex roles is clearly a large force in shaping the way we behave. That's why it is hard to talk about the definitions of masculine and feminine unless we also know the particular country, culture and year.

From this Guide's perspective, any culture's definition of masculine, feminine and erotic is arbitrary, transient and often artificial. Nonetheless, people take these definitions seriously and get really bent out of shape if you ignore their local customs.

France Weighs In

Counterpoint One reader from France writes, "You have done a great job in this chapter explaining cultural differences, yet you blow it with the first sentence of your final paragraph. In my mind, it's a culture's rules and definitions that make it unique. It would be a very boring planet if we were all the same, and especially if we were all like Americans."

73

Men's & Women's Experience of Sex

Men's and women's genitals are generally found in the same location: behind the buttons of a person's blue jeans. But what about the way we experience sex? Do men and women experience sex differently? That's what this chapter is about. But first...

Forget Everything Else!

Forget penises, vulvas and chromosomes. The biggest difference between male and female sexuality throughout the ages has been the fact that men don't get pregnant and women do. Forget the "behavioral influences" of estrogen and testosterone—instead, consider how differently we might approach sex if men were the ones who got knocked up and had to carry a baby inside themselves for nearly ten months, and if men were expected to be the child's primary caregiver for the next eighteen years.

Of course, there are other factors that influence men's and women's experience of sex. While most of these have to do with culturally defined roles and expectations, some reflect differences in biology. For instance, there are subtle differences in brain anatomy which may influence behavior. Consider how the female brain responds to the smell and taste of chocolate. Think of how different life would be if male ejaculate squirted out in ribbons of chocolate, or if the penis tasted like Hershey's Kisses.

There are also claims about differences in the behaviors of male and female newborns. The author of *The Guide* spent a number of years in graduate school holding and studying babies, from two-pound preemies to drug-addicted newborns of crack-smoking moms. He can assure you that the only difference between boy babies and girl babies that means a single thing is how the babies pee. Boy babies have the capacity to wipe out your favorite shirt, tie, glasses and note pad, while girl babies are more forgiving pee-ers. Working with boy babies requires a quickness of hand. Some women report this kind of skill is just as necessary when working with the babies' fathers.

Perhaps a more relevant finding of infant research is that girl babies are every bit as strong and healthy as boys at birth, if not more so. Yet we often treat girl babies as though they were more fragile. Researchers have dressed the same baby as a boy and then as a girl. When caregivers thought that the baby was a girl, they said things like "Aren't you pretty and dainty." When they thought it was a boy, they said, "Aren't you a big one; look at how strong you are." And if you want to know the sex of a baby from ten yards away, just observe how its daddy plays with it; girl babies get an abundance of hugs and kisses while boy babies get the rough 'n' tumble. With such profound differences in the way we raise our children, it's hard to imagine how subtle variations in neurology or genetics even matter.

Note We use the term "opposite sex" when comparing men and women, yet there is not a single psychological test battery that can distinguish male from female test takers. Surveys on attitudes can pick up differences, but those are different. Good luck eliminating the influences of culture on surveys. And as you will see, the differences in attitude decrease when men and women are in mixed groups.

Typical Male Porn vs. The Newer Female Porn

What happens to these babies twenty years later when they are having sex? Do the women's experiences fall into the "pretty and dainty" category? Are the men's "big and strong?" Perhaps not, but our culture does have specific insults that it hurls at women whose sexuality appears to be "big and strong" and at men whose sexuality is "pretty and dainty."

To help illustrate possible differences in men's and women's experience of sex, we have included a few samples of pornographic writing. The following is a typical letter to a male magazine that is commonly used for masturbation. It had a monthly audience of around 5 million people before the Internet took the staples out of its spine.

> It wasn't long before a wet area began to appear in the front part of DeAnne's bikini panties. I slowly started to pull them down, at first revealing a neatly trimmed patch of silken blonde down, then the glistening tip of DeAnne's swollen clit, and finally the rest of her hidden steamy treasure. The mere sight made me so hot I nearly exploded.
>
> DeAnne must have sensed my excitement. Without saying a word, she ripped open my bulging blue jeans and started ravaging my 9-inch

cock with her pleading lips. Within seconds I was filling her hungry mouth with load after load of white hot cum. DeAnne kept sucking and slurping on my throbbing cock until she milked my big balls dry.

Okay, so getting your rocks off is the name of the game in traditional male porn, with the focus being on the particular body parts that get you there the fastest. There's also the premise that within every woman lives a raging nymphomaniac begging to wrap her lips and legs around the teeming bulge of the nearest available guy.

The next two passages are from *Erotic Interludes,* a collection of women's pornography—uh, erotica—edited by Lonnie Barbach, Harper & Row:

J.B. tenderly caressed my breasts until I could feel the space between my legs grow warm and wet. His kisses were different than ever before, long and slow at first, then his tongue licked mine like fire dancing in the dark. His long, slender legs gradually, rhythmically inched mine apart. The tip of his cock played on my belly, and I couldn't resist rising up to meet him, opening my legs as far as the backseat would allow. A soft flash of red filled my vision when he entered me, his kisses wild on my face. I remember only the sense of infinite motion that followed. (Written by Sharon S. Mayes)

Amy groaned with pleasure as his large hand cupped her gently and his third finger came to rest on the one sweet spot he knew so well. As he touched it she felt an electric current flow from his hand into her. His energy swirled inside her till the whole universe seemed to start spinning around…. The spinning sensation rose up and flooded her whole body, pushing at the boundaries of who she thought she was…. Finally, unable to hold the energy back any longer, she let it explode through every cell in her body, cleansing her with light and pulsating out into the room. (By Udana Power)

Blinding light? Infinite motion? This has a different edge than "Within seconds I was filling her hungry mouth with load after load of white hot cum." Still, one female reader says that the samples of women's porn "left me bored," while she found the male passage to be "erotic for me until he wastes his cock in her mouth." Several female readers have echoed this same sentiment, but with phrasing that is more delicate. At the same time, a male reader says that he finds the women's passages to be more erotic. Perhaps it's not so easy to generalize about the preferences of men and women, although the samples could easily be tagged as *typical male* or *typical female*.

Is It Really Different?

Are men's and women's experiences really different, or do they just use different words to describe them?

Researchers asked men and women to write a paragraph describing their experience of orgasm. A panel of judges could not tell the women's descriptions of orgasm from the men's. So much for those charts on orgasm that make men and women look like they come from different planets. Nonetheless, studies have shown that there are some sex-related differences in the attitudes of men and women, but mostly when they are with members of the same sex. These differences decrease greatly when men and women are in mixed company.

This isn't what Madison Avenue wants us to think. Advertisers work hard to make us believe that men and women are very, very different. That's because manufacturers can often charge more for products that are targeted to a specific sex, such as cigarettes, deodorants, and even hemorrhoid ointments which are for one sex only. It's a little surprising that we haven't seen toilet paper that's made just for a man's or woman's "special needs"—although one manufacturer, Kleenex, did try to sell man-sized facial tissues, which really were better for jerking off into than normal-sized tissue.

How Men and Women Experience Visual Pornography

It is often said that women aren't as turned on as men by X-rated movies, but this notion seems to be less pronounced in today's young adults. Research shows that rather than being turned off by visual pornography, women are turned off by the premise of most male pornography, and they are particularly turned off by mainstream pornography where the female actors are faking orgasms. The are plenty of hardcore X-rated movies that women find just as arousing as males. The movies just need be better selected for.

In research on pornography, college students have been hooked up to devices that measure blood flow in the genitals. They are then shown X-rated movies. Although these devices indicate that the groins of the female students were as sexually aroused as the male groins, many of the women were not consciously aware of their arousal. Speculation abounds on why. It could be that women's brains process sexual arousal differently than men's brains, and that pussy status alone is not enough to do the job. We also know that males might not be as conscious of their own arousal if they didn't have a penis that pretty much taps them on the shoulder when it gets hard. However, most guys learn to tell the difference between an erection that is erotically-grounded and one that isn't, so there is more to it than just having a boner.

As for the idea that women's sexual arousal is more relational and more deeply grounded in their emotional feelings about a partner, the latest research shows that this is more true for women who are having sexual difficulties than for those who aren't. For the majority of women, their description of how they experience sexual arousal is the same as most males.

In studies about sex, we tend to ask women a lot more questions about their sexuality than we do men. Maybe the reason why researchers feel that women's sexuality is somehow more complex than men's is because they ask women more questions. Or maybe it's because women tend to be more verbally expressive about their sexual feelings—we notice a huge difference in the length of women's answers to our sex-survey questions on this book's website than the men's answers. The men tend to answer in monosyllabic grunts. Is this a reflection of men's actual feelings, or simply a reflection of how they express their feelings when asked by others?

While brain studies tell us that men's brains are wired in ways that make porn movies more of a turn-on for men than women, a recent study from the UK found that women are looking at porn sites in far greater numbers than was originally assumed. While men might use those images to masturbate with when at the computer, women might have a tendency to call up the images or scenarios at a later time when they are masturbating.

Role Reversal—Fingers up Men's Rear Ends

Getting a finger up the rear during a routine physical exam makes many guys feel like they've been violated, yet they don't think twice about sticking their own fingers up a woman's vagina. It is possible that a woman's experience of sex might feel more private than a man's since her body is the one that is usually being penetrated. One woman reader comments:

> "Even if he's wearing a condom, it still feels like a man leaves something inside of me during intercourse. He's got to have something I really want inside of me, or I won't do it."

One of the few times when a woman gets to stick something of hers inside a man is during French kissing. Some men love the feeling of a woman's tongue inside their mouths, while other men are only comfortable if kissing imitates intercourse. There tends to be more body-cavity equality in couples who are into the kind of anal sex where the woman penetrates the man's rear with her fingers or sex toys.

Intimacy in Men vs. Women

In our society, we often assume that women are better at intimacy than men. Is this true? The answer depends upon how you define intimacy. According to psychologist David Schnarch, women are often better at some levels of intimacy (sharing feelings, talking about how the day went, etc.), but when you get past the small talk, neither women nor men do particularly well with intimacy.

A Final Perspective

Some evolution experts believe that nature has programmed men to ejaculate into each and every available vagina, while women are programmed to couple with males who will offer the best chance to successfully raise a family (relationship material). The people who take these theories most seriously are the evolutionary psychologists themselves. They have a wild propensity to twist facts to fit their theories, and people who question the process are dismissed as fundamentalist quacks. It's interesting how with changes in economics and politics, more women are looking to catch more ejaculations from more men than they did fifty years ago.

In spite of what the evolutionist would want us to expect, a man who is straight and masculine-appearing might experience sex in a way that we would typically expect of a woman—sensitive, monogamous and intimacy seeking, while a very feminine-appearing straight woman might enjoy sex with numerous men, value it for the rush of sensation that it offers, and avoid long-term relationships. It's also possible that what we want at one point in our lives may be totally different from what we want at another.

The most important thing to be aware of about sexual differences is that your partner might experience sex differently than you do. Instead of making silly assumptions about how your partner experiences sex, why not ask, explore, and find out for yourself? Maybe your partner's responses are not as tied to gender role stereotypes as you might think.

74

The Horny Pill & Patch

This chapter is about women's sexual desire when it is at its low ebb. It might seem strange that a chapter on low desire would appear in a book like this. After all, if you are reading *The Guide,* the least of your problems is low sexual desire. Right? Well, maybe.

There are things we can learn about normal desire when we look at the attempts that are being made to woo women with low sexual desire.

Why We All Need To Be Concerned

Drug companies have been spending millions and millions of dollars to find a "cure" for women's low sexual desire, as if it were a disease rather than a communication. They thought they had hit the jackpot when they found Viagra. After all, a woman's genitals aren't that much different than a man's, or so they assumed. If you look at how much blood rushes in when a woman's genitals are aroused, there isn't a big difference between that and an erect penis. Fill 'er up, and she'll be good to go.

In anticipation of the wonderful success they assumed they were going to have with the girl version of Viagra, the drug giants bought themselves—uh, sponsored—studies that discovered that 43% of woman suffer from sexual dysfunction. So for the longest time, you couldn't hear a single report about women's sexuality that didn't begin with the words "43% of women suffer from sexual dysfunction...." Of course, none of the reports bothered to mention the furor that was brewing behind the scenes when some of the country's top sex researchers said, "Your definition of 'dysfunction' seems a wee bit self-serving." We also know that the percentages researchers report depend greatly on the questions they ask, and that different studies ask different questions.

With it being announced that 43% of women are on the verge of sexual breakdown, think of how many girls would be running to their physicians for a prescription of the new pink Viagra. It's that or lose their husbands to some devious babe up the street whose medicine chest is crammed full of the new Prozac for the Pelvis.

But then the drug companies discovered something that they hadn't expected to find—that a puffed-up pussy does not make desire in the mind. While Viagra can increase the blood flow between a woman's legs, it no more makes women want to have sex with their partners than sitting on the washing machine during the spin cycle. The idea that a woman will want to have sex if we can just give her a swollen vulva turned out to be a colossal flop. They would have done much better giving her a trashy novel or a new partner.

And it gets even more complex than that. When researchers were studying the impact of birth-control pills on women's sexual desire, they found different results among women in Scotland and women in the Phillipines. It seems that the women in one country had a different expectation of what they should be getting from sex than women in the other. Although the pill had an equal effect on their bodies, the women in one country were more disappointed by its unwanted side effects than the women in the other. So even culture has an important effect on different groups of women.

But the drug companies aren't about to give up on "low sexual desire." It's really perfect for them. Like depression, low sexual desire is poorly defined, the kind of thing you can convince anyone they have, given the right kind of marketing campaign. And so they have now set their sights on testosterone.

Not long ago, Procter and Gamble (P&G) asked the FDA to approve a new testosterone patch called Intrinsa to cure "low sexual desire" in women, a condition that apparently strikes every woman past the age of 37.

But unlike Viagra, a woman doesn't take a hit of testosterone an hour before sex and she's good to go. Testosterone is a steroid, the kind of drug that helped female swimmers from East Germany achieve that unique, chiseled look. We're talking Arnold Schwarzenegger in women's Speedos.

The interesting thing is that a lot of women who first start taking testosterone really do feel more chipper, more energized. It isn't for a couple of years until Jacqueline starts to sound like Jack when she answers the phone.

The FDA's advisory panel voted seventeen to zero against approving P&G's horny patch. There were issues of increased chances of breast cancer, heart problems, liver ailments, skin inflammation, excessive hair growth and masculinization that P&G didn't sufficiently address. There are also unanswered questions about the impact of testosterone on a woman who is 30 as opposed to 60. How would the extra testosterone affect her fertility or future children? And how would it effect women of different ethnicities?

Then came a report from a task force of the Endocrine Society that strongly recommended against the generalized use of testosterone by women until a number of very important questions are addressed and answered.

You would think if we were going to give women a potent steroid we would have a test to tell if a woman actually needs it. But scientists can't agree what form of testosterone should be measured and what to make of the results. One woman can have a very low reading of free testosterone and be a lioness in bed, while another can have a decent amount and not be interested in sex at all. In fact, there's now a fairly definitive study that shows there is little correlation between a woman's hormones and her level of horniness.

There is no question that supplemental testosterone can be helpful for some women who are experiencing certain physical conditions, such as the loss of their ovaries or after taking hormonal methods of birth control that might have shut down the female body's ability to make its own testosterone.

However, approval for narrow uses like these is what the drug companies will likely use to open the flood gates for off-label use, which their marketing campaigns will quietly encourage. Women may soon be bombarded with a wave of testosterone-containing products in the form of sprays, inhalants, patches and pills. Studies will claim that girls enjoy sex more when greased with the new guy juice. Forget the reality of your life or of your relationship. They will be marketing it for everything from wrinkles to low energy.

This will not be the kind of cautious and measured approach that knowledgeable and conscientious urologists, gynecologists and endocrinologists take when working with a woman to decide if supplemental testosterone might be helpful. Hopefully, women and their healthcare providers will ask serious questions before consuming a drug that promises more than any drug in the history of humankind.

Many years ago, while the author of *The Guide* was still in grad school, he was fortunate to have been under the guidance of one of the most highly regarded pediatric neurologists in the world. He can still remember one of the rare days when he ever saw this doctor express anger. There had been a leadership change (or "coup" as the esteemed physician called it) at the National Institute of Mental Health. He said that much of what we worked for would be over, and that research funding in all areas of medicine and mental health would be focused on finding a pill for everything. He feared this change would have a profound effect on the future.

Time has proven him right. These days, our front-line approach to everything from depression to sexual desire and intimacy is finding "the right" pill to throw at it. It would have given this physician a chuckle if he'd known back then that with all of the devastating diseases left to conquer, drug companies would be spending millions of research dollars on trying to find a pill that would make women want to have sex.

75

I Knew the Bride
Long Term Relationships

This chapter is about marriage and long-term relationships. It doesn't pretend to be comprehensive, but it does speak about weddings, tradition, sex in marriage, fights, make-up sex, kids and divorce.

I Knew the Bride

One of the fun things about weddings is watching the white-laced bride taking her vows of marital bliss and wondering if she has ever handcuffed the groom and done some of the outrageously nasty things to him that she once did to you. The memory puts a smile on your face and maybe even makes you blush. But it's not the kind of question you ask as you are working your way through the reception line—not with everyone's parents standing there with an array of cold, clammy hands hanging out of pastel gowns and rented tuxedos.

Weddings—What's Love Got to Do with Them?

You don't have to go much farther than the average magazine rack to realize that weddings are big business. Plump, glossy zines with names like *Modern Bride* nearly bite your arm off as you walk by. The ads in these magazines reflect the many segments of our society that thrive on marriage-related businesses — bridal-wear shops, tuxedo rental centers, wedding gift registries, boutiques, kitchen appliance stores, caterers, florists, bakers, wedding coordinators, ministers, priests, rabbis, justices of the peace, churches, synagogues, reception halls, hotels, resorts, diet plans, etc.

In our society, traditions like marriage (and Christmas) have become an economic spectacle rather than a symbol of love and commitment. Today's marriages are so choreographed that you seldom get a feeling that two people are making a promise to be there for each other no matter what, and to be inseparable partners on the great climb through life. Instead, what you often get is the familiar bride-to-be psychosis, where the future bride and her mother become so savagely obsessed about things like table centerpieces and bridal gowns that any sense of love is pretty much out the window.

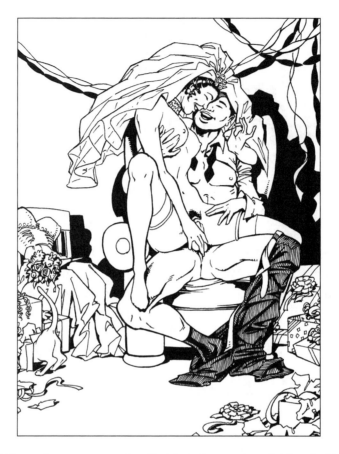

What if couples put as much effort into improving the level of intimacy and fun in their relationship as they do selecting wedding invitations? And what about those bizarre, adolescent feeding frenzies known as bachelor parties? If guys need to see high-priced women getting naked or want to lick whipping cream off silicone-filled breasts, why not just do it? Why use weddings as the excuse?

Marriage is a big step, an important step. Hopefully you won't get caught up in our culture's expectation of marriage as a generator of crippling debt, and will instead work to make your union a safe haven in a world that is sometimes anything but.

And what if couples took the money they spent on weddings and set it aside for one long weekend each and every month, just to be with each other and have fun? No cell phones, no work, just a three-day weekend each and every month where your only laptop is each other?

Styles of Problem-Solving

Besides feeling love and friendship, an important ingredient in keeping a relationship happy is a couple's ability to solve conflicts. Couples with a knack for problem-solving tend to have happier marriages. (Duh!)

Researchers tell us that such couples approach conflicts with a willingness to talk things over and work them out, and we are sure that such couples exist somewhere. The rest of us occasionally resort to sarcasm, name-calling, stubbornness, making threats, automatically giving in, taking blame needlessly, becoming silent or pretending that there is no conflict when all hell is about to break loose.

Contrary to what you may have heard about the value of releasing anger, trying to resolve a conflict when you are still fuming at each other is not always productive. Sometimes it is best to wait until cooler heads prevail. Of course, some people will use this as an excuse to avoid confronting a partner altogether. Then nothing ever gets worked out.

The Good, Bad & Ugly

When you enter into a marriage or long-term relationship, the chances are good that you will discover hidden but wonderful aspects of your partner's character. Cherish, respect and admire these. To deal with the less fortunate parts of your sweetheart's character, consider the following:

Learn how to fight constructively. This means that no matter how nasty or unpleasant your fights might be, try to keep them issue-oriented so you can work your way toward a solution or compromise. This is different from fights that revert to name-calling or rehashing past hurts. These accomplish little, except to degrade whatever dignity you once may have had.

Fighting is preferable to indifference, unless you are getting violent.

Every once in a while, when you feel like wringing your partner's neck, do something really nice for him or her. This could end up being far more satisfying than fighting, and it might even get you laid.

Instead of blaming your partner for things that are going wrong or wishing that he or she would somehow change, try to eliminate ways that you might be setting your partner up to be the bad guy. This doesn't mean that you should stay in a relationship that's no longer working, it just means that the things you control most in a relationship are those that you put into it. If your efforts to change yourself don't inspire changes in your partner, then there's not much more you can do.

Birds of a Feather Get Bored with Each Other

Long-term relationships can sometimes be a challenge to keep fresh and vital unless both partners make a constant effort to enjoy each other.

For instance, think about all the extra things you did to impress each other when you first met; you probably even cut your toenails or trimmed your bikini line. Why would there be any less need for romance and wooing after you've known each other for what seems like forever? Mature relationships require more rather than less effort at romance and improvement—from cards, flowers and special dates to extra attempts at tenderness.

Single vs. Hitched

Being single makes it easier to maintain the illusion that you are a perfect human being. Long-term relationships force you to confront parts of yourself that many of us would rather not. For instance, in a long-term relationship, your husband or wife will probably get fed up with your worst faults and remind you of them at least six times a day. If you are the rigid type who is incapable of change and compromise, then you might not be well-suited for marriage. On the other hand, a reader from San Francisco comments, "It could be just what you need."

Sex after a Fight, aka "Make-Up Sex"

Fights leave most couples worn out or sad. However, some couples enjoy sex after a good fight, given how their neurotransmitters are already fired up and ready for action. On a biological level, the body might confuse a fight with sexual excitement, thus eliminating the need for tender preliminaries. Hopefully, the reasons for the fight have been resolved and the sex isn't simply being used as a cover-up.

Your Partner's Bad Moods

Like colds and flu, occasional bad moods are part of the human condition. In better-functioning relationships, the partner who is in the good mood is sometimes able to maintain a healthy perspective when confronted with a partner's bad mood. He or she might even take steps that will help the other's bad mood to go away. But in difficult relationships, all bets are off.

In a difficult relationship, the partner who is in a good mood experiences the other's bad mood as a personal attack, even if it has nothing to do with him or her. Attempts to help are often filled with so much anxiety that they only make matters worse, and the partner in the bad mood might lash

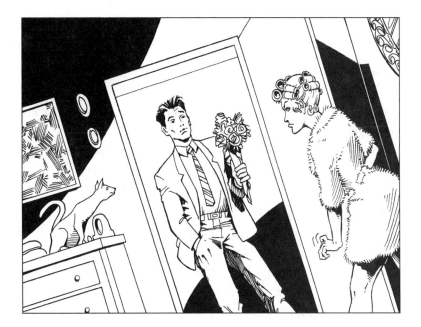

out at the other just for the heck of it. (Why not be nasty to the person who loves you? After all, no one else would put up with you.)

Such couples usually do better if one spouse has a job that keeps him or her on the road for long periods of time.

Sex after the Baby Arrives

Our society doesn't provide many role models for caring parents who are also sexual beings. We sometimes separate the two roles entirely, as though being a good mom or dad precludes your giving great head or loving the feel of your partner's naked body next to your own. Just identifying as a parent may make you feel less sexual than you really are. Hopefully you will take the time to talk this over with your partner before having children, as well as after. There is no reason why you can't be great parents and have great sex—although the latter won't be as spontaneous as it was before the children arrived. A married reader comments: "We had lots of sex during nap time and Sesame Street."

Also, never discount the extent to which exhaustion might erode the desire to have sex, and don't expect to have sex if you aren't doing your fair share of the child care and housework. While you've probably never considered vacuuming and taking the garbage out to be romantic acts, good luck getting laid without doing these sorts of things once the new baby arrives.

One reader who is a prostitute adds, "And for heaven's sake, hire someone to help with the cleaning or wash before you spend the money on a prostitute."

Divorce & Your Children

Don't assume that kids automatically do better if their parents stay together. While some children feel a terrible sadness when their parents get divorced, others feel relief. It usually depends on how bad the marriage was, how bad the divorce is, and whether the kid gets to live with his or her favorite parent, if there is one. The absolute worst arrangement for some children is spending half of a week or a month at one parent's house, and half at the other. This can be the psychological equivalent of cutting the baby in two. On the other hand, it can work if it's being done in the child's best interest as opposed to simply placating two warring parents.

What often destroys kids more than the actual divorce is the parental lunacy for years before and years after. In an emotional sense, children of divorce often end up having no parents at all because their parents are sad, joyless, hateful or frightening to be with. If you are getting a divorce, do what you can to reach through your own pain, remembering that children need to see at least some form of hope reflected in their parents' eyes. And remember that your child's psychological health will in large part be determined by how amicably you and your former spouse are able to co-parent when divorced. It is not possible to emphasize this point too much.

Highly Recommended Resources: *Divorce Busting: A Step-by-Step Approach to Making Your Marriage Loving Again* and *The Sex-Starved Marriage: Boosting Your Marriage Libido: A Couple's Guide* by Michele Weiner Davis.

———————————

Dear Paul,

Friends set me up with a wonderful woman and we've hit it off really well. We have had sex four times and are building a caring relationship. Unfortunately, I went to her place for the first time last night. (Before that, we'd always gone to mine.) Her bathroom looked like it hadn't been cleaned for a year, and some kind of alien life form was growing from the tile in her shower. She appears clean and neat, but this is another side of her that's scary. Just so you'll know, I've never been a neat freak, and don't even buy antibacterial soap. What do I do?

Tyler in Jackson Hole

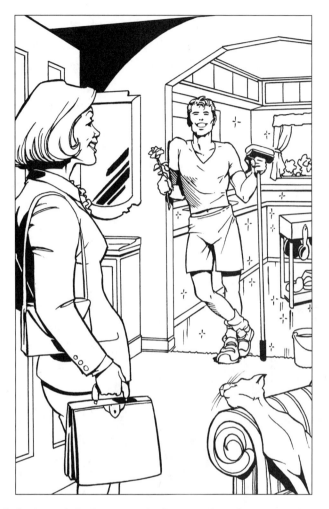

Men who help around the house get laid more often than guys who don't, causing speculation that Windex and Lysol are better aphrodisiacs than oysters and fast cars.

Dear Tyler,

Your letter would have gone straight into the wastebasket if you hadn't mentioned the slimy ooze growing from the grout in your girlfriend's shower.

Let me tell you a story about Bill and Nancy, a couple whom I feel proud and honored to have known for more than fifteen years. Their house has always been immaculate—I'm talking serious sparkle. Even the litter box smells clean. One night a few years ago, we'd been having too much wine and I mentioned how impressed I was with Nancy's ability to keep such a clean house. At that point, Bill started hyperventilating and nearly bled from the ears. He told me about the first time he went into Nancy's bathroom when they were grad students at the University of Chicago. It took him five hours of scrubbing and several gallons of bleach before he could reach terra firma on her shower floor.

My point, Tyler, is the way your lover keeps her bathroom doesn't need to be a deal breaker. What's more important is the way you and she handle the situation. If you say nothing and continue to ignore her wanton disregard for Lysol and Ajax, then I'd say your relationship is in trouble. And if she is unable to handle your spending half of next Sunday scrubbing her bathroom, your relationship is also in trouble. But if you clean her bathroom and don't make her feel bad about it, and she returns the favor with the finest blowjob you've ever received in your entire life, then I think you're onto something good.

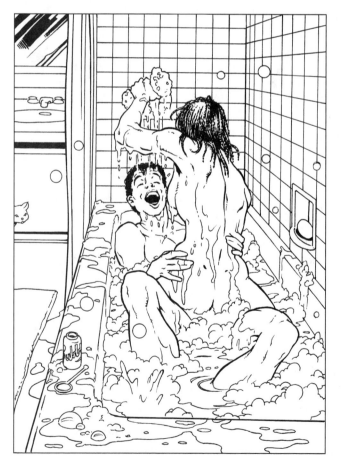

76
Sex in the Military

" Things the military could do to help sex be better?
Make the damn uniforms easier to get out of!"
female, age 19

It's not like soldiers leave their sex drives in their home towns. However, providing helpful information about sexuality for new recruits is not always a top priority of the military. Since the military does not publish reports on the sexual practices of its members, we have put this information together based on clandestine reports from the field. Hopefully, our intelligence is better than that of some governmental agencies.

The Uniform Code of Military Justice prohibits displays of physical affection while you are in uniform. The defense that you were naked and not in uniform while having sex is probably not going to wash. The UCMJ prohibits sex in barracks and sex between people of different ranks. It also prohibits sodomy, which is defined to include oral sex. If that isn't a recipe for "boring," it's hard to know what is.

It's also worth noting that while there are some fascinating aspects to sex in the military, it is really just a cross-section of sex any place where Americans are gathered. So if you are looking for a bizarre expose, you're in for some serious disappointment. On the other hand, there are some interesting dimensions to sex in the military, especially if you are a female G.I. who likes her men well armed and ready to engage.

For soldiers and the partners of soldiers who have been in combat,
*Please see **Sex after Combat** at the end of this chapter.*

The "Guide To Getting It On" Recruiting for the Military?

Before we start on the cultural and sociological aspects of sexuality in the Armed Forces, consider the following observations from two khaki-wearing philosophers:

> "Believe me, its the women in the military that are sex mad, but nobody complains or calls them sluts, because we would all do the same in their situation." *male age 25*

> "I mean it's usually five females living in a building with 100 horny males. The girls pretty much pick who they want to sleep with that night." *male age 23*

Girls, if you really like sex and you decide on college, you will find somewhere around 60 women for every 40 males. In fact, the best advice we have for a young man who wants sex is to go to college. For women, it's to join the military, where there are only 15 women for every 85 males. Plus, if you wanted to have sex with a number of Uncle Sam's finest, you don't have to worry about getting a reputation, as long as you make efforts to be discrete about it. It's not like it's going to follow you 500-guys later, when you settle down in civilian life with the young minister from the First Church of Christ. What happens in the military usually stays in the military.

Now, before those of you who are upstanding military women decide to bomb the offices of Goofy Foot Press, everybody knows that at least half of you are true-blue and not interested in sleeping around—which ups the odds for those who do to 7.5 women for every 100 men. Consider the following words of advice from a reader who knows:

> "For new females—have fun! I was so eager to be the good airman, obey all the rules, etc., that for my first few years I didn't have a lot of fun with the unique situations we can get into. Most of the people you will know will be young men in good physical shape. Take advantage!!!"
> *female age 25*

As for a male's chances of having sex in the military, these sentiments from two experienced soldiers echo what we heard time and again:

> "I thought being in the military would be like taking a vow of celibacy. However, it turned out that there were good opportunities." *male 25*

> "Coming from a smaller town in Iowa I was a little shocked how others showed no concern that someone was married." *male age 37*

Some of the opportunities include young civilian women who have historically found the words "base adjacent" and "Available Men!" to be synonyms. There is seldom a scarcity of them near military bases. Opportunities also abound in ports of call in Europe and Asia, although in Muslim countries, the sex is mostly on base between members of the military.

As for the willingness of some military wives to offer the comforts of a warm bosom to needy soldiers while the wives' husbands are deployed, some do and some don't. We have heard from some military wives that it's not unusual for them to share tender moments with each other rather than with other men while their husbands are away. However, there may be different expectations for the wives of officers than for the wives of enlisted men.

The Culture

Sex in the military is a mirror of sex any place else where Americans live and work. However, there are a few complexities that help define sex in the military as different at times.

There is the never knowing when you will be put in harm's way—but always expecting it and always training for it. This can contribute to a sense of fatalism or cynicism within the culture of the military, or a bit of a *devil may care* attitude when it comes to what you do in your free time.

There's also the emphasis on the body and its abilities, the impact of group living, and constantly being moved from one base to another. This can make for a climate where the sex is catch as catch can. And soldiers are frequently immersed in cultures where sex is perceived differently than it is here. In foreign lands, sexual economies often thrive around military bases. Even here in the states, different bases have different sexual cultures.

These are just some of the factors that help give sex in the military its very own and sometimes unique perspective.

Short Tour vs. Long Tour

"My sister, who is also in the service is married to a serviceman. She recently returned from a TDY (temporary duty) assignment, and while there, engaged in an extramarital affair with another married serviceman. These things happen a lot." *female age 25*

Deployments in the military are often categorized as "short tour" or "long tour." If you are married and you are on a long tour, they will often move your family with you. If it's a short tour (under a year), your family usually stays behind. There are plenty of exceptions, especially if you are going into combat.

The Impact of Your Status

"The base where I received the bulk of my training after basic, Sheppard, is where most of the people are young, first time away from home, and have just undergone an enormous life-changing experience. There's a sudden freedom after basic training. Everyone's hormones are raging. One piece of common wisdom is, 'Don't get married at tech school!' I guess that's because lots of people jump the gun. There are lots of random hookups, some racy stuff going on at the dance clubs, and lots of alcohol. Another base I spent some time at recently, in Florida, has a greater population of 'adult' service members, so there's less of a panicky, gotta-have-it-now attitude." *female age 25*

Members of the armed forces usually fall into two groups: first termers, and lifers:

First termers are often younger and unmarried. They usually have high sex drives, and they are eager to be accepted into the military's macho culture.

Lifers are a different story. The have made the military a career, and they have often sampled many different customs and cultures. Lifers tend to be married and have families, but it is also not unusual for them to spend a good deal time away from home.

Social & Economic Class Distinctions—The Dangers of Sex between Ranks

Since there is currently no draft, there is little equity in the military. Enlisted people are almost all from the middle class and below, while commissioned officers tend to be from the middle class and above.

In addition to the political and economic divisions within the armed forces, there are strictly-enforced prohibitions regarding fraternization among the ranks. People in the military who marry other military people are expected to be in the same or a similar rank. It is a violation of the *Uniform Code of Military Justice* to even socialize with someone not in or close to your own rank. Good luck trying to explain away that little affair between a lieutenant and a private, or a colonel and junior commissioned officer.

No matter how hot that first-class private is, a commissioned officer can get him- or herself into big trouble for fraternizing when their uniforms are on the floor.

Women in the Military

"A female private and myself were going through an abandoned building and on the middle floor she just went crazy and started sucking me off like there was no tomorrow. She even answered her radio in the middle of it then carried on." *male age 26*

"With my coworkers, sex is not an issue—I'm a woman working a job which is, even now, pretty much a 'man's job.' I have a very non-sexual relationship with the boys in my shop. I think it surprises them when I wear civilian clothes and they remember that I'm a real girl. However, I do feel like the females are a bit of a commodity. I know several women who take advantage of the situation and live it up with all the partners they want, and others who are from conservative families/areas who wouldn't dream of it." *female age 25*

Like working women in the civilian world, women in the military often change personas between home and when on duty. Some have said that their military persona is more masculine and aggressive, while their civilian persona can be more relaxed or feminine.

In the past, sexual harassment has been prominent. That's because a woman who wanted to report someone had to report to the officer in charge. She couldn't report to an independent person. The officer would seldom want to lose a good man, and would often ignore the charges.

In the last couple of years, that has begun to change. Reporting is through separate channels, and women's complaints are being taken more seriously. As for the reality of reporting harassment, one female soldier says it will no longer get you demoted, but forget being promoted and forget being treated decently ever again. A female Marine in the Middle East who is quoted in Newsmax.com says, "You have two choices. You can keep your pants on and be miserable and be harassed, or you can take your pants off and you'll still get harassed, but you'll be a little less miserable."

Sex in Different Bases & Ports of Call

"Seemed to be a lot of screwing around going on overseas. Hell, when you are out to sea for 65+ days and come into port and see women offering sex for next to nothing, its hard not to. The Philippines was approximately $5 bar fine for a gal all night. Treat her with respect and she's yours the whole time you're there. Singapore was easy to

get laid. Any cab driver knew were the brothels were located. Be careful of street walkers as many of them were benny boys (transvestites).
Hong Kong–ask cabbies. Perth, Australia. OHhhhh YES! Blonde hair
blue eyed beauties whose parents encouraged the relationships (short
or long term)." *male age 44*

"In Greenland it was an isolated base with only around a hundred or
so military people and some civilians. There was probably a higher
amount of cheating there than most places because it was so remote.
Not much to do but drink and screw." *male age 48*

"For nearly a year in Iraq, I was under constant threat of death with my
work, and I was rarely alone. I didn't have sex at all when I was there."
male age 37

"In Washington, sex seemed more about starting a family, although I
did more easily find sexually-deprived women there willing to forgo
a relationship." *male age 24*

"In ports of call, the official 'off limits' list was usually a liberty battle
plan because the bars had the best booze and the whore houses had
the best broads. Drinking on liberty was expected, getting drunk was
a badge of honor, getting wasted to the point that you can't remember
where you were, what you did, who you did it to, nor how much it cost.
There was honor in being a drunken whore monger." *male age 58*

Saigon Vs. Baghdad

While some members of the military do have sex in Iraq, it's mostly
between male and female soldiers or interpreters, and not in the best of circumstances. This is different from Vietnam, where sex was often available
in bars, hotels, and at "skivvy huts" which were often close to bases. "Skivvy
huts" might have three or four beds next to each other in a 12-by-12 room.
Local women would be having sex with soldiers who had their pants pulled
down around their ankles. There was not much privacy.

Cultures: There was a bit more neon in Saigon than Baghdad. In a country like Iraq, sex outside of marriage is strictly forbidden for women and for
a woman to sell herself for sex is unthinkable. It's a rare day when a soldier
even sees the hair of a local woman let alone make serious eye contact, and
maybe only while on a "knock and talk" and if none of the men are home.

The Military: During the war in Viet Nam, there was a draft. So the average soldier was single and somewhere between 18- and 22-years of age. In Iraq and Afghanistan, the make up of the troops is very different. Many have wives and children stateside. Many of the troops are National Guard or Reserves who tend to be older and married when compared to active duty Army or Marine Corps. Plus, today's military has a much higher percentage of females than was the case in Vietnam. There is more room for intra-armed forces fooling around.

Danger in Different Places: While the local communities in Vietnam were not harbors of safety for American military personnel, at least a soldier could visit the occasional prostitute if he wanted to assume the risk. Even if there were brothels in Baghdad, no Amercian soldier would risk taking off a single bit of armor to liberate a lonesome penis.

Considering the age of the troops and the Muslim culture's attitude toward sex versus that of the Vietnamese, the respective conflicts were in different centuries in more ways than just figuratively.

Korea vs. Europe

Soldiers in Korea often move off base and set up housekeeping in a one room "hooch" with a "Moose." A Moose is a Korean woman who cooks, cleans and provides companionship, including sex. They are quite good at keeping their solider smiling. It was not unusual for a soldier to marry his moose and bring her home to the US as his wife.

Most bases in the Pacific and Asia have their own form of a "moose culture." There might be some bases where the men in a military dorm pool their money and hire a group of mooses to take care of the men's needs, including their sexual needs.

In Europe, prostitutes are plentiful and legal. Contacts can be made through night clubs, bars and online.

Sex in Home Bases with Spouses of Others

"There is one extreme or the other in the military. You either have sex on the casual or you really fall in love with them. Those that I knew that wanted to stay together were completely faithful to each other and some even left the military together." *male age 25*

"I had a lady friend during a remote assignment who was married to another AF member stationed elsewhere, and they seemed to have an understanding that going without sex for a long time apart wasn't a reasonable expectation. Although she and I were never intimate, she made it plain that she was willing if I was. My only sexual encounters while apart from my wife were casual, with no expectations of a lasting relationship." *male age 54*

"Most couples that I know usually ended in divorce or breaking up. I'm not sure that it was because of infidelity or not. But a lot of the women I slept with were married." *male age 23*

"There was an atmosphere couples were fooling around a lot on both ends. There were places you could go if you wanted to pick someone's wife." *male age 24*

While we have heard from plenty of military people who say they remained true blue to their spouse or lover, we have heard from plenty who didn't. It's not unheard of for married couples to have understandings that all is fair in love and war, or when deployed or on tour. Whether these understandings are spoken or merely understood varies with the people involved.

Masturbation

"Most guys after a while would pretty much talk about it openly. From what I gathered everyone was doing it in their bed (rack). It's enclosed on all sides and pretty much offers the most privacy. The only other place I would masturbate is in the shower. Some masturbated in the places they worked at day to day (shops). Although it is tempting because of the access to a t.v. and a computer, I only did this once. A few people I've know over the years were really open about it. So open as to not stop if accidentally walked in on them. They would simply ask you to come back later." *male age 24*

"I would masturbate late at night when the rest of the hooch was asleep, or in the showers. I don't recall being aware of anyone else doing it, but the general attitude was everybody did it sometime."
male age 44

"My roommates and myself were usually pretty good friends and we knew each other rather well. If one of us had to beat off we would usually just ask the other person to leave for awhile or to take their time at the store or wherever they were at the time. Or you just take a walk to the bathroom and stroke it in the stall." *male age 23*

"I did it very quietly. We had curtains on our bunks but you could usually tell when someone was solo pleasuring. You didn't say anything as everyone did it and you wouldn't like it if things were said about you." *male age 44*

E.M.H.O.s

"I don't recall any incidents where a morning erection (E.M.H.O. for Early Morning Hard On) became an issue. We joked about it a lot when coming to the end of midnight shifts. Morning erections aren't just for people waking up, there's something about dawn that seems to bring them on!" *male age 54*

Not a single man in our surveys said that early morning erections were a concern. Some said everyone had them, it was a normal part of being a guy, and no big deal. Another said he suspected the military was putting something in the food to decrease early morning erections during during basic training, because he doesn't remember getting one after the first week. He does remember getting many of them after basic training. Who knows the impact of exhaustion and fear on the spontaneous erection?

Swingers & Nudists in the Military

Swinging and nudism is a fairly prominent activity in the military. This is especially true in bases in Europe or parts of Asia where the social prohibitions against swinging and nudism are not as great as they are in the US.

"Where to find sex?"

"You really don't have to go anywhere. It usually finds you." *male age 29*

"Local clubs known to be meat markets." *male age 37*

"Probably the bars on post. They are usually full of married women looking for someone to play with while their husbands are away."
male age 23

Unlike males, women in the military seldom needed any help in finding partners. For men, the Internet is now being used for finding sex. This echoes its use in civilial life. Where soldiers go online depends on what kind of sex they are looking for. Www.USMilitarySingles.com appears to be a legitimate dating service. It also hooks up soldiers with interested civilians who live in the surrounding communities.

Between Gay and Bisexual

> "It's somewhat expected that everyone will date; if you don't date, co-workers will assume you're a homosexual. While this is very seldom true, it is a stigma." *male age 47*

> "While on ship, I had sex with as many guys as I wanted and as often as I wanted it. I had sex with men and women—in deep corners and heck, even in the barbershop once!" *male age 31*

> "There were very few homos onboard ship. It was never a concern." *male age 43*

> "A lot of military in Washington use Craigslist. You would see men on the site advertise for women at first and then as the day went on and the posting came later and later you would see the same men advertising for any sex. Some of them wanting their first homosexual experience. These were guys in their early 20s, in their sexual prime." *male age 24*

Our survey-takers are apparently not typical, as there wasn't a single one who said he or she felt homosexuals were a concern for them in the military. None reported feeling stared at while in the showers, and none listed homosexuality in others as a cause of concern.

There does appear to be a very well hidden gay and bisexual culture in the military. The men and women who are part of this culture take extreme measures to keep it hidden. It's nothing for them to drive hours from a base to a private gay club, where there is little likelihood that they will be found out.

How you define "homosexual" in the military is interesting. For example, there is the navy term, "It ain't queer unless it's tied to the pier," which indicates a different set of standards for what happens on land, where women are plentiful, and what happens on board ship. There is also an old military joke that defines a "buddy" as a guy who will go off base while you are restricted to base, get himself two blow jobs, and come back and give you one. So it is possible that when you do find same-sex activity, the operative terms should be "bisexual" rather than "homosexual," unless indications are to the contrary.

It can be dangerous for any man or women in the military to not date or have "girlfriend" or "boyfriend," as they risk being perceived as gay. Gay officers have to be particularly careful, as other officers' wives are constantly trying to set them up. A "stunt babe" is a woman who poses as a gay soldier's girlfriend at military events and whose picture he keeps on his desk. She is the military equivalent of a "beard," who is a friend or acquaintance who pretends to be a romantic interest when your parents are in town.

The smarter commanders in the military turn a blind eye to casual reports of homosexual activity. They don't want to deal with it and they don't want to lose some of their more qualified people to a modern day witch hunt. There is even a "queen-for-a-day" exception in legal proceedings if the homosexual conduct is considered to be highly unusual activity for the person who was doing it.

Gay service members are most likely to be outed by homophobic soldiers or groups like the *KKK* or *Aryan Alliance,* which are both active in the military.

Gay Females in the Military

Contrary to what you might think, lesbians can have a pretty rough time in the military, especially tomboyish dykes as opposed to fem-looking lesbians. Everyone is expecting women in the military to be gay, so straight women in uniform can be especially sensitive to this. They consider their gay sisters as a bad mark on the family name, and often display a total lack of tolerance. Lesbians in the military quickly learn this, and constant scrutiny can become nightmarish. While straight girls in the military can have a sexual heyday, lesbians in the military say they won't even risk kissing another woman in "the privacy" of a base apartment, let alone muff-diving when on government-owned real estate. All eyes are on any woman who is thought to be gay.

In her piece *No Ass, No Tail,* Myriam Gurba says that real military dykes aren't getting laid. She quotes one lesbian who said she believed herself to be the only dyke among 60 girls in her basic training outfit. Given the rampant homophobia, she said, "I think living in close quarters with 60 women was actually one of the most dreadful experiences I've had to endure."

While there can be opportunities for homosexual exploration, it would seem to be among women who no one suspects as being gay. Otherwise, they are too well watched for it to be comfortable.

Advice from People Who Have Been There

"I wish that I was told about the sexual reputations of all branches and how much people in military towns resented you before they even met you." *male age 24*

"Military people enjoy sex pretty much the same as everybody else. The dangers of military service, and the travel and deployments, make an active sex life a little more challenging, I suppose. I always appreciated a sexy welcome home, even though I realized that my being away increased my wife's burdens a great deal. Popular culture paints military members as macho types who enjoy rough sex and even rape. The truth is military people are the same as everybody else in the sex department, and what works for civilians works for GIs equally as well." *male age 54*

"Be very careful about propositioning someone for sex. The military is very paranoid about harassment of any kind. The accuser is the one who drives the charges; you will not win any legal dispute. Also, don't record (video, audio, photo) your sex acts; that is called evidence!"

male age 45

"If it's going to be casual sex, make sure you both agree and understand this. Don't talk about any sexual partner with coworkers, ever." *male 47*

"Here in Iraq, it's really hard... I feel too dirty and stinky to talk to girls here, and a lot of times coming back to the fob, we've seen contact with the enemy and are maybe upset, or are not into talking to girls because we've just seen the edge of humanity, like a dead body or dead friend, and the last thing on your mind is having sex. Also exhaustion is a factor." *male age 23*

A Special Salute to MSgt. Glenn B. Knight, USAF Retired for advice & research. Glenn proved just how thoughtful, intelligent and perceptive soldiers can be. Special thanks also to the active military who participated. We feel it is in their best interests not to include their names. One particularly telling account was provided by a military wife: "The military really programs a feeling of distrust toward non-service members. I didn't know how deep it went until I felt like I betrayed them by telling you our dirty little secrets. Very odd, it seems like I should be saying "Well, there isn't much to talk about. It's missionary all the way and affairs are unheard of.""

Sex after Combat

Thanks to better armor and more immediate medical attention, fewer soldiers are being killed in battle, but more are returning home with injuries. Some of the most common problems include traumatic brain injury (TBI), post-traumatic stress disorder (PTSD), burns, amputations and trauma to different parts of the body including the crotch. Many of these injuries are caused by blasts from IEDs.

Unfortunately, the VA does not want to hear about combat-related sex and relationship problems, especially those that can't be treated with pills like Viagra or Prozac.

While the discussion that follows is a brief summary, we have more information at www.GuideToGettingItOn.com. It's free and has the latest on sex after combat for both the vet and his or her partner.

More than 10% of combat vets are returning with PTSD, which tends to keep the body in a hyper state of alertness. This can seriously disrupt your sex life, given that the adrenaline that's surging through your system can make it difficult to kick back and feel like getting it on. Your body is in a permanent "fight or flight" mode, with sex taking a back seat to worries that bad things might happen. Just letting your guard down enough to talk about your feelings can be frightening. Plus, the sounds and sensations that happen during sex can become flashback triggers. Even the way we describe what sex feels like often includes combat imagery, "I started coming so hard it felt like an explosion..." or "There was this blast of light and energy..." Also, the sounds people make at the height of sexual passion often sound like cries of pain.

Fortunately, there are cutting-edge treatments for PTSD. Early reports indicate that they are effective. Since the studies are still being done, we will provide more information about this and other PTSD treatments on our website as the reports become available.

Just under 20% of returning combat vets are showing signs of traumatic brain injury. TBI can impact your ability to connect the dots in every-day life. Things that you used to take for granted can become head-scratchers, especially in relationships. And while it's highly unlikely that TBI is making you more horny, it could be making it difficult to know the appropriate time and place to masturbate, or who to have sex with and when or where.

Even though you seem perfectly normal on the outside, a brain injury could be impacting your judgement. While some of you might be thinking, "Finally, an excuse for some of the dumb things I do anyway," this would not be what you'd think if your brain really was compromised. More likely, you would be having problems expressing emotions and processing feelings.

TBI can be confusing for everyone, especially the people around you who expect you to be the person you were before combat concussed your cabeza. Like any of us, you might be trying to fake it or cover things up if you can. But you probably wouldn't know how to put what's going on into words anyway.

When possible, it's important to sort out traumatic brain injury from PTSD, as TBI symptoms can often look like those of PTSD. A great resource for learning more about TBI is a book written by Bob and Lee Woodruff: *In an Instant: A Family's Journey of Love and Healing*. Mr. Woodruff is a journalist who suffered an extensive TBI as a result of a war-related explosion.

As for burns and other tissue trauma, these can result in skin that is numb or painfully sensitive. Combat-related amputations are common and require huge adjustments to life in general, not to mention problems with keeping your balance during intercourse and having difficulty with thrusting. It's not like Oprah is going to have on the best-selling author of a book on *intercourse positions for the returning vet who has a double amputation*. The good news is, you might actually be able to get into positions that your able-bodied self could never fathom, but there will be a learning curve.

Always lurking behind any disfiguring injuries are problems with how you feel about your body, aka "body image" and "self-esteem." How is your partner going to respond? And if you don't have a partner, how will you find someone who wants to have sex with you? Not only will you need to heal physically, but you'll need to become comfortable with yourself. While you will probably want and need some alone time, isolation can be a devil of its own making.

Of course, to compound all of these problems, the medications used to treat depression and pain can bring their own sexual side effects.

We are just beginning to understand some of the unique problems that today's vets are bringing home with them. We will keep you updated on the book's website. If you have concerns about combat-related sexual problems, please visit: **www.GuideToGettingItOn.com**. Click on "Sex after Combat."

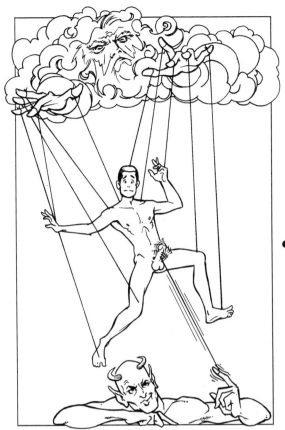

When people ask why I wrote this book on sex, I usually say it was revenge for eight years in Catholic school. But even before I went to school, I had started to appreciate the influence of religion on people's lives—both good and bad.

One of my earliest memories as a child was being at a holy-roller revival in a big tent with people waving their arms in the air and begging the Lord to save their souls. (Our family wasn't evangelical, but the baby-sitter was.) Later, as a teenager, I would revisit the revivals out of curiosity.

Revivals were like the circus. They rolled into town for a couple of days, and then rolled out in the dark of night. The county where we lived was poor, so it was interesting to see the Evangelists arrive in shiny new Cadillacs.

At what seemed like a pre-arranged moment during the revival, one of the women who had arrived in one of the new Caddys would start screaming that she'd had inoperable cancer and had been saved by Jesus. She would then crawl up the aisle to the collection basket, waving serious amounts of cash as she wept and wailed. Sometimes the preacher would lay his hands on her and she would faint, other times not. On the second night of the revival, at the very same moment, this same woman would be wearing a different colored wig and would scream that the Lord had saved her from the ravages of alcoholism and sexual excess. Again, with big bills in each hand. Many in the audience followed, admitting to their own transgressions of the flesh, and asking that Satan be cast from their souls.

The most important thing that I learned at the revivals wasn't that they were well-planned and well-orchestrated. Rather, it was their impact on the people who went to them. Even to my young self, I could see how these events put hope into the lives of people who didn't have much. It's where they went to confess and be saved, until the next time.

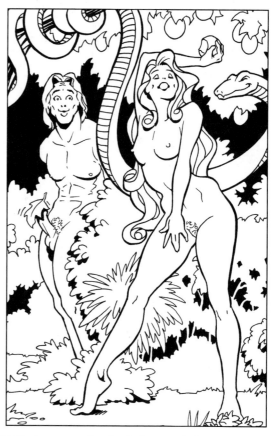

Maybe that's why people would show up at those revival tents and wave their arms in the air and not notice that the woman who started the parade of bill-waving sinners was a ringer from the bank of the preacher. I didn't know then—and I still don't know—if that was such a bad thing. It's hard for any of us to live our lives without hope.

As for my own personal experience with religion and hope, there was a radio evangelist by the name of Brother Popoff who I sometimes listened to on the all-night radio station that beamed up from Mexico. He was on after The Wolfman. If you sent him money, he promised to send you a special prayer cloth. So I taped some dimes and quarters to a card, and sent him what I had.

A few weeks later, a piece of red cloth arrived in the mail. It was about one-foot square, with no seams on the sides. The accompanying note said for me to lay it over anything that was troubling me. So I went to bed every night with that red prayer cloth tucked inside the front of my briefs.

I never did see much of a dividend, but then again, not too many people go on to write 992-page books on sex.

78
Sex in the 1800s

What? The longest chapter in Goofy Foot history is on sex in the 1800s? Perhaps that is because sex in the 1800s was fascinating. So fascinating that the authors of America's definitive text on sexual health have included this chapter in their four-volume set.

So if you bought *The Guide* to learn how to give a better handjob, then get thee to the first half of this book. But if you want to see how Americans enjoyed sex during our nation's own adolescence, you've struck it rich.

In the pages that follow, you will discover how prostitution was a vital part of American culture long before men and women started going out on dates. Time and technology would need to intervene for dating to evolve.

If you had been a young man in the 1800s, you might have had sex with prostitutes on a weekly basis. And unlike today's teenager who works at the mall or at Burger King, if you were a 16-year-old working-class girl in the 1800s, you most likely would have been a maid or seamstress who worked 60 hours a week for pennies a day, or you may have turned tricks in a brothel.

In this chapter, you will also learn about the birth of pornography as we know it today, about high-water condoms that only covered the head of a man's penis, and about oral sex in the century of the Civil War.

Best of all, learning about sex in the 1800s will help you have a better perspective on sex today, and that is one of the things this book is all about.

Note Many of the facts and perspectives used in the pages that follow are from the authors listed below. Without their efforts, we would know little about the incredible richness of America's sexual landscape in the 1800s:

Helen Lefkowitz Horowitz, Timothy Gilfoyle, Elizabeth Haven Hawley, Janet Farrel Brodie, Andrea Tone, Al Rose, James Morone, Sharon Ullman, Alecia Long, David Nasaw, Lewis Erenberg, George Chauncey, Alan Brandt, Anne Seagraves, Ruth Rosen, John & Robin Haller, Karen Lystra, Thomas Lowry Patricia Cohen, John Donald Gustav-Wrathall, Mark Carnes, William Cohen, Elizabeth Reis, Jan MacKell, Anne Butler, James Kincaid and Angus Maclaren.

Bicycle Seats or Live Sex Shows?

There are all kinds of ways to learn about sex, from downloading porn on the Internet to taking your clothes off with someone you love. Each lights up a different part of your brain and feeds a different part of your curiosity.

Of all the ways to learn about sex, the chances are excellent that you've never read about the ways our forefathers and foremothers did it in the 1800s. This chapter invites you into a lovemaking time machine. You'll get to look at how our great-great-great-grandparents got it on when they were young.

Just like today, sex in the 1800s had its contradictory ups and downs. For example, let's take a brief look at two things that you wouldn't think would be happening in the same century at the same time: live sex shows and concerns about women on bicycle seats.

Live Sex Shows If watching live sex shows is what turns you on, it was much easier to find one in the 1800s than it is now. Consider The Busy Fleas, a trio of young women who made up one of New York's City's most famous live sex shows. For $5, you could stand close by and watch the three Fleas get very busy, sexually speaking. Unlike today, there were no windows to look through or booths to enter, and no one carded you at the door. You would watch the girls give each other oral sex, do themselves with dildos, place cigars in their vaginas and rectums, suck on each others' breasts, and lick freshly poured beer off of one anothers' vulvas while their legs were tucked behind their necks. At the show's conclusion, you might be one of the lucky audience members who would get to have sex with one of the performers while the other men in the audience watched and cheered you on. As sexually explicit as this might sound, the Busy Fleas sex show was tame and downright virginal when compared to the live "Sex Circus" shows at Emma Johnson's Brothel in Storyville, the legal red-light district of New Orleans.

Concerns about Women and Bicycle Seats At the same time that there were explicit live sex shows, America's professional journals were waiving flags of caution about American women who were starting to ride bicycles. A number of feminists and medical experts were concerned that the shape of the bicycle seat would leave America's women sexually aroused. They cautioned that the bicycle seat would promote "libidinousness and immorality" in the fairer sex, and that raising a leg in public to get on a bicycle might scandalize a woman of the better classes.

So how do you judge sexuality in America during the 1800s—hardcore live sex shows or concerns about bicycle seats for adult women? For that matter, how do you judge it today—abstinence-only sex education or porn-filled Websites on the Internet? Perhaps it's a bit of both.

"Evil Is Generally Sniffable, Don't You Think?"

Disagreements among the American people about what is and isn't sexually acceptable go back a long way. Consider the following two newspaper reviews from 1896 about a live performance that took place in one of America's popular burlesque halls. While these are reviews of the exact same performance, it would be hard to find two perspectives that differ more, down to the descriptions of the performers' legs.

"I witnessed the performance of the Barrison Sisters and never saw an exhibition in any theatre more suggestive, lewd and indecent. It was disgraceful. The whole aim of these women seemed to be to excite the base emotions of the audience. Their dresses had been constructed with this one object in view, and all their motions were simply vicious and libidinous. Before the curtain went up the ten legs of these Barrisons could be seen by the audience under the edge of the curtain, indecently twisting and wriggling, as they sat upon the floor. This was designed to whet the appetite of the spectators. Then they came out and turned their backs to the audience, lifting up their dresses in a vulgar and indecent manner. Their underclothes had been specially made to excite the spectators, with many parts plain to the feminine eye... The Barrisons exert an immoral influence. A law ought to be passed putting a stop to such exhibitions, and I will make a recommendation of this kind to the Legislature this Winter." *By feminist reformer Charlotte Smith, who, by the way, was no fan of the bicycle seat.*

"As Miss Lona Barrison appeared I began to sniff around for a little evil. (Evil is generally sniffable, don't you think?) Where was her beauty? That was the first question I asked myself. A complexion like boiled veal and a figure that had neither symmetry nor grace of any sort.... After she had left the stage, without any attempt on the part of the defrauded audience to cheer her by applause, she returned with the five Barrison sisters. They showed us their legs first, for they sat with them poked out under the curtain. I like a leg or two occasionally, but it must be a leg in the true sense of the word. The spindle shanks that the Barrisons betrayed were so screamingly funny and so bewilderingly emaciated that I had hard work to keep in my seat. In fact, I don't mind saying that the only things immoral about the Barrisons are their legs. They are an affront to symmetry. They should be sewn up in masses of petticoats and kept from an unfortunate public. Amputation would be justifiable.... And then the poor little Barrisons began to do what they had been taught to do for the delectation of imbeciles. They sat on the stage looking hopelessly ill at ease, and ridiculously cheap, and sang a vulgar but stupid song dealing with the physiology of generation. There was no tune to it, no metre to it, no rhythm to it, nothing latent, nothing chic, nothing clever.... The applause, like the letter, never came. Not a gleam of intelligence gleamed in their eyes. Not a wicked look was cast in any direction. Five little frumps tugging away at a cheap concert hall chason was all we saw. Such utter inanity made you feel that you might as well have left your brains at home." *By Alan Dale, a journalist and popular critic.*

While neither of these reviewers had a single kind thing to say about the performance, you would get a very different sense of sexual standards during the nineteenth century if you read only the first review and not the second.

Perhaps people in the 1800s were even more confused about sex than we are today—especially American women, given how large numbers of them were working in brothels while others were wondering what to do about bicycles. (By 1870, the second-largest industry in New York City was the selling of sex.) On the other hand, the mixed messages about sex may have seemed normal back then, just like they seem normal to us today when conservative TV networks and religious talk shows are just a click away from radio shock jocks and pay-per-view porn.

Layers Upon Layers

Historians who write about sex in the 1800s sometimes present it as having different layers—with The Busy Fleas and Concerns about Girls on Bikes being examples of two very different layers. Here are a few more layers that make sex in the 1800s all the more interesting:

What percentage of American women could even get on a bicycle in the 1800s when our physicians were prescribing large amounts of opium and morphine for everything from headaches and depression to menstrual pain and sleepless nights? By 1872, a half million pounds of opium poppies were being legally processed in America each year, and the morphine that came from them was being used like Tylenol and Prozac are today. By 1898, a new wonder drug called heroin was being billed as a totally safe, non-addictive substitute for opium and morphine.

Narcotics were more often prescribed for women, who took them at home, while men seemed to prefer alcohol, which they consumed in more public settings like saloons and concert halls.

We know today that morphine-based drugs do a serious number on the human sex drive. We also know that between the years of 1886 and 1906 there was so much cocaine in Coca Cola that people who had a second eight-ounce glass risked a cocaine overdose. Hashish was not exactly in short supply, and amphetamines were racing their way into the drug scene. All of this while the average American man was drinking up to a half a pint of liquor daily.

So how do you discuss sex in the 1800s without taking into account how many men and women were under the influence of drugs or alcohol? We'll never have an answer, but good luck understanding sex in the 1800s without considering it. (One of the first questions a sex therapist asks a patient today is if they are taking any drugs that might be impacting their sex drive.)

And how do we handle knowing that sex-for-sale was such a central part of our culture when our country considered itself to be the home of Christian values, a fortress of fundamentalism, and site of frequent Evangelical revivals? Perhaps the drugs and alcohol helped us deal with our contradictions!

Our Sexual Desires—Shaped or Innate?

As we will see, there were many forces that shaped the sexual desires and decisions of Americans in the 1800s. Perhaps there are as many forces that are shaping our sexual desires and decisions today, but we aren't able to see them because we don't have the perspective that a hundred years can offer. We figure we do what we do because we are horny or in love. But what if there were other influences, such as art, religion, science, technology, fashion, television, music, birth control, the law, where you live, how much you make, what you drive, your education, your relationship with your parents, the drugs you take, whether you like your job, the cost of food, rent, and the price of gasoline—just to name a few?

Statistics

A writer can face no greater peril than when his readers expect sex, and he delivers statistics on population and immigration. Take comfort in knowing that sex is on the horizon. But first, we need to look at the population of America in the nineteenth century before we can appreciate what the population did in bed.

The Population of America's Ten Largest Cities in 1800

1.	New York city, NY	60,515
2.	Philadelphia city, PA	41,220
3.	Baltimore city, MD	26,514
4.	Boston town, MA	24,937
5.	Charleston city, SC	18,824
6.	Northern Liberties township, PA..	10,718
7.	Southwark district, PA	9,621
8.	Salem town, MA	9,457
9.	Providence town, RI	7,614
10.	Norfolk borough, VA	6,926

The Population of America's Ten Largest Cities in 1900

1.	New York city, NY	3,437,202
2.	Chicago city, IL	1,698,575
3.	Philadelphia city, PA	1,293,697
4.	St. Louis city, MO	575,238
5.	Boston city, MA	560,892
6.	Baltimore city, MD	508,957
7.	Cleveland city, OH	381,768
8.	Buffalo city, NY	352,387
9.	San Francisco city, CA	342,782
10.	Cincinnati city, OH	325,902

It's hard to compare these two sets of figures without saying "Wow!"

In 1801, America was a small nation of 5,000,000 people. Its home was the Atlantic Seaboard. Only a few people lived west of the Alleghenies, and fewer yet had ever seen the Mississippi. Less than 10% of the population lived in cities.

By 1901, we were a nation of 77,000,000 people living in 45 states that stretched from San Francisco to New York City. Nearly 60% of us lived in cities, including millions of immigrants. Unlike our white, Protestant, old-stock settlers who arrived before 1800, English was a second language for many of our more recent immigrants.

At the start of the 1800s, America had defined herself as a small country on the edge of a boundless frontier. In 1891, the government announced that the frontier no longer existed. In less than 100 years, America had transformed from a sleepy seafaring and farming society of thirteen colonies into a major military power that produced one-third of the world's industrial output. Our rural persona was quickly becoming industrial and impersonal, especially in the North.

As we shall see, these changes resulted in a new social order that would impact our sexuality in many different ways.

Immigration & The New Sperm Glut

Today's social scientists are warning about the growing disproportion of males to females in China, where there will soon be 120 boys for every 100 girls. They worry that this will cause an "inherently unstable" society with increased amounts of violence, prostitution, rape, and warlike aggression.

Imagine what these social scientists would say if they learned that between 1870 and 1910, the male-to-female ratio in some of America's largest cities may have been up to 135 males for every 100 females?

By the end of the 1800s, nearly a million immigrants were entering America every year, and most were settling in the larger cities of the North. As a result, there were almost twice as many foreign-born residents living in the big cities of the North as there were native-born citizens. The bulk of these immigrants were young, working-class males. For example, 80% of the Italians who entered the United States from 1880 to 1910 were males between the ages of 14 and 44. Our largest cities were being filled with young virile male bodies that nature programmed to ejaculate like machine guns.

Worse yet, the already high male-to-female ratio assumes that all of the potential female sperm catchers were as sexually willing as the male sperm hurlers. But think about it. Among the immigrant working class, how many Irish, Italian, German, Greek or Chinese fathers do you think allowed their daughters to cruise big city streets that were slick with the dripping testosterone of working-class stiffs? And how many middle- and upper-class daughters of white, protestant American families during the Victorian era were willing to put out sexually for the swelling ranks of working-class males?

Good luck finding material about our cities from the 1800s that doesn't refer to them as "Satan's slums" or "infernos of vice." There are reasons for this. The demand was swelling for prostitution to flourish.

America's New Sporting Culture

Past generations of Americans who had been craftsman or farmers were suddenly living in big cities and working in large factories. Industry was becoming America's employer; cities were replacing small towns as America's bedroom. In the past, you knew who your neighbors were because you grew up with them. Now, you were living in a large city, and it was likely that your neighbor or your neighbor's parents were born in a foreign land.

A whole new "sporting culture" of young men started to emerge in America—a hard-drinking, hard-working wave of American "boyz" who craved sexual release and wild entertainment. These young men were no longer constrained by small-town mores and middle-class values. The apprenticeship system that had helped to mold young men's lives was collapsing. A factory and corporate culture had taken its place, one that provided few restraints on what a person did when not on the clock.

Men in America no longer had a desire to marry young. They were working 10 to 12 hours a day, 6 days a week. They had no traditional homes to go to. The streets, saloons and brothels became their home away from home. Whoring, gambling, fighting and public entertainment filled their free time.

The penises of millions of American men were up for grabs, and prostitution rose to meet the demand. Whores became cheap and plentiful. They thrived in a society that believed the daughters of the better classes would face grave danger if America's men didn't have outlets to sow their seed.

Equally as important, America's economy during the 1800s was a treacherous landscape of booms and busts, pocked with financial recessions.

Brothels provided one of the few safe, high-yield investments. The rents that brothels paid were at least ten times higher than if the same building had been occupied by a home or business, and the "fees" that were collected from brothels and prostitutes kept the governments of many American towns and cities in the 1800s from going bankrupt.

A Funny Thing Happened on the Way to the 20th Century

Before 1820, when American men were often farmers, craftsmen or artisans, they worked out of their homes, and women had an important role in keeping the household together. But with the creation of factories, a number of important items like food and ready-to-wear clothes could now be bought in stores. Women were not as essential to the running of households as they had been, but it was still important for women of the working classes to contribute to the household economy.

Most of the new factory jobs needed male muscle from the working classes, and many of these jobs were dangerous. The few clerical jobs were mostly filled by males from the middle class. It wouldn't be until the early 1900s that the labor force would want large numbers of women in the form of secretaries, sales girls, clerical workers, and phone operators. As a result, the years 1840 to 1900 were often brutal for women of the working classes. The job market was so bad for these women that prostitution was often the best alternative among a small group of dismal choices.

For instance, after the Civil War, a seamstress might earn as little as 20 cents a day, with $2 to $3 a week being a good wage for a woman who was employed full time. This would hardly pay her rent. The same woman might earn more in a single night of whoring than during an entire week of domestic work. Domestic work was often unsteady, unavailable, and, according to a number of women, much harder on them than turning tricks.

Since this was the first time in our history when women needed to earn income outside of the home, there were no protections against sexual harassment. If a woman had to give in to the sexual advances of her boss to keep her domestic or seamstress job, she might as well get paid top dollar for it.

Another problem with the transition into an industrial economy was that factory jobs for men were often seasonal and lay-offs were frequent. Unemployment benefits didn't exist, and so the survival of the family would suddenly rest on a wife's ability to rustle up quick cash.

As a result, between 5% and 10% of all young women in cities like New York were probably involved in prostitution at one time or another. During harsh economic swings, the number might have been higher, and during boom times it might have been lower. (Like women today, women in the 1800s also traded sex for rent, goods and services in lieu of paying with cash. This has never been considered prostitution.)

We will talk more about prostitution later in this chapter. For now, it's important to realize that there can be no discussion of sex in America during the 1800s without an awareness of how important prostitution was, both socially and economically. While prostitution is still an economic force in America today, it is not nearly as central as it was in the 1800s.

In some ways, the modern porn industry has taken prostitution's place, but even that hardly holds a candle to the importance of prostitution for working class women in nineteenth-century America. Today's porn starlet has many choices for making a living besides helping men ejaculate. This is not to say that the average prostitute in the 1800s would have chosen bank telling over whoring, but today's woman has a range of choices that would have made a nineteenth-century woman's jaw drop.

Honey, Who Shrunk the Family?

In 1800, a healthy, white American female had, on average, 7 children. One hundred years later, she would be popping out only half as many little ones. Among the upper and middle classes, the size of the average family would drop 50% between the years of 1800 and 1900.

There have been suggestions that the decline in family size was due to a Victorian disdain of sex. But as we look at the availability of birth control and the flow of information about sex during the 1800s, it will become obvious that this was highly unlikely.

Also, since there were no sex researchers in the 1800s to ask people what they did in bed, we can only speculate about how often couples had sex. In one of the most complete surviving diaries from the 1800s, the author put a series of Xs on the pages when she and her husband had sex. She apparently did this to help her calculate the rhythm method of birth control which was popular during the day. The frequency of her Xs throughout a marriage that lasted for several decades indicates that she had intercourse with her husband as often as married couples supposedly do today. Her writing also indicated that she looked forward to having sex with her husband, and that it was an important part of her married life. The love letters that were written between husbands and wives during the 1800s tend to corroborate that physical passion was an important part of their relationships.

Advice and Content

There were no movies until the 1890s, and radio and TV were products of the twentieth century. Yet people in the 1800s craved information just as much as we do today. To help answer this need, public lectures became very popular, as did advice books and women's magazines.

The fact that the lectures were often about sex and birth control tells us that sexual enjoyment was no stranger to the masses of women and men from middle and upper classes. In the 1860s and 1870s, "Physiological Societies" also sprung up where birth control and sexual knowledge were often discussed. And some of the most popular books in the 1800s were about sexual enjoyment and birth control.

One modern sociologist who has studied the availability of sex information has speculated that the American woman of 1860 may have known as much or more about sexuality as the American woman of 1960.

Considering all of the pamphlets, books and lectures on birth control and sexuality that were available by the middle of the 1800s, there seemed to emerge a unified voice about sexual pleasure. This voice said that sex was important to both men and women, and that abstinence and celibacy—whether you were married or not—was unnatural and bad for you.

The Cherished Victorian Sex Scandal

Even today, it is not considered proper for TV news anchors to talk about oral sex and male ejaculation. However, when a recent American president was embroiled in a major sex scandal, the American people couldn't get enough of it. First-graders suddenly knew what fellatio was, and who among us hadn't heard about "that woman" and her famous blue dress?

It was no different in the 1800s, when a good scandal or criminal trial was a cherished part of the daily headlines. America loved a sex scandal—from the 1830s murder trial of Richard Robinson, who was the moody, sporting-culture boyfriend of prostitute-victim Helen Jewett, to explicit reports from Oscar Wilde's 1895 trial in England. The more sordid the details, the better. (If comparisons to recent American murder trials are in order, after the Robinson verdict was read, people claimed that he, too, had gotten away with murder.)

During the 1890s, American newspapers reported the grizzly details of America's first—and perhaps deadliest and most gruesome serial killer. Medical schools had marveled at the wonderful condition of the skeletons that H.H. Holmes sold to them. These were the bones of his early victims, who he had gassed in his suburban Chicago chamber of horrors and, whose flesh he removed by hand. It was estimated that 200 men, women and children were murdered by "the archfiend" Holmes before his crimes were discovered by Frank Geyer, a Philadelphia police detective.

In addition to the reporting of the mainstream press, the 1800s had newspapers like the *Policeman's Gazette,* which was the precursor of today's popular police and crime shows. The American appetite for crime-reporting and sex scandals has always been robust. It is not a modern phenomena.

Contraception and Abortion in the 1800s

People who don't have sex don't need contraception. People who value abstinence will "just say no." They won't be buying vast quantities of contraceptives. Yet, in the 1830s, America's largest newspapers had advertisements for contraceptive devices, diaphragms (womb veils), drugs to induce abortions, condoms, aphrodisiacs, and cures for sexually transmitted infections. By the 1870s, more than a third of the advertisements in America's tabloids and sporting papers were for birth control. This is not evidence of a sexually-repressive society.

But would we be able to recognize the content of these ads if we read them today? Consider the following newspaper ad from the 1800s:

> *Ladies. Carter's Relief for Women is safe and always reliable; better than ergot, oxide, tansy or pennyroyal pills. Insures regularity.*

Today, we would assume this was to help with constipation. But after reading this ad, Americans in the 1800s weren't envisioning smoother moves in the outhouse or less time squatting over the chamber pot. Based on the wording, they could tell that the ad was for a drug that was supposed to cause an abortion, which was an acceptable form of birth control in 19th Century America. For instance, the terms "Insures regularity" and "Relief for Women" were expressions that referred to abortion. Other well-known terms for abortion included "remedy for producing the monthly flow," "ladies' relief," "cure irregularities," "ridding oneself of an obstruction," "female regulator," "female pills," "tansy regulator," "uterine regulator" or "female cure." Ads for abortion-inducing pills promised to "bring on the monthly period with regularity, no matter from what cause the obstructions may arise."

The second clue had to do with the herbs that were mentioned: "better than ergot, oxide, tansy or pennyroyal pills." These herbs were thought to induce an abortion. Abortion was legal and common in the United States until the last part of the nineteenth century. It was allowed if performed before the quickening that occurred at approximately 16 to 20 weeks after conception.

Ads for abortion-inducing products sometimes contained "warnings" such as "women who are pregnant should not take them as they would surely cause a miscarriage," or "if a pregnant woman took the pills by mistake and a miscarriage resulted, it would not at all injure her health."

Women in the 1800s could also buy instruments for self-inducing an abortion. There were several different types of uterine probes (also known as "sounds") that were popular for this purpose. These instruments could easily be purchased at drug stores and through catalogues.

In addition to drugs and instruments, abortion clinics freely advertised in America's newspapers before the 1870s.

Types of Contraceptives in the 1800s

Withdrawal (Coitus Interruptus)

Withdrawal was one of the most widely practiced methods of birth control in the 1800s. There were actually two kinds of withdrawal: one was where the man pulled his penis out of the vagina shortly before orgasm, ejaculating outside of the woman's body. The other was partial withdrawal, where he pulled out as far as possible while still leaving the head of his penis inside the vagina when he ejaculated.

Partial withdrawal made sense in the first part of the 1800s, when two ancient theories about conception still prevailed. One was that the sperm had to be forcefully ejaculated against the cervix for conception to occur. The other was that a woman needed to have an orgasm in order to become pregnant. Partial withdrawal became less popular by the middle of the century, as the ability of sperm to swim became known.

Although withdrawal was widely practiced, some physicians and even feminists warned that it was unhealthy for males to ejaculate outside of a woman's body, as if an essential circuit was not being made, and the man's body was being unnecessarily depleted.

Douching

By the 1880s, one of the most common forms of birth control was vaginal douching. This usually happened after intercourse, but sometimes before.

Imagine what it was like for a woman in the 1800s to get out of bed on a freezing night in an unheated room to douche with cold water immediately after making love. Some of the birth control literature in the 1840s suggested that a woman could add spirits to the douche water to keep it from freezing over. Some physicians of the day—males, no doubt—recommended that the douche water be as cold as possible. This echoed the Aristotelian notion that it took heat for conception to occur.

More than twenty different solutions were used as spermicides or astringents, including vinegar and bicarbonate of soda. It may have simply been coincidence, but the average pioneer family who traveled west on the Oregon Trail took eight pounds of baking soda with them.

The instructions in some of the earlier douching kits that were intended for birth control said that women should douche even if they didn't have an orgasm. This was because it was still assumed in the early part of the 1800s that if a woman didn't have an orgasm, conception wouldn't occur.

Rhythm

By the mid-1800s, another "new" form of birth control became popular. It was based on the idea that there was a safe period when a woman could have intercourse without becoming pregnant. There was only one problem: modern science in the 1800s got the timing wrong. Ovulation usually occurs in the middle of a woman's cycle, and not at the start of menstruation as they thought back then.

Condoms

Condoms in the 1800s came in two styles—the full length models, like we have today, and high-water models that fit just over the head of the penis. For a long time, the caps that only covered the head were more popular than full-length condoms.

The better condoms were made from animal intestines that had been processed in lye. They were thin and strong. Large amounts of the material that they were made from—called Gold Beater's Skins—was imported into the United States during the 1800s. It was still being widely imported after 1873 when the Comstock laws made it illegal to import birth-control materials. Condoms made of fish skin and membranes were also available. They were considered better than those made of rubber. (The Comstock laws made it illegal to mail condoms or send information about sex or birth control anywhere in America. They will be discussed in another part of this chapter.)

Even with vulcanization, which made the rubber stretchy instead of brittle, rubber condoms were thick and inconsistent. Their only advantage was cost. By the 1870s, the price of condoms had fallen to $1 or $2 a dozen.

Although they were widely used, condoms were associated with prostitutes. As a result, they had a higher sleaze factor than rhythm, douching, or pills for abortion.

Diaphragms or Womb Veils

When an ad in a newspaper from the 1800s mentioned "Ladies rubber protectors" it wasn't talking about boots for the rain. Just about any woman reading such an ad knew that it was selling diaphragms or douching syringes that were specially made for contraception. Diaphragms were called womb veils, the French Shield for Women, and closed-ring pessaries. They became very common by the 1880s.

The diaphragm was the one contraceptive that a woman could use without her husband's knowledge. This was particularly helpful when the husband's withdrawal abilities were less than stellar, or when he didn't respect the rhythm method's black-out days. She could also use a womb veil when her husband didn't want her to use birth control.

IUDs and Nursing

During the 1800s, there were dozens of different intracervical and intrauterine devices for birth control. Many of these were quite popular, and women usually inserted them by themselves. It was also believed that nursing a baby kept you from getting pregnant. We know today that nursing should never be relied upon as a form of birth control.

The Bigger Issues of Birth Control—Then vs. Now

At the beginning of the 1800s, it was beyond the consciousness of Americans to believe that they could have control over any aspect of their health. Life was fragile. Even if a loved one was healthy, death could whisk him or her away at the snap of a finger. So how could you possibly control something as profound as when you became pregnant? It's hard to imagine today, but the concept of birth control required a shift in consciousness in the early part of the 1800s.

Pregnancy had always been a concern for most women, but the option to do something about it didn't arrive in America until the 1800s. Before then, there was no difference between sex for pleasure and sex for pregnancy.

The option to use birth control was not welcomed by all women. Many of the feminists during the 1800s worried that contraception would rob women of the one effective reason they had for saying "no" to sex—because they didn't want to become pregnant. And men in the 1800s had to digest the idea that if their wives could have sex without becoming pregnant, what would keep them faithful? What would keep their daughters chaste?

Both males and females who were social purity crusaders accused women who advocated for the right to control the size of their families as being proponents of free love. Politicians accused middle- and upper-class women who used birth control of committing race suicide. Yet America's Protestant ministers—the very people who you would expect to be opposed to birth control—seldom spoke out against it.

Our concerns about birth control today are much different than they were in the 1800s. They center around cost, convenience, effectiveness and side effects. The bigger moral and philosophical issues were for our ancestors in the 1800s to work out.

Technology and the Presses of Satan—The Birth of Modern Pornography

The 1800s saw the birth of America's first anti-obscenity laws. Anti-obscenity laws don't just drop from the skies. There needs to be enough indecency floating around to create a fuss, and it needs to have inserted itself far enough into the mainstream to be seen by more than its intended audience. During the 1800s, these conditions were easily met and exceeded many times over. The term "flaunted" would not be an exaggeration.

(Recently, a person with a controversial past and a penchant for media attention tried to open a brothel in Nevada. It would have male prostitutes for female customers. The other brothel owners in Nevada were upset about this, because they feared the publicity would motivate a movement to shut down all of the legal brothels in Nevada. These brothel owners were acutely aware of something that the commercial sex industry in America during the 1800s had no clue about—that "vice" is usually tolerated as long as the citizens are allowed to turn a blind eye to it. It seldom matters whether the sexual "vice" is prostitution, pornography, cross-dressing or homosexual enjoyment, as long as the public isn't forced to trip over it.)

Leaps in technology during the nineteenth century helped it become the temporal birthplace of pornography as we know it today.

First came the modernization of the printing press and new printing technologies. This allowed cost-effective print runs that could be tailored to fit the mass markets for mainstream porn and smaller niche markets for the kinky stuff. Then followed the technology that allowed paper to be made by machine. Before that, sheets of paper were crafted by hand. Handmade paper was often scarce and expensive.

And you can't call it pornography if it isn't captured in a camera's lens. The invention of the photograph in 1839 and the ability to mass produce it by the 1860s not only made the Kodak moment possible, but helped put the N in nasty. Finally, there was the invention of the moving picture in 1877, and the ability to show it to large audiences in 1895.

Pornography that has survived from the 1800s is amazingly explicit and shows most of the same sexual acts that pornography does today. As for written erotica, here are just a few of hundreds of titles that were popular in the 1800s. Some of these titles were best-sellers:

Amorous Adventures of Lola Montes

Aristotle's Master-Piece (an explicit how-to that saw many incarnations)

Awful Disclosures by Maria Monk, of the Hotel Dieu Nunnery of Montreal

Confessions of a Sofa

Curiositates Eroticæ Physiologiæ; or, Tabooed Subjects Freely Treated. In Six Essays, viz.: 1. Generation. 2. Chastity and Modesty. 3. Marriage. 4. Circumcision. 5. Eunuchism. 6. Hermaphrodism, and followed by a closing Essay on Death.

Exhibition of Female Flagellants, in the Modest & Incontinent World, Proving from indubitable Facts that a number of Ladies take a secret Pleasure in whipping their own, and Children committed [sic] to their care, and that their Passion for exercising and feeling the Pleasure of a Birch-Rod, from Objects of their Choice of both Sexes, is to the full as Predominant as that of Mankind.

Fanny Greeley: Confessions of a Free-love Sister

Marie de Clairville; or, The Confessions of a Boarding School Miss

Male Generative Organs

Physiology of the Wedding Night

Romance of Chastisement; or Revelations of the School and Bedroom. By an Expert.

Scenes in a Nunnery

Six Months in a Convent

The Amours of a Musical Student: being A Development of the Adventures and Love Intrigues of A Young Rake, with Many Beautiful Women. Also Showing The Frailties of the Fair Sex, and their Seductive Powers.

The Amours of Sainfroid and Eulalia: being the intrigues and amours of a Jesuit and a Nun; developing the Progress of Seduction of a highly educated young lady, who became, by the foulest Sophistry and Treachery, the Victim of Debauchery and Libertinism

The Bridal Chamber, and its Mysteries: or, Life at Our Fashionable Hotels.

The California Widow; or Love, Intrigue, Crimes, & Fashionable Dissipation.

The Child of Nature; or, the History of a Young Lady of Luxurious Temperament and Prurient Imagination, ...

The Intrigues and Secret Amours of Napoleon

The Lady in Flesh Coloured Tights

The Marriage Bed—Wedding Secrets Revealed by the Torch of Hymen

The Wanton Widow

The Lustful Turk

Venus' Album; or, Rosebuds of Love

Oral Sex in Another Time

In the 1800s, the medical experts of the day claimed that oral sex was an unnatural act because a woman couldn't become pregnant from it. However, oral sex was present in pornographic photos from the nineteenth century and it was no stranger to the erotic literature of the day, where it was sometimes referred to as "gamahuching." This rolls off the tongue as smoothly as "cunnilingus" and "fellatio," which begs the question of how things that feel so good can sound so bad.

As for cunnilingus, references to it appear in nineteenth century erotic literature and in pornographic photos as well. Woman-to-woman oral sex was one of the favorites in the live sex-shows. If a man paid to watch one woman give another oral sex, it seems that he might be inclined to try it on a woman himself, if he was allowed the opportunity.

Unlike today, a man in the 1800s who wanted to receive oral sex from a prostitute needed to find a brothel or a girl with a reputation for giving it. The buzz words to look for were "French," "French talents," "French-house," "unnatural practices" and "indecent dances and dinners." This means that when a man encountered a prostitute with the name "French Blanche LeCoq" or "French Marie," he was safe to ask for oral sex, especially if she spoke with a Midwestern accent.

In New Orleans's famous red-light district of Storyville, there was a brothel known as Diana and Norma's. This was a so-called French house, which means that fellatio was the specialty. Because blow jobs were all that Diana and Norma's offered, the rooms could be smaller (they didn't have to fit a bed) and the men didn't need to take off their shoes and pants. Due to the faster turnover and smaller space, Diana and Norma's was able to take advantage of the economies of scale and offer oral sex for the same price as intercourse. This was unusual during the 1800s, when blow jobs were considered kinky sex and usually cost more.

The best known "French House" in Storyville was that of Mme. Emma Johnson, who called herself the "Parisian Queen of America." Rather than being born in Paris or Versailles, French Emma was a native of Louisiana's Bayou country. Her oral skills were so renowned that even though she was notoriously long in the tooth, she offered a "sixty-second plan" where any man who could handle more than a minute of her ministrations without ejaculating did not have to pay. Emma Johnson's brothel offered more than oral sex, including live sex circus shows where the male performer had a mane, four legs, hooves and a tail. (It goes without saying he was hung like a horse.)

In his 1961 interview with former Storyville prostitutes, author Al Rose recorded the following words of a black woman who had worked out of a small row house known as a crib:

"Mos'ly for plain fuckin' on a weekday night, I use' t' get twenny-fi' cent. Ten cents in d' daytime. We chawged fifty cent, mos' alway fo' suckin' off and' seven'y-fi cent fo' lettin' d' prick come in our ass.... Good weeks I could take fo'ty dolluh, Big money dem days... Dey [black men] come fo' fuckin'. Dat's all day hawdly done. White boys?... Shit! Dey come fo' everyt'in' else. Mos'ly dey come fo' suckin' off. Sometime' dey come fo', fi', six at one time, all jam in dat po' li'l crib an' pay me a dime to let 'em watch me suck 'em. Shit! Carrie don' caiah!"   —From *Storyville, New Orleans: an Authentic, Illustrated Account of the Nortorious Red Light District* by Al Rose, University of Alabama Press, (1978).

Another Storyville prostitute interviewed by Rose was proud to recall that the madam of the house she worked in required the girls to give oral sex only when they were menstruating. She was disgusted to say that at some of the brothels, the women didn't do much else but give oral sex all of the time!

(Beginning in 1933, the American Social Health Association began doing a survey of the kind of sex acts that were requested of prostitutes. Only 10% of the requests in 1933 were for sex acts other than intercourse. By the end of the 1960s, nine out of ten requests of prostitutes were for oral sex or a combination of oral sex and intercourse.)

As for oral sex in New York City, during the 1880s there were a dozen brothels in close proximity to the newly-opened Metropolitan Opera House. Since a number of these brothels were "French-run," it is likely that the prostitutes performed arias the likes of which these opera goers had never known. Anti-vice investigators reported that because the girls in these French-run houses performed oral sex, other prostitutes would not associate or eat with them. But it is unlikely that one group of prostitutes cared about the sexual talents of another. If there was rivalry, it was for other reasons.

The Great Masturbation Panic

With many wonderful puns that were not lost on readers in the 1800s, Charles Dickens' famous novel *Oliver Twist* (1837-1839) refers often to the male body and its sexual maturation. Consider the following passage:

"I suppose you don't even know what a prig is?" said the Dodger mournfully.

"I think I know that," replied Oliver, looking up. "It's a th—you're one, are you not?" inquired Oliver, checking himself.

"I am," replied the Dodger. "I'd scorn to be anything else." Mr. Dawkins gave his hat a ferocious cock, after delivering this sentiment, and looked at Master Bates, as if to denote that he would feel obliged by his saying anything to the contrary.

The word "Prig," which was a term for thief, sounds very close to the word "frig" which was a well-known slang word for masturbation. Then we have a "ferocious cock" which is followed by "Master Bates." The puns and references to masturbation keep getting better, as Master Bates produces four handkerchiefs to clean up the mess that his name suggests will occur.

In spite of masturbation being well known and practiced in the 1800s, a serious anti-masturbation panic arose in the middle of the century. There are many reasons why masturbation started being described as such an evil at that time. One factor was the creation of the modern insane asylum in the early 1800s. The physicians at these harsh facilities discovered that patients often masturbated. Instead of viewing masturbation as one of the few pleasures that inmates of these dungeon-like asylums could give themselves, physicians published scientific articles claiming that masturbation had caused the insanity of the poor wretches who were under their care. In other words, the patients had masturbated themselves into the looney bins.

These reports helped fuel the fires that were being stoked by fanatics of the day like John Kellogg and Sylvester Graham, who wrote that more than 40 ounces of blood were lost during each male ejaculation. They believed that this huge depletion of blood led to horrible diseases such as cholera and the plague. In order to save a man from such a terrible fate, they declared that he was to have sex no more than once a month, and that he was to totally abstain from masturbation. This tied in nicely with religious prohibitions against any kind of sexual release that could not result in conception.

Understanding more about this panic helps us see why organizations like the Young Men's Christian Organization (YMCA) worked so hard in the 1860s and 1870s to pass anti-obscenity laws. These laws targeted any materials that might cause a young man to masturbate. There is a bit of irony in this, as it wasn't too many years later that if a young man in America wanted to find a place where he could masturbate with other young men, the YMCA was often at the top of his list.

Prohibitions against masturbation in America reached their climax in the second half of the 1800s. People today assume that these prohibitions must have scared young men and women into not masturbating. They also

THE NATIONAL POLICE GAZETTE: NEW YORK

PROPRIETY ARTICLES | MEDICAL

FREE CURE

I was quickly and Permanently cured of nightly emissions, complete impotency, varicocele, and small, wasted and shrunken organs, caused by self-abuse. Thousands have been fully restored though me. I will mail the means of this UNFAILING SELF-CURE (sealed) FREE: Inclose stamp. C.C. Crane, Narengo, Mich

---

Dr, Fuller's Youthful Vigor Pills. For lost manhood, impotence and nervous debility. By mail $2. Office, 429 Canal Street, New York

---

MONEY RETURNED IN CASE OF FAILURE

Certain parts of the body enlarged, Sexual power increased. The effects of youthful errors removed and manly vigor and full development guaranteed. For one dollar I mail a sealed box of MAGETINE for external use, also a guarantee, stating if parts are not Enlarged, and sexual power increased, I will return $1. Geo. Yates, Box 52, Jersey City, N.J.

BIG G

Cure Yourself! If troubles with Gonorrhea, Gleet, Whites, Spermatorrhoea or any unnatural discharge ask your druggist for a bottle of Big G. It cures in a few days without the aid or publicity of a doctor. Non-poisonous and guaranteed not to stricture. The Universal American Cure. Manufactured by The Evans Chemical CO. Cincinnati, O. U.S.A.

CERTAIN PARTS

of Body Enlarged, Beware of Bogus free cures. Send for the common sense method. Surest and safest developing tonic known! Cures all weaknesses. Increases sexual power. Sealed information *Free. Address:*
Albion Pharmacy Co. Albion, Mich. Box 18

MANHOOD RESTORED

A victim of youthful impudence, causing Premature Decay, Nervous Disability, Lost Manhood, etc. have tried in vain every known remedy, has discovered a simple means of self-cure, which he will send you (sealed) FREE to his fellow sufferers. Address, J.C. Mason, P.O. Box 3179, New York City

FREE TO MEN

We have a positive cure for the effects of self-abuse Early Excesses, Emissions, Nervous Disability, Loss of Sexual Power, Impotency, etc. So great is our faith our specific we will send one full month's medicine and much valuable information FREE address G.M. Co. 835 Broadway, New York

---

Results of Errors of Youth completed removed: Health and Manhood restored by the Nervous Debility Pills. Address N.E. Med. Institute, Boston

---

McQueen's Matico Injection. A preventative and specific cure for Gonorrhea. Gleet and all urinary troubles, without the unpleasant results from swallowing nauseous medicine. Price $1. All druggists.

SYPLILIS

A SPECIALTY.

Primary, secondary or tertiary syphilis permanently cured in 30 to 90- days. We eliminate all poison from the system, so that there can never be a return of the disease in any form. Parties can be treated at home as well as here (for the same price and under the same guarantee)

90 DAY'S TRIAL

DR. DYE'S

ELECTRO VOLTAIC BELT and other electrical appliances. We will send on 90 day trial to men, young or old, who are suffering from nervous debility, lost vitality, and those disease of a personal nature resulting from abuses and other causes speedy relief and complete restoration to health, vigor, and manhood guaranteed. Send at once for illustrated pamphlet free. Address. **VOLTAIC BELT CO. MARSHALL, MICH.**

MAY 28, 1892

1892...

Doctor Discovers Pill For Male Enlargement!
PRO+PLUS PILLS WILL WORK FOR YOU!
WE OFFER A 100% MONEY BACK GUARANTEE!!!
Doctor Approved Pill Will Enlarge Your Penis up to 5 inches!
You Will Have These Penis Gains In A Few Weeks!!!

• • DO YOU WANT • •
A LARGER PENIS?

If having a small penis makes you self-conscious, you can now add up to 3" in just minutes. No matter what size you are, you can add inches & make it thicker & firmer. An amazing new product! Not a pill or drug: not weights or a pump but a natural way to prosthetically increase your penis to its maximum potential. Increases your power & makes you the stud you always wanted to be.

REGULAR
&19.95

$8.95 each

NOW ONLY
Plus $1.00 postage & handling

TO ADD 8" TO YOUR PENIS SEND $14.95
Plus $2.00 postage & handling

• • *Rush to:* **LIBERTY LABS** • •
P.O. Box 2088 • GA72
Toluca Lake, CA 91610

SMALL PENIS?
ERECTION PROBLEMS?

LINGA-100 is the pure, natural laboratory blend designed to actually enlarge the penis and induce & maintain multiple, long term erections. LINGA-100 allows a more intense, deeply satisfying male climax while developing sexual power, physical strength and mental awareness. LINGA-100 was developed by top Swiss scientista involved in natual sex hormone research. Thousands of European men have experienced dramatic results. Impotency overcome. Increases in organ size of one-to-two inches not uncommon. LINGA-100 is perfect for the older man's problems. Studies reveal women definately consider the penis as the real measure of the man. Let LINGA-100 increase your sexual power and size. Only $9.95 plus $2 p/h. Order now!

SWISS LABS
Dept. A62, Box 276, Torrance, CA 90507

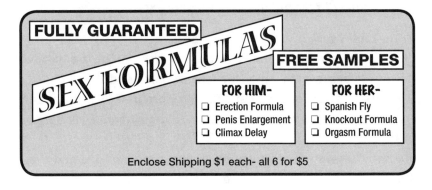

FULLY GUARANTEED

SEX FORMULAS

FREE SAMPLES

FOR HIM-	FOR HER-
❑ Erection Formula	❑ Spanish Fly
❑ Penis Enlargement	❑ Knockout Formula
❑ Climax Delay	❑ Orgasm Formula

Enclose Shipping $1 each- all 6 for $5

...Today

assume that there must have been serious prohibitions against masturbation in America before the 1800s, and that anti-masturbation zealots like Sylvester Graham and John Kellogg were giving voice to long-standing fears. None of these assumptions are true. At best, the bizarre prohibitions made people feel guilt or shame, but they didn't seem to stop many from masturbating.

Anti-masturbation fanatics like Graham and Kellogg were the first to admit that there was hardly an adolescent boy in America who didn't masturbate or know about masturbation. While the anti-masturbation fanatics weren't as concerned about masturbation among girls as among boys, this wasn't because they thought that girls didn't suffer horribly from it. It had more to do with their initial focus, which was saving the bodies and souls of white, middle-class Protestant youths who they believed were in grave danger from sexual excess of any kind, including masturbation.

The fires of masturbatory panic struck a chord in the minds of middle-class urban parents. Self-help and advice books were becoming hugely important, and the bogus medical advice of people like Sylvester Graham and John Harvey Kellogg may have found an audience among the new middle class who was consuming these books. Of course, these couples didn't take seriously the prohibitions against intercourse in marriage. The only prohibitions they may have taken seriously regarded their children's masturbation. And it's unlikely that children heeded their parents' concerns about sex any more than today's children do.

Sex writers today tend to make too much of zealots like Graham and Kellogg. While these men were not without influence, they hardly defined sex or the sexual climate in America during the 1800s.

Sex & The Civil War

The thirty-year span from 1846 to 1876 was one of the bloodiest in our history. It began with America's war against Mexico and ended with Sitting Bull's massacre of Custer at Little Big Horn in 1876. In between were Gettysburg, Chickamauga, Chancellorsville, Fredericksburg, Vicksberg, Shiloh and Appomattox.

Today, most Americans know about the attacks of 9/11 and the wars in Afghanistan and Iraq as images on a TV screen or computer monitor. In the 1860s, the Civil War impacted Americans in a much more personal way. Instead of fighting an enemy on foreign soil, we were fighting each other.

Among the nearly 60,000 books that have been written on the Civil War, there is only one currently available whose focus is sex.

Today, when we talk about a woman having access to the military, we mean that she is able to join and rise within the ranks. In the time of the Civil War, having access to the military meant that a woman got to sexually service men in the ranks. And there was no shortage of prostitutes who did just that. There were entire camps of prostitutes who followed the military divisions.

For instance, much has been written about how the word "hooker" may have come from the large camp of prostitutes who General Hooker allowed to be located near his division in Washington, D.C. While General Hooker was known to have had a personal fondness for whores, the slang term of "hooker" predated the Civil War by many years.

An interesting story about prostitutes in the Civil War emerged when the Army ordered 150 whores from Nashville to be placed on board a brand new passenger ship named the *Idahoe*. As was reported in the *Nashville Dispatch* on July 9, 1863: "Yesterday a large number of women of ill fame were transported northward.... Where they are consigned to, we are not advised, but suspect the authorities of the city to which they are landed will feel proud of such an acquisition to their population."

The city where the women were supposed to be let off was Louisville. The trip should have taken a few days at most. But neither Louisville nor any other ports along the Mississippi would allow the load of whores to come ashore. The *Idahoe* became famous and was called "The Floating Whorehouse." Its cargo of prostitutes nearly trashed the entire boat. They were finally returned to Nashville in August of 1863.

Love letters between Civil War soldiers and their partners are often poignant reminders that sexual intimacy was seldom forgotten in the face of tragic circumstance:

From a soldier to his wife: "I anticipate unspeakable delight in your embrace and look forward to your volumtuous touch." In her reply to him, she wrote: "How I long to see you... I'll drain your coffers dry next Saturday, I assure you." From the diary of a soldier who had just returned to duty after a short leave with his wife—"We didn't sleep much last night... The reunion so buoyed up our affections that we had a great deal of loving to do." From

General Weitzel to his lover—"My darling Louisa, I have pinched your picture and it does not holler. I have bitten it and it does not holler. I have kissed it and it does not return my kisses. I have hugged it and it does not return my hug. So just consider yourself pinched, bitten, hugged and kissed."

One thing we often forget about the Civil War is how the absence of men at home impacted traditional sex roles. This was studied at length during World War II, when Rosie the Riveter ran our heavy industries while men were away at war. It is likely that similar role reversals occurred during the Civil War, impacting how men and women related both at home and in the world of business. These role reversals contributed to the nineteenth century woman's growing sense of independence.

The Civil War & Proposed Constitutional Amendment

A fascinating by-product of the Civil War was a constitutional amendment that was proposed in 1863. Its wording affirmed "Almighty God as the source of all authority and power in civil government, the Lord Jesus Christ as the Ruler among the nations, and His Will, revealed in the Holy Scriptures, as of supreme authority."

You would think that such an amendment would have been a backlash against so much commercial sex in America. However, sexual excess was not the primary motivator. The main reason for the proposed amendment was because politicians feared that God was angry with the Union government, and that's why the North had been doing so badly in the Civil War.

A number of state governors supported the proposed amendment, and William Strong, the man who headed the organization that spearheaded it, was appointed to the United States Supreme Court. He would be instrumental in helping Anthony Comstock get his anti-sex legislation through Congress.

The Civil War and Rape

War is often associated with an increase in rape. While there were certainly rapes during the Civil War, the numbers were low compared to wars in Europe. Perhaps that's because the soldiers who committed rapes were often court marshaled and hanged or shot—sometimes the same day they were caught. Perhaps American soldiers had more respect for women than their European counterparts.

The rape victims of both Union and Confederate soldiers tended to be slave women. It is a sad irony that the Union soldiers who were supposed to be liberating slave women were raping some of them. But these women were the property of Southern men, and "destroying" their property may have been a way of humiliating the slave owners. Black women were also thought to have been more sexual than white women.

Slaves and Sex

For slaves, "family" had a different meaning than for most whites. The black family could be forever separated because a master wanted it that way, or because an auctioneer had placed family members in different lots. Black men were not allowed to protect their wives and children.

Sexual relations between white masters and black slave women were frequent. Some of these relationships were tender and caring, while others were rape and exploitation. The resulting mixed-race children drew particularly poor lots in life. Their presence could be a reminder to the white wife of the owner about her husband's adultery with the slave.

Before the Civil War, it was not unusual for free black women to have long-term relationships with white men. Between 1870 and 1894, it was even legal for white men and black women to marry in Louisiana. But that was an exception. After the Civil War, white America convinced itself that there was an epidemic of black men raping white women. Affairs between white women and black men threatened the social order and were no longer tolerated.

It is a myth to think that the North was any less racist than the South. Few people in the North were willing to tolerate the idea of blacks as neighbors or as lovers, except for visits to black prostitutes. After the Civil War, the few protections that society had afforded blacks all but disappeared.

Prostitution in the 1800s

Here lies Charlotte
She was a harlot
For 15 years she preserved her virginity
A damn good record for this vicinity.

–from the graveyard plaque of a nineteenth century prostitute in Colorado

In the bigger cities of the North, between one-in-ten and one-in-twenty women were at one time working as prostitutes. For most of these women, it was an occasional job. Some would do it exclusively for a couple of years, while others would do it only as the need arose.

Brothels were plentiful, and prostitutes could be found in almost every neighborhood of every city. Prostitutes also worked out of restaurants called Lobster Houses, concert saloons, or dance halls where they might take a trick to an upstairs room for a quick drop of the drawers. Big-city hotels were hubs of whoring, with the finer hotels having separate entrances for "respectable" women so there was no risk they would be confused with the prostitutes.

It was unusual for a man to walk down a street in a big city and not receive offers for sex. The offers came from women who appeared classy and from girls sitting half-naked in open doorways. A man could pick up a woman on the street and have sex in an alley, or he could find a whore working out of a small market, liquor store or cigar store.

If he were in a miner's town in the West, a man's only opportunity for sex might be to wait in a long line in front of a tent. This would get him a soggy poke with the area's only whore—not that his experience would be any worse than if he'd been with a prostitute in New York. Even garrisons on the frontier offered whores along with food and water for your horse. There were also Native American women who danced with more than wolves.

How the Whores Lined Up

Prostitution had its pecking order. At the top were the courtesans or mistresses to the wealthy. These select, educated, charm-school graduates could turn a phrase as elegantly as they could turn a trick.

Then were the Parlor Girls who worked in the upscale brothels or parlor houses. They were followed by the girls who worked in the public houses. These ladies didn't earn as much per poke, but turned more tricks per night.

Next were the cribs, which were rows of tiny shacks that were rented to prostitutes. Cribs were the horse stalls of commercial sex, often populated by former brothel girls who had grown too old or who were in poor health, or who didn't have the minimal looks or social graces to work in a brothel.

Lower yet in the ranks of whoredom were the streetwalkers. Streetwalkers were the dregs of commercial sex. They lived in sleazy hotel rooms or wretched apartments. They were not known for their cleanliness or good health. Life for streetwalkers was difficult.

At the very bottom of the whore barrel were the signboard girls. These girls lived on the streets and did their tricks in back alleys or behind billboards or large street signs. They didn't have a single good thing going for them.

Some of the occasional prostitutes in the cities ran in packs of teenage girls. They would hook up with men for a quick hit of cash or for a date to see the kinds of entertainment that they couldn't otherwise afford. These young women became such a visible part of popular culture that they earned the name "charity girls."

Economics and Inclination

When Dr. William Sanger did his study of prostitutes that was first published in 1858, he had expected to find poverty as the main reason for why a woman would do this kind of work. What he didn't expect to find was that the second most common reason the women gave for why they were working as prostitutes was "inclination" or sexual desire. In the minds of white Christians from the better classes, this was a frightening and perplexing finding. They wanted to believe that a woman's place was in the home, with her husband supporting her. They were also trying to convince themselves that women weren't interested in sex. To realize that thousands of prostitutes were not only supporting themselves financially, but weren't exactly hating their jobs, was a curve ball that threatened their very view of the world.

It's a Whore's Life

A full-time prostitute's best chance of finding friendship was from a fellow whore. But how many prostitutes had rewarding relationships with other prostitutes—either as friends or as sexual partners—is not known. For instance, there were plenty of brothel customers who paid to watch two prostitutes have sex with each other. Some of these situations evolved into same-sex relationships, but actual accounts are rare.

For many full-time prostitutes, the main source of companionship was their pets or their children. Long hours and boredom made for high rates of alcoholism and drug addiction. Some prostitutes did themselves in with overdoses of morphine, opium, cocaine and/or laudanum. Pregnancies were frequent, and venereal disease went with the territory as did abuse from police, pimps, customers and fellow whores. Tuberculosis, pneumonia, infected tonsils and poisoning from abortion-causing drugs were not unusual.

Prostitutes were sometimes a jealous, competitive, socially challenged lot whose only chance to feel good about themselves was at the expense of the women they were working with. Arrest records from the 1800s show that more whores were arrested for public drunkenness and fighting among themselves than for pandering.

Also, before 1885, the average age of consent for American girls was ten to twelve. It was not unusual for brothels to have young girls working as full-time whores. Most girls in the 1800s did not begin to menstruate until they were fifteen years of age. So a young prostitute of twelve to fifteen years of age had "the advantage" of not having to worry about pregnancy.

As for America's concern about its teenage girls, Alexis de Toqueville wrote in 1835 that there was no country in the world where he had seen girls turned out at such a young age. There was also a high demand for virgins. A virgin could get as much as $50 to $500 for her first time, which was a tremendous incentive when you consider that she might only make $1 to $2 a day for full-time employment, if she could find it.

Sex in Brothels

By the end of the 1800s, the brothel in America was a one-stop multiplex of sexual excess. To put it in perspective, there were at least as many neighborhood brothels as there are neighborhood gyms today. The main difference is in the body parts that were being exercised.

Brothels were dedicated centers of prostitution and were run by madams. They tended to be one of two kinds—private or public.

Private houses, which were also known as parlor houses, were the forerunners of today's upper-end country club. Only the wealthy could afford them. Membership was restricted to regular, well-known customers of the better classes. The furnishings were finely appointed, and everything from the food to the women were five-star. Members of private houses might be influential businessmen or lawyers, puffing on the finest cigars from Cuba and drinking the best whisky.

Public houses were the Pizza Huts of prostitution. The average stiff was welcome. There were often long, loud lines of drinking and drunken men, especially from Saturday night to Monday morning, given how this was the only time that men from the working classes had off from work.

The better of the public houses were known as dollar-houses, where men from middle class dropped their drawers. There were also fifty-cent houses that catered to the working class. These places often smelled bad and were infested with cockroaches and rats. In the working-class brothels, there might be a bench in the waiting area where men lined up next to each other. A voice from another room would yell, "Next!"

The one sex venue that a man absolutely wanted to avoid was called a panel house. A panel house was a room designed to help prostitutes rob their customers. There would be a false wall or panel that another prostitute or pimp would hide behind. Once the customer had his pants off, the accomplice would quietly relieve his wallet of all cash. Good luck finding a sympathetic policeman when you'd been robbed while doing business with a whore.

The Madam

The person who ran and sometimes owned the brothel was the madam. Madams were often former prostitutes who knew the business from their bottoms up.

The madam was one of the best management positions a woman could hold in the 1800s. Put in today's terms, she was a combination of hotel and restaurant manager, personnel director, head of marketing and publicity, nurse, counselor, bookkeeper and director of customer relations.

Besides being venues for sex, the better brothels were often places where business deals were made and where political wheeling and dealing occurred. When a well-known businessman or politician suffered a coronary at the brothel, the better madams would have the still-warm corpse moved to a more respectable location before the authorities were notified.

Storyville, the Sinful, Sexual Sapphire of the South

"In 1897, New Orleans city officials, acknowledging their belief that sins of the flesh were inevitable, looked Satan in the eye, cut a deal, and gave him his own address."

—Alecia P. Long, author, *The Great Southern Babylon: Sex, Race, and Respectability in New Orleans, 1865-1920*, LSU Press, (2005)

By the late 1800s, city governments all over the country were talking about establishing legally-controlled red-light districts. Prostitution would be allowed within these districts, but nowhere else. The most famous and longest enduring of the municipal vice districts was in New Orleans. It was called Storyville, and it was the nineteenth century's most successful attempt at harm reduction.

By 1890, the city of New Orleans was becoming a massive, municipal gumbo of sexual excess. To help save the city, a reform-minded, classical-music loving alderman named Sidney Story drafted an ordinance to create a red-light district at the edge of New Orleans' French Quarter. This was to be the only place in all of New Orleans where prostitution was allowed. The concept worked well for more than fifteen years. Naturally, "Storyville" was the last place on earth that a man like Sidney Story would want as his namesake.

By 1900, only two years after its official creation, Storyville housed more than 2,000 prostitutes in 230 brothels and houses of assignation. It was also home to a generous number of dance halls, concert saloons, gambling dens and firing ranges.

Particularly popular in Storyville were the brothels that promised girls who were octaroons and quadroons. These were light-skinned, mixed-race beauties. They were the product of "almagamation" or sex between the white and negro. An octaroon was theoretically one-eighth black, while a quadroon was one-quarter black.

Octaroons were thought to be the genetic superstars of Southern whores. They had just enough black in them to make them drip with a primitive, unrestrained, animal desire for sex that people believed the negro possessed, but with enough white to have the supposed intelligence, personality, creativity and beautiful physical features of the Aryan races. Sex with an octaroon was thought to win a man the best of both worlds, and he often paid more to fulfill his racist fantasy.

As the rest of America has recently become aware, Storyville and New Orleans were built over a swamp. Indoor plumbing and sewer pipes were rare in Storyville. The streets were flats of mud mixed with excrement from freshly-emptied chamber pots and the remains of decaying rodents. The smell was putrid, but a nose for whoring could ignore the wicked odors that steamed up from the streets below.

The sounds of Storyville were not tranquil. Trains ran along the main street, shooting galleries operated at all hours and music blared from the dance halls and concert saloons. A loud chorus of barkers, pimps and whores wooed the wads of the passersby.

Storyville did big business during winter, when tourists from the North could warm themselves before the fires of Satan. They could gamble, bet on horses and go on sexual rampages that made the offerings of their hometown red-light districts look like church socials.

At the height of Storyville's existence, the possibilities for excess ranged from visits to expensive, elaborate brothels and bars that were the Las Vegas casinos of their day, to tiny, dark, foul-smelling cribs, which were little more than livestock pens with beds in them.

In addition to selling sex, some claim Storyville was the birth place of jazz. But jazz was born long before Storyville. What Storyville did, however, was employ as many as fifty musicians a night, including some of the early jazz greats like Clarence Williams and Jelly Roll Morton.

Jelly Roll Morton played piano at Emma Johnson's during her notorious, live sex-circus shows. And in addition to tickling the ivories, Clarence Williams was a cabaret manager who invented the "Ham Kick." The Ham Kick was a contest for willing females. A ham was suspended from the ceiling, and if a woman was able to kick it, she got to take it home. But it needed to be obvious to the audience that the woman wasn't wearing any underwear.

Did the Customer Always Come First?

According to the few lasting memoirs from nineteenth-century madams, the men who arrived at their brothels were often lonely, feeling like aliens in a changing society that offered few comforts. Their hope was to find a moment of connectedness with a kind and caring woman. But even in the rare situations when a prostitute did pretend to be kind and caring, she was often getting ready to service her next customer before the man had finished his final thrust.

When Al Rose (author of *Storyville, New Orleans*) interviewed men who had been frequent customers of the prostitutes of Storyville, similar stories were told in different words:

> "She'd take hold of your prick and milk it to see if you had the clap. I think the girls could diagnose clap better than the doctors at that time. She'd have a way of squeezing it that if there was anything in there, she'd find it.... Then she'd fill the basin with water and put in a few drops of purple stuff—permanganate of potash, it was... Then she'd wash you with it. She'd lay on her back and get you on top of her so fast, you wouldn't even know you'd come up there on your own power. She'd grind so that you almost felt like you had had nothing to do with it. Well, after that, she had you. She could make it go off as quickly as she wanted to—and she didn't waste any time, I'll tell you. How did I feel about it?... I was never satisfied. I don't mean that I thought that the girls of the district had cheated me... They'd drain me off. I'd be depleted and enervated—but I never had the feeling of satisfaction that I

was always looking for. The truth is that a man wants something more from a woman than that... No, I can't say I have happy memories of the District. I just had a weakness for those whores—and they were so easy to get."

The next Storyville veteran interviewed by Rose had frequented the more expensive brothels in Storyville and had the added perspective of comparing American prostitutes with those in other parts of the world:

"She approached me and seized my genital organ in one hand, wringing it in such a way as to determine whether or not I had the gonorrhea. She did this particular operation with more knowledge and skill than she did anything else before or after.... She washed me with some foul-smelling disinfectant and lay down on the bed, inviting me to mount her. This I proceeded to do, and the mechanical procedure that followed endured for perhaps a minute.... I've been in whorehouses all over this globe. I've been in the cheap brothels of Montmartre and in the House of Seven Stories in Tokyo. I've been fucked in Singapore, Kimberly, San Juan, Buenos Aires, and Calgary... The foreign whores, somehow, manage to feign an attitude that leads you to believe, at least for the moment of intercourse, that you have their attention and that they are interested in seeing that you have a pleasant time. While they never do it free, they always seem just a little surprised when you hand them the money—as though they'd forgotten about this crass detail... Storyville whores, no matter how well-dressed or how gaudily expensive the whorehouse, were avaricious, greedy, and uncouth.... No house in the District could, with their practices, survive for a month in Paris.... It took much time and trouble to seduce the young ladies of our social circle, though I sometimes took the time and trouble. These experiences, few and far between, were much more satisfying—but it was difficult to make the effort with the District so near."

From the Belle of the Ball to Pussy Non Grata—
Dating Does the Whore In

While talking about prostitution's decline in America is more academic than erotic, it helps us understand about the birth of dating and sex as we know it today. By the time the 1800s are over, prostitution is in decline and sex in America is starting to assume its current shape.

You would think that in the history of sexual relations in America, dating would have come before prostitution. But in reality, it happened the other way around. Prostitution was a mighty force in America from the 1830s until the end of the century, when dating started to take its place. While dating by no means boarded up the brothel door, it was one of the things that helped drive a stake through the heart of the harlot as a central figure of sex in America.

By the 1900s, the "new" American woman was becoming the standard bearer of sexual release, and she didn't work in a brothel or bear the stigma of women who did. Women now had the option of more jobs and better wages, including white collar jobs in sales and in the service sector. They were also gaining more sexual freedom.

The winds of favor that had made prostitution the centerpiece of popular culture started changing direction. Young men and women started expecting sexual enjoyment to be the reward of relationships rather than the result of pulling a dollar from a wallet. Dating and "stepping out" became the new darlings of our market economy, helping to ease prostitution into the shadows.

For instance, in the 1890s, the average age of a New York City prostitute was as young as fifteen years. By 1915, the average whore was twenty-five with some being as old as thirty or forty. Prostitution was no longer an entry-level position for young girls in America.

There were many reasons for prostitution's decline, few having to do with reformers, anti-vice crusaders, or sexual repression. As New Orleans Mayor Martin Behrman lamented shortly before World War I when the Secretary of War forced him to shut down Storyville, "You can make it illegal, but you can't make it unpopular."

One of the reasons for prostitution's decline was the failure of prostitutes to put the satisfaction of the customer ahead of their own greed. Prostitutes also refused to operate within socially acceptable boundaries. Prostitution in America had become like a neighbor who never turned his stereo down.

Downtowns started to grow and become centers for shopping and commerce. Good taste dictated that they needed to be protected from the antics of whores who couldn't keep from lifting their skirts in the faces of men on the street. Whores in the nineteenth century knew no subtlety, not that those in the current day are models of modesty and good taste. Changes in real estate, jobs and technology were making the in-your-face type of prostitution of the 1800s a liability instead of an economic plus.

During the 1800s, brothels were the most lucrative tenants for real-estate owners. However, in the 1900s, this was starting to drastically change. Land was badly needed for skyscrapers and high-rise apartments. Factories and office buildings needed space to expand, with nowhere to go but the land occupied by brothels.

Many city governments in the 1800s would have gone bankrupt without the fees they collected from their whores. However, with the start of the twentieth century, the revenue base of America's cities grew stronger, and politicians had their fingers in more pies than just the prostitute's. Close ties to prostitution were no longer worth the political repercussions, and politicians were finding cleaner ways to get dirty money. Due to citizen demands for reform, corruption in police forces was decreasing. Policeman could no longer collect large stashes of cash from prostitutes, and so the incentive to protect them was evaporating. All of these factors helped make the climate for whoring less favorable.

By the 1900s, telephones were widely available. A man could phone a prostitute and arrange a meeting for sex rather than needing public spaces for the transaction to occur. The telephone also helped make gambling and numbers-running more profitable than prostitution.

There had always been a close association between alcohol and prostitution. What made the throat wet also helped to quiet the protests from the mind. Also, it was easier for a prostitute to relieve a drunken trick of his money than a sober one. But with the start of Prohibition, the availability of alcohol in social settings became limited to speakeasies. Whores followed the shot glass, and speakeasies became America's new brothel. While speakeasy sex could be notoriously brazen, it was also hidden, allowing the rest of society to turn a blind eye.

A major source of demand for prostitution in the 1800s had been the huge waves of immigrants, led by younger males who left the old world to find their fortunes in America. However, by 1933, the number of immigrants to America had fallen to 23,000, down from nearly a million a year during parts of the 1800s. Male-to-female ratios no longer favored the prostitute.

While settling the West had often been the job of male pioneers and gold prospectors, America's railroads were making travel safer and more sensible for women. During the covered-wagon days of the 1800s, small towns often had ratios of one woman to every 10 to 100 men. These numbers started to even out by the 1900s. The long lines in front of the whore's tent were becoming a thing of the past.

With the invention of photography and leaps in printing technology, pornography was becoming a lucrative business. Resources that had gone into prostitution during the 1800s started shifting into pornography during the 1900s—to the point where adult films, magazines and X-rated Websites would one day rival the market domination that prostitution once held. The porn starlet of today may have well been the parlor girl of the 1800s.

Brothels and concert saloons were the command centers of prostitution after the Civil War. But by the 1900s, movie theaters were becoming the hubs of entertainment. The new movie theaters offered social legitimacy and dark balconies—providing a new set of sexual possibilities. Rather than being haunts for beer, burlesque and whores, the movie theaters were a place to take a date, find entertainment, eat popcorn, enjoy fine confections, make out and cop a feel. They provided places where a respectable girl could go with the approval of her parents and be sexual but not scandalized.

While the whereabouts of the sporting man's penis in the 1800s was controlled by the number of bills in his wallet, after the 1900s it became fashionable for him to surrender control of his sperm wagon to his sweetheart. The single man's sexual expectations were changing. He and his partner were exploring sexually while keeping the head of his penis on his side of her hymen. Since intercourse was increasingly tied to serious relationships, men and women started marrying at a younger age than they had in the 1800s.

Around the time of the Civil War, sex between whites and blacks was a gray area. While people certainly noticed, their protests were often limited to searing stares and mumbled expletives. In many of the commercial sex venues throughout the country, interracial sex was not uncommon. However, by 1900, segregation was becoming the law of the land. The new segregation laws were impacting commercial sex districts, like the nation's number-one address for vice, Storyville in New Orleans. (Storyville had originally been set up as two separate, segregated vice districts, one for white whores and one for black whores, but this was ignored until its final years.)

A fascinating motivator for the move to close the brothels was not so much the feminist or religious outcry, but the growing sentiment that sperm was a bad thing to waste. For instance, camp whores had been seen as an important way of providing Civil War soldiers with a much-needed sexual release. But by World War I, Americans felt that prostitutes posed a great danger to our soldiers—both with venereal disease and physical depletion.

With America's approaching involvement in World War I, we believed that the best way to protect our boys was to keep their khakis on. Harsh new laws were enacted to protect our troops from the dangers they might encounter when their private parts were in a whore's hands—as if mustard gas and the trenches of Western Front could not compare. Cities that didn't aggressively hide their red-light districts faced losing their war-related expenditures. In the case of Storyville, the Secretary of War told the City of New Orleans that if it didn't shut down its famous vice district, they would send in soldiers to do it. Where prostitution used to be a financial lifeline, it now threatened the wartime gravy train.

Ransacked Hymens & Myths about the American Woman

During the first half of the 1800s, people believed that sexual enjoyment was just as important for women as for men. But as the latter part of the century ticked away, some very bizarre theories emerged about women's sexuality and about women in general.

For instance, in 1881, the *New York Times* claimed that the reason for the falling birth rate among the better classes was because women were addicted to the "purse-destroying vice" of shopping. According to the *Times,* promiscuous and unrestrained shopping was destroying the fabric of American life. Even the head of the Women's Christian Temperance Union cried out against "the love of finery," which she said was one of woman's greatest temptations.

A popular public-health manual warned about the physical cost to women of higher education: "Great mental exertion is injurious to the reproductive power" and "college produces women with monstrous brains and puny bodies." Not to be outdone, some of America's best-selling books in the latter part of the 1800s claimed the place of a Christian woman was in the home, where she could excel at cleaning, cooking, mending and having children.

An editorial in America's leading medical journal in 1911 lamented the new trend of women choosing careers over marriage. America's physicians, it said, should always encourage marriage.

As for getting down'n'dirty in a sexual way, so-called medical experts began to claim that women were pure and free from sexual desire or excess. Women were starting to be described as innocent of the faintest ray of sexual pleasure, and it was said that they never experienced feelings of physical pleasure or yearning.

Of course, America's streets were lined with prostitutes, and our newspapers were overflowing with ads for birth control, so the people who concocted the new propaganda about women's natural state of purity added the caveat that if a woman was exposed to wanton sexuality, she could easily be lost to sin and hopeless vice. Vice was apparently more robust than purity, considering the scores of ransacked hymens it had left in its wake.

It is likely that these bizarre theories emerged as a backlash to the social and economic advances that women in America were beginning to make by the end of the 1800s. For instance, more teenage girls from the middle class were going to school, and they often outnumbered boys in high school. Instead of going straight home after school, the new breed of American girls socialized with each other and with boys. Instead of cooking, sewing, and caring for younger children, they were reading books and thinking thoughts that were previously restricted to men. By the end of the 1800s, a more independent, modern American woman was being born, and this was disturbing to both women and men from prior generations.

Worse yet, between 1870 and 1920, the divorce rate in America increased 1500%. The size of the middle-class American family had plummeted, and an increasing number of women were choosing careers over marriage. More and more, women were being seen as assassins of the white, middle-class family.

As for notions of women being pure and avoiding sex, the new invention of the moving picture begged to differ. The most popular titles shortly after the turn of the century showed American women as being sassy, seductive, and very much in control.

Technology Gives America a New Nightlife

Technology can change a culture in many ways. For instance, think of how the television changed America. And what about the car, radio, telephone, record player and iPod?

The influence of technology was particularly profound after the 1870s, when Thomas Edison's invention of the light bulb may have done more to liberate American women than the day's feminists and social activists.

Before Edison brought us the light bulb in 1879, America's downtowns after dark were dangerous and scary places. They were lit by gas lights which cast dark, ominous shadows. However, the electric street light helped transform America's downtowns into places that were bright and inviting. America's women no longer needed to stay behind closed doors after dark, and our modern concept of the nightlife was being born. The scene was set for America's women and men to start going out and "steppin' out."

When we think about how the electric light helped change the way that Americans socialized, the invention of the telephone had an even greater impact. For instance, in 1848, it took upwards of a month to get a letter from coast to coast. Good luck casually checking in on a friend who lived only five miles away. Fifty years later, Americans were talking to each other on nearly a million telephones. The new telephone industry not only created thousands of jobs for women as telephone operators, but the young women who now had good jobs were able to call each other and say, "Let's go to the movie" or "Meet me at the soda shop." And what would modern dating be without the first generation of young men who called young women at the start of the 1900s to say, "Would you like to go out dancing with me?"

Technology not only changed how we spoke to each other, but how we could meet each other. For instance, in April of 1846, the Donner party began their famous journey west. If you wanted to go west, the covered wagon was the only game in town. But that drastically changed in May of 1869, when the final spike was hammered into the first of five transcontinental railroads that would connect East and West. What used to be a perilous journey in covered wagons now took less than five days by rail. By 1880, railroads criss-crossed the entire country. Not only did they provide a safe and convenient way for men, women and their families to populate new parts of the country and to visit each other, but the railroads allowed goods produced in one part of the country to be sold in another. Completing the railroads was no less of an engineering feat than putting a man on the moon—which occurred exactly 100 years after the completion of America's first intercontinental railroad.

Soon after the railroads were built, Americans turned to building public transportation in our cities. Public transit helped America's downtowns and new amusement parks become centers of social activity. Not only would young men and women have places to go for socializing after work, the new networks of public transportation would give them a way to get there.

Technology also transformed how long we lived. For instance, from 1800 to 1870, the average white American could expect to die at the ripe old age of 39. But suddenly, between 1880 and 1900, our life expectancy leapt to almost age 50. Infant mortality dropped in half. Why the sudden change? Cities began installing sewer and water systems between 1880 and 1900.

Imagine how bad our cities smelled before the installation of sewers and the diseases we suffered due to the lack of sanitation and potable water? It was the new sewers and plumbing, rather than advances in medicine, that added ten more adult years to the lives of Americans. Ten more years for romance and sex!

What Used to Happen in Private Becomes Public

It wasn't until the very end of the 1800s that dating and the social mixing of young men and women started becoming a normal part of popular culture. Before then, males socialized with males, and females with females. And when young males were allowed to be with young females, there was often a chaperone.

The segregation between the sexes was so great that during the last third of the 1800s, nearly one-in-every-five men in America belonged to a male-only fraternal order—from the Freemasons and Odd Fellows to the Knights of Pythias, Modern Woodmen of America and Improved Order of Red Men. These secret fraternal organizations required men to be at the lodge many nights each month for the initiation rites that were held when a member rose from one level in the fraternal order to the next. Membership in fraternal orders began to decline rapidly as technology helped transform American popular culture into a dating culture at the end of the 1800s. To survive, the fraternal organizations had to trim their elaborate initiation ceremonies.

Only a few years after the invention of the electric light bulb and the telephone, the moving picture arrived. This marvelous invention would herald in the era of the majestic movie theater—yet another public place where males and females could meet and date.

At the same time, magnificent events called "world's fairs" and "expositions" were awing millions of Americans. 14 million people attended the Chicago World's Fair of 1893. By 1904, another 19 million people would attend the great expositions in Atlanta, Nashville, Omaha, Buffalo and St. Louis. These events impacted their hosting cities like the Olympics do today.

In 1895, there had been no amusement parks on New York's Coney Island. By 1904, three newly-built amusement parks were attracting more than 4 million visitors to Coney Island each year—many of them young couples on dates. One of the first amusement parks on Coney Island was lit up by 250,000 of Edison's miraculous light bulbs.

After the first years of the 1900s, almost every city in the country had amusement parks. Some of the new amusement parks were as amazing as Disneyland and Disney World are today. They became popular venues where millions of American couples and families would spend the day or evening.

Visitors to these story-book amusement parks could marvel at exhibits such as "Streets of Cairo and Mysterious Asia." They could see the latest in technology in the great halls, or listen to the new phonographs and view the new moving pictures. Visitors could enjoy the carnivals with their magnificent carrousels, roller coasters, skating rinks, and even "Blowhole theaters" where jets of air would blow women's dresses up into the air.

Some of the most popular attractions in America's amusement parks were their dance halls and ballrooms where single men and women could meet—men and women who didn't know each other beforehand and who were not chaperoned. Before then, unsupervised meetings of single males and females were often in sleazy surroundings, where it was assumed that the women were prostitutes and the men their customers.

Until the end of the 1800s, much of America's nightlife had centered around the hard-drinking, whore-loving, sporting culture of males. The new amusements prided themselves on having no beer gardens and on quickly removing any thugs or drunken patrons. They were some of the first places in America where members of all genders and economic classes could mix and mingle, and they helped transform the way that Americans socialized. They marked the beginning of dating as we know it today.

Beyond the Boundaries of Home

During the 1800s, the American woman of the middle and upper classes had prided herself on being the anchor of the home. She provided her man with a refuge against a working world that was difficult and demanding. The home was where he went to escape the gambling, whoring, and bawdy street life of the lower classes.

However, as one author put it, "God Bless Our Home" never meant "God Make Our Home Happy." By the end of the 1800s, the American woman's options were evolving. It was becoming safe for women of any social class to be out in public, laughing and dancing with men they didn't know—without having to worry so much about their reputations. There were now places where young Americans could meet, and the public transportation to get them there and back.

Venereal Disease in the Time of Victoria

No discussion of sex in the 1800s would be complete without a look at venereal disease.

An interesting thing happened to venereal disease over the course of the 1800s. In the mind of physicians, syphilis and gonorrhea went from being no more serious than a headache or cold, to a social and moral plague that was worse than cancer or leprosy. The truth was somewhere in between.

It wasn't until 1837 that scientists discovered that gonorrhea and syphilis were two distinct diseases. Even then, there was little awareness that syphilis could cause blindness, heart failure, insanity and death. The more devastating forms of the disease that did not occur until years after the initial infection were not understood to be parts of syphilis until the late 1800s. Before then, physicians thought that these were separate diseases that had nothing to do with sexual infection.

As for gonorrhea, physicians believed that it was a benign infection, often resulting from too much sexual activity. Well into the 1870s, many physicians believed that it was normal for women to have gonorrhea and that there was no reason for concern. It wasn't until the latter part of the 1800s that we learned gonorrhea was a cause of sterility in women, and could cause blindness in a child who was born to a woman with an active case.

Once physicians started becoming aware of how dangerous venereal diseases could be, the pendulum swung far in the other direction. A moral panic ensued in the ranks of our medicine men. Although they had no clinical tests to confirm the presence of venereal disease, leading physicians made bold, unfounded declarations that venereal diseases caused more death and destruction than all other diseases combined. They made outrageous claims that as many as 80% of American men had a venereal disease. They declared that we could get venereal diseases from cups, kisses, pens, pencils and toilets.

Cases of vaginitis among school girls were said to be gonorrhea, and people had to be especially wary of contact with America's immigrants, who, physicians warned, were naturally disposed to moral and physical degeneracy.

Once the medical community became aware of the danger of venereal disease, they did not treat it as a medical matter, but as a problem of morality. When they did provide "education" about venereal disease in the 1900s, it was fear-based and shame-based. And when some states started requiring proof of no venereal disease before issuing a marriage license, it was only the man who was examined. Such examinations were thought to be disrespectful for a proper woman.

America's physicians, who were starting to view themselves as the new high priests of morality, stated that venereal disease posed an even greater threat to the American family than birth control. Perhaps, they wrote, the decreasing size of the American family wasn't the fault of selfish women who were practicing birth control, but of philandering husbands who were bringing home venereal diseases that were making their innocent wives sterile!

These ideas fit nicely with the sentiment of America's finer minds that women were constitutionally weaker than men. Not only were women's bodies being emaciated by foolish pursuits such as attending college, but America's leading physicians were now declaring that our women were being cheated from their sole purpose and destiny in life—to bear and raise children—by the venereal diseases of an immoral society.

Just how much the general population paid attention to our physicians' hysteria is not known. While popular newspapers and magazines were happy to accept paid advertisements for quack venereal-disease cures, they were terrified to actually report on the subject. In 1906, the popular *Ladies' Home Journal* became one of the first magazines in the country to publish articles on venereal disease, and it lost 75,000 subscribers as a result. As late as 1912, the U.S. Post Office seized Margaret Sanger's pamphlet *What Every Girl Should Know* because it talked about syphilis and gonorrhea. It was declared obscene under the Comstock Law.

Even if the general population did know about the physicians' fears, history shows that this might not have altered their behavior. For instance, in the 1840s, physicians started declaring that masturbation caused insanity, but there is no evidence that their dire warnings stopped a single person from masturbating. Even today, when we know that unprotected anal sex can cause AIDS, the practice of barebacking remains epidemic in large parts of the gay community. And good luck getting more than a small percentage of Americans who are having intercourse with a new partner to use condoms—at least at the time of this volume's publication.

It is difficult to know how extensive venereal disease was in America during the 1800s. Since the more devastating secondary and tertiary phases of syphilis were thought to be caused by other diseases, we don't know how many people died from them in the 1800s. And once the connection to syphilis was understood, physicians would often change the cause of death to protect the reputation of the family. Also, the diagnostic criteria for venereal disease was so broad that many people who did not have it were diagnosed with it.

What we can assume is that venereal disease was a significant problem and that many people died from it in the 1800s. We also know that the "cures" for syphilis were often toxic and could cause as much pain and suffering as the disease itself. However, because the initial symptoms of syphilis usually became dormant as a natural part of the disease's progression, even the strangest of the quack cures were thought to cure it.

While prostitution was often blamed as the source of venereal disease, it is unlikely that fear of catching the disease caused the decline in prostitution in the United States. The decline in prostitution started in the last decades of the 1800s, while awareness of the true dangers of venereal disease had not become part of the nation's consciousness. Even then, the newfound knowledge did not stop people from visiting prostitutes.

Anti-Obscenity Laws of the 1800s

The 1800s brought us the light bulb, telephone and magnificent railroads that tunneled through mountains and spanned rivers and gorges. The 1800s also brought America its first anti-obscenity laws.

By the end of the 1800s, our government had given itself the authority to throw people in prison for up to ten years at hard labor for mailing information about condoms or for printing or receiving a romance novel that was declared obscene by postal inspectors—men whose sole basis for expertise was their membership in the Young Men's Christian Organization or the Society for the Suppression of Vice.

A name that has become synonymous with anti-obscenity laws in America is that of Anthony Comstock. The anti-obscenity laws of 1872 that were nicknamed after him were the most far-reaching of any in our nation's history. Yet America's first federal anti-obscenity laws were enacted in 1842, when Anthony was a mere twinkle in the eyes of his evangelical Christian parents.

These laws were part of the Tariff Act of 1842. This might seem strange, given how tariff acts are supposed to regulate foreign imports. But that was the point. Our politicians assumed that the indecent materials that were circulating in America in the 1840s were imported from abroad, particularly from Satan's country of birth, France. America's first federal anti-obscenity law attempted to stop "the importation of all indecent and obscene prints, paintings, lithographs, engravings and transparencies."

It was beyond the comprehension of American politicians that some of the erotica that was starting to flood our cities may have been homegrown. From their perspective, the new wave of printed filth must have followed the immigrant aliens from Europe who were landing on the sacred shores of our forefathers.

The second round of anti-obscenity laws were enacted in 1865. These were an expansion of the Tariff Act of 1842. Again, Anthony Comstock had nothing to do with them, as he was still a prostheletizing and unpopular Civil War soldier stationed far from combat in Florida.

By 1865, the newer printing presses had the ability to mass produce photographs, particularly those of Victorians doing nasty things. As a result, dirty books were fast replacing the Good Book as the mainstay of the Civil War soldier's napsack. Special X-rated booklets were made in smaller trim sizes that allowed them to conveniently accompany the Civil War soldier. While it was fine for a soldier from New York to kill a soldier from Virginia, our government believed it was morally unacceptable for a soldier to keep a picture of a naked woman next to his spare ammo.

The crowning jewel of American anti-obscenity legislation came in 1872. It was the brain child of the conservative power elite from the Young Men's Christian Association. This unusual legislation was passed during a last-minute, late-night session of Congress. It is unlikely that members of Congress understood its implications any more than Congressmen understand the laws they pass today. But at least with today's laws, there is usually a quorum in the House of Representatives before a vote is cast, and legislation seldom passes the Senate without the vote being recorded. Neither condition was met when the anti-obscenity legislation was passed in 1872.

Comstock's law, which was nearly identical to one written by members of the YMCA a few years prior, was quite deceptive. Its stated purpose was to close loopholes in legislation that prohibited the interstate sale of obscene literature and materials. It's title was "The Act for the Suppression of Trade in, and Circulation of Obscene Literature and Articles of Immoral Use."

But buried in the text of Comstock's law was the inclusion of "any article whatever for the prevention of conception, or for causing unlawful abortion." Not only had Comstock managed to make it a crime to send contraceptive devices in the mail, but he made it illegal to send information about birth control as well. The highly repressive laws that he and his cohorts got through Congress helped breed a number of state laws that made it a crime for a physician to even discuss birth control with his patients.

The Comstock law made it illegal to give away, exhibit in any manner, publish, write, print or have any card, circular, pamphlet, book or notice of any kind, any drug, medicine or article for the prevention of conception or for causing abortion.

Before 1872, contraception in America was neither obscene nor illegal. For the next hundred years, it would be. It was not until 1965 that the courts would declare it illegal for a state to prohibit the use of contraceptive devices, and it wasn't until 1971 that it became legal to send information about birth control in the U.S. mail.

Thanks to the Comstock legislation, the federal government now controlled the reproductive behavior of its citizens.

Anthony Comstock was rewarded for his efforts by being appointed the nation's chief postal inspector. Not only did his new law give him the power to seize material, but to arrest those sending it, as well as those who received it. That might not be such a big thing today, when many alternatives to the U.S. mail exist for sharing information. But in the 1800s, the US mail was the main artery short of telegrams for getting information from point A to B.

As America's first czar of the chaste mind, Comstock believed that the minds of the young were delicate and easily corruptible. He believed that any materials that could generate impure thoughts were obscene. This included information in leading medical journals about birth control.

Allowing Anthony Comstock to police the U.S. mails was like allowing an abortion-clinic bomber to have oversight of Planned Parenthood. Remarkably, it is difficult to find evidence that Comstock and his anti-obscenity crusade helped stem the flow of pornographic materials that might be considered obscene. He may have inconvenienced the producers of pornography, but he was unable to check them.

Comstock did his damage by stemming the flow of information about reproduction and birth control. In 1913, after searching some of the biggest libraries in America for information about contraception, birth-control crusader Margaret Sanger could find virtually no medical information about birth control anywhere in America. This had not been the case in America before the 1870s, when information about birth control had been freely available. (The stance of America's physicians against the use of contraception did little to help check Comstock's influence. Physicians, who were mostly white, male, Protestant and from the better classes, were trying to position themselves as guardians of the American family. Many of American's physicians in the late 1800s believed women should be at home, having and raising children.)

While it is easy to make blanket condemnations of people like Comstock, we need to remember that Congress and the courts could have stopped him. Instead, they usually did the opposite. It is also important to remember that the purity groups of the late 1800s occasionally had an important battle on their hands. It was not unusual for twelve-year-old girls to be turning tricks in houses of prostitution. This, and the out-of-hand nature of prostitution and pornography, was often at the center of their concern.

Fairies, Wolves, Trade and Loop-the-Loop

An important starting point for our modern categories of straight, gay, and bisexual occurred at end of the 1800s. This is when the notions of heterosexual and homosexual first got off the ground. Before then, males in America tended to socialize with males, and females with females. Men could sleep in the same bed without eyebrows being raised, and two men who had a caring relationship did not usually pay a large social price for it as long as they did not flaunt what they were doing or appear to be effeminate. And it was perfectly normal for women to live together and share the same bed for much of their adult lives. Author Lillian Faderman chronicles these *romantic friendships* in her book "Odd Girls and Twilight Lovers," Columbia University press (1991).

Until the end of the 1800s, an American male was not usually ostracized for having sex with another man as long as it seemed like he was maintaining the normal male role in the sexual act. It was only the guy on the receiving end of male-to-male sex who was considered a "fairy," "queer," "invert" or member of the "third sex." For instance, a masculine-appearing sailor who let it be known that he enjoyed having sex with a male prostitute lost no social standing because people assumed that it was the male prostitute who was taking the "woman's role" in sex. The effeminate male was called a "cocksucker," "pogue," or "two-way artist," depending on whether he liked to give oral sex, receive anal sex, or do both.

Even when the government set up a sting operation to entrap homosexuals in the Navy in 1919, the male decoys who allowed themselves to receive oral sex and who were the inserting partners in anal sex did not consider themselves to be homosexual—nor did the Navy. Only the sailors who performed oral sex or received anal sex were charged with criminal activity.

By the end of the 1800s, same-sex activity could be found at social clubs, baths, beaches, parks, tearooms (washrooms and comfort stations where men were known to meet for same-sex activity) and rooming houses. The larger cities in America had masquerade balls where men dressed as women, dance halls where same-sex couples danced, and certain buildings and public parks that were known for their cruising and pick-up opportunities. By the time the 1900s rolled around, a young man wanting to explore sex with other men couldn't go wrong by getting a room at the local YMCA, as the Y would soon become the vortex of same-sex relations for males in America. Lesbian enclaves were forming as well by the end of the 1800s.

On the commercial side of same-sex relations, there was no shortage of "fairy prostitutes," such as Loop-the-Loop, who wore women's dresses and borrowed his name from a popular ride at Coney Island. Sailors in the 1800s had a full range of sexual possibilities, from female prostitutes who crowded naval ports, to interested males who would wine and dine sexy seamen in exchange for being able to give them oral sex or share anal maneuvers.

Only as the social order started to change in the late 1800s and early 1900s did the notions of "homosexual" and "heterosexual" come into play. Women were suddenly getting high-school and college educations, and they were beginning to compete with men for jobs in the workplace. Middle-class males found their world being invaded by women. One way these men coped with the increasing social status of women was to see themselves as having distinctly different roles from women—or to appear to be the opposite of women. This had never been necessary because men's and women's roles in society had been so different. It may have been the origin of our modern-day notion of masculinity, which rests upon the premise that a man's feminine side needs to be well-hidden. This also corresponded with a time in the late 1800s when physicians and psychiatrists were trying to invent the notion of psychopathology. Men who were attracted to men became excellent targets for modern psychiatry, as did women who were defying the social order by choosing careers over motherhood.

Then and Now

This is as good a place as any to end our look at sex in America during the 1800s. While it is sometimes difficult to see the forces that are guiding our sexual choices of today, that is certainly not the case as we peek under the sheets of generations past.

Whether it's 1850 or today, our sex drives have always been present. They are the engines that entice us to be naked together. But how we get there and what we do when we get there often depends on the time and culture.

Today's young couples might wonder about techniques for giving each other better oral sex. In the 1800s, there were no articles in books or magazine about oral sex. But modern technology in the 1800s became a vehicle for delivering pornography just like modern technology has today. Consider the invention of the phonograph recording in the late 1800s. The brand-new technology of Thomas Edison and Alexander Graham Bell was being used to delight listeners with the sounds of vulgar conversations, dirty songs, simulated sexual encounters, and even a "secret" recording of a husband's verbal advances to the family maid.

We could fill an entire book talking about the impact of the Model T on dating and relationships in America. It was just around the corner from where this chapter stops. And we could compare the impact of the railroads in the 1800s with the Internet today, or the obscenity laws of the 1800s with the latest attempts of the FCC to levy massive fines for indecency.

As we look back over the evolution of sex and the different twists and turns it has taken, hopefully we will appreciate that it continues to twist and turn today. As our great, great-great-grandparents were its guardians in the 1800s, so we are its guardians today.

Within each of us lies a sexual heritage that includes prostitution and explicit sex acts on the one hand, and fears about everything from birth control and masturbation to bicycle seats on the other. As we look at the sexual landscape in America today, it's difficult to see how any of that has changed. The issues might be different, but the duality remains.

The Gold Rush, The Automobile and Beyond

In 1846, there were only 40 miles of telegraph wire in the entire US. It was a test system set up by Morse between Baltimore and Washington DC. By 1852, there were more than 23,000 miles of telegraph cable in the US, with another 10,000 miles under construction—the precursor of today's cellphone.

We leave off in the early 1900s, as the automobile is about to change the landscape of America and the Alaska-Yukon gold rush was giving prostitution in North America a new frontier and a new face. In the next chapter, we turn the clock ahead 100 years, to look at Sex on the Interstate.

A Bit of Sex Slang from the 1800s

CRIB GIRLS—prostitutes who lived in tiny row houses or shacks that were known as cribs. Crib girls were often former brothel whores who had grown old or were in poor health. They often had to pay high rent to a landlord, pimp or madame.

CRUISERS—prostitutes in New York City who gathered in small groups along Broadway. If these girls had a sense of subtlety or reserve, it was hidden well.

FRENCH LOVE—when a prostitute was willing to give a man oral sex.

GAMAHUCHE—to have oral sex with, "she gamahuched me with her warm lips."

GASH—vulva

GROG SHOPS—term for bars or taverns that often had rooms in the back or upstairs that were rented to prostitutes in order to service customers (1790 to 1820), aka "slop shops" and "tippling houses"

GUIDEBOOKS—in most cities around America, small guidebooks were printed that listed the brothels and their specialties. These books were often made in a size that could easily fit into a coat pocket.

HAVE YOUR ASHES HAULED—for a man to be sexually serviced.

LEMON—stealing the money of a man when he was focused on the sexual favors of a woman.

Terms for Prostitutes in the 1800s

charity girls	female Bacchanals	jezebell
cockyneys	femmes d'amour	lorettes
Corinthians	frail sisters	nymphes de paves
Cyprians or "Cyts"	gay figurantes	perter misses
daughters of vice	gay nymphs	soiled doves
dirty loafers	gay sisters	strumpet

Terms for a Whore House

brothel	female boarding house	lust palace
bawdy house	French house	palace of perdition
Corinthian haunt	house of assignation	parlour house
den of infamy	house of bad fame	public house
den of iniquity	house of infamy	

MASQUERADE BALLS—masked balls which were often sponsored by the madams of the leading brothels. These became popular in the 1840s and remained so for the rest of the century. Dress for these often elaborate and elite affairs ranged from masks and magnificent costumes to masks and the costume you were born in. By the end of the night, the line between a masquerade ball and a drunken orgy was sometimes thin.

PANEL HOUSE—a room used by prostitutes with a false wall that an accomplice could hide behind. He or she would quietly rob the customer's wallet once his pants were off.

PUBLIC HOUSES—brothels where the average man was welcome. Often had long, loud lines of drinking and drunken men, especially from Saturday night to Monday morning.

SIGNBOARD GIRLS—prostitutes who lived on the streets and did their tricks in back alleys or behind billboards or large street signs. These were women who didn't have a single good thing going for them.

SOLDIER'S DISEASE—drug addiction to morphine by Civil War veterans. Morphine was frequently used as a pain-killer during the Civil War. A number of soldiers became addicted as a result.

SPORTING CULTURE—generations of hard-drinking, whore-loving, gambling, fighting American males who abandoned traditional mores for a social life that was lived on the streets and in the back alleys of nineteenth century America.

STORYVILLE—located in New Orleans between 1898 and 1917, the nation's most notorious and famous legally-mandated red-light district.

THIRD SEX—people who preferred to have sex with same-sex partners.

TRADE—manly or "normal" males who allowed or invited the sexual advances of "fairies" or effeminate-appearing males.

TWO-WAY ARTIST—a man who gave other men oral sex and received anal sex, e.g. "a two-way artist is a cocksucker and a pogue."

VAGINAL TENTS—diaphragms for birth control

RESOURCES

Alexander, R. M. (1995). *The Girl Problem: Female Sexual Delinquency in New York, 1900-1930. Cornell University Press.*

Becker, R., & Selden, G. (1985). *The Body Electric: Electromagnetism and the Foundation of Life. Harper Paperbacks.*

Belenko, S. R. (2000). *Drugs and Drug Policy in America: A Documentary History. Greenwood Press.*

Bleser, C. K., & Gordon, L. J. (2001). *Intimate Strategies of the Civil War: Military Commanders and Their Wives. Oxford University Press.*

Brandt, A. M. (1987). *No Magic Bullet : A Social History of Venereal Disease in the United States Since 1880 (Oxford Paperbacks). Oxford University Press, USA.*

Brodie, J. F. (1997). *Contraception and Abortion in Nineteenth-Century America (Cornell Paperbacks). Cornell University Press.*

Butler, A. M. (1987).n *Daughters of Joy, Sisters of Misery: Prostitutes in the American West, 1865-90. University of Illinois Press.*

Caren, E. C. (2000). *New York Extra: A Newspaper History of the Greatest City in the World from 1671 to the 1939 World's Fair.*

Carnes, M. C. (1991). *Secret Ritual and Manhood in Victorian America. Yale U. Press.*

Census, U. S. B. o. t. (1974). *Catalog of Publications: 1790-1972.*

Chauncey, G. (1995). *Gay New York: Gender, Urban Culture, and the Making of the Gay Male World, 1890-1940. Basic Books.*

Cohen, P. C. (1999). *The Murder of Helen Jewett (Vintage). Vintage.*

Cohen, W. A. (1996). *Sex Scandal: The Private Parts of Victorian Fiction (Series Q). Duke University Press.*

Hawley, E. H. (2005). *American Publishers of Indecent Books, 1840-1890.*

Erenberg, L. A. (1984). *Steppin' Out : New York Nightlife and the Transformation of American Culture. University Of Chicago Press.*

Gilfoyle, T.J. (2006). *A Pickpocket's tale: The Underworld of Nineteenth-Century New York*. W.W. Norton & Company.

Gilfoyle, T. J. (1994). *City of Eros: New York City, Prostitution, and the Commercialization of Sex, 1790-1920*. W. W. Norton & Company.

Gustav-Wrathall, J. D. (1998). *Take the Young Stranger by the Hand: Same-Sex Relations and the YMCA (The Chicago Series on Sexuality, History, and Society)*. University of Chicago Press.

Haller, J. S., Jr., & Haller, R. M. (1995). *The Physician and Sexuality in Victorian America*. Southern Illinois Univ Pr (Tx).

Hodgson, B. (2001). *In the Arms of Morpheus: The Tragic History of Laudanum, Morphine, and Patent Medicines*. Firefly Books.

Horowitz, H. L. (2003). *Rereading Sex : Battles Over Sexual Knowledge and Suppression in Nineteenth-Century America (Vintage)*. Vintage.

Long, A. P. (2005). *The Great Southern Babylon: Sex, Race, And Respectability in New Orleans, 1865-1920*. Louisiana State University Press.

Lowry, T. P. (1994). *The Story the Soldiers Wouldn't Tell: Sex in the Civil War*. Stackpole Books.

Lystra, K. (1992). *Searching the Heart : Women, Men, and Romantic Love in Nineteenth-Century America*. Oxford University Press, USA.

Marsden, G. M. (1982) *Fundamentalism and American Culture : The Shaping of Twentieth-Century Evangelicalism, 1870-1925*. Oxford University Press.

McLaren, A. (1999). *The Trials of Masculinity : Policing Sexual Boundaries, 1870-1930 (The Chicago Series on Sexuality, History, and Society)*. University Of Chicago Press.

Morgan, Lael (1998). *Good Time Girls of the Alaska-Yukon Gold Rush*. Whitecap Books.

Morone, J. A. (2004). *Hellfire Nation: The Politics of Sin in American History*. Yale U. Press.

Nasaw, D. (1999). *Going Out : The Rise and Fall of Public Amusements*. Harvard U. Press.

Reis, E. (2000). *American Sexual Histories (Blackwell Readers in American Social and Cultural History)*. Blackwell Publishers.

Rose, A. (1978). *Storyville, New Orleans : Being an Authentic, Illustrated Account of the Nortorious Red Light District*. University Alabama Press.

Rosen, R. (1983). *The Lost Sisterhood : Prostitution in America, 1900-1918*. The Johns Hopkins University Press.

Seagraves, A. (1994). *Soiled Doves: Prostitution in the Early West (Women of the West)*. Wesanne Publications.

Tone, A. (2002). *Devices and Desires: A History of Contraceptives in America*. Hill & Wang.

Ullman, S. R. (1998). *Sex Seen: The Emergence of Modern Sexuality in America*. University of California Press.

79

Sex on the Interstate
& In the Woods

For some people, there's nothing like cruising down a deserted highway with one hand on the wheel and the other on their lover's sweet spot. It doesn't matter if you are rich or poor, mongrel or blueblood, this is one time when our motor-driven culture nips you in the rear and makes you feel good all over.

Acts described in this chapter may be illegal or dangerous in many parts of the world, including the United States. Local, State and National ordinances should be your guide, in addition to common sense. Goofy Foot Press does not condone nor encourage any acts that might be dangerous or illegal.

The Rolling Monotone of a Nebraska Back Road

It might be particularly nice when your brain's in a narcoleptic funk and your sweetheart slyly grabs your free hand and slips it into the warm, wet space between her legs. Or maybe you're taking that long drive from Texas to Washington D.C. and the wind's not the only thing that's doing the blowing.

Ten years after the fact, one of you will occasionally say, "Honey, remember that time going 'cross Kansas..." and you'll both stop whatever you are doing, smile, and shut out the rest of the world for a precious moment.

The best way to use a car for sex, besides for driving to your sweetheart's house to get some, is when parking at a romantic spot and seeing how quickly you can steam the windows up. People who live in the inner city often don't have cars, so they sometimes find a favorite rooftop or "tar beach" with a romantic view where they can make love. Just be sure it's not a spot where junkies like to shoot up; you don't want to roll over on someone's stuff.

Winnebegos on the Continental Divide

While it's important to do things that inspire fond memories, it's also nice to stay alive so you can enjoy them. Keeping your bearings on the road while sharing certain types of physical pleasure is a talent that few people should ever attempt. Also, your state might have laws about sex behind the wheel. Call your State Trooper, State Police or Highway Patrol and ask.

As for other driving risks, driving with your head up the tailpipe is probably safer than driving while talking on a cellular phone, and thousands of people die each year from falling asleep at the wheel. We'd love to keep you as readers of future editions, so please, if you find yourself feeling sleepy, get some coffee or pull far off the road and take a nap.

Sex on the Rail of the Hoover Dam & Beyond

Some people like to have sex in public places where other people will see. While this might be a fine form of release for all parties involved, it is not what this section is about. What's being described here is that rare moment in life when you and your partner get to make love in a natural setting which is so magnificent that nature's sweet vibration nearly explodes inside of you. What transpires can be so expansive that it's difficult to think of it as just sex, or maybe it's what sex was meant to be before we started living in high rises and condominiums.

There are natural settings where you don't have to be too cautious about getting it on, like in a meadow filled with wildflowers, on a deserted beach, or under a god-sized rainbow in the Montana Big Sky. But there are other equally compelling locations, like dams, bridges, trains, planes, and various national monuments, where a well-honed sense of cunning and mischief is absolutely essential. The following are but a few suggestions about sex in the outdoors that you might find helpful:

Bug Repellent Don't forget the bug repellent if you are baring your all next to some humid bog or any place where the average mosquito would take one look at your naked butt cheeks and think it had died and gone to heaven.

Dress for Sex For sex in public places, it can be more than helpful if the woman wears one of those full 1950s-type dresses or sundresses. It's the equivalent of wearing her own private dressing room. She won't need to take a single thing off except for her underwear, unless she's not wearing any. That way, if she leans over the rail at a vista point, her partner can stand behind her and indicate objects of interest with his private pointer.

Beach Blanket Bingo If you are doing it at the beach or on a sandy river bed, be sure to take two large blankets. There's something about being on

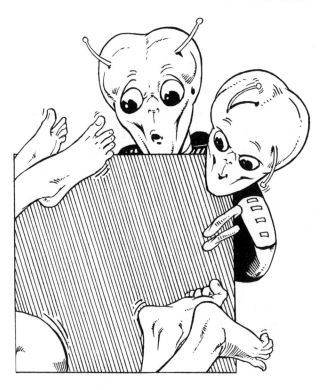

This couple enjoys having sex while camping near Area 51.

top of two blankets instead of one that helps keep sand from getting in your crack. Extra lube might help take the abrasive edge off any sand that makes its way inside a vagina or other places of intimate pleasure.

Wet Sex Sex in water provides its own set of challenges, given how water washes away natural lubrication. Try coating your genitals with a silicone-based lube ahead of time. Also, according to Luann Colombo, author of *How To Have Sex in the Woods,* intercourse in the water tends to pump the vagina full of water, so women will save themselves embarrassment if they will squat to let their crotches drain as they are emerging from the deep.

Condoms & Wet Spots in Sleeping Bags Ms. Colombo recommends carrying your condoms in a thermal cooler bag to keep them from freezing or frying. Using condoms when having sex in a sleeping bag will help decrease the drip factor and will help keep your sleeping bag dryer. (There's not a lot of room in a sleeping bag to avoid sleeping on the wet spot.) Consider packing a pet pee-pad or a disposable blue hospital pad for when you are doing the nasty in a sleeping bag. They are absorbent on one side, but waterproof on the other. Ms. Colombo says that for sex in a sleeping bag, more "in" and grinding results in a smaller wet spot than lots of in-out.

Highly Recommended *How To Have Sex In The Woods,* by Luann Colombo, Three Rivers Press. In addition to being wise, practical and lots of fun, this book makes a great gift for friends who like to hike and pack. Some of Ms. Colombo's other books include *Dead Guys and Gals of Science, Make Your Own Superballs, Sleepover Madness* and *Gross But True Germs.*

Public-Sex Caution

One reader comments, "A close friend of mine went to jail for having sex in public; it was her first arrest and very traumatic." So please be aware that while it's perfectly legal for a couple to have a really loud and nasty fight in public, having sex in public (or maybe even in your backyard) is likely to break local, state and federal statutes and might get you arrested. For some people, the risk is half the fun.

CHAPTER

80
Kink in the Animal Kingdom

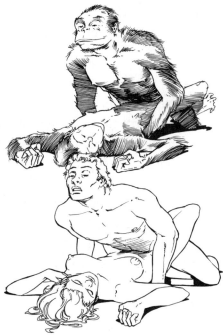

Are humans the only animals who have sex just for pleasure? Do the others only have sex for reproduction and dominance? Is there no kink in the rest of the animal kingdom? Until recently, that's what the biologists had told us.

Fortunately, some biologists have been reconsidering the party line that humans are the only animals who have sex just for the heck of it. So for the rest of this brief chapter, let's pretend you are a biology professor who wants to study sex in the jungle.

Sex in the Jungle (No, Not Manhattan)

After spending years of applying for grants, you have finally gotten your project funded. Your plane is about to set down in a third world country where you hope to observe bonobos in the wild.

Discovered in 1929, the bonobo is one of the Great Apes. The bonobo's genes are closer to human genes than most other living creatures; closer than even savanna baboons and chimpanzees. It's not that bonobos are identical to humans, but they are found swinging on 98% of the same limbs of the evolutionary tree. Girl bonobos don't give birth until they are 13 or 14 years of age, reaching full maturity by age 15. When they do have babies, bonobos nurse and carry them around for up to five years.

While they don't ride skateboards, play Guitar Hero or have iPhones, it can safely be said that bonobos are more like humans than, say, white mice or pigs.

Your Lab in the Bush

You are finally able to set up camp in an area where you can watch bonobos do what bonobos do. You write in your notebook that you have successfully paid off the local officials, and you feel relieved that insurgent rebels haven't captured, killed or raped you. (You think we're kidding?)

And then it happens—your first sighting. Not only do you see bonobos having heterosexual sex, but you notice one big male has his hand on the erect penis of another male and he's giving his bonobo buddy a handjob. Eventually you see two bonobo women rubbing their genitals together, like in lesbian porno flicks. You also observe two males rubbing their penises together in a pleasurable way, and you then you see a male and female having face-to-face intercourse.

After your first year of observing bonobos, you decide that they're certainly not sex maniacs, but that sex appears to be an essential part of their social interactions.

After spending two years in the jungle watching bonobos, you find yourself desperate for a little sea air, so you apply for another grant that will allow you to watch dolphins and whales have sex.

After two more years at sea, you long to go back to the jungle, only this time you apply for funding to watch giraffes have sex. By now, people at the various foundations are saying, "We'll be darned if we're going to give any more money for that pervert professor to watch another species have sex." So instead of funding your project, they spend millions of dollars trying to teach sexual abstinence to students in inner-city high schools, and then they build a bridge to nowhere. Fortunately, your great aunt Clarice recently died and left you enough money to return to the jungle to watch giraffes have sex.

After a few more years, you sit down and try to make sense of all your findings. There's simply no way around it—your years of research tell you that the sexual encounters you have described were not limited to acts of sperm competition, aggression and dominance. The same animals who one day were having a homosexual tryst might be enjoying heterosexual loving the next. And in spite of years of being told this can't possibly be, you get the sense that these animals were having sex for the mere pleasure of it, spilling sperm with a devil-may-care indifference to the tenants of evolutionary good-housekeeping. Good God, you say to yourself, I'll never get tenure now. So in order to make your findings more palatable to your colleagues, you report that animals have sex in order to resolve conflict, for tension regulation, and as appeasement behavior. There, you didn't use the words "fun" or "pleasure," even if that's what you've been watching for the past six years.

Your findings show that not only does a full range of pleasure happen, but animals don't spend a lot of time having an identity meltdown because they were trying out their finest mating behavior on a member of the same sex. Nor did you notice any animals with white collars and bibles who were telling their fellow animals that they would burn in hell for their ungodly sins. That kind of behavior is only found on the highest branch of the evolutionary tree.

RECOMMENDED For more on bonobos, see the writing of Frans B. M. de Waal.

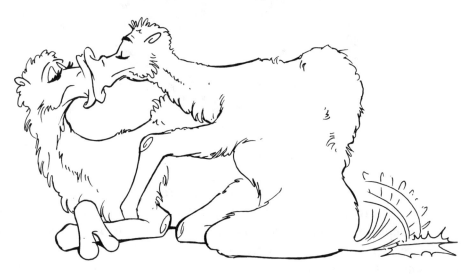

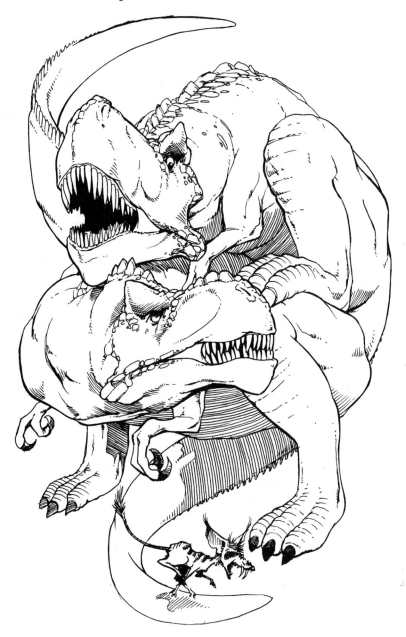

Tyrannies Having Sex

This is an artist's conception of how the tyrannosaurus had sex. While tyrannies were clearly meat eaters, it is difficult to imagine them giving or receiving oral sex. In the Mesozoic Era, the term "I got some tail last night" was more descriptive than misogynistic. (Special thanks to brilliant dinosaur artist Luis Rey for inspiration.)

81

Vaya Con Dios!

This is the final chapter of the *Guide to Getting It On!* It talks about things like hippies, cash flow, meaning and integrity, and then it says goodbye.

What Puff the Magic Dragon's Tears Were Really All About

Two generations ago, a small group of hippies suddenly appeared in this country. These hippies didn't think like the rest of us and probably arrived from another planet. The nation became infatuated with them.

After the arrival of the real hippies, there suddenly appeared millions of hippie wannabes. These were often college students who didn't have to work because they were getting money from home. They spoke a great deal about love and peace, but they didn't know much about either. They were going to save the world from anything that was even remotely like their moms and dads.

In time, the hippie wannabes started getting degrees in fields like law, business and medicine. Guys started cutting their hair and women stuffed their breasts back into bras, all in preparation for an important American ritual called "the job interview." Words like "marketing" and "standing to sue" took the place of "bitchin" and "groovy." Designer labels became more important than flowers and beads.

There was the constant specter of work, often sixty hours a week, with a person's whole life mapped out according to which rung of the corporate ladder he or she planned to hang from.

It may seem strange that a book on sex would mention things like jobs and money, but in the course of our lifetimes most of us will fret more over money than love. The people at MasterCard will probably know more about us than our sex partners do. Yet no matter how much money or social status you acquire, you can never leave who you are or what you have become on the floor at the edge of the bed. Sex may be a wonderful thing, but it can't make up for an existence that has little integrity, value or meaning.

A Better Place

This Guide was not intended to be radical or reactionary. It was written with the hope of giving something back to the world, trying to leave it a little better than how we found it.

This Guide may not have the head rush of good drugs, and it doesn't pretend to have many answers. But it is a more advanced view of sex than many of us had when we first started getting it on. Thank you for being patient with its efforts to be more than just another how-to manual on sex.

There are so many more dimensions to sex than just huffing and puffing while the bedsprings squeak. This book is 992 pages long, and it still can't define sex. Hopefully you will be able to define it on your own, or at least have a beautiful time trying.

Vaya Con Dios!

About the Illustrations

While readers for the most part ask for more illustrations, some do wonder why all of the characters in our illustrations are so darned thin, buff and kind of perfect. So we thought we'd include some background for you about the illustrations, including how one of the new illustrations in this 6th edition of *The Guide* came to be.

The line-art in *The Guide* is particularly challenging to do, because the illustrator has so little to work with—a simple black line on white paper. He doesn't use any of the usual tools that bring art to life: the shadows, texture and colors. As a result, to give the line-art its feeling, the illustrator has to be a master of exaggeration. Without the exaggeration, line-art quickly becomes flat and boring.

Notice how cut and buff the males in the book's drawings are, while the women are soft and smooth? Without those exaggerations, it's hard to distinguish males from females in line art. Plus, there's the comic-book tradition where the males were werewolves, monsters and Supermen.

One of the challenges is in pulling the exaggeration back just enough so the illustration is still fun and has life, but doesn't put you off because it seems so outrageous. So each illustration is often worked and reworked, with a lot of give and take between Daerick, the artist, and Paul, the author:

> **Paul:** Her breasts are humongous and his penis looks like it's 16 inches long! And can't you put some weight on her? She looks like she hasn't eaten in two years.

> **Daerick:** OK, but you're going to hate how this one looks if I make them normal.

The Anatomy of a Drawing

While the concept sketch of illustration on the next page looks promising, it is still in sketch-form where the illustrator has used shading to deliver the concept. Getting it from there to line-art form can be fraught with peril. Fortunately, the illustrator for *The Guide* is one of the finest in the world, and if anyone can make it work, it is he. Sometimes just a tiny tweak at the edge of a character's mouth can be the difference between an illustration that works really well and one that doesn't.

Another huge benefit in working with Daerick Gross is the humor, parody and detail that he is able to create within his line-art drawings.

1

THE CONCEPT

Paul to Daerick: I'm looking for a commentary on the connected couple who gives the impression the world will end if they aren't constantly checking their laptop or cellphone for messages. So I'd like you to try creating an illustration with a couple having intercourse doggie style–she's on her elbows and knees, and he's kneeling behind her. At the same time, she has a laptop open on the ground in front of her, working the keyboard with the fingers of one hand, while perhaps texting on her cell with her other hand. Her male partner has his laptop open on her back while he's texting someone with a Blackberry in his other hand.

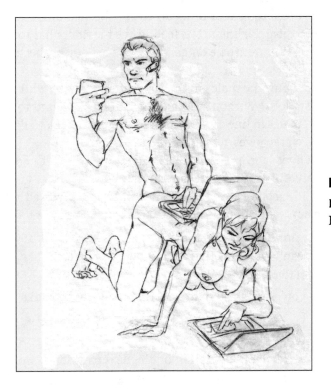

2

FIRST DRAFT
Daerick to Paul:
How's this?

3

CRITIQUE OF FIRST DRAFT

Paul to Daerick: Fascinating—if they weren't using laptops and headsets, it would be obvious they were having sex. But given the technology that's key to the concept, it's confusing. The sex needs to be way more obvious; perhaps more of a sideways POV. Also, can you reel in her chest and make it a little less gravitationally challenged?

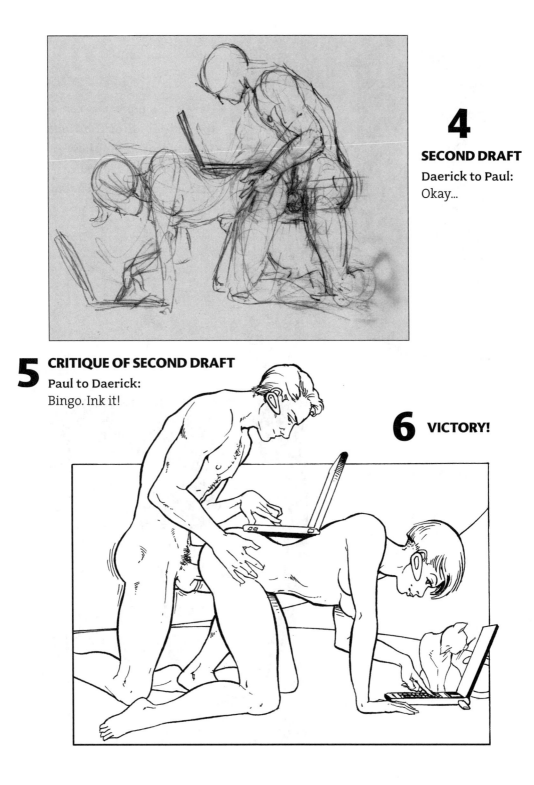

4

SECOND DRAFT
Daerick to Paul:
Okay...

5 **CRITIQUE OF SECOND DRAFT**
Paul to Daerick:
Bingo. Ink it!

6 **VICTORY!**

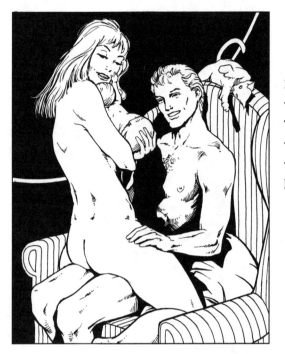

Here's an illustration from the 2nd edition of *The Guide.* The concept was to show that sex brings a lot more than just orgasms, including hope and new life.

Naturally, someone complained, claiming we were showing a couple having intercourse while holding a little baby. So for the 3rd edition...

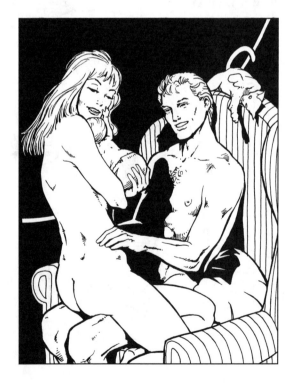

Thanks! Thanks! Thanks!

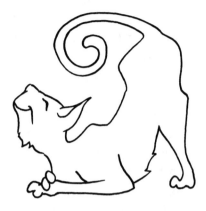

A special thanks to Mr. Jed Lyons and his staff at National Book Network who have been a safe harbor during a hellstorm. You made it possible for *The Guide* to stay independent and strong.

A sad and heartfelt goodbye to what was Publishers Group West, who took this book in and helped it to grow, and grow, and grow.

Thanks and appreciation to:

Mr. Dan Poynter, Tracy Fortini, Kidder Kaper, Bill Hazeltine, Liz Brody, Cory Feldman, Kim Wylie, Sheri Lent, Rich Freese, John Cabral, Sarah Rosenberg, Heather Cameron, Melissa Fonseca, Kevin Votel, Elise Cannon, Cathy Vancik, Judi Baker, Mary Skiver, Kent Anderson, Sue Ostfield, Charles Gee, David Dahl, Eric Green, Keith Arsenault, David Ouimet, Kat Mulkey, Bill Richter, Michelle Fisher, Andrea Tetrick, Betty Redmond, Bill Getz, Eric Kettunen, Cindy Heidemann, John Masjak, Jon Mayes, Kristen Keith, Mike Katz, Ron Shapiro, Roy Remer, Graham Fidler, Sarah MacLachlan, Jill Kamada, Chris Schrader, Sabrina Young, Lance Tilford, Charlie Winton, Jerry Delaria, Becky Kaapuni, Cyndy Perlich, Chris McKenney, Sandra Patterson, Betty Redmond, Patricia Kelly, Harry Kirchner, Matthew Chilcott, Lina Hines, Roni Gallimore, Mr. Paul Rooney and Gary "started the whole thing rolling!" Todoroff.

Renee Lane, Jeff Ochs, Jill Esch, Carleen Rogers, Vickie Jedele, Kerwin Leader, J.P. Stando, Dave Hite, Dave Fleming, Mike Vezo and the fine staff at McNaughton & Gunn who print *The Guide*.

Angela Hoffman, Kara Wuest, Bob Francoeur, Bill Taverner, Sue Palmer, Joe Marzucco, Rich Siegel, Jennifer Ashley, Theresa McCracken, Scott McCann, Bev Cutler, Cyrus Farivar, Kayla Strassfeld, Adrienne Benedicks, Inger Klekacz, Ryan Hanson, Todd Hawley, Dan Cullinane, Trena Jayne, Leslie Rossman, Michael Meller, Franka Schmidt Zastrow, Anke Vogel, Ralph Bolton, Dmitri Siegel, Denise Westmoreland, Harry Gilmartin & Karen Kummerfeldt, Janet Hardy, Jay Wiseman, Matt Torrey, Dan Culliane, Kirk Groeneveld, David Hoffert, William W. Young, Claire Yang, Alessandra Rellini, Marca Sipski, Marilyn Milos, Stanley Althof, Violet Blue, Braxton Sherouse, Annie Bradford, Joe Pittman.

Matt Comito, Rose Reed, Janice Hamilton, Larry Hedges, Barbara Keesling, Debra Hanson, Steven Wales, Avedis Panajian, Bill Young, Rob Hill, John & Miss Kelly, Nancy "Professor B" Carmel Eyes, Carol Bee, Ron, Steve, Linda & Jeanette at Old Town Printers (RIP), Martha and the staff at the Newport City Library.

Jon Westover, Morgan & Burce Yarrosh, Suzanne LaPlacette, Mike Fischler, Wanda Moore, Veronica Monet, Monte Farrin, Dixie Marquis, Mike Conway, Karen Saliba, Carol Tavris, Michael Kogutek, Katherine Almy, BJ Robbins, Ken Sherman, Bob & Kim Otto, Duncan Rouleau, Bill Applebaum, Nancy Reaven, Bruce Voeller, Andre Deuschanes, Meridith Tanzer, Roan Singh Sidhu, Evan Rapostathis, Kenny Wagner, Ross Rubin, Paula Samuels, Daphne Rose Kingma, Cathryn Michon, Diane Driscoll, Billy Rumpanos, Ben Fiorino, Ray Calabrese, Diana Heiselu, Judy Seifer, Randi Lockwood, Breta Hedges, Brent Myers, Ron Goosen, Pat Lincoln, Alison Rosenzweig, Marty Gilliland, Val Littou, Mat Honig, Sheryl Palese, Chip Rowe, Kathy Herdman, Jack McHugh, Pat Patterson, Dana Smart, Laura Corn, Elizabeth Olsen, Pam Winter, Judy Linnan, Theresa Benedick, Joe Sparling, Carol Queen, Lily & Bill & Louie at Sir Speedy, Monte at Input/Output, Joe Marsh at the Earthling (RIP), Juliann Popp, Jason Aronson, Bill & Beryl Johnson, Karen Seemueller, Christianna Billman and Lisa Blai , Glenn Knight, Emily Gudhe, Barbara Seamen.

Connie Overholser, Phil Bruno, Pam White, Jan Nathan, Terry Nathan, Peter Handel, Carol Fass, Eda Kalkay, Leslie Rossman, Patricia Holt, Adrienne Benedicks, Heidi Cotler, Babs Adamsky, Kevin Samsel, Mark Collins, Vince Darkangelo, Jon Cooper, Kris Lorret Rourke, Ben Saltzberg, Whitney Thomas, Stacie Herndon, Genanne Walsh, Rachael Cart, Joanie Blank, Constance Claire, Gretta, Christophe and Heather Shaw from Blowfish, John Davis, Leonore Tiefer, Marian Dunn, Michael Metz, Julian Slowinski, Katherine Hall, Helen Fisher, Dodie Ownes.

Andrea Best, Adam Moore, John Money, Rob Hardy, Kristen Kemp, Nooshin Thorpe, Carol Briezke, Esther Crain, Julia Gaynor, Carol Edington, Paul Harrington, Ed Alcocer, Diane Morrison, Elizabeth Lee.

William Erwin, Donald Marcus, Verne Graham, Brett Miller, Joe Casella, Anne Katz, Donna Coomer.

Glossary of Sexual Slang in Popular & Unpopular Culture

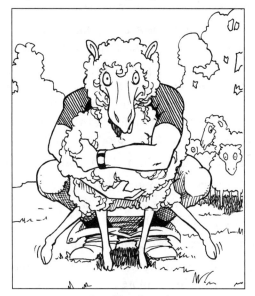

animal husbandry

A2M—means "ass-to-mouth." Sucking on a partner's penis after it has been up your butt or someone else's.

AARDVARKING—term for sexual intercourse coined by B-movie-reviewer extraordinaire Joe Bob Briggs, e.g. "Absolutely no plot to get in the way of the story. Thirty-four breasts. Multiple aardvarking. Gratuitous hot-tubbing. Man in a cheesy lizard suit. Sorority hosedown. Gratuitous topless dancing at a radio station. Slapstick Fu. My kinda movie. Two stars."

AC/DC—1. a bisexual; enjoys bedding members of either sex; "ambisexterous," "switch-hitter," or "versatile." 2. Very successful metal band, now geezer-rock.

ADULT GRAPHICS COMMUNITY—3-D adult erotic art, comics and animation created by graphic artists in programs like Bryce, Carrara, Curious Labs Poser, DAZ, 3D Studio Max and Photoshop. Premier website: www.renderotica.com.

AFRODESIAC—sexy-looking black man.

AFTER MARKET—a biological female whose genitals have been surgically constructed to appear male, as opposed to "factory-equipped" or "original equipment;" aka: "F2M transsexual."

AFTERNOON DELIGHT—sex in the afternoon; "a nooner."

AGE PLAY—sexual role-playing where one partner pretends to be older and in control while the other pretends to be much younger.

AIRHEAD—in a discussion on the effects of global warming, an airhead would want to know how it would affect her tan lines; "bimbo."

AIRPLANE BLOND (US) OR AEROPLANE BLOND (UK):—a woman who has dyed her hair but still has a black box. When the carpet doesn't match the curtains.

AMATEUR—a genre of porn that's supposed to be the real deal, allegedly created at home by real-life, red-blooded, horny housewives, hubbies with hard-ons, naughty neighbors, slutty sorority sisters, and sinful swingers (according to one porn review site). Prides itself in putting the grass back into grassroots by being free of the gloss, glitter and high production values of studio porn.

AMERICAN CULTURE—refers to traditional, missionary-position intercourse.

AMERICAN BOYZ—"an organization which aims to support people who were labeled female at birth but who feel that is not an accurate or complete description of who they are." See "transgendered."

AMPALANG OR PALANG—a horizontal piercing through the head of the penis.

ANAL STRETCHING—what you do if you are into body modification and want your anus to be nearly 12 inches or more in diameter.

ANABEL CHONG—convent-school student turned porn starlet, whose claim to fame is having intercourse with eighty different men on the same day.

ANAL—a blanket term for anal sex, anal play and rimming. Also refers to a person who struggles with orderliness and perfectionism to a point of not being able to complete things. Tends to be rigid and stubborn. People need to be at least somewhat anal to succeed in life, but more than that and they drive everyone around them crazy with their anal compulsiveness.

ANAL BEADS—worry beads for the rectum, to be pulled out as orgasm is beginning. Since the anus has an extreme number of nerve endings, pulling out the beads can help intensify the feelings of orgasm. They come in many sizes and configurations; "pearl string."

ANAL BLEACHING—rather than an attempt to turn the rectal mustache blonde, this is an attempt to bleach the dark skin that anal hair grows out of. Some porn stars apparently slather skin fade cream on their brownish anal openings to make them pink. Makers of age-spot creams haven't included "anuses" on their list of body parts that are safe to bleach.

ANALINGUS—kissing or licking ass; "rimming."

ANDRO DYKE—a lesbian who is neither butch nor fem, "butch lite."

ANDROGEN INSENSITIVITY SYNDROME (AIS)—a genetic anomaly where an embryo with XY chromosomes is not sensitive to androgens. Adrogens are the masculinizing hormones that push a male embryo out of its natural female state and result in male genitals and a masculinized brain. (That's how guys get to be guys.) There are different kinds of AIS, including complete, partial and mild. With complete AIS, the baby is born a female, with a feminized brain and a vulva. Her vagina can be a bit short, and she doesn't have a cervix or uterus. As for appearances, she can be as plain or beautiful as any other woman, and she is a woman in almost every way except for a short bit of code on one of her chromosomes. A lot of women with AIS don't even find out until their late teens, when they go to a gynecologist because their periods haven't started. AIS is known as an intersex condition.

ANDROGYNOUS—not really masculine or feminine. Can you name three androgynous rock'n'roll musicians?

ANIME—animated art or cartoons from Japan with a distinctly Japanese style. It is sexualized and is aimed at a more mature audience than American cartoons; characters have large eyes and wild expressions; women have multi-colored hair and breasts so big they look like they are going to pop. Often has nudity and violence, but stops short of being considered porn in Japan; "Japanimation." Amine that crosses the line into porn is "hentai."

ANGEL FOOD—a gay pilot.

APADRAVYA—a vertical piercing through the head of the penis.

APHRODISIAC—substance that is given (or taken) to increase sexual desire. Be wary of anything that is called an aphrodisiac because it is usually people, and not chemical concoctions, that turn other people on.

ARSE—British for ass, e.g. "piece of arse," "up your arse," "arse wipe," "Tom's an arse," "arsing about," "arse-over-tit" (a bad fall), or "tight as a duck's arse."

ASS BLOW—sticking your tongue into the anus; "rimming," "tossing salad."

ASS PLAY—when the focus of erotic activity is on the buttocks or bum, especially focusing on the anus.

ATROPHY—1. scientific term for "use it or lose it." 2. a fear that many guys have concerning their penis, especially when they haven't had sex for an epoch or two. Atrophy happens to muscles; the penis is not a muscle. The penis often gets a better workout from jerking off than from intercourse, so if you are worried about atrophy...

AUSTRAILIAN SEX—licking your partner's back, starting at the neck and taking almost an hour to reach his or her rear end; "cat bath."

AUTOFELLATIO—to suck one's own penis. Requires a long penis and nimble spinal column.

AUTOPEDERASTY—when a guy can stick his partially-erect penis into his own anus; not the sport of short-dick men. "Pederasty" is when an old guy has sex with a young guy, so why this is called "autopederasty" makes no sense.

AVN—Adult Video News, official organ of the adult-video trade. Started in 1982 as an 8-page newsletter to adult stores, its reach now extends far and wide.

BABE RATIO—ratio of people you find sexually attractive to the total number of people in the room.

BAD LESBIAN—among politically stiff lesbians, a bad lesbian is a gay woman who has sex with a man or fantasizes about it. Writer Carol Queen attributes this kind of rigid thinking to "the lezzie thought police."

BAGGER—male who attempts to partially asphyxiate himself while masturbating. Has resulted in deaths that are mislabeled as suicides.

BALL—to have intercourse with; past tense is "balled."

BALL GAG—a mouth gag. The BDSM version of Croakies, with a round rubber ball where the glasses should be. The ball is put in the submissive's mouth.

BALLS TO THE WALL—a state of mind where one powers through a situation with tenacity and guts; origin: the Air Force.

BANGER—British for sausage or penis, with a "banger hanger" being a vagina.

BAREBACKING—anal intercourse without a condom.

BARE-BALLING—when a guy isn't wearing underwear.

BARTHOLINS GLANDS—two small glands at the bottom part of the vaginal opening which help secrete lubrication; explains why you should reach to the bottom of the vaginal opening to bring lubrication up to coat the clitoris.

BASHFUL BLADDER SYNDROME (PARURESIS)—when you can't urinate in a public bathroom, or when someone else is present. Can be very debilitating. Shows how severely the mind can mess with the body; "pee-shy."

BATTERY-OPERATED BOYFRIEND—a vibrator.

B-BOY—short for "butt-boy," a man who enjoys taking it up the rear.

BBW—means "Big Beautiful Women."

BDSM—umbrella term for erotic power play including bondage, discipline, spanking, and certain types of fetish play. The term BDSM started on the World Wide Web, and encompasses the older acronyms of BD (bondage & discipline) and SM (sadism & masochism) and DS (dominance & submission). While BDSM is sexual, genital orgasm and stimulation is not its focus.

BEAR—large, mature male with masses of body hair and a fondness for other males. Used in gay porn and ads for sex or dating to describe big hairy guys.

BEARD—date or marriage arranged for a person who is gay to make them appear straight. Important for when mom and dad are in town, or when you are in the Armed Forces, where a beard is known as a "stunt babe."

BEARD BURN—inner-thigh hazard to women who receive oral sex from men with five o'clock shadow. Can be prevented by draping the woman's thighs with towels or plastic wrap, or by a quick shave on Thor's part.

BEER GOGGLES—alcohol-impaired vision that casts a beautiful glow on all that walks, often resulting in feelings of dread upon waking in the morning.

BEAT OFF or BEAT YOUR MEAT—when a male masturbates; "wank," "jerk off."

BEAVER—someone who attends Oregon State University. Refers to the female sex Oregons. See "split beaver."

BEEFCAKE—idealized nude male body in photos and drawings that appeared in muscle magazines whose stated purpose was to extol the virtues of exercise and nutrition. The giants of the beefcake magazines were Bernaar MacFadden's *Physical Culture,* started in 1908, and Bob Mizer's *Physique Pictorial* which he founded in the 1950s. Its brother publication, *Athletic Model Guild* was wildly popular from the 1960s until 1993. Tom of Finland's famous drawings were highly stylized and overtly gay versions of the beefcake.

BEN WA BALLS—a pair of metallic balls that are inserted into the vagina for sexual pleasure while the woman rock back and forth or squeezes her thighs together; more hype than reality since they don't work for most people.

BESTIALITY—when your sexual partner has four legs and a tail; "farm sex," "K-9" and "animal training." The Spanish called it "the Italian vice."

BICURIOUS—someone who is interested in exploring sex with a member of hir or her own sex, but hasn't gotten around to it yet.

BIDET—oval-shaped porcelain bowl that is plumbed with a fountain of water over which a person squats to clean and sometimes stimulate the genitals; found in traditional European bathrooms; also be used for anal hygiene.

BIKINI—a type of low-cut panties or swimwear that were originally for women. The bikini has been a fashion staple of the Western world for the past fifty years. The modern bikini was born in 1946. It was named after the island Bikini Atoll, which is part of the Marshall Islands in the Pacific Ocean where nuclear-weapon tests were done. It was so daring that the only model who would originally wear it was a nude dancer. It did not become popular in the U.S. until Brian Hyland's song *Itsy Bitsy Teenie Weenie Yellow Polka Dot Bikini* hit the charts, and women suddenly started gearing up, or down, in bikinis.

BIKINI LINE—how girls in modern America define their vulvas, on the basis of what needs to be plucked or shaved in order to look good on the beach.

BIO-BOYS—transgender term for males who were born as males and who remain males.

BIOLOGICAL CLOCK—refers to a procreational urge or crisis that overwhelms some people between the ages of 35 and menopause.

BISEXUAL—person who is able to feel sexual arousal for both sexes.

BLADDER INFECTION—when bacteria with a painful kick establish residency in the human bladder; "cystitis." A person so affected would be willing to pawn her great-grandmother's wedding ring for a hit of antibiotics. Bladder infections are more common in women because the passageway from the bladder to the outside of the body is much shorter, allowing bacteria easier access.

BLENDED ORGASM—popular-culture term for an orgasm that is thought to be from both clitoral and G-spot area stimulation.

BLIND DATE—aptly-named social event where two people who don't know each other have been set up by others.

BLOOD SPORTS—extreme BDSM play where the skin is broken and/or blood is drawn, such as such as piercing, whipping, cutting and vampire games.

BLOW—cocaine.

BLOWJOB—oral sex that's done on a guy; "hummer," "give head," "go down on him," "fellatio."

BLUE BALLS—refers to a condition where a male has been sexually stimulated but not to orgasm. Sometimes actually hurts and is rumored to cause a blue tint to shroud the scrotum. Is easily cured by jerking off. At one time, blue balls was thought to cause physical damage, but recent evidence does not support this fear. Get used to it, dude.

BMS—acronym for "baby-making sex."

BODY SHOTS—when doing tequila shooters, suck the salt from whatever part of your lover's body he or she puts it on, and then suck the lime from his or her mouth. Somewhere in between, gulp down the shot of tequila.

BODY MODIFICATION—things people do to change their bodies in primitive ways, including piercing, tattooing, branding, binding, cutting, castrating, nullification or corset training. The Rome is www.bmezine.com.

BOFF or BOINK—to have intercourse.

BONDAGE—when someone gets a sexual high from that which the rest of us try to avoid.

BONE—a less than delicate reference to intercourse; e.g., "to bone a babe." Also the dominant partner in a prison relationship, or a penis.

BONEYARD—area in prisons where conjugal (sex) visits occur with spouses.

BOOSTER SHOT—a one-night stand.

BOOTH TROLL—a male who cruises for sex with other men in the video booths at the cheesier adult sex stores. If successful, anonymous sex occurs, often while viewing straight porn flicks to give the appearance of being straight. Has the added excitement of potentially being busted by the vice squad.

BOOTY—means "rear end," "bum" or "caboose." Can refer to having sex, but not anal sex; go figure.

BOOTY CALL—late-night text message or phone call for sex, often cryptic, as in "R U busy?"

BOOTY CHECK—prison slang for "rectal cavity search;" "finger wave."

BOTTOM—means "sexually submissive," a BDSM term; see "top and bottom." Can also be the receiver of the penis during anal intercourse; "catcher."

BOTTOM'S DISEASE—BDSM term for when a submissive takes the role too far.

BOTTOM SURGERY—when a transgendered person has their genitals surgically reassigned, as opposed to "top surgery" which refers to everything else.

BOXERS OR BRIEFS?— a question every guy ponders at one time or another, but often ends up wearing whatever his mother originally dressed him in. Or maybe he'll settle on the hybrid boxer-briefs.

BOY SHORTS—see "hipsters."

BRA HOOK—no single device known to humankind has caused more guys (and some women) more angst than the hook of the bra. Legend has it that Obi-Wan Kenobi originally taught Luke Skywalker about "the force" to help him unhook Princess Leia's bra. Given that they turned out to be brother and sister, it's fortunate that Leia's bra hook proved even tougher than the force.

BRAZILIAN—differs from a usual bikini-area waxing because it goes all the way back to the butt, including deforestation of the asshole. People mistakenly think that a Brazilian has to do with the vulva being bare, but the key element in a Brazilian waxing is that the perineum and butt are plucked, as well as the sides of the labia. The mons pubis is the wild card: it can be bald or left with a landing strip, as long as your kitty's whiskers don't hang out the sides or top of your thong.

BREATH PLAY or BREATH CONTROL—erotic asphyxiation. When the oxygen supply is cut off as part of a sexual turn-on. It is done during masturbation or couple's play, but is a health hazard and should never be done under any circumstances. The danger cannot be controlled or minimized, even if a cardiologist were monitoring the act.

BREEDER—a gay term for a straight person.

BREMELANOTIDE—originally tested as a sunless tanning lotion, imagine the surprise when 9 or 10 men who were test subjects got boners in addition to their tans. Women test subjects wanted to jump the male test subjects, and it was off to the races. Development was stopped in 2008 due to side effects including high blood pressure. The company will apply for approval to use bremelanotide for another application (think of the off-label potential once this drug is approved for anything!), and they will try to develop a related compound that does not appear to cause elevated blood pressure.

BRO JOB—oral sex between two guys who consider themselves to be straight, often alcohol aided.

BROKEBACK MOUNTAIN—closeted cowboy extravaganza. Now, for the truly important commentary about the butt-fucking scene in the pup tent: *Get over it!* The sex was symbolic. No self-respecting gay man is going to throw spit on his penis and shove it up the butt of some cowboy who hasn't had a shower since he was 10 and has been eating nothing but beans by the campfire. Butt-fucking requires preparation and lube, or at least some bacon drippings, given the quaint campfire setting. So the pup-tent scene was just symbolic. Symbolic of what? It depends on who you are and what your life experiences have been. (Thanks for the excellent imagery, www.Nightcharm.com!)

BROWN SHOWERS—when being crapped-on is a sexual turn on as opposed to a normal life condition; "scat," "coprophilia," "brown session."

BROWN SUGAR—refers to a sexy black woman or to having sex with her.

BUCK WILD—rap term, meaning to have wild sex or to act crazy; "buckwildin." An example of proper usage is provided by *Body Count*: "Get buckwild with the white freaks, show 'em how to work the white sheets."

BUDDY BOOTH—booth in an adult sex venue where there's a window to the next booth. There are curtains in the windows and buttons that raise them. This lets you watch the person in the next booth stripping or doing whatever, as long as you both raise each other's curtains.

BUDDY SEX—see "fuck buddy."

BUFF—having well-developed muscles, often the result of spending an ungodly amount of time at the gym. While the buff look on men is sexy today, that might not have been the case in 1900, when buff men tended to be members of the working class and were slaving at factory jobs. Back then, the pot belly may have been an indicator of opulence and sexual desirability.

BUGGERY—an academic tradition. Also, anal sex that's done to boys and young men in boarding schools as well as other places where men are warehoused.

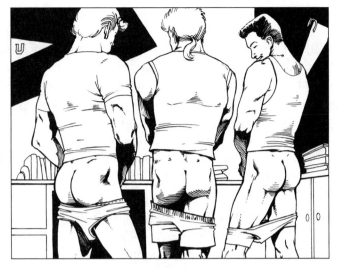

Boys Will Be Boys

BUKKAKE—a Japanese term that refers to showering the face of the receiver with the ejaculate of many men. Legend has it that in ancient Japan, a woman who was unfaithful was tied up in the town center where the male citizenry ejaculated on her face to show their distaste. Perhaps they were angry because the adultery happened with some other Samurai and not them. Has since become a fetish with some Japanese porn featuring it; aka facial.

BUM—British term for "rear end."

BUNK-BED SEX—an agony forced on college students who live in dorms. Sex is the main reason to avoid bunking your beds, but get the bottom bunk if you have no choice. Sure, the whole thing will shake each night when your roommate in the upper bunk is jerking-off, but imagine trying to get you and your drunken hook-up to the top bunk? With the way a lot bunk beds shake, it will be like trying to shag while sitting on top of an ocean buoy. What about overhead clearance? Do you get her a helmet if she's feeling like doing a cowgirl? And if one of you falls out of bed from the lower bunk, we're only talking a broken clavicle at worst. Fall out of the top bunk, & all bets are off.

BUSH—female pubic hair or genitals.

BUTCH—a lesbian who has adopted the male role and run with it. An exaggerated form of manliness.

BUTCH-FEMME—an alluring woman who combines the no-nonsense strength of a stone butch with the steamy "make your crotch drip and throb" attraction of a femme fatale. This is a woman who can ride into town on a hog wearing tattoos and leather, and ride out with men and women tripping over themselves to get her in bed. She blurs sex and gender boundaries, yet you would never use the word "androgynous" to describe her. The butch-femme is played well in some movies by actress Angelina Jolie. Butch-femme also refers to the community of women who describe themselves as being butches, femmes, stone butches, stone femmes, TGbutches, transmen and FtMs.

BUTT PLUG—toy for the rectum that's diamond-shaped or shaped like a Christmas tree with a stand, minus the holiday cheer. The base is specially flared so the anus can grasp and pucker around it, while the stand-part keeps the rectum from sucking it all the way inside. Gives a feeling of fullness. Can be made of silicone, rubber, metal, tempered glass or acrylic and sometimes vibrates and shoots fluid.

C2C—when used as a sexual term, it means "cock-to-cock," as in two men rubbing their erect penises together.

CAMEL TOES—when a woman's clothes (pants, shorts, bikini bottom) dig into her crotch and you can see her labia bulging along the sides of the crease; "crotch cleavage." Is occasionally used to describe a man's genitals.

CAMGIRL/CAMBOY—someone who spends from a few minutes a day to fulltime broadcasting images of themselves or their living space in front of a webcam. The vast majority of people who are doing this throw in a lot of sex and personal diary entries, enticing viewers to ante up a monthly fee for the privilege of watching. But now, it can include anything from exhibitionists to lifecasters to kids from Japan who spend a few seconds a day live but pull in hundreds of thousands of viewers; "camwhore."

CAM WHORE—person who spends hours in front of his or her webcam, sometimes with clothes on, sometimes with clothes off.

CANDIDA ALBICANS—a yeast growth or yeast infection.

CAN ENTERTAIN—swinging term, signifies you are able to host the sexual activity in your home.

CASTING COUCH—entertainment-industry term referring to a process where a director or producer receives sexual favors in exchange for casting an actor/actress in a production or show.

CATHETER—in medicine, a tube that goes up the urethra to allow the draining of urine from the bladder. Used for sexual play in some parts of the fetish/kink/BDSM world; see "urethra play."

CBT—cock'n'ball torture.

CERVICAL CAP—birth-control device approximating a small rubber beanie that sits on the cervix to discourage male ejaculate from entering. Differs from a diaphragm in several ways: it is smaller, stays in longer, is usually not filled with birth control jelly, and is not as effective, especially for women who have had prior pregnancies.

CERVIX—the bottom part of the uterus found in the back of the vagina. It can be as small as a cherry in a woman who has not delivered a baby through her vagina, or it can be much bigger. Mucus passes through the cervical opening ("os") and bathes the vagina. Sperm enters the uterus through the os of the cervix. The diaphragm birth control device is placed over the cervix to prevent the sperm from passing through it. The cervix feels softer during ovulation and its secretions change at that time. This is an important indicator for couples practicing natural birth control.

CFNM—means "Clothed Female, Nude Male" where male strippers walk around naked and clothed female party goers grab their penises, blow them, etc. Think of a bachelorette party gone wild. Can include domination and submission, and can occur in a variety of sexual venues or situations. To find CFNM websites, just enter the four letters in your search engine.

CHAKRAS—an eastern concept (India, not New Jersey): makes up the fuse box of the body whose seven points are said to regulate energy.

CHERRY—virginal or like new. Also refers to the hymen or maidenhead (in case you read Shakespeare).

CHEW TOY—refers to a person you are having sex with, usually on the Q.T.

CHICKEN & CHICKEN FOX—a "chicken" is a boyish-looking younger man who wants to be cruised, cared for, or paid for by an older man or "chicken fox."

CHICKEN OF THE SEA—a young gay sailor.

CHICKS WITH DICKS—persons who appear to be women in many ways except for the genital region. Usually a gender-bending or transsexual MtF man who would like to have bottom surgery but hasn't, or he loves his breasts, estrogen, female exterior in addition to his penis; "she-he," "she-male" or "he-she." Could possibly be a woman whose clitoris was enlarged prenatally due to a late dose of male-type hormones bathing a female fetus (an intersex condition), but that's not how the term is usually used.

CHIGGER—a small mite. You are more likely to get them from walking through infested areas. Can cause reddish welts and intense itching. Unlike scabies, they don't burrow into the skin and they don't drink blood. Their saliva causes a small wound in the skin, which becomes a welt. The chigger then drinks the body fluids which are in the welt. They usually drop off the skin in a couple of days. Under a microscope, they look like a small spider as opposed to scabies which look like small June bugs or tiny sand crabs. They are not as much of a medical problem as scabies. See "scabies".

CHLAMYDIA—called "the silent sexually transmitted infection" because women often don't know they have it, although men often have symptoms. There are about three to five million cases each year. Although often without symptoms, chlamydia can cause sterility and also increases the chances of having an ectopic pregnancy. Sexually active people, especially adolescents, should get a test for it every year. Women can easily have the test done during pelvic exams. The test is inexpensive and doesn't hurt. Treatment involves giving antibiotics to both sexual partners, not just the one with symptoms; otherwise, it won't work. You can carry chlamydia for years before displaying symptoms of the infection.

CHOCOLATE—one of the few substitutes for sex. Traditionally used in the wooing process, chocolate lights up the same part of the brain as heroin. May have anti-depressant properties for women.

CHORDEE—downward curvature of the penis, congenitally caused.

CIRCLE JERK(S)—guys masturbating together. Also a semi-notorious punk band of the 1980s.

CIRCUIT OR THE GAY CIRCUIT—a series of same-sex dance parties. A cool concept in its early years, some say the circuit still sizzles, others say it has become commercialism at its worst, catering to the cookie-cutter masses.

CIRCUMCISION (GOYIM)—an often unnecessary medical procedure where the foreskin of the penis is sliced or chopped off. The foreskin comprises up to a third of the skin on the entire penis. It was originally done in this country to prevent masturbation. More recently it has been done to enhance the profits of the physicians who perform the surgery. There is no scientifically valid reason that justifies routinely circumcising young males, nor does it prevent the spread of HIV (the "studies" claiming it does are mostly rubbish).

CIRCUMCISION (JEWS)—"the way a Jewish mother lets her son know who's in charge"—jmw. What if Jewish males were required to wait until they were old enough to phone the mohel themselves so it could be a young man's conscious expression of his faith?

CLAMPS—see "nipple clips."

CLAP—gonorrhea. One of the old timers in the field of sexually transmitted infections. Can cause a burning sensation during urination as well as an unusual discharge. Is easily treated, but can do damage if not attended to.

CLINTON'S LEGACY—when someone who's had oral sex doesn't think they've had sex at all.

CLITORIS—1. Latin for "darned thing was here just a second ago." 2. the only organ in either the male or the female body whose sole purpose is pleasure—which from a biological perspective might indicate that female genitals are more highly evolved than males'. 3. sometimes regarded as the Emerald City of women's orgasmic response. 4. not to be approached in haste. 5. sometimes wants to be caressed with vigor, other times can hardly tolerate being breathed upon. 6. while the clitoris is a fine organ to lavish huge amounts of attention upon, qualities such as tenderness, playfulness and respect also contribute largely to orgasmic response. 7. in Ebonics, it is called a "click." 8. UK slang for an aroused clitoris includes the term "budgie's tongue." Please see the illustrations in the "What's Inside a Girl" chapter to appreciate how much more there is to the clitoris than meets the eye. (The part you see is only the glans, which is little more than the crater at the top of the volcano.)

CLITORAL PUMP—a suction device placed over the glans of the clitoris in hopes that it will increase the blood flow and create more sensitivity.

CLOCKED—when a stranger has identified an MtF transsexual as being a biological or factory-equipped male; "read."

CLUBBING—a term that is sometimes used in porn-movie making, when the person who is receiving a blowjob uses his penis to whack the side of the face of the person who is giving the blowjob. For most couples, this would not be a big deal, but with the size of the average porn star's penis, facial trauma can occur; aka a "danza." Also refers to trendier version of bar hopping, as clubs often have a bouncer or gatekeeper who determine which people get in.

CLUSTER FUCK—army term for being in a bad situation. Also, three-way sex.

COCK-AND-BALL TOYS—small harness-like assemblies that snap around the base of the male genitals to pull the testicles up and apart. Some men hang weights on their CBT toys to stretch or pull down the scrotum.

COCK AND BALL TORTURE—For the man who can't get enough abuse from life, involves being hit or slapped in the genitals as part of a sexual turn on. Can include being zapped in the testicles with electric devices, having the testicles placed in big vices, or having the genitals tied up until they swell and look like they are going to pop; CBT." Add an extra "T" (CBTT) and you get "Cock and Ball and Tit Torture."

COCK RING—a ring made of rubber, steel or leather that fits tightly over the base of a hard penis or over the penis and testicles like a halter. The purpose is to help maintain an erection when the mind and body are otherwise unwilling, or to make the male genitals appear larger. In BDSM, a cock ring can be used on a submissive to denote ownership. Can also be worn as jewelry when hung from a chain around the neck. See "Cock-Ring Ken" in the chapter on Barbie. Cock rings hold shut the veins near the surface of the penis so the penile blood pressure does not escape. They are of somewhat dubious value, and should not be worn for more than 20 or 30 minutes without being taken off for a few minutes. Otherwise, there is a risk of permanent damage. Regarding rings made of steel, if it gets stuck on your swollen penis, you will have to go to a hospital to have it removed. What if they have to call in a locksmith or welder? This is why it is best if the ring is made of rubber or leather, or if it is made of metal it should have a hinge for easy opening.

COCK SOCK—slang for a condom. This term is also used in gender bending: if a girl decides to go out dressed as a guy, or has FtM fever and wants to become a guy, she will probably wear a "cock sock" or jock-like harness which is made to hold a soft pack (artificial penis and balls) between her legs; see "packing."

COITUS—scientific term for sexual intercourse, taken from the root word "coit," which is a carpet- and drapery-cleaning business in Northern California.

COJONES—Spanish for "testicles." Often misspelled as "cajones," which means "big boxes."

COKE WHORE—person who is so strongly addicted to cocaine that he or she will do anything (or anyone) to feed the habit; also "meth whore."

COME CUP—a device that attaches to the head of a vibrator and fits over the glans of the penis. Be sure to use lots of lube.

COMING TOO SOON—definitions vary, one is when a male sexual partner consistently comes in less than two minutes and both he and his partner are distressed that he doesn't last longer. The "average" male lasts between 3 and 8 minutes. "Premature ejaculation," "PE" or "rapid ejaculation." See the chapter "Dyslexia of the Penis" which covers the subject in depth.

COMPUTER BULLETIN BOARDS (BBS)—a place in early cyberspace for interchanges including porn; predated today's chat and Internet forums.

CONDOM—another name for a rubber.

CORNHOLE—means the anus or anal sex. The term probably originated from the use of dried corn cobs in the place of toilet paper.

COTTONTAIL—term that nude sunbathers sometimes use for a person who wears a bathing suit; see "textile."

COWGIRL—intercourse position where the girl is on top in a face-to-face orientation with the guy. See "reverse cowgirl."

COWPER'S GLANDS—tiny structures near the urethra inside the base of the penis which produce the clear, silky drops of fluid known as "precum."

COYOTE GIRLS—Sexy dancers in Thailand who wear just enough to keep their nips and lips covered, but not much more. Inspired by the 2000 movie *Coyote Ugly*, this brand of sex dancers claim they are not prostitutes, but are working to pay their way through medical school and the like.

CRABS—what people often see on Card 10 of the Rorschach (ink blot) test. Also, sexually transmitted lice that live on pubic hair and can sometimes make you itch to the point of near insanity. They have six legs, with two of them looking like the claws of a crab. They live on your blood. Crabs will die within a day or two of leaving a body; they can't live without the body's warmth or food supply.

CRACK A FAT—Australian term for "have an erection."

CRAMPS—abdominal pains women sometimes have during their period, related to the beginning of labor pains. Our gyno goddess says the key to using Midol-like pain relievers is to begin taking them a day or two before your period and cramps start. Also, orgasms can help relieve cramps. See the chapter "Surfing the Crimson Wave."

CRANK—speed (methamphetamine). The nasal decongestant propylhexedrine is often used to get a quick crank-like rush.

CREAMPIE—noun: a woman's vagina with male ejaculate dripping out of it; "a wet deck." verb-like: porn-speak for when a man comes inside a woman's vagina or rectum instead of doing the standard "money shot" where he pulls out and shoots his wad on her body. As reassurance that the actor has truly ejaculated, viewers often see a close-up of ejaculate oozing out of whatever orifice it was shot into.

CROSS-DRESSER—when a man gets joy from wearing a woman's clothes and make-up; "transvestite."

CROSSDRESSING—when a person of one sex makes a serious attempt to dress like a member of the other sex—and not a woman simply wearing her boyfriend's shirt or boxer shorts.

CRUISING—primarily a gay term, when guys are on the prowl for a quick sexual encounter; aka "jonesing for bone." Cruising spots can include parks, parties, bars, baths, or where ever it's known that guys are looking for sex. Besides the thrill, cruisers risk being robbed, beat up or busted by the vice squad. In traditional cruising, there is no conversation or small talk; business is business. In many ways, the cruising of the '70s, '80s and '90s is now being replaced by making contact on Craigslist or Internet chat rooms, and then meeting in person twenty minutes later for sex.

CRUMPET—British term for sexual activity. Also a bakery product.

CRUSH—intense romantic feelings unencumbered by the burden of good judgment. See "Dicknotized."

CRYPTORCHIDISM—Greek for a "hidden gonad." See "undescended testicle."

CRYSTAL DICK—impotence caused by taking crystal meth. Men who use crystal as a party drug sometimes take Viagra to counter crystal dick, which can create its own health hazard.

CUM (COME)—male ejaculate, the majority of which is produced by the seminal vesicles and prostate gland. Most males fill a teaspoon or two per ejaculation. Varies in consistency and taste among different men. Contains sperm, hormones, polyamines, prostaglandins, PSA and other substances. According to www.nightcharm.com, slang terms include: Splooge, Man Chowder, Spunk, Population Paste, Manthrax, Gizzum, Jizz, Love Juice, Baby Gravy, Pearl Necklace, Wad, Baby Batter, Pimp Juice, Dong Water, Man Jam and Number 3.

CUM SHOT—see "money shot."

CUNNILINGUS—"cunnus" is Latin for vulva (the part of a woman's genitals that is on the outside) and "lingere" means to lick—put 'em together and see what you get; "muff diver," "go down on her," "carpet munching," or "eating her out." Has any living human being ever used the term "cunnilingus" outside an academic setting?

CUNT—from the Latin "cunnus" (meaning vulva).

CUNT TORTURE—cock'n'ball torture for the BDSM-babe who has everything but a cock and balls. Intense stimulation that may or may not include pain.

CUP—see "Shock Doc."

CUPID'S HOTEL—a vagina.

CURVED DICK—a penis that curves as it gets hard, most likely due to a tight ligament. This is perfectly normal unless it causes physical pain, or becomes increasingly worse with time, in which case it should be taken to a physician for consultation. Since some guys with curves feel self-conscious, consider the following pearl of information: one highly experienced woman explained that the best sex she ever had was with an Italian guy who had a curved penis. If you've got a curve, experiment with different intercourse positions that might provide an advantage over guys who don't have a curve. If your curve is a new occurrence, see "Peyronie's Disease."

CUT—refers to a male who has been circumcised. Also a weightlifting term for muscles that have great definition.

CYBERSEX—when two people in a chatroom or live multi-person environment pretend to have sex, usually consisting of two males, with one claiming to be a female while the other doesn't know or doesn't care, aka "tinysex" or "cybering." Differs from "meatsex," which is sex in real life.

CYBERTRANNY—a man who goes into chatrooms and pretends to be a woman. "I was having the hottest sex of my life for three months on the Internet with this hot babe from Harvard who turned out to be a 50-year-old cybertranny with a beard."

CYSTITIS—see "bladder infection."

DAIRY QUEEN—a gay guy who likes to suck on men's nipples.

DARKROOM—designated place in clubs, bars, baths, parties where men who enjoy sex with men can have orgy sex.

DAISY CHAIN—sex involving multiple participants where the crotches are being pleased in a multitude of ways.

DATE—without this event, men might never cut their toenails.

DATE RAPE—when a woman is raped by someone she knows or someone who won't stop with sexplay after she indicates that she wants to stop.

D/D—in sex ads this means "drug and disease free."

DELIVERING THE WOOD—to have intercourse with.

DEPILATORY—cream for removing body hair.

DEPTH PLAY—refers to liking your dildo placed deep inside of your favorite orifice. Requires an extra-long dildo, maybe even a foot or more and perhaps one with a special shape.

DHAT SYNDROME—an excessive preoccupation with semen loss. This is a fairly common obsession in India and Pakistan where the belief exists that semen is a perfect and powerful body fluid and to lose it robs the body of its vitality.

DIAMOND CUTTER—the mother of all erections. It is so hard it feels like you could cut diamonds with it. Thank goodness not all erections are diamond cutters, because the pressure inside the penis gets so intense it can actually hurt. At the other end of the erection spectrum from a "half-master," "chubbie," "softie" or "floppy dog."

DIAL-A-PORN—phone sex at the rate of $2 or more a minute. Masturbation enhancement for those who like their stimulation over the phone; "dial-a-fuck." The women who give phone sex usually work with the caller to create his favorite role-playing fantasy, often something he is too embarrassed to act out with a real-life partner. A massive source of income for phone companies.

DIAPHRAGM—a contraceptive barrier device that holds contraceptive jelly against the cervix. A cross between a condom and a frisbee.

DICK FLICKS—movies with lots of guns & violence, as opposed to "chick flicks."

DICKNOTIZED—when a girl has a serious crush on a guy, and her life becomes defined by wanting to hold him, touch him, talk to him and be with him. Brain researchers are actually able to see the specific brain structures being lit up when a lover looks at a picture of his or her idealized lover. The parts of the brain that help us to have good judgment are actually being shut down, while the reward parts that are involved with things like drug addiction are having their own little fireworks display.

DIESEL DYKE—a manly lesbian; "bull dyke" or "butch." Opposing terms are "lipstick lesbian," "diamond dyke" and "femme."

DILDO—sex toy that brings much happiness. Can be used freestyle, or when mounted in a harness. Also slang for a person who is being a jerk or a moron.

DILDO HARNESS—a rig that holds a dildo in place at the same angle as a penis. Puts the strap in "strap-on." Gives a dildo penis-like properties of suspension and thrustability, but without the maneuverability of the real thing.

DILDONICS—think of a robotic droid in the form of a dildo, and have it controlled by someone in cyberspace. You now have a flavor of what dildonics could someday be. For now, dildonics is little more than a vibrator that someone at another computer controls with a mouse or joystick. Can also be when people on a webcam control each other's electronic sex toys.

DOCKING—when an uncircumcised male pulls his foreskin over the head of another man's penis There is no reason why it can't be pulled over a woman's nipples. Also can be cyberslang for "having sex;" "to dock."

DOGGIE STYLE—intercourse from behind, not to be confused with intercourse in the behind. More popular than the missionary position in some parts of the world. Often results in better stimulation of the vaginal roof, which some women prefer. Can also refer to anal intercourse, but not usually.

DOGGING—formalized voyeurism, where couples who like to be seen having sex log onto special dogging forums and announce the time and place where they will be having sex in their car. Spectators who show up get watch. Takes most of the risk and long hours of waiting out of being a voyeur. Started in the UK. The term originally referred to peeping Tom action, which was not necessarily done with the consent of the couple. Then came the Internet!

DOG'S BOLLOCKS—an expression in the UK which means "The best!" such as "Marty's new car is the dog's bollocks!" or "The mutt's nuts."

DOM—a dominatrix. For advice on hiring a dominatrix, see the kink chapter.

DO-ME QUEEN—in BDSM, a bottom whose entire existence revolves around getting the attention of others, while giving little in return. In the entertainment industry, an actress or actor.

DORK—a whale's penis.

DORMCEST OR HALLCEST—having sex with someone who lives on the same hall or in the same dorm. Does not always turn out well.

DORMGASM—trying to stay very quiet when having sex or masturbating while your roommate is present, or if the contractor was over-budget and didn't put any insulation in the walls.

DORMROOM SEX—see "bunk-bed sex," "sexiled," and "dormgasm."

DOUBLE ANAL—simultaneous penetration of the anus by two penises.

DOUBLE BAGGED—wearing two condoms at once. Not a good idea.

DOUBLE DILDO—dildo that seats two. See "Feeldoe dildo."

DOUBLE PENETRATION—penises in the vagina and rear end at the same time; "sandwich." Can also be two penises in the same vagina at the same time.

DOUCHE BAG—less-than-complimentary term for a woman or prissy man. Also, a gravity-driven device for feminine hygiene. Women who douche three times a month are three times more likely to develop pelvic-inflammatory disease than women who don't douche at all.

DOWNLOW—slang term in the black community for a gay or bisexual black man who is not out but who has sex with men. Often he can be married or have a girlfriend but the man-to-man sex is kept quiet so he isn't kicked out of the straight part of the black community.

DRAG—when a man wears women's clothing.

DRAG KING—a factory-equipped female who is dressed like a dude. Judith Halberstam divvies the drag kings into two groups: the *butch drag king* who's such a natural at it that not even the manly guys mess with her, and the *femme drag king* who has to work really hard at it. Can include anyone of any gender who makes hyper-manliness an act, performance, or parody.

DRAG QUEEN—men who love to dress up and become female characters. A drag queen often refers to her female character as if she were another person: "Cynthia had a bad day and is feeling like a total bitch" or "Crystal was dressed to the nines tonight!" Drag queens tend to be a bit more boisterous about their gender identities than either transsexuals or transvestites; when you are in a room with a drag queen you often know she's there because she so loves giving life to the female character she is playing. Mind you, just when you think you've got gender classifications such as "drag queen" sorted out, someone comes along and proves you to be totally wrong.

DRAINING THE WEASEL—taking a leak.

DRESSED TO THE RIGHT OR LEFT—guys who wear boxer shorts have to make a decision in life: on which side of the fly to rest their genitals. This is no big deal (sorry) unless you get your Wrangler's tailor-made, in which case the tailor will inquire, "Sir, do you dress to the right or to the left?" He will then leave extra denim on whichever side you indicate. Deciding which side your package should rest on is usually a no-brainer for most guys, since it naturally feels better on one side or the other, unless you are amballdexterous.

DRUNK DIAL—calling or texting after you've had way more alcohol than is good for you, usually with regrettable or embarrassing results, especially when it's an ex- who you contacted.

DRY HUMP—traditional sport of young couples, where pubic regions are feverishly rubbed together while both participants are fully clothed. Can result in chafing, irritation, orgasm or all three; "frottage."

DRY SEX—intercourse where the woman tries not to lubricate, practiced in parts of Africa. If she lubricates as much as a Western woman, she risks having bad things thought about her character.

DVDA—means "double vagina, double anus." This porn-movie silliness refers to the penises of four men simultaneously penetrating a woman's vagina and rectum. It is not possible, but was alluded to in the B-movie satire *Orgazmo*.

DYKES ON BIKES—an all-girls motorcycle club.

DYSPAREUNIA—a persistent or recurrent genital pain associated with sexual intercourse. May have multiple causes and can be a bear to treat. Associated terms are vulvarvestibulitis and vaginismus.

ECTOPIC PREGNANCY—a pregnancy in which the embryo implants into the wall of the Fallopian tube instead of the uterus. A very dangerous condition which can result in maternal death.

EDGEPLAY—in the world of BDSM, there's your mainstream whip, chain and collar play, and then there's the edge, which refers to the edge of what is safe. People into edgeplay are willing to take the extra risk of permanent harm or death for the added rush or thrill.

ELBOW GREASE—a brand of lubricant often used for masturbation or anal play, well known in the gay community.

ELECTROPLAY—using different types of electrical current on the genitals and other body parts. Requires special equipment and can be dangerous in the wrong hands. Some kinds of electroplay use the current in an attempt to enhance pleasure. Other forms of electroplay are used to administer pain, which people who are into BDSM can perceive as pleasurable. See "e-play."

EMERGENCY CONTRACEPTION—see "morning-after pill."

EMERGENT SEX—when cybersex occurs in games that were not designed for players or avatars to have sex in. Can range from simple avatar-avatar flirting in an MMORPG like *World of Warcraft* to entire sexual economies in an MMO such as *Second Life*. While it might feel safer because it is not real life, emergent sex can take on some of the emotions that accompany real-life sex.

ENDOCRINE DISRUPTERS—see "phthalates."

ENDORPHINS—hormones secreted during exercise, laughter and orgasm. These hormones are pain-relieving and share similarities with morphine. Endorphins are also secreted when the body is being stressed or when pain is applied, such as in BDSM, which is said to result in pain reduction and euphoria.

ENGLISH CULTURE—refers to being turned on by spanking or caning.

ENURESIS—peeing in your sleep. Happens to almost as many girls as guys and can last until adulthood. It can be a really lousy thing to have and is sometimes very difficult to shake. Modern pee-absorbing underwear makes it less embarrassing.

EPHEBOPHILIA—where an older man has a sexual obsession for teens who are approximately 15 to 18. The term "Lolita" is associated with straight men who have this desire, and "twinks" with gay men, where the boy's genitals are fully adult, but his beard hasn't come in and he looks young for his age.

EPIDIDYMIS—tightly coiled tube that sits on the top and back of the testicles; a storage space where the sperm can mature. The scrotal version of oak barrels where wine or whiskey mellows and ages.

EPIDIDYMITIS—when your epididymis gets an infection.

EPISIOTOMY—an incision made in the bottom of a woman's vaginal opening to increase its size so she can deliver a baby without tearing herself.

EPISPADIAS—a developmental problem where the urethra comes out the top of the penis. Related to hypospadias but different and much less common.

E-PLAY—using electricity in a way that is sexually exciting. Can be mild (e-stim or e-jo, electrical jerk off), or painful for BDSM. See "electric play."

EROTICISM—state of tension fueled by sexual desire.

EROTOPHILIC—refers to people who have positive feelings about sex.

ESCORT— fancy term for a prostitute, although some provide social as well as sexual services.

EUNUCH—man without balls, literally; sometimes without a penis as well. It can be a self-administered fetish or is done at the man's request. In past centuries, it was done to slaves and choir boys. Eunuchs could rise to positions of influence or power, given how they were not seen as the kind of threat that a man with sexual urges might be. In the later Roman Empire, the "real power" was thought to be in the hands of the Emperor's Chief Eunuch. In the Byzantine era, it was not unusual for parents to have one of their sons castrated, with the hope that he would rise to a trusted position, and would then be able to offer help and aid to his other family members. In the modern era, parents don't have this done to their sons, but it doesn't mean they haven't thought about it.

FACE SITTING—when a woman straddles the face of the person who is giving her oral sex; see "queening."

FACIAL—when a male ejaculates on his partner's face. A staple of traditional male porn; may we suggest you not try it at home without discussing it first.

FAG HAG—a woman who hangs out with gay men and claims to want sex with straight men, but seems to fear intimacy with them; "fruit fly."

FARANG—Thai term for whites or Westerners, from the Thai term "farangsayt" which means "French;" also a Thai word for "guava." "Farang prostitution" refers to the flesh trade that revolves around the pocketbooks and penises of Westerners. It wouldn't be unusual for the Thai to say, "These are Farang sex tourists on a two-week shagging spree."

FARMER TED—term for an undesirable male who is trying to make a move on you; from a character in the movie *Sixteen Candles*, "Oh crap, it's Farmer Ted."

FAYGELEH—Yiddish term for gay male.

FANNY—in Britain and Australia, the vulva or vagina; in America, the arse.

FANNY MAGNET—British for something that attracts swarms of women, "You should see his brother's Aston Martin, a right fanny magnet!"

FAUXMOSEXUAL—man who appears gay by his mannerisms but who sleeps with women; aka "metrosexual."

FEELDOE DILDO—a two-headed dildo that stimulates both the "doer" and "receiver." In many circles, the Feeldoe has bypassed the Nexus model as the double-dildo to beat. If a woman is beefy enough, she might get away wearing it without a harness. Has a bulb-like end that goes in the vagina of the wearer that helps it stay put. The company makes a model with a smaller dildo end, which is preferred by male-female couples in 'bend over boyfriend' situations. The model with the bigger dildo end is preferred when the receiver has a vagina.

FEEL UP—to touch or stimulate a partner's genitals with your hand; "grope."

FELCHING—when a man sucks or licks his own ejaculate out of whichever of his partner's orifices he shot it into.

FELLATIO—from the Latin "fellare" meaning "that which stops after marriage."

FEMBOT—a droid commissioned by Dr. Evil to do in Austin Powers.

FEMDOM—a term born from the fusion of "female" and "domination," where a woman has control or dominance in a relationship because it fits the emotional chemistry of both partners, and they want it that way. Femdom can be as extreme as a full-time mistress/slave arrangement including serious cock'n'ball torture, or it might include only occasional role-playing and perhaps a bit of foot worship, bondage or queening.

FEMALE EJACULATION—some women squirt extra fluid as part of having an orgasm. Traditionally known as "the wet spot," this varies in volume and frequency. See "gusher."

FEMALE MASTURBATION—"she bop," "diddle," "frig," "jill off," "muffin'buffin'," "slam the clam."

FEMORAL INTERCOURSE—when a lubricated penis slides between the labia like a hot dog sliding up and down the length of a hot-dog bun.

FEMME—feminine-looking lesbian as opposed to butch; aka "lipstick lesbian."

FETISH—a particular prop (leather, rubber, underwear, shoes, etc.), body part (feet, hair, breasts, etc.), or a scenario that a person relies on to get off sexually; "a paraphilia." The prop can be fantasized or exist in actuality. One philosopher has described a "fetish" as when a hungry person sits down at a dinner table and feels full from simply fondling the napkin. Also a lucky charm or object that is believed to have special or magical powers.

FIFTY-FOOTER—someone who looks hot from across the room, but starts looking less inviting with each approaching step.

FIGGING—When a peeled piece of ginger is inserted into the anus as you would a suppository to create a burning feeling that is said to increase sexual enjoyment. Why "figging" and not "gingering"? The term probably comes from the 19th century expression "feague" or "feaguing" which meant to put a piece of peeled ginger up a horse's arse which caused the horse to march with its tail held high—a popular practice among mounted military regimens.

FIGMO—military term meaning "fuck it, got my orders;" used when someone wants you to do something but you are already doing something else.

FIST FUCKING (FISTING OR HANDBALLING)—placing a fist into the rectum or vagina, hopefully with lots of lube. It can be a male fist or a female fist, but if you hold the average male hand against the average female hand, some people might prefer the woman's while those with a skosh more room in their orifices might prefer the male hand. The term is a misnomer, since the hand goes in with the fingers extended and fingertips bunched together rather than in a fist. However, once it's inside, all bets are off.

FLAGGING—at one time there was supposedly an elaborate set of codes in gay and BDSM communities where potential partners wore flags or hankies in their pockets to denote their particular kink. For instance, a yellow hankie hanging out of the left pocket meant you liked to be on top for golden showers, while the same hankie hanging from the right pocket meant you liked to be peed on (you'll never guess what a brown hankie meant). Theoretically, you could have all sorts of hankies hanging from various pockets.

FLAMING—term for an effeminate male; "nellie," "a nancy boy," "fem," "queen," the opposite of being butch. In the cybersphere, flaming is an extreme and perhaps pointless argument in a chat room or forum; aka "flaming out."

FLAPPER—term used to describe a sexually liberated woman during the 1920s who flaunted her unconventional approach to life.

FLIP & FUCK—a cheap fold-out chair made out of large foam cushions that easily turn into an imitation futon. Comes in handy for couples as a quick place for sex in college dorm rooms and student apartments.

FLOG THE LOG—to masturbate.

FLUFFER—a person who keeps male porn stars erect when they are not on camera. Fluffers aren't used as much these days, as today's male porn star either has trained wood (erects on cue), takes lots of Viagra, or is out of a job.

FORCED MILKING—A term borrowed from our friends in the BDSM community, where a male is made to ejaculate repeatedly.

FORESKIN—male equivalent of the clitoral hood. A sensitive flap of skin with thousands of nerve endings that extends from the shaft of the penis over the glans to keep the latter moist and safe; aka "lace curtain." Also allows the penis to more easily glide during intercourse, and makes lube unnecessary for jerking off and hand jobs. The part that gets chopped off during circumcision.

FORNICATION—intercourse between people who are not married.

FOUCAULT—a French philosopher who philosophized about sex. What's more fun and exciting, reading Foucault or Lacan?—get back to you on that one. One of the things Foucault believed: Once the church decided we needed to confess our sins to a priest in order to save our souls, we needed to find ways to put our sins into words. And so we started describing sex, which was sinful, with words, and this gave governments and religions ways to regulate it, and sex became a way of having power over someone, even in intimate relationships. Got that? And unless you've just drained a six-pack of Jolt or two cans of Rockstar Punched, be very wary of paragraphs containing the names of both "Foucault" and "Nietzsche."

FRAZIER—manliest lion to ever live in captivity; once had intercourse more than 160 times in three days. Died shortly thereafter.

FREEBALLING—when a guy isn't wearing any underwear.

FRENCH—term for oral-genital contact, not to be confused with "French kiss," although one often leads to the other.

FRENCH EMBASSY—place where there's lots of gay sex going on.

FRENCH KISSING—kissing with mouths open as opposed to closed. Usually involves transfer of tongues (in the nonbiblical sense); "suck face."

FRENCH TICKLER—any form of condom that has bumps, projections or ridges that are marketed to increase a woman's sexual pleasure. Spend the extra money on flowers, and you'll both be happier.

FRENULUM—sensitive part of the penis just below the head on the side of the shaft that faces away from the abdomen when the penis is erect.

FRESHMAN 15—urban myth that college freshmen put on 15 pounds their first year. Research shows it's actually 5 pounds for girls and 6 pounds for guys. How much of it is from beer and how much from dorm food has not been determined.

FRIG—British for "jerk off," "wank," "five-against-one."

FROG KISSER—person who believes that she can turn a loser into a winner.

FROT—when aroused males rub their erect penises; "C2C," "bone-on-bone."

FROTTAGE—see "dry hump."

FSD—stands for "Female Sexual Dysfunction." Beyond that, all bets are off as to the specific meaning, or as they say, "The definition and correlates of female sexual response and female sexual dysfunction continue to evolve."

FUCK BUDDY—friend or acquaintance you occasionally (or often) have sex with. While the sex might be serious, the relationship isn't; "buddy sex," "hooking up," "friends with privileges."

FUN AND GAMES—in the swinging lifestyle, a term that refers to having sex.

GANG BANG—when a woman enjoys having intercourse with several men in rapid succession, at her invitation; "pulling a train." This is something that women who are in the swinging lifestyle can do without much fuss.

GANG BANGER—member of a street gang.

GAPE OR GAPE SHOT—the flower of Gonzo Porn, where the camera does a close-up interior shot of a woman's anus right after intercourse. The hallmark of the gape shot is that the woman's anus is still open and is dripping with male ejaculate. Can be of a vagina as well. See "Gonzo Porn."

GAYBORHOOD—a neighborhood primarily populated by gays, such as the Castro in San Francisco, Boystown in the Lakeview part of Chicago, South Beach and Key West in Florida, Asbury Park in New Jersey, Le Village in Montreal, Washington West in Philadelphia, West Hollywood in Los Angeles, and according to Fox News, almost all of New York City. While there used to a handful of prominent gayborhoods in the major cities around the world, there has been a strong move in the last decade toward decentralization resulting in smaller gay enclaves in more cities.

GENDER-BENDER—person of one sex who has become, is becoming, or fantasizes about being the other sex. Requires a person with a fluid sexual identity; see "transgendered."

GENDER DYSPHORIA—when the genitals you have and the genitals you wish you had are not the same. This is when a guy seriously wishes he were a girl or a girl seriously wishes she were a guy. May lead to taking feminizing or masculinizing hormones of the desired gender, and sometimes sex-reassignment surgery (SRS).

GENDER FUCK—mixing and matching gender attributes, such as wearing a lacy bra with an athletic supporter, having a beard and wearing a dress, or wearing a hard hat with high heels. A watered-down version is when a woman wears a frilly dress with Carhartt boots or Doc Martens. While this was originally a gender fuck, it is now an acceptable part of fashion and no longer has the defining elements of being a gender fuck (in most cases).

GENDERQUEER—when the usual gender roles and terms don't work for you. People who are gender queer can identify as both male or female, or mostly one and not the other, or neither. So genderqueer has become a blanket term for all things having to do with gender and transgender when the normal definitions of male and female don't quite do it for you.

GENITAL ACNE—a condition caused by the eruption of small glands on the labia and scrotum called apocrine glands. Looks like zits, but isn't really.

GENITAL BEADING—a form of body modification where beads are implanted under the skin that's on the shaft of the penis.

GENITALS—the part of yourself that you play with under the covers; in the UK, the term "bits" is often used, especially for female genitals.

GETTING OFF—coming or having an orgasm; "getting your rocks off."

GFE—stands for *The Girlfriend Experience,* which is when a prostitute goes that little extra and acts like a girlfriend for the night, including kissing, hugging and holding hands. BFE is *The Boyfriend Experience.*

GIVE HEAD—to perform oral sex; "a blow job." The term "give head" usually refers to performing oral sex on a male, as opposed to "going down" which can involve either sex, or "munching carpet" or "eating out," which are specific to doing oral sex on a female.

GLANS—head of the penis.

GLORY HOLE—a crotch-high hole in a partition between two enclosed areas that a penis can be stuck through. Located in places where gay guys cruise: the baths, video booths, tea rooms, etc. The penis can be sucked or played with by whoever is on the other side of the glory hole, or the other person can look through the glory hole to watch what you are doing with yours. Can also be used for anal sex if the giver is long enough. It is not wise to ask a guy on the other side of a glory hole to go outside and have sex in your car, as sex in cars that are parked anywhere but your garage is illegal in most municipalities and why would you want to invite someone you've never said two words to into your car? (Some people would ask why you would want to have sex with someone who you've never said two words to, but that's a different discussion for a different time.) Also, don't assume that the glory hole is legal—it depends on the location. Origin of the term might be from British ships, where a "glory hole" was a small storage space between decks where treasure or unwanted items were hidden or stored. See "cruising" and "glory-hole protocol."

GLORY-HOLE PROTOCOL—one shouldn't indiscriminately stick his penis through a glory hole and hope for the best. He might try looking through it first. If the person on the other side is hard and stroking, he might then poke a finger through. If a finger from the other side returns the gesture, it's time to play ball. Or he might stroke his own penis as a sign of availability until a guy on the other side bites. All is nonverbal. There is no room for small talk in the world of cruising and glory holes. And whatever you do, next time you are at the Minneapolis-St. Paul Airport, don't tap your shoes under the stall.

GOATSE.CX—a bit of cyber-history and perhaps the most famous of the Internet shock sites, contained the infamous Hello.jpg which shows the rear end and dangling penis & testicles of a skinny man who is reaching back and spreading his rectum wide. Did we say "wide"? Put a flashlight beam up that man's gaping anus and you could see the roof of his mouth. Hello.jpg is part of a photo series of the Goatse.cx man pushing a butt plug up his rectum which appears to be at least 6 inches in diameter. (Do you speak in past tense when images on the web are pretty much forever?)

GO DOWN ON—to perform oral sex on.

GOLDEN ENEMA—kinky enema where the "nozzle" is a peeing penis.

GOLDEN DOUCHE—kinky douche where the "nozzle" is a peeing penis.

GOLDEN SHOWERS—peeing on or being peed on as a sexual turn-on; "water sports." Silviculturally speaking, a tree of the legume family that's native to India whose Latin name is *cassia fistula*.

GONAD—sex gland, "nads," "wank tanks," "testicles " or "ovaries."

GONZO PORN—a style of adult movie making that intentionally appears to be low budget and over the top. It is filled with close-up shots and has even more sex and fewer attempts at cheesy plot lines than the usual fare. The actors are often brash, highly enthusiastic and playing to the camera. The camera angle is frequently from the male point of view (aka "POV"). The term "Gonzo" is associated with Hunter S. Thompson's tendency to be over the top and in your face, not that Mr. Thompson ever directed porn. One of the more unfortunate twists of Gonzo porn is that it has become particularly disrespectful and increasingly violent toward the female actors. Names often associated with Gonzo porn are directors Seymore Butts and John "Buttman" Stagliano.

GREEK—usually refers to anal intercourse.

GROMMET—a young, rookie surfer who often substitutes gumption for intelligence, and hyperactivity for poise; "grom," "surf rat." Sex is a matter of great concern and mystery for the young grom: "What does one do?" "For how long?" "Is it all right if I don't get completely naked?"

GROT SITE—a term used in the UK for a porn site. In the UK, "grot" is a similar term to "filth," but not quite as strong, e.g. in the same way you could say that something is "filthy," you could also say it's "grotty."

GROUP SEX—see "swinging," "Roman culture" or terms with "poly" in front.

G-SHOT—the latest sex scam where a so-called healthcare professional gives a woman a shot of collagen in what they claim is her "G-spot" to somehow make it bigger and miraculously increase her sexual pleasure. Do not be naive or dumb enough to fall for this inane and potentially dangerous scheme. What if it causes long-term damage inside of your vagina?

G-SPOT—area of potential sensation on the roof of the vagina named after the lucky man (Grafenberg) who claims to have discovered it.

G-STRING—about a quarter of a bikini bottom. See "thong."

GUICHE—a piercing on the male perineum.

GUSHER—term for when a man has an orgasm at the same time that his prostate is being stimulated. For some men, it feels spectacular; others find it is annoying. Refers to female ejaculation when large amounts of fluid squirt out just before or during orgasm.

GYNECOMASTIA—when boys appear to be developing breasts; happens to about 20% of boys during puberty and usually goes away in two years.

HANDBALLING—see "fist fucking."

HAND JOB—bringing either yourself or a partner to orgasm with your hand.

HAND WARMERS—Australian term for breasts, perhaps explaining something about the way Australian men regard Australian women.

HAPPY ENDING—if you are in Thailand getting a massage and your Thai masseuse asks if you want a happy ending or "han-mei," smile, and say, "Yes, please!" After she's done, be sure to remember the *Guide To Getting It On!* in your prayers.

HARD-ON—when the penis becomes erect; "wood," "trouser tent." For a rap variation on the term, Dr. Dre might say, "Ya dick's on hard." In the UK: "stiffy" or "pitch a tent." In Australia: "crack a fat."

HAVING IT OFF—British slang for having sex, "My roommate and his girlfriend were having it off while they thought I was asleep;" aka, "Have a naughty."

HEART—that which contains all love, caring, passion, tenderness, happiness, courage, loyalty, gentleness, awe, hope, beauty, feeling, play, laughter, trust, charity and joy. An important thing to have.

HEBEPHILIA—this is when an adult man is sexually attracted to pubescent children and teens, roughly between the ages of 11 to 14, which is different from pedophiles who are attracted to younger children. While some men are both pedophiles and hebephiles, they usually tend to be in one camp or the other, with the majority of incarcerated offenders being hebephiles. A true hebephile who cherishes 11-year old boys might find little arousing about the same boys when they are sixteen, and nothing arousing about young children. Another category called ephebophilia is where an older man has an obsession for teens who are approximately 15 to 18.

HELLO.JPG—see "goatse.cx."

HENTAI—animated Japanese pornography. Includes Japanese cartoon porn, or graphic novels in the anime, manga, or doujinshi forms. Can be described as amine with all female orifices occupied by large penises. Huge breasts unaffected by the forces of gravity are obligatory. In Japanese, hentai means "pervert" or "abnormal." See "anime."

HERMAPHRODITE—A misleading term that is hopefully going out of usage. See "Intersex." In spite of what your friends tell you, you are probably not.

HERPES—a virus that affects the mouth and/or the genitals with a rash, lesions or canker sores. Herpes is usually harmless when dormant or hibernating inside the body, but it occasionally surfaces with a vengeance. It hibernates deep in the nerves that surround the mouth and/or genitals. If you have herpes, spend time reading up on it and learn as much as you can; that way you become the master of it rather than it becoming the master of you. Start by reading the free and fine *The Updated Herpes Handbook* by Terri and Ricks Warren. It is one of the best resources on herpes you will ever find. You can now read the entire book online at www.westoverheights.com. Click on "free herpes handbook." The authors are great about keeping it updated.

HERSHEY HIGHWAY—refers to "anal sex" or specifically to the anus or rectum.

HETEROFLEXIBLE—a person who identifies as straight but is not beyond the occasional same-sex hook-up after having enough beers.

HICKEY—love bite resulting in a bruise. A source of embarrassment for some, a badge of honor for others. For how to cover a hickey, see the Kissing chapter.

HIPSTERS—low-rise briefs that offer full coverage without looking like granny panties. Close cousin to "boy shorts." Hipsters stop higher on the thigh while boy shorts have the start of a leg. Materials range from cotton to lace.

HIRSUTISM—male-pattern hair growth in women.

HIT A HOME RUN—to have intercourse.

HOBBYIST—slang term for a man who likes to visit prostitutes and makes it a bit of a lifestyle. Prostitution is referred to as "the hobby" and the Johns prefer to be known as "hobbyists." One of the more famous websites for hobbyists that rates "the providers" in various cities is www.TheEroticReview.com.

HOLMES—wanna-be ganster talk for "dude."

HO CAKE—rap term for "vagina."

HOOCH—illegal liquor. A hut or shack, often where a prostitute lives. Also slang for "vagina."

HOODED CLITORIS—when the hood of the clitoris is either bonded to the surface of the clitoris or does not retract easily. This is not uncommon, and it frequently causes no problems. If it makes sexual enjoyment difficult, speak to a gynecologist. Surgery should be avoided if at all possible, as the results are not always good. If surgery is recommended, get a second or third opinion.

HOOKING-UP SEX—a one-night stand; sex without expectations (or with very low expectations), usually where neither party has any plans to become emotionally involved with the other. Drinking is generally the foreplay. Marks an interesting shift in the idea that sex should be part of a relationship, and that it's the man who wants the sex while the woman carefully regulates access to it. Hooking up is usually done for the pleasure and excitement of both partners. It can sometimes also be an attempt to gain status or to one-up someone else, as when one of our readers hooked-up with the fiance of a co-worker who she didn't like.

HOOKING UP (prison)—prison slang for when a jocker, daddy or pitcher enters a relationship with a punk. The daddy controls the relationship and provides protection for the punk who provides anal and oral sex at the whim of the dominant daddy jocker. Even if the punk is 100% straight and masculine, the jocker may want him to act more feminine so he can deny the punk's masculinity. The jocker sometimes shares the punk with others or can keep him all to himself. Hooking up can sometimes evolve into a loving, protective and caring experience, given the unusual world of prison culture, or it can be an extension of life in hell; see "punk."

HORNY—having the sexual urge. The term in Australia is "randy."

HOSE MONKEY—fireman, although this term can be used in a less charitable way when referring to someone who isn't a fire fighter.

HO STRO—rap term which means "whore stroll," which refers to a street or neighborhood where prostitutes work.

HOT COFFEE MOD—an interactive sex mini-game that allowed players of *Grand Theft Auto: San Andreas (GTA:SA)* to go inside with CJ when a woman invited him to "have coffee." Without the mod, players could only hear love-making sound effects. This mod created a huge scandal and moral outrage in 2005, which is amazing considering how technologically crude the portrayal of sex in the mod was, although the "excitement meter" was pretty interesting.

HOT-PILLOW TRADE—slang used in the hotel business for people who rent rooms just for sex. Best when the parking lot is not visible from the street.

HOTWIFING—when a man and his wife get off by her having sex with other men. The husband either watches, listens, or has sex with her afterward while she tells him the details; can include him orally tidying her up while the other man's trail is still fresh.

HPV—human papilloma virus; has more than seventy different forms. Hangs out in moist genital skin. Some strains are the cause of cervical cancer, other strains cause genital warts. (The forms of HPV that cause genital warts are not the ones that cause cervical cancer.) Sudden presence of HPV doesn't mean your partner cheated. It can stay dormant for years. If you are a woman who has HPV, please, please, please get annual pap smears. Condoms can help but won't stop the spread of HPV. The HPV vaccines remain controversial.

HUMAN VITAE—the pope's master plan for semen, where every act of intercourse must be open to conception. Sex that can't result in conception is wrong, including oral sex, intercourse with birth control and masturbation.

HUNG—refers to a male whose sex organs displace more space than most. Usage might include: "Melvin is hung" instead of "Melvin is hung like an elephant" which would be redundant. On the other hand, saying "Melvin is hung like a mouse," would not be redundant.

HUSTLER—male prostitute, usually gay; "rent boy," "joy boy" or "escort" with a client known as a "John."

HYMEN—a small collar or ring of tissue located just inside the opening of the vagina. You can't see it unless you pull the labia or outer lips apart. The hymen is located where the vulva and vagina meet. The hymen probably formed because the vulva and vagina were made from two different kinds of embryonic tissue. As for the idea that the hymen or cherry gets "popped" or is torn to shreds after the first intercourse, it's just a myth. As a girl approaches puberty and her body produces more estrogen, her hymen starts to change. The ring of tissue becomes more elastic. After puberty, the hymen often becomes more like an o-ring or a collar of tissue rather than a barrier, almost as if it is changing in anticipation of intercourse. Way more than 50% of our survey takers said they had no bleeding during their first intercourse, and researchers often have trouble distinguishing between the hymens of teenage girls who are sexually active and hymens of teenage girls who are still virgins. That wouldn't be the case if hymens were like pop-bottle caps or cherries that pop. While the hymen may become less prominent with age, it never goes away. (Read more about the amazing hymen in Chapter 8: "The Hymen" which is on pages 107 - 114.)

HYPOSPADIAS—a developmental anomaly where the urethra does not go all the way to the end of the penis, but exits on the lower shaft.

IMPOTENCE—when a guy can't get it up on a regular basis, or can get it up most of the way but it isn't rigid or hard enough to get it in.

INCEST—sex among immediate family members or blood relatives.

INCOMPETENT CERVIX—when a cervix is weakened and can't hold the fetus in the uterus to term. No doubt, named by a male.

INDOOR SPORTS—swinging.

INFIBULATION—the process of piercing the male foreskin or female labia and stringing jewelry through it to prevent sexual intercourse.

IRIE—rasta or reggae term meaning cool, relaxing, calm, and collected; how you hopefully feel after making love.

INTERSEX—term for a variety of conditions in which a person is born with a reproductive or sexual anatomy that doesn't fit the typical definitions of female or male. See the chapter "Intersex."

INTERSTITIAL CYSTITIS—pain or discomfort in the pelvis that is related to the bladder. Symptoms often include a persistent urge to pee or the need to pee frequently, as often as a couple times an hour. This is not called "painful bladder syndrome" without good reason, as the urge can feel quite extreme and it can be accompanied by spasms and pressure. People can have pain while urinating, pain while driving, and pain while having sex. In men, there can be painful ejaculation. The cause is not known, although a number of theories are on the table, and it could be there are different things that cause it. There are a number of different treatments, with one of the main goals being in decreasing the pain. People with this disorder are often very depressed as a result, in part due to the pain and discomfort, and in part because it causes such incredible interference in their lives.

JACKING OFF—stroking your genitals in ways that cause fine sensations; other terms include jerking off, choking your chicken, beating your meat, wanking, masturbating, cranking the shank, blowing your load, dishonorable discharge, flogging your log, massaging your muscle, pud whacking, rubbing one out, playing with yourself, sending out the troops, spanking your monkey, stroking it, and Code 20 (prison slang–Texas Dept. of Corrections Offense Code).

JACK'N'JILL PARTIES—gatherings of sexually uninhibited men and women who attend in their underwear and masturbate in front of each other. A by-product of concern about AIDS.

JADE STALK—Chinese Taoist term for penis.

JANEY—lesbian slang for vagina.

JELLY ROLL—jazz term for female genitals.

J-LUBE—a powdered lube that veterinarians mix with water that helps them slide their hands up the vaginas and rectums of livestock. Is said to work great for fisting, anal sex and for jerking off, except for that little matter about how an 1,100 lb horse will drop dead within a few hours of very small amounts of J-Lube getting into their peritoneal cavity. You might find that there is no such warning on the sides of cans of vegetable shortening, and it is renowned for its fisting-friendly properties.

JOANI'S BUTTERFLY—a small vibrator that can be strapped in place for use during intercourse or when out on the town.

JOCKSTRAP—jog bra with only one cup.

JOHN—someone who pays a prostitute for sex, "trick."

JOHNSON—old-fashioned term for penis.

JOHN THOMAS—British term for penis; "old fella."

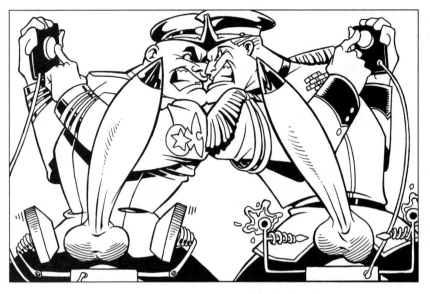

The Cold War. Hopefully gone but not forgotten.

JUNKIE—a heroin addict, as well as anyone who's infatuated with someone or something; not necessarily a negative term.

KEGEL EXERCISES—genital aerobics—when you squeeze or contract the muscles surrounding your genitals in a way that would stop the flow if you were taking a leak. Some people claim that these exercises will fix everything from a floppy penis to an unhappy vagina. Research results do not always support these claims. The exercises can be useful in becoming more aware of genital sensations, and some people say they result in stronger orgasms as well as being helpful for certain incontinence issues and for improving vaginal as well as male genital tone. Kegels have never been proven to help nonorgasmic women start coming, although there is much mythology that they do.

KILLER PUSSY—vintage rock'n'roll group who sang the cult classic *Teenage Enema Nurses in Bondage* as well as *Pepperoni Ice Cream, Pocket Pool* and *Bikini Wax.* Also a term guys occasionally use to refer to a truly memorable vagina or to steamy-looking women as in, "There's some killer pussy at Kittredge, but I'd still rather live at Will Vill."

KINK—beyond vanilla.

KINSEY AVERAGE—about two-and-a-half minutes. The amount of time sex researcher Alfred Kinsey estimated that it takes the average American male to come during intercourse.

KNICKERS—British for "panties." Historically, undergarments worn by your great-great-grandmother. What your great-great-grandfather dreamed of getting into; "granny panties."

KNOCKED UP—pregnant.

KNOCKING BOOTS—rap term for "having intercourse;" the "boots" part means "booty," and the "knocking" refers to the slapping sound that a man's hips make when hitting the woman's thighs while doing it doggie style. Can also mean "anal sex." See "lay pipe."

KY JELLY—a brand name of a water-soluble lube that people have historically used to help increase the slip'n'slide coefficient during intercourse. They have newer KY Personal lubes for sex as opposed to the old tube of lube that's still used for medical procedures. If it starts to dry out during use, add a few drops of water, not more KY.

LABIA MINORA—the inner lips of the vulva, which also attach to the underside of the clitoris. Along with the glans, shaft crus and bulbs of the clitoris, the labia minora are the most sexually reactive parts of female sexual anatomy. Contain different tissue than the larger lips or labia majora.

LABIOPLASTY—cosmetic surgery of the inner labia.

LADYBOYS—term for transsexuals in Cambodia.

LANDING STRIP—medium to severe form of bikini waxing where the pubic hair is done in a small rectangle.

LAPAROSCOPY—visual examination of the ovaries, Fallopian tubes and uterus with an instrument that's inserted just below the navel.

LAWRENCE V. TEXAS—2003 Supreme Court decision declaring it constitutional for one man to suck the cock of another man in their own home in Texas; ditto for anal penetration. If you have ever been anywhere in Texas outside of Austin, you will immediately appreciate the magnitude of this decision. Since the court's majority decision focused on the right of liberty rather than on the right of privacy, we must assume that the court was speaking directly to the liberties that Mr. Lawrence was taking with Mr. Garner's rear end. How this decision is being interpreted by lower courts in other decisions is interesting. While it appears that it is no longer a crime for a woman to use a vibrator in Alabama, it may still be a crime to sell one.

LAY PIPE—rap term for having sex, "I lay pipe with all the lonely bitches while da husbanz hard at work." Also: "to freak," "bag up with," "bag up bitches," "get busy."

LEFT HAND—what a right-handed person sometimes uses to masturbate with so it feels like someone else is doing it.

LEG SPREADER—a bar with ankle cuffs on each end that keeps a woman's legs spread open; "spreader bar." Also can be a type of mixed drink, although no two recipes for it are even remotely the same; often includes some or all of the following: Bacardi 151, Wild Turkey, Jack Daniels, tequila, vodka, sweet vermouth, and a cherry.

LESBIAN—woman who prefers sex with women.

LESBIAN BED DEATH—the lesbian equivalent of when straight couples are married, have kids and both are working full time.

LIBIDO—what Freud said is the fuel for our desire to make an emotional connection with others; he did not limit the term to erotic or horny feelings as is often done in the present day and age.

LICHEN SCLEROSUS—a chronic inflammatory disorder of the skin that affects women far more often than men, usually impacting the vulva and greater crotch area but also the breasts and upper arms. The exact cause is unknown.

LIFESTYLES ORGANIZATION—a large organization for couples who like to have sex with other couples (thousands of couples belong), based in Anaheim, California, pride of Orange County, home of God, Country and eating your apple pie between someone other than your wife's legs. If you went to one of the weekly dinners or dances sponsored by this organization, you might be surprised at how many police, members of the military and teachers belong.

LINGAM—Sanskrit term for penis.

LIPSTICK LESBIAN—feminine-appearing woman (in a traditional sense) whose choice in sexual partners is other women.

LONG FLANNEL NIGHTGOWN—very effective birth-control device.

LOSING YOUR V-CARD—losing your virginity.

LOVE—a very special way that we have of relating to one another.

LUCKY PIERRE—a gay or bisexual term, referring to three-way sex; lucky Pierre is the person in the middle.

LUG—means "Lesbian Until Graduation."

M2M—means man-to-man, and is used to signify same-sex attraction or sex between men. Take away the penises, and you've got "machine-to-machine," which in telemetry systems means data-sharing between two machines.

MAGIC WAND—Hitachi's contribution to women's sexual pleasure; has two speeds, a big round head and vibrates like a Federation freighter at warp 9.

MAINTAIN—product you slap on your penis to numb it out and supposedly help it last longer during intercourse. Also what you try to do when parents or authority figures are around.

MAKE A MILK RUN—gay term for cruising.

MAN'S SHIRT—object of male clothing which girlfriends often lay claim to and love wearing, especially to bed. The feel and smell of it gives the girl comfort. Any man who had a similar attachment to a piece of woman's clothing would be called weird, kinky or a paraphiliac, but who's complaining?

MAP OF TASMANIA—slang term in Australia for "women's genitals" or "vulva."

MASOCHIST—a person who invites pain and passively controls others in the process; "bottom" or "submissive." The term "masochism" was coined by Havelock Ellis and named after Leopold Von Sacher-Masoch, a nineteenth-century author who begged his wives to whip and humiliate him. An ideal day for Leopold began with a good whipping; otherwise, he struggled to get into a productive groove.

MASTURBATION—a date with your own genitals; for males, see "jacking off."

MATANUSKA THUNDERFUCK—a medicinal with a distinctive, burning-rope smell that is sometimes used to enhance the enjoyment of sexual relations. Grown in Alaska's Matanuska Valley, an area known world wide for its legendary herb production as well as being home to the town of Wasilla.

MDMA—ecstasy.

MEAN QUEEN—a drag queen who is into BDSM.

MEATOTOMY—a form of body modification where the penis is sliced in half.

MEATSEX—real-live sex as oppposed to cybersex.

MENAGE A TROIS—(sounds like "may-naj-ah-twa") when three French people are sharing sexual intimacy. Includes either two men and a lucky woman or two women and a lucky man; "threesome."

MENSTRUAL CUP—a soft, flexible container made of soft silicone rubber or latex that is inserted into the vagina to collect menstrual fluids. It looks a bit like a small, upside down funnel, although the stem is not hollow and the body of the cup is more rounded than a funnel. There are from six to eight different kinds of menstrual cups, such as the Lunette, Diva, Moon Cup, Lady Cup, Femmecup, Miacup Keeper and Pink Cup. Most are made of medical grade silicone, with each having a slightly different length, softness, rim, stem and color. Once it's in place, a menstrual cup forms a seal against the wall of your vagina which allows it to collect the flow. Unlike a tampon which also absorbs your vagina's natural secretions, a menstrual cup holds only your period flow until you remove it and wash it out. As a result, it won't dry out your vagina.

MERCY FUCK—intercourse done from a sense of duty or pity rather than burning desire.

MERKIN—wig for the pubic area; supposedly originated in past centuries to hide syphilis lesions. Was held in place by toupee glue or a small G-string.

MILE-HIGH CLUB—to have had sex in a plane while it is airborne.

MILF—acronym for a "Mother I'd Like to Fuck," which is when you have lust in your heart for a PTA mom, a soccer mom, or any mom; "yummy mummy." Used in the movie *American Pie* where the term refers to having a hard-on for a friend's mom, but its origin may have been the movie *Milk Money*. More recently brought into the mainstream by the choice of an MILF as a U.S. vice-presidential candidate in 2008. See "Matanuska Thunderfuck."

MISSIONARY POSITION—an intercourse position where the man and woman are horizontal and face to face, usually with the man on top. The term was possibly coined by savages who associated this position with conquering missionaries.

MISTRESS—formerly "the other woman," now is BDSM-speak for "dominatrix."

MONEY SHOT—the heart of traditional porn movies, where the male unloads a wad of white splooge somewhere on his partner's body; "cum shot."

MONILIA—type of vaginal yeast infection that can be very uncomfortable for the woman. Can cause thicker discharge than is normal, extreme itching, and painful intercourse.

MONS PUBIS—fleshy mound at the top of the vulva where pubic hair grows.

MONTGOMERY NODES—little bumps that often form on the nipples after puberty, especially prominent when you feel a chill or are sexually aroused.

MORNING-AFTER PILL (PLAN B)—pill that can be taken up to 72 hours after unprotected intercourse which greatly reduces the chances of pregnancy. Especially helpful if the rubber broke; "emergency contraception."

MORNING-AFTER PILL VS. ABORTION PILL—let's say you didn't use birth control, or your method failed (the condom broke, you forgot to take the pill for a few days or because you were raped). The morning-after pill or emergency contraception does not cause an abortion. It can reduce, though not eliminate, the likelihood of pregnancy. There are two kinds of emergency contraception: 1) insertion of an IUD, and 2) emergency contraceptive pills. An IUD can be inserted up to 5 days after sex, but is more expensive and is mostly used in women who want a long-term method and want to start it at that time. The brand name for the pills that are regularly prescribed is "Plan B," which is a very concentrated dose of progestin-only birth control pills given as two pills.

A woman should take one pill no later than 120 hours after unprotected sex. The second pill is then taken 12 hours later. The sooner the medication is taken (hopefully within the first 12-24 hours after sex), the more effective it is. The 72-hour mark is the official FDA approved time span, but 120 hours is commonly used by most practitioners. Some medical providers have the woman take both pills at once, which leads to better adherence. Plan B and emergency contraception are not the same as a chemical abortion, and emergency contraception does not alter or terminate an existing pregnancy. Plan B also does not cause a woman to bleed or have a period. Plan B works the same as regular birth control pills: to prevent ovulation if it has not occurred, to thicken the cervical mucus to make it harder for sperm to swim through, and to alter the uterine lining to make it less likely for a fertilized egg to implant. Plan B has been shown to be extremely safe, even if taken multiple times. This is why the FDA panel recommended that it be sold over the counter a few years ago. People often confuse Plan B with Mifepristone which causes an abortion. (Mifepristone was known as RU-486 during clinical trials, and in the US it is called Mifeprex.) Mifepristone causes an abortion, as opposed to providing emergency contraception. It must be taken under a doctor's care within 49 days of conception, and does carry medical risks. As of presstime, the greatest risks for Mifepristone appear to have been when doctors administered it vaginally as opposed to orally. Only oral administration has been approved by the FDA. Whether it remains on the market will be determined by further studies.

MOTHER FIST AND HER FIVE DAUGHTERS—British masturbation term; the equivalent American term is Rosie Palm and her five sisters. In Australia, one would say, "Mrs. Palmer and her five daughters."

MOUSE POTATO—person whose whole social life occurs while he or she is online; "compusexual" or "A-O-Loser."

MTF—transgendered term, means "male to female," or changing your genitals and physical appearance from male to female. The order designates which way the sex is changing, as FTM is a bio-girl changing sex to become a male.

MUFF DIVING— going down on a woman; lip service. See "cunnilingus."

MUNCH—purely social events in the swinging and kink communities which are held in neutral locations where no sex occurs. These meetings allow people who are interested but not active to meet with experienced members of their respective lifestyles. They also allow regular members to meet in an environment that does not include overt sexual play.

MYSPACE WHORE—a girl who spends way too much time on Myspace.com, is obsessed about having thousands of Myspace "friends" and will post slutty pictures and change them often in an attempt to get even more Myspace friends. She'll post all kinds of bulletins saying "NEW PICZZZ! OMG, they are sooo hoTTTT. PLZZZZ comment!!!" or "I have 5K friends, click my button and whore me!" (Thanks, Urban Dictionary!) There are plenty of Myspace boy whores, as well.

NAPPY DUGOUT—slang for "female genitals." "Nappy" refers to the pubic hair, and the "dugout" is the recessed part of a baseball stadium where the players sit. In rap, this term refers to what a woman will do sexually, e.g. "Those hoes give up the nappy dugout."

NASCA—the North American Swing Club Association. One "r" short of going to the races.

NATURAL FAMILY PLANNING (NFP)—has taken the place of the old rhythm method as a means of birth control that determines when it safe to have intercourse with the risk of pregnancy. When used correctly, can be as effective as any other form of birth control. NFP is a fertility-awareness method of birth control that is used by people who abstain from intercourse during a woman's fertile period. In other forms of fertility awareness, couples use barrier methods of birth control during their fertile period.

NATURIST VS. NUDIST— think of your average birdwatcher without his or her shorts on. That's a naturist. You won't find much that is sexual going on at a place with the word "naturist" in the title, as being naked is considered natural, but sex isn't. You'll find a lot more sexual possibilities at a "nudist beach" or location with the word nudist in the title, not that walking around with a hard-on is going to be tolerated at either.

NELLY—an effeminate male.

NIPPLE CLIPS—variation of a roach clip that is placed on each nipple as part of sex play aka, "nipple clamps." Used by people who like to have their titties tweaked. Can apply varying degrees of pressure, depending on the type of clip used. There are many styles, including vibrating and electrified nipple clips. Some people like them on their labia or scrotum.

NOCTURNAL EMISSION—sexual dream of the male that includes ejaculation; aka "wet dream." A lot of guys don't have wet dreams, and they can be scarce for those who do. Most will occur in the mid-teens. There is also no reason why a sex dream has to include an ejaculation, as plenty are dry.

NONOXYNOL-9—active ingredient in most contraceptive foams and jellies that renders the male ejaculate infertile by changing its pH (acid-base balance). Should only be used by monogamous couples who are not worried about the spread of STIs, as it has been known to irritate tender tissues, making them more vulnerable to STIs. Not recommended for tooth brushing, but if you happen to swallow some during oral sex you're not going to die.

NPVA—acronym for "No Practical Vertical Application," which refers to a person who is good for sex but not much else.

NSU (NONSPECIFIC URETHRITIS)—common infection of the urinary tube.

OFF PREMISE—in the swinging lifestyle, a place where swingers meet socially but don't have sex, "a social."

ONANISM—means "masturbation," named after the Bible's Onan who spilled his seed (pulled out and came on the side). However, Onan was doing coitus interruptus rather than jerking off.

ONE-EYED—slang terms for the penis in the UK and Australia often begin with "one-eyed," such as "one-eyed wonder worm," "one-eyed trouser snake," "one-eyed pant python," "one-eyed willie," etc.

ON THE OTHER BUS—UK slang term for "gay."

ON THE RAG—means to be having your period. Before tampons and sanitary napkins were invented, rags were used to catch menstrual flow.

OPEN SWINGING—having sex with others in the same room as opposed to "closed door," which is one couple per room.

OTPHJ—stands for "Over-The-Pants-Handjob." Done when it's private enough to fool around but public enough that unwrapping the salami would be unwise, or just because it's what she wants to do. Talk about a gross feeling afterward, unless you manage to pop a napkin over the head in time.

OUTING—a vicious process where gays publicly expose gays who aren't out of the closet, supposedly to show the straight world that some of its biggest heroes and stars are really gay, as well as to slap down a gay person who remains in the closet. Used more benignly when referring to yourself, as in "I outed myself to my family and friends, and couldn't believe they weren't more surprised."

PACKING—when a woman who is cross-dressing wears a penis-shaped object in her pants to make it look like she is well hung. More realistic when made of a soft material rather than silicone (a good packing device does not make a good dildo). Done by some male rock'n'roll singers.

PANDERING—pimping.

PAPERVINE— drug injected into the penis that causes it to get hard.

PARAPHILIA—kinky stuff. See "fetish."

PARTY CLOTHES—when used in the swinging lifestyle, has a somewhat different meaning than what you might wear to a church social.

PASS—if you are transgendered, means being able to walk through the market or go to work without being clocked, which means people don't recognized that you are a TS. You'll know you pass if they hold the rest-room door open for you without giving it a second thought.

PDE5 INHIBITOR—short for phosphodiesterase type 5 inhibitor, aka Viagra, Cialis, Levitra. Works by inhibiting cGMP specific phosphodiesterase type 5, which is an enzyme that regulates blood flow in the penis. Was originally to be a drug for hypertension. It's most interesting use to date, other than the obvious, is among track and field athletes, and not just the pole vaulters. Athletes are using it to increase blood flow to the lungs and muscles. They call it Vitamin V, and the World Anti-Doping Agency (WADA) is thinking about adding PDE5 inhibitors to its list of illegal substances.

PEARL NECKLACE—coming on a woman's chest.

PECKER CHECKER—prison slang for a guy who looks at others guys' genitals in the shower; "shower shark" or "peter gazer."

PEDERAST—man who has sex with boys or young men; "chicken fox." See "hebephilia."

PEEING WITH A HARD-ON—a misery inflicted on the human male in the morning, though much worse when he's a teen. Peeing with a hard-on is a difficult act to achieve, since the passageway to the bladder is closed off when a male gets an erection. Even if you can pee when it's hard, what do you do—stand back three feet and hope the arc ends in the toilet? A phenomenon that originally caused Hindus to invent meditation, with the earliest mantra being "Lord, let this hard-on subside before my bladder bursts."

PEGGING—when a girl does her guy in the rear. See "strap-on" and "Feeldoe."

PELVIC INFLAMMATORY DISEASE (PID)—inflammation of the female reproductive organs, often the Fallopian tubes, usually caused by a bacterial infection.

PERINEUM—demilitarized zone of the human crotch. The area between the bum and genitals in men and women. Interestingly, it's a lot longer (2x) in males than in females. Taoist types get all weak in the knees about the perineum, which they consider to be quite sensitive. See "taint."

PERIOD PANTIES—formerly favorite or less than 100% underwear that women reserve for period duty, can also be budget wear. Or some women just wear dark panties during flow days, so they don't have to worry about stains.

PERSISTENT GENITAL AROUSAL DISORDER (PGAD AS OPPOSED TO EGADS!)—when a woman's genitals are physically aroused for hours, days, weeks or even years—but she doesn't feel any desire to have sex. Having sex provides no relief, and orgasms don't help her arousal to reside. This would be like if a man had an erection for weeks at time, where he desperately wanted the thing to go down, but the most earth-shaking orgasm and ejaculation would not bring a smile of satisfaction or a dent in the tent in the front of his pants.

PEYRONIE'S DISEASE (PD)—a condition that results in a curving or bending deformity of the penis that can range from mild to so severe that intercourse is not possible and there can be pain with erection. PD results from plaques forming on the tunica albuginea of the penis, but what causes that to happen is not fully understood. The only effective treatment seems to be surgery, with the results being from very good to not great. While there is spontaneous repair in some cases, these would be in the minority. Men who have moderate to severe cases often experience clinical depression, and often describe themselves as "feeling like a freak." The depression can take its toll on a relationship.

PHTHALATES—esters of phthalic acid that are added to plastics to make them more flexible. Used in everything from baby bottles and detergents to shower curtains, certain glues, and jelly rubber sex toys. These are endocrine disruptors which cause genital abnormalities in the fetus. The distance between the scrotum and anus in baby boys born to mothers with higher levels of endocrine disruptors are often shorter than normal, which is highly significant because this distance in females is only half as much as that of males. This shorter distance would indicate that the male's genitals may not have been as fully masculinized as nature intended. There are indications that sperm counts are in peril, as well. As you might have guessed, phthalates and endocrine disruptors pose a huge environmentas hazard. There is concern that they are contributing to a lower birth rate of males and an increase in undescended testicles.

PIERCING—placing jewelry, a safety pin or facsimile through a person's nose, lip, nipples, navel, genitals, or anywhere skin grows; a form of body mod.

PINK PEARL—pink, bullet-shaped vibrator; can be inserted into the vagina.

PILLOW BITER—refers to anal sex, or when receiving anal sex is painful.

PISTON SHOT—in porn, when the camera is doing such an extreme close-up that you can see the woman's inner labia slide in and out with each stroke of the penis; related terms: "gyno shot" and "P&P (pimples & penetration)."

PITCHER—partner who is doing the inserting in anal sex; "top."

PIT JOB—intercourse using the armpit as a vagina.

POCKET POOL—rubbing the testicles or penis when you have your hands in your pockets. It often looks like a guy is doing this when he's just rubbing coins or his fingers together.

POLYAMORY—in this form of lifestyle, people have sex in more than one committed relationships that are ongoing. It is different from swinging, where you have sex with other swingers but aren't in a committed relationships with them. Can include everything from open marriage to polygamy.

POLYCYSTIC OVARY SYNDROME (PCOS)—a hormone imbalance that can result in irregular periods, unwanted hair growth, acne, extra weight gain, baldness, and patches of dark skin on the back of your neck and inner thighs that weren't caused by some guy giving you a hickey. Nearly 1 of every 10 to 20 women have it, and it tends to be especially common in young women. Cases can be mild or severe. Researchers still don't know what causes PCOS, but they suspect that insulin resistance plays a factor in many cases. The symptoms of PCOS start when your pituitary makes too much leutinizing hormone (LH) and/or your pancreas makes too much insulin. This causes your ovaries to make more testosterone than your body needs, which helps explain the extra acne and body hair. Too much testosterone can also cause cysts in your ovaries which aren't so much cysts as they are immature follicles which started to develop but stopped before they could release an egg. The most common treatment for PCOS is the birth control pill, which lowers testosterone in a woman's body, as well as diet and exercise. PCOS is also associated with diabetes and obesity, and can result in making it difficult to conceive. Consultation with an endocrinologist who specializes in PCOS is highly advisable.

POLYMORPHOUS PERVERSE—kinky

PON FARR—the Vulcan mating cycle, which causes logic to crumble and the normally stoic Vulcan to become an emotional mess. See "Star-Trek sex."

POONTANG—word of dubious origin that refers to a woman's genitals, or what one received from them if he is a male.

PONY BOY—BDSM-speak for a man who pretends to be a horse while his master or mistress rides him, hopefully with crop in hand. There are specially made halter gags, pony tail butt plugs and leather pony-feet trainers for Pony Boys & Pony Girls. "Pony training" is BDSM-speak for schooling a submissive.

POOFTER—British term for a gay male; "anal amigo," "bum chum," "starfish trooper," "sausage jockey" or "on the other bus."

POP A COD—to seriously injure a testicle.

POP A SQUAT—when a woman has to pee outside; often refers to when she's in college and has been drinking at a party.

POPPERS—sold over the counter as a liquid air deodorizer, poppers were originally made of amyl nitrate (which is for heart patients). Then the formula was switched to butyl nitrate because the amyl formulation could no longer be legally sold over the counter. When butyl nitrate was outlawed, popper makers switched the formula to a type of isopropyl alcohol which is fairly dangerous, but legal nonetheless. Poppers are very popular in the gay community. Popper vapors are inhaled immediately before orgasm with the resulting sensation described by some as amazing and indescribable. One problem with poppers is that the current formulation can kill you if you have hidden heart problems. It is especially dangerous to combine poppers and Viagra, as both lower blood pressure. Some people feel that popper usage might weaken the immune system, but there's no research on the matter.

POSER PORN—generic term that refers to 3-D adult erotic animation. Some of the first and best software for creating 3-D erotic animation was Poser from Curious Labs, and this is how the entire genre came to be called Poser Porn; "renderotica;" see "adult graphics community."

POV PORN—a type of porn that is filmed from the male actor's perspective or "point of view." The camera is either placed behind the male actor or he holds the camera while performing. Allows the viewer to imagine he's *the man*.

PRECUM—slick, clear fluid that drips out of the penis when it is excited. Most people assume it is nature's own form of sex lube. Precum also helps to neutralize or deacidify the urethra. This makes it easier on semen during ejaculation. Precum also makes the walls of the urethra more slick so the wad has less resistance. It helps you get your girlfriend pregnant. It also helps the foreskin slide more easily over the head of the penis; see "Cowper's glands."

PREPUCE—the foreskin.

PRIAPISM—a hard-on that won't quit. Not good. Having an erection for more than four hours straight without its going down can result in permanent penile paralysis. Not a common occurrence, but emergency room visits should be planned accordingly. Priapism is named after Priapus, son of Aphrodite and Dionysus, god of male reproductive power. It can occur in boys between the ages of 5 and 10 (causes include leukemia, sickle-cell disease, or physical injury), as well as in older males, where causes can range from drugs or black-widow spider bites to bicycle injuries, disease, or a kick in the crotch while martial-arts sparing. In many cases, the cause is not determined. There are two types of priapism, low-flow and high-flow. It is very important for the physician to diagnose which type it is, as this can help determine proper treatment and follow-up. Low-flow is often more dangerous. In some types of priapism, the glans or head of the penis is not erect, though the shaft is.

Priapism often has little to do with sexual arousal.

PRIMARY ORGASMIC DYSFUNCTION—when a woman is able to feel sexually aroused or sexually excited, but has never been able to have a toe-curling orgasm, either with masturbation or with a partner. Directed masturbation exercises are often successful in helping women with primary as opposed to secondary orgasmic dysfunction. See "secondary orgasmic dysfunction."

PRINCE ALBERT—male genital piercing where the ring goes in through the urethra and comes out on the underside of the penis. Allegedly named after the husband of Queen Victoria, who had it done so he could strap his rather well-endowed penis to his leg to keep it from showing through the tight-fitting trousers that were in fashion. But this is probably more rumor than truth. Queen Victoria never mentioned it in her state papers. See "showerhead effect." Also, there's an entire chapter in this book on piercing.

PROMISCUOUS—term for a person who is having more sex than you, often said with a tone of moral superiority.

PROSTATE—walnut-shaped gland located on the floor of a man's rectum nearly a finger's length up his bum. It generates about 30% of the fluid in each ejaculation. The prostate contracts seconds before orgasm, resulting in a fine feeling. It enlarges with age, sometimes making it difficult to pee. Some men (straight, gay—it doesn't matter) enjoy the feeling that results from having the prostate rubbed; others would sooner die.

PROSTATITIS—according to the excellent Prostatitis foundation, "Prostatitis is an inflammation of the prostate gland, often resulting in swelling or pain. Prostatitis can result in four significant symptoms: pain, urination problems, sexual dysfunction, and general health problems, such as feeling tired and depressed." Less than 5% of cases of prostate pain are from infection. The problem often isn't in the prostate itself, but from the tissues and muscles that surround the prostate. For more information, go to www.prostatitis.org.

PSA—abbreviation for "prostate specific antigen," which is made by the prostate and helps liquefy semen after it's been ejaculated. (Come in a glass, and see what happens to your thick wad in about 25 minutes or less. That's PSA doing its job.) The liquefying action of PSA is what makes male ejaculate so easily drip down women's legs after intercourse, as well as contributing to the wet spot on the mattress. PSA tends to be elevated in men who have prostate cancer. Can be checked via a routine blood test, but is never definitive by itself. PSA is present in very small amounts in breast milk and amniotic fluid. PSA is also what Southwest Airlines used to be called.

PUDENDA—anatomical term for women's external genitals (vulva); from the Latin word "pudere," which means "to be ashamed."

PULLING A TRAIN—see "gang bang."

PUNANNY—rasta or reggae term for sex; "I wan' punanny!"

PUNK—a prison term for a submissive and often younger male who is on the receiving end of anal sex; "catcher." The punk is seldom in the relationship because he is gay or because it is his choice; see "hooking up (prison)." Musically speaking, the term "punk" was adopted in the late 1970s to describe a movement within rock'n'roll. Punk bands had a rougher and more immediate edge than mainstream bands.

PUSSY POSSE—the vice squad.

PUSSY WHIPPED (PW)—a mental illness whereby the male grovels and begs in excess of what is normally required to have sex.

PUSSY WHIPPER—a sexual partner who is controlling and rarely satisfied. She often wishes aloud that her man would be more aggressive, yet would annihilate him the second he dared.

QAF—*Queer As Folk*, the ground-breaking television series about the lives of six gay men and a lesbian couple. A wildy-successful American-Canadian production that ran from 2000 to 2005.

QUEEF—a vagina fart.

QUEENING—when a woman straddles a man and rubs or grinds her vulva into his face; "face sitting."

QUEER EYE FOR THE STRAIGHT GUY—A very successful TV show that ran from 2003 to 2007 where "five gay men transformed a style-deficient and culture-deprived straight man from drab to fab."

QUIM—very dated British term for "vulva," "vagina," "fanny," or "twat."

RANDY—Australian term for horny.

RAPE—sexual bodily assault. Because the developmental arrest is so profound and the capacity for empathy is so diminished, rapists rarely seek psychotherapy. There are men who are capable of committing rape and an hour later going home to have what appears to be normal sex with their wives. Most rapists don't view their acts as being criminal or brutal and are apt to justify themselves by saying that the woman wanted it, needed it or deserved it. The only good news on this front is that juvenile sexual offenders can often be helped. This is one of many reasons why they should never be placed with hardened adult offenders. See Chapter 46: "Good Sex after Bad."

RAPE FANTASY—a common fantasy where a person is aroused by the thought of being raped, but would not want it to happen in real life. The "rapist" in rape fantasies is often a person whom the "victim" would very much like to have sex with, although sometimes not. A person having a rape fantasy is in full control of her fantasy, while a real rape victim has no control at all. As a result, a better name for this would be "pseudo-rape fantasy."

RAW DOG IT—to have intercourse without protection.

REACH AROUND—when someone is doing a guy in the rear with a strap-on dildo or a penis and wraps her hand around to the front to stroke his penis.

REAM JOB—licking the anus; "rimming," "reaming," "tossing salad." Also what a conscientious plumber does to the inner lip of pipe that's just been cut.

RED WINGS—what a man earns when he's performed oral sex on a woman who is having her period. Also the name of Detroit's team in the National Hockey League.

RENDEROTICA—see "poser porn" or go to www.renderotica.com.

RENT BOY—male prostitute, usually a gay male, but sometimes staight.

REPARATIVE THERAPY—during the early 1900s, the testicles of straight men were transplanted into the scrotums of gay men to help the latter become heterosexual. Today, conservative Christian therapists aim for a similar outcome but without the surgery.

RETARDED EJACULATION—when a guy's sexual hang time is so long that his partner has mentally filled out a year's worth of shopping lists before he comes; "delayed ejaculation."

RETROGRADE EMISSION—when an ejaculating penis backfires. Can be caused by prostate problems, diabetes, MS, spinal-cord injury, and because a man clamps the end of his penis shut when he's jerking off—to name a few. An important reason why socks, Kleenex and toilet paper were invented was so guys could have something to shoot their wad into when masturbating. Otherwise, some men who don't have the luxury of leaving a wad on site will clamp the penis shut when they come so nothing shoots out. Ouch. Intentionally causing a retrograde emission can cause severe plumbing problems and should only be done in the most dire of circumstances unless you want to end up at the doctor's office doubled over with pain having to answer some really embarrassing questions.

REVERSE COWGIRL—intercourse position where the female is on top, facing the man's feet. Since the woman is on top and facing south, this allows her to watch her partner's toes curl with delight each time she squeezes the muscles in her crotch; she might also get to see his testicles rise up and hug the shaft of his penis when he begins to ejaculate or she can reach down with her hand and feel them do this (in some guys this is more pronounced than in others). This is also a good position for her to massage her clitoris or for using a vibrator during intercourse.

RIMMING (RIM JOB)—kissing ass, literally, "ass-blowing," "tossing salad" or "E-coli pie" (a term from supervert.com).

RING TOSSING—when your NuvaRing comes out during sex or when you are having a bowel movement. No problem. It can be out for three ours with no decrease in effectiveness. Longer than that, you should put it back in but check with your healtcare provider as soon as possible.

ROAD ERECTION—unwanted wood can happen any time to a guy who is sitting in a vehicle that vibrates (bus, car, tractor, etc.). It is caused by a combination of the vibration, which sends extra blood into the penis, and sitting, which tends to shut the veins that carry blood out of the penis.

ROMAN CULTURE—refers to swinging and group sex.

ROOFIES—refers to any number of drugs that are used in date rape, sometimes rohypnol, sometimes GBH, maybe even ketamine. While a concern, also a bit of media hype when you consider that the vast majority of women who experienced date rape had been drinking lots of alcohol with the moron who committed the felony. It is a sad and unfair fact: if you want to lower your chances of date rape, don't drink at parties or in places where bad things might happen.

ROID RAGE—unpleasant mood occurring in some people who take steroids.

RU-486—the name given to mifepristone when it was in its testing phase, this is the drug that causes an abortion if taken within 49 days of conception. See "Morning-after pill vs. Abortion pill."

RUBBERS—common name for condoms; origin: before the invention of latex, condoms in this country were made of vulcanized rubber. In the UK, a rubber is an eraser, which can make for some amusing translational instances.

SADOMASOCHISM—where people find it erotic when there's an imbalance in power in a relationship and one person submits while the other dominates.

SAFE—prison slang for "vagina" or place to hide drugs or contraband.

SAME-ROOM SEX—the swinger's equivalent of the family room. A dedicated space where couples have sex together.

SANGER, MARGARET—(1883-1966) famous birth-control advocate at a time when dispensing information about birth control was illegal in America.

SAPPHO—poetess on the island of Lesbos noted for her use of nonphallic imagery.

SAFE WORD—BDSM-speak for a special prearranged word or gesture that the bottom can say to the top that means to stop.

SAUSAGE FEST—an event or gathering where the men greatly out number the women; "brodeo." The opposite might be "clam bake," but it's rarely used.

SCABIES—small mites that burrow under the skin, causing a rash a month after infestation. Since it takes a month for symptoms to form, it is likely that other family or living-group members are infected and require treatment. Should be treated by a physician; be sure to follow instructions carefully. Soften your skin by taking a bath before applying pesticide treatment. Since scabies can't live away from human skin for more than 24-hours, you don't need to nuke your surroundings. However, do wash your clothes and sheets at the time of treatment. They look a little like beach crabs when magnified. See "chiggers," which are mites of a different sort.

SCAT—when brown is a turn-on and the phrase "Look at that sexy shit!" means just that; "coprophilia."

SCHLONG—Jewish term for penis.

SCUM BAG—a condom. Also, a term for someone you don't like.

SEA FOOD—a gay sailor.

SECONDARY ORGASMIC DYSFUNCTION—when a woman has been able to have orgasms in the past, but is unable to now although she is able to feel sexually aroused and excited. There can be numerous reasons, from illness to a change in partner.

SEMEN ALLERGY—an immune response against allergens contained in male ejaculate. Symptoms include vaginal burning, swelling and itching occurring approximately ten minutes after intercourse. While not rare, not overly common. Can develop right away, or quite suddenly after a few years with the same partner. To differentiate from chronic vaginitis, see if using a condom stops the problem. (You might try a polyurethane condom, as a latex allergy could possibly mimic semen allergy symptoms.) Aside from a complete gynecologic exam, diagnosis should include intradermal testing, where a tiny bit of the semen is injected under the skin. Treatment under the supervision of an allergist or immunologist can include a "graded challenge" where dilute solutions of semen are placed in the vagina every 20 minutes until the patient can tolerate undiluted semen. The downside is that the couple has to have intercourse at least once every 48 hours to maintain the desensitization. Darn! As is the case with food allergies, the semen allergy might go as fast as it came.

SERIAL MONOGAMY—sounds like a dangerous criminal activity when it really means getting married, then divorced, then married again.

SEVEN-OF-NINE—a former member of the Borg, one of the most sexually alluring female characters in the history of the *Star Trek* series, can be seen on reruns of *Star Trek Voyager.*

SEX—stands for "sign extend," an assembly language mnemonic used in the venerable DEC pdp-11s.

SEX BEFORE THE GAME—refers to masturbating or having sex fewer than twenty-four hours before taking part in a major sporting event. Mirkin and Hoffman in *The Sports Medicine Book* have looked into the topic and found there's no correlation between sex before the game and decreased athletic performance. They report that in a recent Olympics that an athlete had sex approximately one hour before the event and won a gold medal; another Olympian had sex right before his event and ran a sub-four-minute mile. Mirkin and Hoffman quote Casey Stengel on the matter: "It isn't sex that wrecks these guys, it's staying up all night looking for it." Ansell International, the official supplier of condoms for the 2000 Olympic games, originally stocked the village where the athletes lived with 50,000 condoms. Halfway through the Olympics, they discovered that there were only 20,000 condoms left and had to do an emergency restocking. Durex, official supplier of condoms for the 2004 Olympics in Athens stocked the village with 130,000 condoms and 30,000 tubes of lubricant. For 2008, the Chinese government stocked their Olympics Village with only 100,000 condoms, but they made up for any shortages by stocking local hotels in Beijing with another 400,000 condoms. The condoms were made by a company called Jissbon. Honest. The Jissbon mascot is a condom-covered banana wearing sunglasses. The 2006 Winter Olympics in Turin marked the first time when the Olympic Village provided free female condoms in addition to those for males.

SEX DREAMS—nature's way of making sleep more interesting.

SEXILED—to be kicked out of your room while your roommate is having sex.

SEX MESSAGING OR SEXTING—using mobile devices for foreplay or taking explicit pictures of yourself and forwarding them to a lover.

SEX-ON-THE-BEACH SHOOTERS—on the West Coast, a drink consisting of vodka, peach schnapps, OJ, and cranberry juice. On the East Coast, a drink consisting of melon liqueur, raspberry liqueur and pineapple juice.

SEXTASY—refers to when people combine ecstasy and Viagra; aka "trail mix." The ecstasy is not good on wood, so Viagra is used to help. No one knows the long-term effects of this combination, nor what's really in the ecstasy or Viagra that you get on the street.

SEXUALITY—an altered state of mind that's often quite enjoyable. Includes various degrees of erotic or sensual feelings.

SEXUAL ORIENTATION—term that describes who you are interested in sexually. It's funny how sexual orientation is often based upon your preferred genital pairings. If it's penis-vagina, then your orientation is probably hetero-sexual. If it's penis-penis or vagina-vagina, then your orientation is probably homosexual. If it's both, then your orientation is described as bisexual. There are some indications that the range of sexual interests are more flexible or fluid among women, and less flexible and more rigid among men, although recent research is indicating that this might be due to the fact that we don't always ask males what they are feeling, but instead assume we know.

S.F. JACKS—notorious men's jerk-off club in San Francisco. A by-product of extreme horniness, a desire to socialize, and concern about AIDS.

SHAGADELIC—someone who looks good enough to shag; a person you'd like to have sex with; vintage Austin Powers, who might say, "She shags like a minx, baby!"

SHAKE 'N' BAKE—to make love; do the wild thing.

SHE BOP—female masturbation song by vintage rocker Cindi Lauper. Became popular enough that "she bop" is now a synonym for female masturbation.

SHE-HE, SHE-MALE, or HE-SHE—see "transgendered."

SHOCK DOC—a popular brand of a cup, which is a device that guys wear to protect their genitals from dick-high line drives, bad hops, elbows, lacrosse implements, kicks & whatever. Which cup you wear depends on the sport and position in that sport that you play, e.g. a goalie or catcher is looking for protection over mobility, where a shortstop or attackman is going to value mobility, as will someone in the martial arts. Cupwise, the new king of the crotch is the Shock Doctor Flex Cup, with other entries including the Warrior Nut Hut, the XO Pro Cup, and the traditional Bike cup. Huge improvements have also come in the design of compression shorts, which are like a cross between bicycle short and an athletic supporter. While it used to be you wore compressions shorts over a jock that was holding your cup in place, they now have compression shorts that do it all.

SHORT-ARM INSPECTION—military term for examining an enlisted man's penis. Supposedly for the detection of VD.

SHORT HAIRS—pubic hair

SHOT MY WAD—ejaculated, came, popped, splooged or blew a load. See "cum."

SHOWERHEAD EFFECT—when a piercing like a Prince Albert or an apadravya goes through the urethra, it tends to make urine spray like a showerhead instead of a stream. While a guy can try rotating the head of his penis or pushing up against the leaky part of the piercing, often the only solution is to pee while sitting down. He will also tend to ooze rather than shoot when he ejaculates.

SISTERS OF PERPETUAL INDULGENCE—a rather spirited, benevolent organization of drag queens who delight in taking the "convent" out of "conventional." Their mission statement: *The Sisters devote ourselves to community service, ministry and outreach to those on the edges, and to promoting human rights, respect for diversity and spiritual enlightenment.*

SIXTY-NINE (69)—when a man and woman perform oral sex on each other at the same time. When French people do 69 they call it "soixante-neuf."

SIZE QUEEN—a woman who likes guys who are seriously well-hung; best to avoid if you are not. Also a guy who likes guys who are seriously well-hung.

SKANK—a person who is short on physical and social graces; hard or harsh.

SKIN FLICK—porn film.

SLICK—refers to male or female genitals that have been shaven. Some people enjoy the look or feel of being slick as a sexual turn-on. Women often shave to accommodate thongs and bikini bottoms, men to make their units look bigger or to make them more inviting as objects for oral sex.

SLOPPY SECONDS—intercourse when you are not first in line.

SLOW DANCING—an event that sometimes causes guys to get erections, especially during the teenage years. When girls congregate in the women's restroom during dances, do they tell each other things like, "Billy got a raging boner while we were slow dancing" or do they limit themselves to mundane stuff like, "This new bra is killing me" or "Damn, Flo just arrived"?

SMEGMA—cheesy stuff that forms beneath the foreskin and under the hood of the clitoris; "knob cheese." Calling someone "smeg" is an insult.

SNAP-ON TOOL—slang term for a dildo that some women wear in a harness and use as if it were an erect penis.

SNAP QUEEN—a gay male where the "snap" refers to the snap of fingers that's done with an exaggerated spin-and-prance attitude, such as that of Laine and Antoine, the film reviewers in reruns of *In Living Color.*

SNOWBALLING—when a man swallows his own ejaculate after it's been somewhere else; for instance, his partner gives him oral sex, he ejaculates in his partner's mouth, and then he kisses his partner and his partner transfers the ejaculate back into his mouth.

SNOW QUEEN—slang term for a gay black man who only dates white men.

SOAPY MASSAGE—one of those Thai sex experiences where the girl undresses and bathes you, massaging your body with her wet soapy body.

SOAPY TIT WANK—masturbating between a woman's well-lubricated breasts.

SOCIAL SWING CLUB—think of a local YMCA for people who like to have sex in groups. A private membership organization for couples who swing.

SODOMY—any kind of sex that is declared illegal by local statute. In some areas, it can be oral sex or regular intercourse, in others, specifically anal sex.

SOFT SWINGERS—nope, not guys in the lifestyle who need Viagra. It means a couple who enjoys sex with others except for intercourse, which they only do with each other.

SOUNDS—special medical instruments used to help dilate the urethra. Used in "urethra play." There are different types of sounds with different shapes and thicknesses, including the Pratt, Van Buren, Hegar, Hank and Dittel.

SOUTHERN COMFORT—sex with someone from the south.

SPANISH FLY—alleged aphrodisiac made from powdered blister beetles; causes severe irritation of the bladder and urethra (peehole) and can be very toxic. Women have died from it. The effect is not dissimilar to drinking Draino. Giving her roses and a foot rub will get you much further and won't endanger anyone's health.

SPASM CHASM—a vagina or "gristle gripper."

SPECTATORING—sex therapist-speak: describes what happens when a person is worried or obsessing about his or her sexual performance instead of being able to enjoy it. Can result in performance anxiety.

SPIT ROASTING—in a threesome, when the person in the middle is on all fours and is being penetrated from behind while sucking on the penis of the person in front. When viewed from the side, it gives the appearance that the person in the middle is a chicken on a two-penis rotisserie. While the middle person gets basted from both ends, it is unlikely that she or he actually rotates.

SPLASH CONCEPTION—getting pregnant from doing anal sex without a rubber, after the male ejaculate oozes out of the woman's rear end and drips into her vagina. Are people conceived in this way doomed to be anal retentive?

SPLIT BEAVER—porn-speak for when a woman spreads her labia wide open.

SPLOSHING—Smearing yourself or a partner with wet and gooey things such as raw eggs, paint, mud or whatever as part of a fetish or sexual turn-on. Became a bit popular in the late 1980s in the UK, growing out of the fetish wank mag Splosh! A related term is: "WAM" or wet and messy. Does not include excrement, which is a fetish of a different color, or smell.

SPREADER BAR—see "leg spreader."

SQUIRT.ORG—one of the more famous gay cruising-for-sex websites. There are also sites like Cruisingforsex.com and Craigslist, to name but a few.

SRPE—SLEEP-RELATED PAINFUL ERECTIONS—results in waking with painful erections. This understudied problem may occur more often than is reported, and can result in serious pain and loss of sleep. Waking erections are not painful for these men, only those that occur during sleep. While the erections occur during REM sleep, which is when erections during sleep usually occur, it appears that the pain from the erections may actually be the result of either spasms or ischemia. Oral baclofen currently appears to be the experimental treatment of choice, but that may change when more is learned about SRPEs.

SSRIs—a class of highly prescribe and overly prescribed antidepressants which include Prozac, Zoloft, Paxil, Luvox, Celexa, Lexapro, Effexor, Serzone and Remeron. According to the Journal of Sexual Medicine (January, 2008), any person who has been given a prescription for an SSRIs should be given a warning such as the following: *There is a high probability of sexual side effects while on SSRI medications. There are indications that in an unknown number of cases, the side effects may not resolve with cessation of the medication and could be potentially irreversible.*

STAR-TREK SEX—*Denobulans:* Denobulans practiced polygamy. Each Denobulan had three partners, and each of these had two other partners. Denobulans were liberal about sex, with sex occurring during Denobulan mating cycles. *Deltans:* Deltans were so highly sexed that they were forbidden from having sex while in Starfleet. Deltan sex was such an intense activity that a member of another species who had sex with a Deltan could go insane as a result. *Vulcans:* Vulcans were ruled by strict logic except every seven years during pon farr, which was the Vulcan mating cycle when a Vulcan lost all emotional control. *Klingons:* There is not a single thing about Klingon sex that could ever be described as "gentle."

STONE BUTCH—A lesbian who displays male gender role behavior; as described in Leslie Fineberg's book *Stone Butch Blues*.

STONEWALL—refers to the 1969 Stonewall Riots, when New York City police raided a gay bar in Greenwich Village and large numbers of gay people resisted arrest. A landmark event in the gay-rights movement; epochs of time are often divided into "pre-Stonewall" and "after Stonewall."

STRAP-ON—abbreviation for "strap-on dildo," usually worn and used by women on men or on women, but can also be worn by men for double penetration or if their own penis can't get hard; "bend over boyfriend" or "pegging."

STUNT BABE—a woman who poses as a gay soldier's girlfriend at military events and whose picture he keeps on his desk.

SURFER—person who has sex with waves.

SWEDISH CULTURE—using hands & massage to sexually stimulate each other.

SWEET DEATH—literary term for intercourse.

SWINGER—partner swapping, enjoys having sex with lots of people.

SWING LOW—rap term for "oral sex."

SWINGERS—couples in committed relationships who enjoy having sex with a variety of sexual partners.

SWITCHES—people into BDSM who enjoy alternating between the top and the bottom roles.

TAINT—perineum, the area between the genitals and anus that *taint his balls or ass*, or *taint her vagina or ass;* see "perineum."

TAR BEACH—rooftop of a tall building in large urban setting where people do things like sunbathe, grow plants, make out or shoot up drugs.

TEA-BAGGING—when a man lowers his testicles into a partner's mouth.

TEA ROOM—public rest-room where gay men go to have sex; in Britain they are called "cottages." In Australia they are known as "beats."

TEDDY—women's lingerie that is a combination of tank top and panties, sometimes snaps at the crotch, usually made of silk, lace, acetate, or leather.

TENTACLE SEX—the full name is Tentacle-Hentai Sex, where monsters and octopuses wrap their well-endowed tentacles around the bodies of shocked and surprised Hentai female characters, who then feel the kind of intense sexual sensations that any woman might feel if a horny octopus slid its slimy tentacle inside of her vagina. Probably no different than going to a sushi bar while taking strong hallucinogens. See "Hentai."

TEXAS TWO-STRAP—highly regarded brand of dildo harness.

TEXTILE—term that nude sunbathers sometimes use for a person who wears a bathing suit; see "cottontail."

THE GAY SEAT—the empty seat that teenage boys and college bros tend to leave between them when they are in a theater, what with the social and possibly emotional dangers of sharing an arm rest.

THIGHBROW—pubic hair that's sticking out from the sides of a bikini or thong.

THIRD-DEGREE CLEAVAGE—refers to breasts that are quite large.

THONG—a narrow piece of material that passes between the legs and up through the butt where it attaches to a waistband. Thongs have traditionally been the underwear of strippers. Different types of thong include the "G-string" or "T-back," which are the underwear equivalent of dental floss, the "Tanga," which has more material in the seat, and the "Rio" which has straps on the sides. Thongs are even popular for some guys to wear. Our gyno-consultant warns about thongs causing vuvlar irritation. They also provide highway (or low-way) for bacteria from your anus to visit your vagina.

THREESOME—sex with two women and a man or two men and a woman. See "menage a trois" or as we misspelled it in earlier editions, "manage a trois." Hopefully, having a menage a trois is not as complicated as spelling it.

THRUSH—vaginal infection caused by candida or monilia fungus. Men can also get it, but not in the vagina.

TICKET—for a guy in the swinger's lifestyle to show up without a woman is like arriving at a church potluck without a tuna casserole. Single men usually aren't allowed. To get around this dilemma, single males will occasionally invite females who aren't necessarily into swinging—just to get through the door. Such a woman is known as a ticket. This is seriously frowned upon.

TIJUANA BIBLES—pornographic pulp parodies that were popular in America from the 1920s until after World War II. These 8-page booklets were printed on cheap paper and often found themselves in the knapsacks of soldiers and schoolboys. The crude little booklets (approximately 4" by 6") often poked fun at actors, politicians, and public figures, although their main focus was another kind of poking. They were irreverent, usually humorous, and always dirty—featuring sex-starved characters from Popeye and Donald Duck to baseball heros, with their pants down and penises proud. They were eventually put into paper graves by glossy magazines such as *Playboy*. The pin-up powerhouse *Esquire* probably served a death notice or two as well.

TINY.SEX—refers to various kinds of cybersex. The term once meant cybersex on a tinymud, but technologies have expanded, taking the term with them.

TIPPED UTERUS—a woman's uterus is usually parallel to her spine; a uterus that is tipped points somewhat toward the back. Can make rear entry or doggie-style intercourse uncomfortable.

TIT-FUCKING—when a well-lubricated penis is thrust back and forth between a woman's breasts; aka "Russian." See "soapy tit wank."

TOOTHING—a media hoax that claimed people were using their Bluetooth devices for proposing sex or hooking up with strangers in their immediate vicinity, such as at a cafe or on the train. It sounded so convincing that it got wide airplay and became part of modern urban legend.

TOP AND BOTTOM—a top is someone who prefers doing, and a bottom is someone who prefers having it done to them. In BDSM, the top is the master, mistress or dominator; the bottom is the servant, submissive or slave. In anal sex, the bottom is the one who is catching or receiving.

TOSS or TOSSING SALAD—licking a lover's anus, aka "rimming." Can also be a UK term for masturbating, "to toss off" or "toss oneself off."

TOXIC SHOCK SYNDROME—very rare and sometimes lethal infection sometimes associated with tampon use. See the "Surfing the Crimson Wave" chapter.

TRAINED WOOD—necessary requirement of a male porn star, meaning he can pretty much get an erection on cue. Failure to get it up on cue means you've got "untrained wood," which puts you and your big bulge in the same unemployment line as most of the legit actors in town.

TRAINING BRA—training wheels for the waking chest.

TRAMP STAMP—a lower back tattoo that rides on the pants line. It peeks out at you when the owner—usually a woman—wears low-rise jeans and/or a cropped T-shirt that shows her midriff, or she bends over and her pants go low or her shirt goes high. The tattoo is often v-shaped and points down in a way that signifies the anatomy below. Designs range from flowers, butterflies, dolphins and tribal art to unusual symbols and geometric art.

TRANNY—that which helps give your car its go. A transsexual, aka "tranny boys," "drag kings" and "transmen." See "transgendered."

TRANSGENDERED—when the sex you were born as is different from the sex you want to be. People who are transgendered challenge notions of what it is to be male and female or masculine and feminine. See "genderqueer."

TRANSSEXUAL—person who uses surgery, makeup, electrolysis, and hormones to correct mother nature's assignment of sex.

TRANSVESTITE—see "crossdresser."

TRAUMA QUEEN—person who is highly skilled at finding or creating chaotic scenes, then feeds on it and fans it, complaining the whole time.

TRIBADISM—two women rubbing their vulvas together, resulting in sexual pleasure; aka "tribbing." The way they shake hands on the island of Lesbos.

TRICK—customer of a prostitute; "john" or a sexual act as done by a prostitute; "turning a trick."

TRIPLE PENETRATION—porn-film term for where there's a wealth of penii and only one taker; "triple play."

TROLL—when someone gets on the Internet and posts messages that are designed to enrage people. Examples of trolling listed on Wikipedia include posting cat-meat recipes on a pet-lover forum, posting "I think *2001: a Space*

Odyssey is Roman Polanski's best movie" on a movie-lover's forum, or posting messages about how all dragons are boring in the usenet group alt.fan.dragons. To those who respond, the reply will sometimes be YHBT.YHL.HAND which means *"you have been trolled, you have lost, have a nice day."*

TROPHY WIFE—physically stunning woman who is the ultimate entertainment-industry or corporate wife. The relationship between a trophy wife and her husband is sometimes described as consensual parasitism. Trophy wives are often involved in charities for dying children when they are not messing up their own. Some trophy wives are complex people, capable of more than abusing maids, caterers, florists, and gardeners. Trophy wives can be warm and kind to others who are able to help their husband's career. Sexually speaking, it's possible that some trophy wives feel sensation between their legs, but this is frowned upon because allowing sexual feelings might result in sloppy decisions when selecting a mate. Trophy wives view wealth, power and security as the ultimate orgasm, as do the men who bed and wed them.

TUBAL LIGATION—female sterilization where the Fallopian tubes are sealed.

TUGGING—when a guy tries to restore his foreskin without surgery.

TURKEY DUMP—when a freshman in college comes home for Thanksgiving and breaks up with his or her high-school sweetheart, or any breakup that happens right before or during the Thanksgiving break.

TWINK—a young and cute gay guy who is often blonde, appears to be somewhat helpless or is not the brightest bulb in Boystown. While twinks used to be young, white and without body hair, the category is now being broadened. Also a gaming term that refers to a new player or character who's been outfitted with better gear than would usually be expected.

UHSE, BEATE—giant German porn and erotica chain founded and run by Beate Rotermund, a formerly destitute woman who, with her young son, stole a plane and cleverly escaped the Russians as they were pulling into Germany at the end of World War II. She funded one of the finest museums of sexuality.

UM-FRIEND—according to the people at Boston Poly, this is a person no one else knows you are having sex with: "This is Dan, my–um–friend."

UNCUT—not circumcised.

UNDERWEAR SWAPPING or TRADING—in Japan, there is such a large market for unlaundered teenage girls' underwear that the legislature outlawed the sale of used underwear by teenagers. Japanese teenage girls could go to small stores called "burusera" and sell their soiled knickers for $20, $30 or more per pair (the more fragrant or soiled, the higher the price). In other parts of the world, some gay or straight guys enjoy swapping underwear of the desired sex as a turn-on or fetish, and only clueless neat-freaks would launder them.

UNDESCENDED TESTICLE—testicles are not formed in the scrotum, but in the abdomen. Before birth, they usually descend into the scrotum. When this doesn't happen, the boy is born with an undescended testicle. About 3.5% of males are born with an undescended testicle, the majority of which descend on their own within the first year. Also known as cryptorchidism which is Greek for "hidden gonad."

UPSKIRTING—porn shot up a supposedly unsuspecting woman's dress. Upskirting is supposedly carried out by men carrying hidden cell phone or mini-cams in bags. They stand close to unknowing women wearing skirts and film their underwear or thighs. Often, the images are then posted on websites. However, if you do a Google search of upskirting, the first hundred or so results are for news reports on upskirting rather than some of the thousands of alleged websites. Seems like a big waste of time—you get a better view going to the beach!

URETHRA PLAY (U.P.)—stimulating the urethra by sticking something down it, usually with instruments called sounds and occasionally a catheter. The feelings can range from an immediate need to orgasm, to pain and discomfort. According to Foz at Fozzie's Den, there are three types of UP persons: probers who do it just for the feel of something in their urethra, stuffers who want to stick the thickest possible rod down their own rod to stretch it out, and plungers who want to go deep, past the prostate and even into the bladder.

URETHRAL SPONGE—cushions and protects the female urethra; is associated with G-spot area stimulation, but may not be what the sensation is all about.

VAGINISMUS—is a tightness in the vagina that causes discomfort, burning, pain, penetration problems, or complete inability to have intercourse. The muscles surrounding the vagina can close so tightly that they won't allow anything to go inside. The reaction can be so severe that a woman can't even insert a tampon. Vaginismus can result from many different things from chronic pelvic pain that is unrelated to sex to psychological trauma to a bad experience at the gynecologist's office. The absolute best source of information and help for vaginismus is Lisa and Mark Carter's phenomenal website and online community at www.Vaginismus.com.

VAJAYJAY—what the women on Grey's Anatomy have between their legs.

VAL (VALLEY GIRL)—San Fernando Valley (Southern California) version of a bimbo or airhead, unique in that this particular species has evolved its own tribal dialect, perhaps caused by the added weight of lip gloss and braces, or it is possible that tanning-booth rays adversely affect the speech center of the brain. Immortalized in song by Moon Unit Zappa and icon dad Frank.

VANILLA SEX—how some people describe sex that doesn't include kink.

VARICOCELE—clump of varicose veins in the scrotum. This causes a swelling in the top and back of the testicle, and results a warmer scrotum which isn't good for sperm production. In 85% of cases, it occurs in the left testicle and is the leading cause of infertility in men.

VASECTOMY—snip, snip.

VASELINE—that which melts condoms, because both Vaseline and condoms are made of petroleum by-products. The Vaseline acts as a solvent and dissolves the latex rubber.

VERSATILE—sex-ad term for "goes both ways" or bisexual.

VERTICAL REENTRY—a difficult but important surfing trick that involves coming out of the wave and doing a skateboard-like maneuver to get back in. A similar maneuver is used during intercourse when a guy pulls out too far.

VIBRATOR—electrical device that makes some women very, very happy.

VIBRATING SLEEVE—soft, tubelike device with a vibrator in the end which men stick a lubricated penis into. A male-masturbation device.

VIRGINITY PLEDGE—a promise to not have vaginal intercourse before marriage, causing great urgency in the part of the lap over which your clenched hands lay during church services. Fortunately, no persons taking a virginity pledge have ever broken it, but just in case, why not keep a condom handy?

VISIBLE PANTY LINE (VPL)—when panty lines show through pants, dresses, or skirts. Considered by women to be one of the more serious of the female fashion felonies. The biggest cause is panties that are too tight. In some cases, thongs or boy-shorts can help, but not if what you are wearing over it is extremely tight or transparent. Interestingly, VPL isn't seen as a negative by most men.

VOYEUR—person who enjoys watching people undressing or having sex.

VOYEUR'S ROOM—swinger's equivalent to the observation tower. A room with lots of mattresses where some enjoy having sex for show, and others enjoy watching.

VULVA—the external female genitals. People often say "vagina" when they are referring to the vulva. The vulva is what you are looking at when you cop a beaver shot; aka "beaver," "snatch," and in the UK, "fanny."

VULVAR VESTIBULITIS—a form of vulvodynia where the pain or discomfort is localized to the vulvar vestibule, which is the part of the vulva that's between the inner lips. In some cases, the pain has been there since their first tampon or intercourse, in others it started long after. Could be from any of a number of different causes, including the use of oral contraceptives. See "vulvodynia."

VULVODYNIA—this would be Latin for "a great big pain in my pussy." Symptoms include discomfort or burning pain the vulvar area of unexplained origin, which means that no infections or neurological disorders appear to be present. Often described as a chronic burning or knife-like pain, this disorder is very complex and can be a serious challenge to treat. Most healthcare providers throw their gloved-hands up in despair, which means that the patient will need to do a lot of research and find a specialist who works with vulvodynia. To give you an idea of the complexity, vulvodynia can be broken down into pain that is generalized or localized, and these categories are further broken down into pain that is provoked, unprovoked or both provoked and unprovoked. While few physicians who specialize in treating vulvodynia believe it is the result of psychological problems, a lot of patients and their healthcare providers mistakenly do. This isn't to say that stress and anxiety can't make the symptoms worse, but the are unlikely the cause. For an excellent brief summary, see "Vulvodynia" by Goldstein & Burrows, *Journal of Sexual Medicine,* January 2008, pages 5-15, and "The Vulvar Dermatoses" in the February issue. Also see "vulvar vestibulitis."

VULVITIS—an inflammation of the vulva. There can be as many causes as there are vulvas.

WAD—male ejaculate; see "cum."

WALK OF SHAME—walking back to where you live in the morning after having had hooking-up sex, wearing the same clothes you wore the night before, sometimes looking sheepish and disheveled, sometimes with your panties in your purse, trying to avoid eye contact with others or trying to avoid the light of the early morning because you're seriously hung over and it just plain hurts. However, if it was an exceptional experience or you're a guy and can brag to your friends so they won't think you are gay, it would be called the *Stride of Pride.*

WAKING WITH A HARD-ON—here are possible reasons why guys often wake up with erections: 1. during REM (dream) sleep, males usually get erections and female genitals swell and lubricate; since we humans have a much greater proportion of dream sleep toward the morning, men frequently awaken in the morning with REM-related hard-ons. 2. when a male has an erection, the entrance to the bladder is clamped shut so his ejaculate can squirt out of his body instead of backfiring into his bladder. Erections may serve double-duty, keeping a sleeping man with a full bladder from peeing on himself; but then, why don't sleeping girls pee on themselves? 3. many males awaken with elevated levels of sex hormones in their blood; while this doesn't necessarily make them hornier, it is possible that it contributes to morning erections; aka "morning glory;" see "peeing with a hard-on."

WANK—UK term for masturbation. Has many uses, such as, "I'm desperate for a wank," "I don't give a wank!" or "He kept wanking on about Marxist theory until the whole class nodded off;" "to toss off."

WANKER—name that the Queen of England calls Andy and Charlie when they are being lazy or bad, e.g. "Go suck on a pig's nose, you little wankers!"

WANK MAGS—UK term for porn; a hidden stash of porn is a "wank bank."

WATER SPORTS—when taking a leak does not signify a break in the love-making action, but is what you came for; see "golden showers."

WEBCAM—with all of the people on the Internet who are watching naked people in front of their webcams, you would think that the webcam would have been invented by voyeurs. Not so, according to Will Judy. The first webcam was built in 1993 by Cambridge University computer science students who didn't want to walk several flights of stairs to see if there was coffee in the building's only coffee maker. So they devised a cam that allowed them to spy on the coffee pot from any terminal in the building, proving that laziness is the mother of ingenuity!

WEST HOLLYWOOD—a gayborhood in Southern California where buff construction workers wear cock rings and hard hats and actually mean "cat" when they say "pussy."

WET DREAM—sex dream; isn't totally accurate because people often have orgasms in their sleep without ejaculating. See "nocturnal emission."

WET SPOT— a wet patch on the sheets or mattress caused by a mixture of male and female sexual fluids. Couples sometimes go through very complex negotiations to determine who sleeps on the wet spot.

WHISKEY DICK—had too much to drink and can't get it up.

WOOD—an erection. "How did Pinocchio find out he was made of wood? His hand caught fire," attributed to Hunter S. Thompson.

YEAST INFECTIONS—group of party-hearty fungi (yeasties) that live in warm, wet places like vaginas, between toes and sometimes in the folds of your skin if you are a buffet junkie. When environmental conditions get out of balance, the yeasties go nuts, causing major discomfort.

YIFF—Internet slang that refers to sex or something that is sexy, e.g. "Wanna

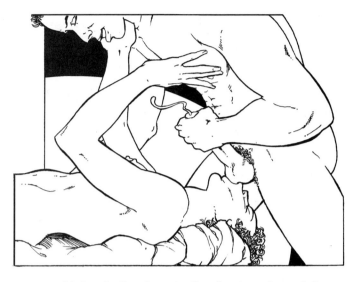

Would that be "teabagging" or "string of pearls"?

A VERY SPECIAL THANKS TO THESE INCREDIBLE RESOURCES
A Glossary of the Low Life
A Prisoner's Dictionary/dictionary.prisonwall.org
Australian Slang/koalanet.com.au
Brainy Dictionary/brainydictionary.com
Boyz Behind Bars/boyzbehindbars.com
Journal of Sexual Medicine
Matt & Andrej Koymasky's Gay Slang Terms/andrejkoymasky.com
Online Dictionary of Playground Slang/odps.org
Probert Encyclopaedia/probertencyclopaedia.com
PseudoDictionary/pseudodictionary.com
Roedy Green's Gay & Black Glossary
Roger's Profanisaurus
Swingers Board Dictionary/swingersboard.com
Strafe's Guide to Streetspeak/strafe.com
The College Humor Guide To College/collegehumor.com
The Peevish Dictionary of Slang for the UK/www.peevish.co.uk/slang
The Sex Dictionary/thesexdictionary.com
The Urban Dictionary/urbandictionary.com
Wikipedia/wikipedia.org

Index

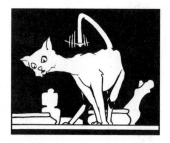

www.GuideToGettingItOn.com